Nutritional Strategies, Predictive Models, and Sustainable Policies

Nutritional Strategies, Predictive Models, and Sustainable Policies

Edited by

Sandeep K. Panda

School of Biotechnology, Kalinga Institute of Industrial Technology (KIIT) (Deemed to be University), Bhubaneswar, Odisha, India

Ursula Gonzales-Barron

Centro de Investigação de Montanha (CIMO)-Mountain Research Center, School of Agriculture, Polytechnic Institute of Bragança (IPB), Bragança, Portugal

Surekha Routray

KIIT-Technology Business Incubator (TBI), Kalinga Institute of Industrial Technology (KIIT) (Deemed to be University), Bhubaneswar, Odisha, India; Aashdit Nutritech Pvt. Ltd., Bhubaneswar, Odisha, India

ELSEVIER

ACADEMIC PRESS

An imprint of Elsevier

elsevier.com/books-and-journals

Academic Press is an imprint of Elsevier

125 London Wall, London EC2Y 5AS, United Kingdom
50 Hampshire Street, 5th Floor, Cambridge, MA 02139, United States

ISBN: 978-0-443-23671-6

For Information on all Academic Press publications visit our website at https://www.elsevier.com/books-and-journals

Publisher: Mara Conner
Acquisitions Editor: Nicole Denis
Editorial Project Manager: Manvi Sharma
Production Project Manager: Supali Acharya
Cover Designer: Raman Kumar

Typeset by Aptara, New Delhi, India

Contents

Contributors

M.W.S. Barbosa, Laboratory of Microbial Process in Foods, Department of Food Engineering, Federal University of Paraíba, João Pessoa, Brazil

Md. Latiful Bari, Center for Advanced Research in Sciences, University of Dhaka, Dhaka, Bangladesh

Vasco Cadavez, CIMO, LA SusTEC, Instituto Politécnico de Bragança, Bragança, Portugal

A.D. Carboni, Center for Research and Development in Food Science and Technology (CIDCA, CCT-CONICET, La Plata), La Plata, Argentina

Rashmita Das, School of Biological Sciences, National Institute of Science Education and Research, HBNI, Jatni, Odisha, India

Sharmin Zaman Emon, Centre for Advanced Research in Sciences (CARS), University of Dhaka, Dhaka, Bangladesh

Lekshmi Gangadhar, NanoDot Research Private Limited, Nagercoil, Tamil Nadu, India

A. Gomez-Zavaglia, Center for Research and Development in Food Science and Technology (CIDCA, CCT-CONICET, La Plata), La Plata, Argentina

Ursula Gonzales-Barron, Mountain Research Centre (CIMO), School of Agriculture, Polytechnic Institute of Braganza (IPB), Portugal

Chandan Goswami, School of Biological Sciences, National Institute of Science Education and Research, HBNI, Jatni, Odisha, India

Luna Goswami, School of Biotechnology, Kalinga Institute of Industrial Technology (KIIT) (Deemed to be University), Bhubaneswar, Odisha, India

Arezoo Haghighian-Roudsari, Department of Community Nutrition, Faculty of Nutrition Sciences and Food Technology, National Nutrition and Food Technology Research Institute, Shahid Beheshti University of Medical Sciences, Tehran, Iran

Abebe Haile, Center for Food Security Studies, CDS, Addis Ababa University, Addis Ababa, Ethiopia

M. Magnani, Laboratory of Microbial Process in Foods, Department of Food Engineering, Federal University of Paraíba, João Pessoa, Brazil

Dam Sao Mai, Institute of Food technology and Biotechnology, Industrial University of Ho Chi Minh City, Ho Chi Minh City, Vietnam

Ipsa Mohapatra, Department of Community Medicine, Kalinga Institute of Medical Sciences, Bhubaneswar, Odisha, India

Soumya R. Mohapatra, School of Biotechnology, Kalinga Institute of Industrial Technology (KIIT) (Deemed to be University), Bhubaneswar, Odisha, India

Sohini Mukherjee, School of Biotechnology, Kalinga Institute of Industrial Technology (KIIT) (Deemed to be University), Bhubaneswar, Odisha, India

Francis Aila Oketch, Department of Health, County Government of Homa Bay, Homa Bay, Nyanza, Kenya

Susan Atieno Onyango, Programmes, The Healthy Woman, Homa Bay, Nyanza, Kenya

Sandeep K. Panda, School of Biotechnology, Kalinga Institute of Industrial Technology (KIIT) (Deemed to be University), Bhubaneswar, Odisha, India

Tithi Parija, School of Biotechnology, Kalinga Institute of Industrial Technology (KIIT) (Deemed to be University), Bhubaneswar, Odisha, India

Subarno Paul, School of Biotechnology, Kalinga Institute of Industrial Technology (KIIT) (Deemed to be University), Bhubaneswar, Odisha, India

M.C. Puppo, Center for Research and Development in Food Science and Technology (CIDCA, CCT-CONICET, La Plata), La Plata, Argentina

Surekha Routray, Aashdit Nutritech Pvt. Ltd., Bhubaneswar, Odisha, India

Adrija Roy, Department of Community Medicine, Apollo Institute of Medical Sciences and Research, Hyderabad, Telangana, India; Achutha Menon Centre for Health Science Studies, Sree Chitra Tirunal Institute of Medical Sciences and Technology, Trivandrum, Kerala, India

Saranyadevi S, Computational Biology and Therapeutics Lab, Saveetha College of Physiotherapy, Saveetha Institute of Medical and Technical Sciences (SIMATS), Saveetha University, Thandalam, Chennai, Tamil Nadu, India

M.V. Salinas, Center for Research and Development in Food Science and Technology (CIDCA, CCT-CONICET, La Plata), La Plata, Argentina

Meghna Sarkar, School of Biotechnology, Kalinga Institute of Industrial Technology (KIIT) (Deemed to be University), Bhubaneswar, Odisha, India

Raju Sasikumar, Department of Agribusiness Management and Food Technology, North-Eastern Hill University, Tura, Meghalaya, India

Shruti Senapati, R&D Department, Aashdit Nutritech Pvt. Ltd., Bhubaneswar, Odisha, India

F.A. Silva, Laboratory of Microbial Process in Foods, Department of Food Engineering, Federal University of Paraíba, João Pessoa, Brazil

Abhishek Singh, School of Biotechnology, Kalinga Institute of Industrial Technology (KIIT) Deemed to be University, Bhubaneswar, Odisha, India; School of Biological Sciences, National Institute of Science Education and Research, HBNI, Jatni, Odisha, India

Paramasivan Sethuraman Sivakumar, ICAR – Central Tuber Crops Research Institute, Thiruvananthapuram, Kerala, India

Selva Kumar T, Vel Tech Rangarajan Dr. Sagunthala R&D Institute of Science and Technology, Chennai, Tamil Nadu, India; Department of Agribusiness Management and Food Technology, North-Eastern Hill University, Tura, Meghalaya, India

Aoife Ward-Gahlawat, German Cancer Research Center (DKFZ) and National Center for Tumor Diseases (NCT), Heidelberg, Germany

Sabina Yeasmin, Department of Genetic Engineering and Biotechnology, University of Dhaka, Dhaka, Bangladesh

Foreword

The growing burden of malnutrition, food insecurity, and nutrition-related disorders continues to challenge both developed and developing nations alike. In an era marked by rapid urbanization, demographic transitions, pandemics, climate change, and sociopolitical instability, the need for innovative, evidence-based, and sustainable nutritional approaches has become more urgent than ever. Against this backdrop, *Nutritional Strategies, Predictive Models, and Sustainable Policies* presents a timely and comprehensive contribution to the evolving field of global nutrition and public health.

Edited by Sandeep K. Panda, Ursula Gonzales-Barron, and Surekha Routray, this volume brings together multidisciplinary perspectives from scientists, academicians, and policy experts working across diverse geographical and thematic domains. The book addresses the intricate relationship between nutrition, predictive science, and sustainable policymaking, while emphasizing the need for region-specific and population-focused interventions.

One of the notable strengths of this volume is its global perspective on nutritional status and strategies. The chapters examining continent-wise nutritional comparisons, nutritional models in India and the Middle East, and nutritional assessments across South America and South-East Asia provide valuable insights into regional disparities and common challenges. By highlighting nutrition across different age groups and socioeconomic settings, the book effectively demonstrates that nutritional concerns are deeply interconnected with culture, economy, healthcare access, and public policy.

The inclusion of chapters dedicated to vulnerable populations further enhances the significance of this work. Discussions on child nutrition in Bangladesh, nutritional challenges during the COVID-19 pandemic in low- and middle-income countries, aging and nutrition, and the nutritional status of women and children in North-East India underscore the pressing need for targeted and inclusive interventions. These contributions reflect the reality that nutritional well-being must be addressed through life-course approaches that recognize the unique needs of children, women, and elderly populations.

Another distinguishing feature of this book is its emphasis on predictive modeling and quantitative assessment. The chapters focusing on cancer-protective nutrition, women's health, and microbiological food safety in tropical countries illustrate the transformative potential of predictive analytics in nutrition science and public health. Such approaches can aid in risk prediction, policy planning, and evidence-based intervention strategies, thereby strengthening the scientific foundation for future nutritional programs.

Equally important is the book's engagement with sustainable nutritional policies in challenging environments. The discussions on policies for war-affected countries, Kenya, and Ethiopia provide critical reflections on the role of governance, international cooperation, and sustainable development in combating malnutrition and ensuring food security. These chapters reinforce the understanding that nutrition is not merely a biological concern but also a social, economic, and humanitarian issue requiring coordinated global action.

The editors deserve special appreciation for assembling a volume that integrates scientific rigor with practical relevance. Their collective expertise in food science, predictive modeling, sustainability, and public health is reflected in the coherent structure and interdisciplinary scope of the book.

This book will serve as a valuable resource for nutrition researchers, healthcare professionals, food scientists, policymakers, and students seeking a broader understanding of contemporary nutritional challenges and emerging solutions. By combining regional perspectives, predictive methodologies, and sustainable policy frameworks, *Nutritional Strategies, Predictive Models, and Sustainable Policies* contributes meaningfully to ongoing global efforts toward improved health, nutrition security, and sustainable development.

I am confident that this volume will stimulate further research, foster interdisciplinary collaborations, and inspire actionable strategies for building healthier and more resilient societies worldwide.

Dr. Ramesh C. Ray
ARS (Retd.), FNAAS
Formerly, Principal Scientist and Head,
ICAR-Central Tuber Crops Research Institute
(Regional Centre),
Bhubaneswar, Odisha, India
Formerly, Project Manager,
International Potato Center, Odisha, India

Preface

Nutrition lies at the heart of human health, societal development, and economic progress. Yet, despite significant advances in science and technology, the world continues to grapple with multiple forms of malnutrition: undernutrition, micronutrient deficiencies, and the rising prevalence of diet-related noncommunicable diseases. These challenges are further compounded by global crises such as climate change, pandemics, population growth, and geopolitical instability. Addressing such complex and interlinked issues requires not only innovative nutritional strategies but also predictive tools and sustainable policy frameworks that are responsive to regional and population-specific needs.

It is within this context that *Nutritional Strategies, Predictive Models, and Sustainable Policies* has been conceptualized. This edited volume aims to provide a comprehensive and interdisciplinary platform that integrates global nutritional assessments, targeted intervention strategies, advanced predictive modeling approaches, and critical policy analyses. By bringing together contributions from diverse geographical regions and thematic areas the book seeks to bridge the gap between theory, research, and practical implementation in the field of nutrition and public health.

The first section of the book offers a global overview of nutritional status, presenting continent-wise comparisons and region-specific insights from India, the Middle East, South America, and Southeast Asia. These chapters highlight the heterogeneity of nutritional challenges across different socioeconomic and cultural settings, emphasizing the need for context-driven strategies. The discussions extend to age-wise nutritional assessments, reflecting how dietary needs and vulnerabilities evolve across the life course.

A significant portion of the book is devoted to vulnerable populations, including children, women, and the elderly. Chapters focusing on child nutrition in Bangladesh, the impact of the COVID-19 pandemic on children in low- and middle-income countries, aging and nutrition, and the nutritional status of women and children in Northeast India underscore the importance of targeted and inclusive approaches. These contributions aim to identify gaps, propose improvements, and reinforce the importance of equitable access to nutrition.

Recognizing the growing importance of data-driven decision-making, the book also explores predictive modeling as a transformative tool in nutrition science. The chapters addressing cancer-protective nutrition, microbiological food safety in tropical countries, and women's health demonstrate how quantitative models can support risk assessment, optimize interventions, and enhance policy planning. These approaches represent a shift toward precision nutrition and evidence-based public health strategies.

The final section of the book examines nutritional policies within complex and often challenging contexts. By analyzing policy frameworks in war-affected regions, as well as in countries such as Kenya and Ethiopia, the book provides critical insights into the role of governance, international collaboration, and sustainable development in addressing nutritional challenges. These discussions highlight the importance of integrating scientific knowledge with policy action to achieve long-term and sustainable outcomes.

As editors, we are deeply grateful to all the contributors for their valuable chapters, thoughtful analyses, and commitment to advancing the field of nutrition. Their collective expertise has made it possible to present a volume that is both comprehensive and forward-looking. We also extend our sincere appreciation to the publisher, Elsevier, for their support and guidance throughout the development of this book.

We hope that this volume will serve as a useful resource for researchers, academicians, students, healthcare professionals, and policymakers. By fostering interdisciplinary dialogue and encouraging innovative thinking, we aspire for this book to contribute meaningfully to global efforts aimed at improving nutritional well-being and building sustainable, healthy societies.

Sandeep K. Panda
Ursula Gonzales-Barron
Surekha Routray

Section I

Current nutritional strategies

Introduction and overview of nutritional strategies

1

Sandeep K. Panda[a], *Surekha Routray*[b] *and Ursula Gonzales-Barron*[c]
[a]School of Biotechnology, Kalinga Institute of Industrial Technology (KIIT) (Deemed to be University), Bhubaneswar, Odisha, India, [b]Aashdit Nutritech Pvt. Ltd., Bhubaneswar, Odisha, India, [c]Mountain Research Centre (CIMO), School of Agriculture, Polytechnic Institute of Braganza (IPB), Portugal

1.1 Introduction

The nutritional status is dynamic throughout the world and has large variations, as per geography, age demographics, political stability, and class. Geopolitical scenarios and pandemics further contribute to the intensity of the dynamics. Geographical location and climatic zone influence crop production, leading to unequal availability of food products around the globe. Land, which contributes 29% of the area on the planet, has many variations in the fertility of soil, rainfall, and temperature, making several places unsuitable for crop production. Per capita consumption of nutrients is significantly reflected by the economic status of the countries. Availability of nutrients for the vulnerable groups, such as pregnant women and children, is one of the critical aspects of the nutritional strategies in low- and middle-income countries (LMICs). Conflicts and forced displacement further worsen nutrition disparity. Malnutrition is observed in three types of conditions: (1) undernutrition, reflected by wasting, stunting, and underweight; (2) noncommunicable diseases represented by overweight and obesity; and (3) micronutrient deficiencies/excess. It is important to revisit the problem statements associated with nutritional requirements and access for every individual and review the strategies for the provision of nutrients as per the recommended dietary allowance (RDA).

1.2 Global malnutrition scenario

Around 390 million adults in the globe are underweight, and 2.5 billion suffer from being overweight. Among the children under 5 years, 149 million children were suffering from stunting, and 37 million lived with overweight or obesity during 2022 (WHO, 2024). Alarmingly, undernutrition contributes to approximately half of the deaths among children under 5 years. The at-risk group in malnutrition includes infants, children, adolescents, and women. The risk amplifies with global conflict and forced displacement. Economic turbulence and climatic extremes also significantly contribute to the malnutrition risk. In 2023 around 281 million people across 53 countries faced acute hunger, which rose to around 295 million in 2024 (UNICEF, 2025). The areas of concern for malnutrition were Gaza Strip, Mali, Sudan, and Yemen. Considering

Nutritional Strategies, Predictive Models, and Sustainable Policies. DOI: https://doi.org/10.1016/B978-0-443-23671-6.00005-0

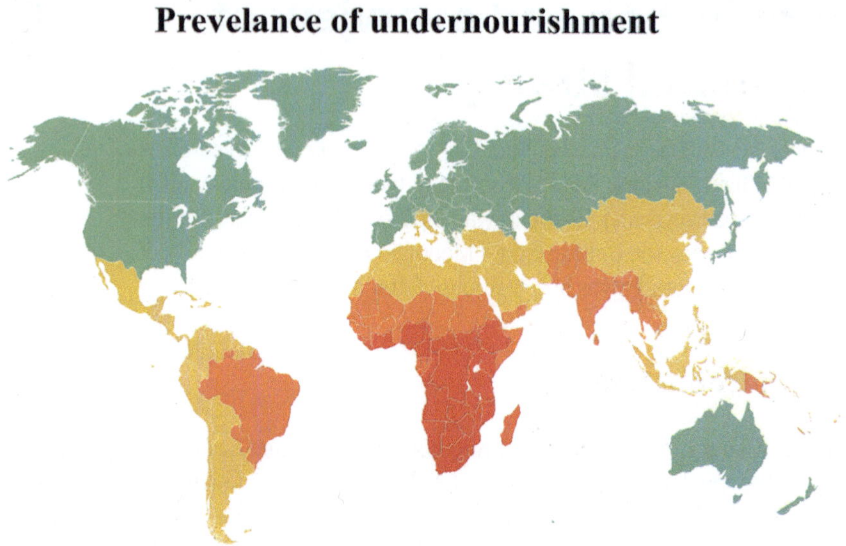

Figure 1.1 Undernutrition map of the world. The map illustrates the prevalence of undernourishment as a percentage of the population, categorized by color to represent different severity levels. Countries shaded in green indicate a low prevalence (0%–4%) of undernourishment, while those in *yellow* represent a moderate prevalence (5%–14%). *Orange* shading denotes a high prevalence (15%–29%), and *red* indicates a very high prevalence (≥30%) (Bentley, 2015; FAO et al., 2024, FAO, 2025; Global Change Data Lab, 2025; Ritchie & Roser, 2023).
Map lines delineate study areas and do not necessarily depict accepted national boundaries.

the latest report of Yemen (during May 2025 and August 2025), approximately 4.9 million people are in crisis for food security (phase 3 + status) of the Integrated Food Security Phase Classification (IPC), and 1.5 million are in IPC phase 4, i.e., emergency. Nigeria, Sudan, Congo, Bangladesh, and Ethiopia are among the countries with the highest population experiencing acute food insecurity (FAO, 2025). In 2023, 604.8 million people were living with anemia, in contrast to 505.7 million in 2012. The global anemia cases recorded during 2023 were mainly contributed by Africa (129.9 million) and Asia (394.3 million). In 2024 the global prevalence of undernutrition was 8.2%, compared to 20% in Africa. During the same year the number of severely food-insecure people was estimated at 828 million worldwide, with Africa and Asia contributing 336.9 million and 417.5 million, respectively. In 2024 23.2% of <5 years children suffer from stunting, and 6.6% of the same age group suffer from wasting, worldwide. The prevalence is 150.2 million and 42.8 million for stunting and wasting, respectively; out of which Africa and Asia contribute 64.8 million and 76.8 million for stunting, and 11.7 million and 30 million are contributed for wasting by Africa and Asia, respectively. Fig. 1.1 presents the world map with undernutrition status. The global situation of malnutrition is a complex and persistent challenge that continues to draw the attention of multiple international and national agencies. Organizations, such as the World Health Organization (WHO), the Food and Agriculture Organization (FAO), UNICEF, and several nongovernmental bodies, are actively engaged in addressing this crisis. Their combined efforts highlight that malnutrition is not merely a matter of food scarcity but also involves issues of poverty, inequality, access to healthcare, education, and sustainable livelihoods (WHO, 2024).

The strategies adopted for different continents and regions are different; further, the policies vary from one age group to the other. Table 1.1 describes the important schemes in operation across different regions of the world. In the Indian context the problem of nutritional deficiencies is tackled through a collaborative framework involving both state and central governments, as well as international organizations that support and monitor progress. India has implemented several flagship programs, such as the Integrated Child Development Services (ICDS), the Mid-Day Meal Scheme, Anaemia Mukt Bharat, and the Poshan Abhiyaan, which aim to improve maternal and child health. These initiatives emphasize not only providing food but also ensuring dietary diversity, nutritional awareness, and access to fortified products. The involvement of state governments allows region-specific tailoring of these schemes, whereas the central government provides overarching policies and funding support (IBEF (India Brand Equity Foundation), 2025; IMPRI (Impact and Policy Research Institute), 2024). The book aims to bring the 360-degree view of nutritional status and strategies across geography, position, and special nutritional needs for women, children, and other vulnerable groups; developments in predictive models on the different categories of nutrition; and policies related to nutrition in the sensitive regions.

1.3 Overview of the book

In detail, the book has 4 sections and 15 chapters. Section 1.1 covers status and models of nutritional strategies in different geographical locations. Chapter 2 describes the nutritional status of India, the second most populous country in the world, and strategies and national policies for combating malnutrition. National surveys reveal persistent high levels of stunting, wasting, and underweight among children, although there has been modest improvement in recent years in India [NFH (IMPRI (Impact and Policy Research Institute), 2024; MoHFW, 2021)]. Chapter 3 categorizes the Middle East countries into three groups based on their stage of nutrition transition: (1) advanced nutrition transition countries, including Bahrain, Saudi Arabia, Kuwait, Oman, Qatar, and the United Arab Emirates (UAE), which exhibit high rates of overweight and obesity alongside a moderate prevalence of malnutrition and micronutrient deficiencies; (2) countries in the early stages of nutrition transition, such as Egypt, Jordan, Lebanon, and Iran, which show medium levels of both overweight/obesity and malnutrition with associated micronutrient deficiencies; and (3) countries with a high burden of malnutrition, including Iraq, Syria, Yemen, and Palestine (Gaza Strip), where acute and chronic malnutrition, widespread micronutrient deficiencies, as well as overweight and obesity remain prevalent. The policies for nutritional improvement in the region have been concisely discussed. Chapter 4 examines the current nutritional status of Brazil and Argentina, the two most populous countries in South America. It analyzes

Table 1.1 Important programs and schemes operated worldwide for mitigation of malnutrition.

Agency/organization	Scheme/program	Location of implementation	Outcomes/impact	References
World Food Programme (WFP)	Emergency Food Assistance and Nutrition Support	80+ countries: Sudan, Yemen, Afghanistan, Syria, Haiti	Reduced acute malnutrition rates, improved food security in conflict zones, school feeding programs reaching 15 million children annually	Deconinck et al. (2014)
UNICEF	Community-Based Management of Acute Malnutrition (CMAM)	Sub-Saharan Africa, South Asia, Horn of Africa	Treatment of severe acute malnutrition in children under 5; recovery rates exceeding 90% in supported programs	Deconinck et al. (2014)
WHO	Global Nutrition Targets 2025	Global (194 Member States)	Monitoring and policy guidance on reducing stunting, wasting, anemia, and low birth weight; country-level policy integration	WHO (2014)
FAO	Hand-in-Hand Initiative	47 priority countries, including Ethiopia, Bangladesh, and Guatemala	Increased agricultural productivity, improved rural incomes, enhanced food system resilience	Food and Agriculture Organization (2023)

(*continued on next page*)

Global Nutrition Cluster	Nutrition in Emergencies (NiE)	Crisis-affected regions: Ukraine, Gaza, Myanmar, South Sudan	Rapid deployment of therapeutic foods, micronutrient supplements, and infant feeding support during conflicts and disasters	Global Nutrition Cluster (2022)
Bill & Melinda Gates Foundation	Nutrition-Sensitive Agriculture Programs	Nigeria, India, Ethiopia, Bangladesh	Improved dietary diversity, increased biofortified crop adoption, reduced micronutrient deficiencies	Bill and Melinda (2025)
International Rescue Committee (IRC)	Integrated Health and Nutrition Services	Refugee camps in Kenya, Uganda, Jordan, Bangladesh (Cox's Bazar)	Reduced child wasting by up to 50% in targeted areas, improved maternal nutrition	International Rescue Committee (2023)
Action Against Hunger	Nutrition and Food Security Programs	Mali, Somalia	Treatment of acute malnutrition, water and sanitation integration, livelihood support	Action Against Hunger (2024), Action Against Hunger (2025)
European Commission (DG ECHO)	Humanitarian Aid for Nutrition	Global emergency response (Sahel, Central America, Pacific Islands)	Funding and coordination of nutrition interventions in acute crises, multisectoral response	European Commission DG ECHO (2023)

and compares the nutritional strategies adopted in both nations to address malnutrition and curb the rise of overweight and obesity, while also discussing key issues related to food labeling. Chapter 5 describes the nutritional status of various age groups in Southeast Asian countries—Brunei, Burma (Myanmar), Cambodia, Timor-Leste, Indonesia, Laos, Malaysia, the Philippines, Singapore, Thailand, and Vietnam—highlighting the underlying factors, current challenges, and ongoing intervention initiatives aimed at improving the situation. Regional initiatives and policy interventions in different age groups have also been highlighted in the chapter.

Section 1.2 of the book has covered the status of the vulnerable groups, children, and pregnant women, and the nutrition disruption because of COVID 19, in different geographic locations. The section highlights the strategies and approaches for special nutrition of children, pregnant women, and patients in different countries and continents. Chapter 6 explores the nutritional status of young children in Bangladesh, with a focus on contributing factors, current trends, existing interventions, and recommendations for improvement. The discussion is grounded in empirical evidence and supported by relevant studies. Chapter 7 provides a concise overview of the molecular relationship between nutritional habits, dietary choices, and the bioactive components present in specific foods, in relation to the aging of tissues, cells, and subcellular organelles, which may be influenced by TRP ion channels. Notably, certain bioactive compounds found in diets or food supplements can modulate TRP ion channels either instantaneously or over prolonged periods. The chapter further elaborates on the role of TRP ion channels in aging and their interactions with dietary factors that shape these processes. Chapter 8 provides a critical account of the disruption of children's nutrition and key nutritional status indicators of malnutrition in LMICs as a consequence of the COVID-19 pandemic. In India, COVID-19 significantly disrupted regular nutrition services. A study focused on children aged 0–5 years showed worsened nutritional status during the pandemic period because of interrupted health services, restricted access to food, and reduced growth monitoring (Vora & Mathur, 2024). Chapter 9 presents the current nutritional status of women and children in Northeast India, encompassing its eight states, Arunachal Pradesh, Assam, Manipur, Meghalaya, Mizoram, Nagaland, Sikkim, and Tripura, characterized by difficult and hilly terrains. It emphasizes the need to improve nutrition outcomes while addressing the social, cultural, and policy-related factors that influence the nutritional well-being of women and children in the region.

Section 1.3 of the book is based on the advancement of predictive modeling with nutrition on the outcome of cancer prevention, progression, food safety, and women's health. Chapter 10 delves into predictive modeling tools and their potential applications in linking nutraceuticals to cancer prevention. Chapter 11 provides an in-depth review of predictive modeling tools and their applications in ensuring microbiological food safety in tropical countries. It highlights key applications and the integration of predictive modeling with emerging technologies, while also explaining how the use of predictive microbiology and quantitative risk assessment presents both significant potential and inherent challenges in tropical and subtropical regions. Chapter 12 reviews current research on the application of machine learning (ML) to predict women's health and nutritional outcomes, with particular focus on methodologies, data integration, and existing research gaps. The chapter also highlights the capacity of ML to integrate diverse data sources such as clinical biomarkers, socioeconomic factors, genetic profiles, and behavioral patterns to forecast health risks and nutritional status. These models demonstrate significant potential in supporting proactive diet planning, early detection of cardiovascular disease, cancer, mental health disorders, arthritis, postpartum complications, menopausal symptoms, and other reproductive health conditions in women.

Section 1.4 describes the nutritional scenario of the war-affected countries and the sensitive countries. The strategies undertaken to improve the nutritional status of the countries have been described. Chapter 13 elucidates the nutritional disruption in countries affected by war. The chapter has provided case studies of countries such as Ukraine, Afghanistan, and Iraq. Chapters 14 and 15 decipher the status of nutrition in Kenya and Ethiopia, respectively. The chapters have examined the implementation of strategies and policies for alleviating malnutrition at the national and international levels in both countries. The pandemic, war, famine, and dislocation not only affect immediate nutritional status but also have lifelong consequences. For pregnant women, malnutrition can cause low birth weight and impede fetal growth; for children, stunting or chronic undernutrition hampers cognitive development, immunity, and productivity (National Human Rights Commission (NHRC), 2024). The book, therefore, makes it clear that tackling malnutrition requires not only immediate relief but also systemic, sustainable solutions that integrate food security with health, education, and social welfare systems.

1.4 Conclusion

The global situation of malnutrition is addressed by multiple agencies. The book provides a detailed and region-wise analysis of the nutritional scenario of the different corners of the world. It examines the prevailing dietary practices, deficiencies, and the health outcomes that arise from them. In addition, it compiles currently adopted strategies and policies that are being implemented by governments and organizations to combat malnutrition. What makes this work particularly valuable is the inclusion of critical perspectives and comments from reputed scientists and authors belonging to multiple countries and continents. Their insights enrich the discourse by offering comparative lessons, highlighting successes as well as gaps, and suggesting ways forward based on scientific evidence and global best practices. Another significant dimension addressed in the book is the impact of global crises such as the COVID-19 pandemic, ongoing wars, recurring famines, and forced dislocation of populations on nutritional security. Each of these crises has disproportionately affected vulnerable groups, particularly women and children.

References

Action Against Hunger. (2024). Mali: Improving food and nutritional security, WASH integration, and livelihoods. Retrieved October 6, 2025, from https://www.actionagainsthunger.org/location/africa/mali/.

Bentley, J. (2015)."Mapping food insecurity. Blog. https://blog.education.nationalgeographic.org/2015/04/17/mapping-food-insecurity/.

Bill & Melinda Gates Foundation. (2025). *Nutrition—Improving food systems, policy, & advocacy.* https://www.gatesfoundation.org/our-work/programs/global-growth-and-opportunity/nutrition.

Deconinck, H., Kiviat, L., Patel, A., & Johnson, M. N. (2014). Effectiveness of community-based management of acute malnutrition in sub-Saharan Africa: Case studies from Ghana, Malawi, and Zambia. *Food and Nutrition Bulletin, 35*(2 Suppl), S34–S38. https://doi.org/10.1177/15648265140352S105.

European Commission Directorate-General for European Civil Protection and Humanitarian Aid Operations (DG ECHO). (2023). Nutrition: Humanitarian aid in emergencies. Retrieved October 6, 2025, from https://civil-protection-humanitarian-aid.ec.europa.eu/what/humanitarian-aid/nutrition_en.

FAO, IFAD, UNICEF, WFP, and WHO. (2024). *The state of food security and nutrition in the world.* FAO https://www.fao.org/publications/fao-flagship-publications/the-state-of-food-security-and-nutrition-in-the-world/en.

FAO. (2025). *FAO hunger map.* https://www.fao.org/interactive/hunger-map/en/.

Food and Agriculture Organization. (2023). *The state of food security and nutrition in the world 2023.* FAO.

Global Change Data Lab. (2025). Prevalence of undernourishment. Our World in Data. https://ourworldindata.org/grapher/prevalence-of-undernourishment.

IBEF (India Brand Equity Foundation). (2025). *Mission Poshan Abhiyaan. Data as of Feb 2025.* IBEF Beneficiary registration, scheme goals (support during the first 1,000 days, convergence with other services).

IMPRI (Impact and Policy Research Institute). (2024). *Poshan Abhiyaan 2.0: India's* nutrition revolution. IMPRI Reports performance between 2021-2024, including participation rates, NFHS-5 data showing stunting at 35.5 %, wasting at 19.3 %, underweight at 32.1 %.

International Rescue Committee. (2023). Integrated health and nutrition services in refugee settings: Impact assessment report. International Rescue Committee. https://www.rescue.org/topic/health.

National Human Rights Commission (NHRC). (2024). *The impact of COVID-19* pandemic on the state of food security and nutrition *in India.* NHRC *Discusses effects on women, children, maternal nutrition, stunting, socio-economic factors, etc.*

MoHFW. (2021). *National Family Health Survey (NFHS-5) 2019–21*, Ministry of Health and Family Welfare, Govt. of India. https://mohfw.gov.in/sites/default/files/NFHS-5_Phase-II_0.pdf.

Ritchie, H., Rosado, P., & Roser, M. (2023). "Hunger and undernourishment." Our World in Data https://ourworldindata.org/hunger-and-undernourishment.

UNICEF. (2025). *Acute food insecurity and malnutrition rise for sixth consecutive year in world's most fragile regions.* UNICEF https://www.unicef.org/press-releases/acute-food-insecurity-and-malnutrition-rise-sixth-consecutive-year-worlds-most.

Vora, A. A., & Mathur, R. (2024). Impact of COVID-19 pandemic on nutrition in children in the age group of 0-5 years. *Wadia Journal of Women and Child Health, 2*(3), 150–151 Shows how the pandemic disrupted nutritional services and worsened child nutrition indicators in India.

WHO, (2014). Global nutrition targets 2025: policy brief series. https://www.who.int/teams/nutrition-and-food-safety/global-targets-2030 (Accessed on 05.06.2026).

WHO, (2024). Malnutrition. https://www.who.int/news-room/fact-sheets/detail/malnutrition (Accessed on 05.06.2026).

Nutritional models in India for tackling malnutrition

2

Paramasivan Sethuraman Sivakumar
ICAR – Central Tuber Crops Research Institute, Thiruvananthapuram, Kerala, India

2.1 Introduction

India's nutritional security strategy has shifted in dealing with postindependence caloric insufficiency to an all-encompassing approach targeting undernutrition, micronutrient deficiencies, and the rising prevalence of overweight and obesity (Fig. 2.1). This change is caused by increased consumption of ultraprocessed foods (Monteiro et al., 2019), more sedentary lifestyles, and greater stress levels (Ruel et al., 2017). These factors have increased susceptibility to nutrition-related noncommunicable diseases, including diabetes, hypertension, and coronary heart disease, in both children and adults. While early interventions focused on food availability, current challenges require integrated solutions that address both the quantity and quality of diets across the life course (Wells et al., 2021).

2.2 The burden of childhood malnutrition in India

2.2.1 *The Indian scenario: Stagnation and severity*

Despite decades of multisectoral interventions, recent evidence indicates that a persistent nutritional crisis persists (Table 2.1).

The National Family Health Survey (NFHS-5, 2019–21) (International Institute for Population Sciences (IIPS) & IIPF, 2021) reports only marginal reductions in undernutrition: 35.5% of children under 5 are stunted, 19.3% are wasted, and 32.1% are underweight (Table 2.1). These figures indicate slight improvements relative to NFHS-4. The prevalence of overweight has increased from 2.1% to 3.4%, showing a growing double burden. Regional inequalities persist, with Meghalaya (46.5%) and Bihar (42.9%) recording the highest stunting rates and Maharashtra and Gujarat exceeding 25% for wasting rates. Childhood obesity is rising in Union Territories such as Ladakh (13.4%) and Lakshadweep (10.5%). The Comprehensive National Nutrition Survey (CNNS) detects significant micronutrient deficiencies, including vitamin A deficiency (17.6%) and concurrent iron, folate, and B-12 deficiencies among children aged 1–4. Multiple indicators exceed the 20% public health threshold, underscoring the urgent need to revise intervention strategies. This is consistent with the Sustainable Development Goals (SDGs), which aim to eliminate all forms of child malnutrition by 2030 (FAO et al., 2025).

Nutritional Strategies, Predictive Models, and Sustainable Policies. DOI: https://doi.org/10.1016/B978-0-443-23671-6.00006-2

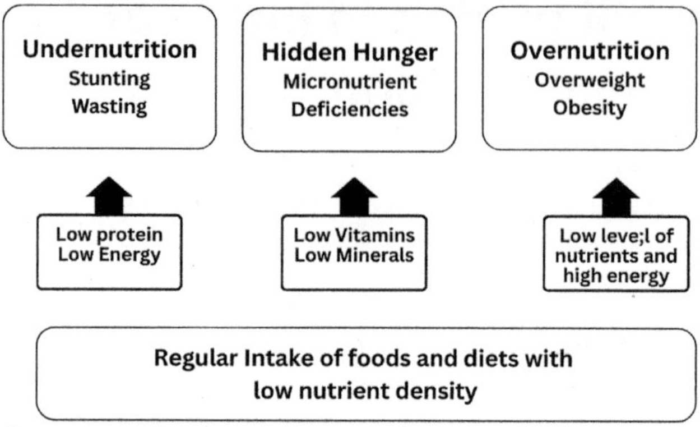

Figure 2.1 Triple burden of malnutrition (Prentice, 2023).
Adapted from Prentice, A. M. (2023). The triple burden of malnutrition in the era of globalisation. *Annals of Nutrition and Metabolism, 79* (Suppl. 1), 1–12. https://doi.org/10.1159/000529514.

2.2.2 Developmental and economic consequences

Malnutrition occurs when essential nutrient intake is inadequate or when the body cannot absorb nutrients from food (Saunders & Smith, 2010). The clinical and socioeconomic impacts are significant:

- Undernutrition: Leads to short stature (stunting), weakened cognitive and educational performance, and significantly lower adult wages (De Sanctis et al., 2021; Soni et al., 2021).
- Overnutrition: In addition to physical health risks, obesity severely impacts children's social and mental well-being and self-esteem (Sahoo et al., 2015).
- Micronutrient deficiencies: The deficiencies of iron, zinc, vitamins A, B-12, and D raise predisposition to infections, cause blindness, reduce physical growth, and damage mental functions (Ji et al., 2024).

These developmental consequences reduce adult productivity and contribute to major economic losses in India. Malnutrition is estimated to cost 4% of India's GDP annually, mainly because of lost productivity, higher healthcare costs, and premature mortality (Assochas, 2017). Research indicates that every dollar spent on nutrition interventions in India can yield a benefit of 19.35 dollars (Kumar & Joe, 2020).

2.3 Toward a systems approach to nutrition—Nutritional models

Nutritional models employ a systems approach to explain how malnutrition develops and persists within social systems. Extensive models are needed because child malnutrition and morbidity are not directly observable and require multilayered analysis to guide efficient interventions (Sharn et al., 2025). These models show how factors such as food access, economic conditions, social norms, health services, sanitation, and

Table 2.1 Key childhood nutritional indicators in India.

Indicator	Prevalence (%)	States with high prevalence
Malnutrition		
Stunting (height-for-age) (<5 years)	35.5	Meghalaya, Bihar, and Jharkhand
Wasting (weight-for-height) (<5 years)	19.3	Maharashtra, Gujarat, Jharkhand, Odisha, and Rajasthan
Underweight (weight-for-age) (<5 years)	32.1	Bihar and Jharkhand
Overweight (weight-for-height > 2 standard deviations)	3.4	Ladakh, Lakshadweep, and Mizoram
Severe acute malnutrition (<5 years)	7.7	Maharashtra, Gujarat, and Jharkhand
Micronutrient deficiencies		
Anemia—hemoglobin level (g/dL) (Children <5 years)	67.1	Gujarat, Madhya Pradesh, and Jammu & Kashmir
Folate deficiency (children 1–4 years)	22.8	Nagaland, Andhra Pradesh, and Assam
Iron deficiency (serum ferritin <12 μg/L) (1–4 years)	31.9	Punjab, Haryana, and Gujarat
Vitamin A deficiency (serum retinol <20 μg/dL) (1–4 years)	17.6	Jharkhand, Mizoram, and Madhya Pradesh
Vitamin D deficiency [serum 25(OH)D concentration <12 ng/mL (30 nmol/L)] (1–4 years)	13.8	Punjab, Uttarakhand, and Manipur
Vitamin B12 deficiency (serum B12 < 203 pg/mL) (1–4 years)	13.8	Gujarat, Uttar Pradesh, and Uttarakhand
Zinc deficiency (serum zinc <65 μg/dL) (1–4 years)	18.9	Himachal Pradesh, Jharkhand, and Assam

Adapted from Comprehensive National Nutrition Survey (CNNS) 2016–2018; National Family Health Survey (NFHS-5), 2019–21.

environmental conditions interact through biological, behavioral, and socioeconomic processes to produce malnutrition (FAO, 2016; UNICEF, 1990). Through analyzing determinants and outcomes, nutritional models help assess how underlying, immediate, and basic causes influence nutritional status (Black et al., 2013). They enable researchers and decision-makers to understand causal mechanisms, predict outcomes, and design or evaluate interventions inside complex systems (Gillespie et al., 2013; Ruel & Alderman, 2013). Although conceptual models map the causes and pathways of malnutrition, intervention models turn this knowledge into executable protocols intended to address identified vulnerabilities.

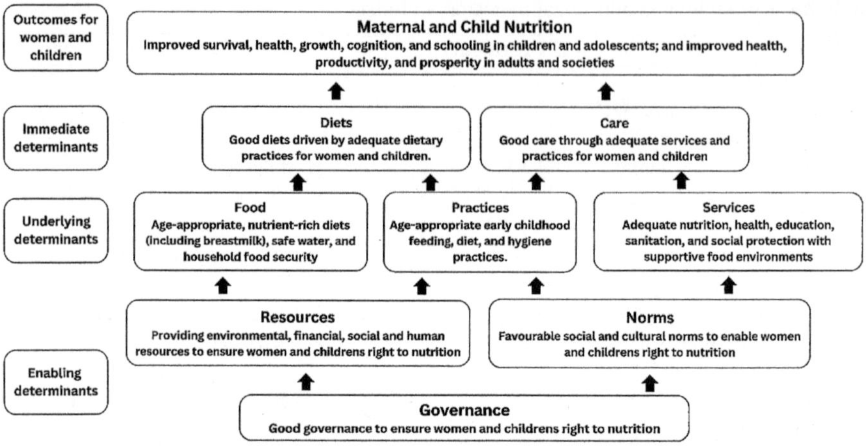

Figure 2.2 UNICEF Conceptual Framework on the determinants of maternal and child nutrition.
Adapted from UNICEF. (2020). *Nutrition, for every child: UNICEF nutrition strategy 2020–2030*. United Nations Children's Fund. https://www.unicef.org/reports/nutrition-strategy-2020-2030.

Nutrition models targeting childhood malnutrition are widely categorized by the determinants they target and the outcomes they seek to achieve.

2.3.1 UNICEF conceptual framework for maternal and child nutrition

The UNICEF conceptual framework (1990, updated 2020) is the most widely used model for addressing child malnutrition. The 2020 update (UNICEF, 2020) builds on the first model, identifying the triple burden of undernutrition, micronutrient deficiencies, and overweight. It details the determinants of malnutrition at three levels: immediate, underlying, and basic/enabling (Fig. 2.2). The UNICEF framework is widely regarded as the global standard for comprehending and tackling the complex causes of malnutrition.

2.3.2 Immediate causes

The immediate causes of childhood malnutrition are inadequate dietary intake and inadequate care and services. These factors generate a cycle in which disease reduces appetite and nutrient digestion, whereas poor nutrition increases the risk of infection.

2.3.2.1 Inadequate dietary intake

Inadequate dietary intake is a primary cause of child undernutrition. Poor-quality diets, characterized by insufficient energy, low nutrient density, and restricted nutritional diversity, combined with infrequent meals, raise vulnerability (Sharma et al., 2020). Suboptimal breastfeeding and complementary feeding practices, such as delayed introduction of foods and infrequent feeding, further reduce nutrient intake (Makwela & Mashaba, 2025). These factors lead to high rates of stunting, wasting, and underweight among young children.

2.3.2.2 Inadequate care and services

Inadequate care practices and weak health services contribute to childhood malnutrition by limiting timely prevention, early detection, and effective management of growth faltering and illness (Nambiar & Arunachalam, 2025). Common infections, especially diarrhea and acute respiratory infections (ARIs), are strongly associated with undernutrition (Macallan, 2009). Diarrheal episodes predict stunting, while ARIs are linked to underweight (Sinha et al., 2018). Recurrent diarrhea worsens undernutrition by reducing appetite, increasing metabolic demands, and impairing nutrient digestion, strengthening the cycle of disease and malnutrition (National Research Council (US), Subcommittee on Nutrition and Diarrheal Diseases Control, 1985).

2.3.3 Underlying causes

2.3.3.1 Inadequate household food security

Poverty and food insecurity: Poverty and food insecurity are major drivers of child undernutrition. Low-income households regularly rely on cereal-based diets with low micronutrient content because of limited access to a diverse range of foods (Raghunathan et al., 2021). NFHS-5 analyses show household wealth is a strong predictor of stunting, wasting, and underweight (International Institute for Population Sciences (IIPS) & IIPF, 2021). Food insecurity reduces food availability and compromises feeding practices, increasing both chronic and acute undernutrition among young children (International Institute for Population Sciences (IIPS) & IIPF, 2021).

2.3.3.2 Inadequate care and feeding practices

Maternal feeding, food preparation, and cleanliness practices during early childhood are critical for child nutrition outcomes.

Infant and young child feeding (IYCF): Steady adherence to IYCF practices, including exclusive breastfeeding for 6 months and the timely introduction of a diverse range of complementary foods, is essential for child nutrition (Black et al., 2013). Maternal education, health, nutrition, and financial decision-making influence the adoption of appropriate IYCF practices.

- Maternal education is a key determinant of child nutrition, showing a caregiver's ability to access healthcare, interpret health information, adopt cleanliness practices, and ensure prompt care and fair food allocation (Black et al., 2013; Cleland & Van Ginneken, 1988; Hasan at al., 2016; Smith & Haddad, 2015). Low-maternal literacy is strongly associated with poor IYCF practices—such as delayed breastfeeding initiation, prelacteal feeding, and nutritionally inadequate complementary foods—causing high levels of stunting and wasting in India (Verma & Singh, 2021). Maternal health and nutrition are central to breaking the intergenerational cycle of undernutrition. Low-maternal BMI, short stature, and chronic anemia strongly predict child growth faltering and stunting, mainly by increasing the risk of low birth weight and impaired growth (Paul et al., 2022; Victora et al., 2021).

- Maternal autonomy affects household nutrition decisions. Limited financial control often prevents mothers from prioritizing nutrient-dense foods, such as eggs, dairy, and fruits, thereby exacerbating micronutrient deficiencies in children (Gupta et al., 2025; UNICEF, 2023).

2.3.3.3 Unhealthy household environment and inadequate health services

Child malnutrition is influenced by inadequate food intake, poor living conditions, and scarce access to medical care. Lack of safe sanitation and faulty waste disposal increase the risk of stunting and underweight (Dahir et al., 2026; Mulyani et al., 2025). Poor WASH conditions cause recurrent infections that impair nutrient digestion, even with adequate diets (Shivakumar et al., 2025; Rachmadi et al., 2024). Limited access to immunization and micronutrient supplements, such as vitamin A, increases the risk of growth faltering, especially among partially or nonimmunized children (Khan & Mohanty, 2024; Purwanti et al., 2025). These risks are greater in areas with weak health systems, where programs such as POSHAN 2.0 and Integrated Child Development Services (ICDS) face coverage gaps because of staff shortages and vaccine stockouts (Prasad, 2025).

2.3.4 Basic causes

The basic causes of childhood malnutrition stem from deficiencies in governance and enabling environments that affect access to resources, service delivery, and equity. Weak political, financial, social, and institutional systems limit women's and children's right to adequate nutrition, making competent governance essential for resource mobilization, service quality, and social inclusion (Nguyen et al., 2021).

2.3.4.1 Financial, physical, and environmental resources

Child malnutrition in India is rooted in socioeconomic inequality and geographic disadvantage. Children from marginalized castes, religious minorities, and poorer regions confront persistent barriers to nutrition and healthcare (Borooah, 2012). Rural and economically disadvantaged districts have a higher risk of malnutrition than urban areas. Climate change and environmental degradation further reduce access to arable land and safe water.

2.3.4.2 Quality of services

Despite initiatives such as POSHAN Abhiyaan and ICDS, the impact is often limited by last-mile delivery challenges, including inadequate local financing, shortages of trained Anganwadi workers (AWWs), and weak monitoring (Sahoo et al., 2016).

2.3.4.3 Social and cultural norms

Maternal autonomy and intrahousehold decision-making strongly influence child nutrition outcomes. Gender-biased food allocation and medical care access persist in many settings, with female children and adolescents experiencing poorer nutritional variety and higher anemia prevalence than males (Mazumdar & Roy, 2025). Harmful practices such as early marriage and adolescent pregnancy further increase the risk of low birth weight and intergenerational undernutrition (Menon et al., 2019).

2.3.5 Application of the UNICEF model in India

The UNICEF Conceptual Framework underlies India's nutrition strategy, providing the rationale for POSHAN Abhiyaan, Saksham Anganwadi, and Mission Poshan 2.0. It has enabled a shift from a food-centric approach to a multisectoral systems approach, tackling immediate, underlying, and basic causes of malnutrition (NITI Aayog, 2019).

In practice the framework guides sectoral convergence using linking nutrition to water and sanitation (the Jal Jeevan Mission and the Swachh Bharat Mission), health, and social protection. It functions as the analytical basis for ICDS, Anaemia Mukt Bharat, and State Nutrition Missions. It supports district-level identification of nutrition gaps through District Nutrition Profiles and Poshan Tracker analytics (Ministry of Women and Child Development, 2021):

- At the immediate level, interventions focus on the first 1000 days through ICDS and the National Health Mission, combining supplementary nutrition, micronutrient supplementation, immunization (Mission Indradhanush), and take-home rations.
- At the underlying level, behavior change is promoted through Jan Andolan activities (e.g., Annaprashan, Godh Bharai) and WASH interventions that reduce diarrheal disease.
- At the enabling level, governance convergence is operationalized through district convergence plans, digital monitoring via the Poshan Tracker, and women's empowerment initiatives targeting adolescent education and delayed marriage, with oversight from NITI Aayog.

Overall, India's application of the UNICEF framework illustrates a systems approach that integrates food, health, WASH, data, and social norms to address the structural drivers of malnutrition.

2.3.6 The Lancet framework—Nutrition-specific versus nutrition-sensitive interventions

The Lancet Framework for Maternal and Child Nutrition (The Lancet, 2013) is one of the most influential approaches to dealing with undernutrition among mothers and young children. This system builds on the UNICEF Conceptual Framework of Malnutrition (UNICEF, 1990) and was further refined by the Lancet Maternal and Child Nutrition Study Group, which developed it through a series of influential papers in The Lancet in 2008, 2013, and 2021. This system assimilates biological, social, and structural determinants of malnutrition into a coherent causal pathway. The key aspect of the Lancet framework is the evidence-based roadmaps developed to tackle

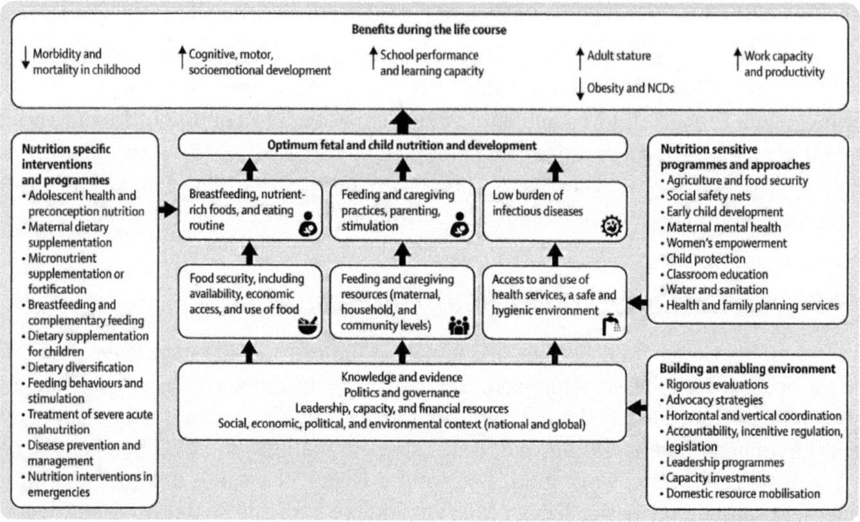

Figure 2.3 The Lancet Framework for actions to achieve optimum fetal and child nutrition and development.
Adapted from The Lancet. (2013). *Maternal and child nutrition: Executive summary of The Lancet Maternal and Child Nutrition Series*. The Lancet.

undernutrition through a critical "1000-day window" from a mother's pregnancy to a child's second birthday.

2.3.6.1 Theoretical roots

The Lancet framework builds on the "20/80 hypothesis," which suggests that even with near-universal coverage of nutrition-specific interventions (e.g., micronutrient supplementation and breastfeeding promotion), about 90% (i.e., 20% reduction in stunting) can be achieved (Bhutta et al., 2013). The remaining 80% of the burden is attributable to nutrition-sensitive factors, including household food security, mothers' caregiving practices, community-level health services, sanitation, mothers' education, and women's empowerment, which address the underlying and basic causes of malnutrition.

This system classifies interventions as nutrition-specific or nutrition-sensitive (Fig. 2.3). Although nutrition-specific interventions directly address the immediate determinants of undernutrition, e.g., inadequate dietary intake and disease, nutrition-sensitive interventions target the underlying determinants, including food security, caregiving practices, health services, water and sanitation, women's empowerment, and social protection.

2.3.6.2 Nutrition-specific interventions

These interventions directly address the immediate causes of malnutrition—poor dietary intake and infectious disease—by focusing on the *first 1000 days*, from conception to birth, during which deficits can cause irreversible cognitive and physical damage. These interventions seek rapid biological effects through health and community platforms.

Core actions include promoting optimal IYCF practices, particularly early initiation and exclusive breastfeeding for 6 months, followed by timely, diverse, and nutrient-dense complementary feeding (Victora et al., 2016; WHO & UNICEF, 2003).

Micronutrient interventions, such as vitamin A for children and iron–folic acid or multiple micronutrient supplements for pregnant and lactating women, address hidden hunger and reduce risks of low birth weight and preterm birth (Bhutta et al., 2013). Large-scale food fortification enhances micronutrient intake at the population level (Das et al., 2013).

2.3.6.3 Nutrition-sensitive interventions

These interventions address the underlying environmental, social, and economic determinants that sustain malnutrition. Rather than treating individuals alone, these interventions strengthen systems—food, health, WASH, education, and social protection—to create enabling conditions for sustained nutritional gains. The 2020 UNICEF Framework increasingly conceptualizes these actions through a systems approach (UNICEF, 2020).

Key nutrition-sensitive pillars include agriculture and food systems that promote access to multiple, nutrient-rich foods (e.g., biofortified crops and homestead gardens); social protection measures that reduce poverty-related food insecurity; WASH interventions that prevent infection-related nutrient losses; and women's empowerment, including education, financial autonomy, and maternal psychological health support (FAO, 2017; Ruel et al., 2013). In India, programs such as POSHAN Abhiyaan integrate both approaches by combining direct nutrition delivery through Anganwadi services with nutrition-sensitive actions, including women-led nutri-gardens, livelihood support, and behavior change, thereby enabling both immediate impact and sustained resilience (Ministry of Women and Child Development, 2022).

2.3.7 Community-based management of acute malnutrition

The community-based management of acute malnutrition (CMAM)—also referred to as the integrated management of acute malnutrition (IMAM)—is a dedicated approach to treating acute malnutrition. Developed by Valid International in 1999, this intervention approach was adopted by the WHO and UNICEF to replace the traditional way of managing acute malnutrition through rehabilitation centers (World Health Organisation, World Food Programme, UNICEF, & United Nations Standing Committee on Nutrition, 2007). This system has been used by many governments and nongovernmental organizations (NGOs) as a long-term program for managing severe acute malnutrition (SAM) and moderate acute malnutrition (MAM).

2.3.7.1 The approach

The CMAM approach works on the assumption that most of the children with acute malnutrition can be successfully treated through a nonhospitalization approach implemented through a community-based system. This approach includes identifying acute malnutrition in its early stages and providing treatment at the community level, thereby averting medical complications in these children. The model rests on four interlinked components—community outreach for early detection, outpatient therapeutic care for uncomplicated cases, inpatient care for children with medical complications, and community participation to secure adherence and follow-up (NITI Aayog, 2023). A critical innovation underpinning CMAM is the use of ready-to-use therapeutic foods (RUTF), which enable safe and effective home-based nutritional rehabilitation without refrigeration or water, thereby substantially reducing caregiver burden and improving program coverage (Collins et al., 2006). Empirical evidence from multicountry implementations of CMAM demonstrates that most children with SAM can be successfully treated as outpatients, achieving recovery rates exceeding international Sphere standards while maintaining low mortality (<5%) and default rates (Collins et al., 2006). Research conducted throughout varied geographic settings consistently shows that CMAM is not only clinically effective but also highly cost-effective compared with conventional inpatient-only models.

2.3.7.2 Community-based management of acute malnutrition in India

CMAM in India follows a hybrid community–facility model, which integrates outpatient community-based care with referral-based institutional care. Under this approach, children identified with SAM and medical complications are referred to Nutrition Rehabilitation Centres (NRCs) for facility-based stabilization, whereas children without complications are managed through community-based protocols. Evidence from India's first large-scale conventional CMAM program implemented by Médecins Sans Frontières (MSF) in Bihar demonstrated that community-based treatment of uncomplicated SAM can achieve low mortality (<1%) and acceptable cure rates among nondefaulting children, supporting the feasibility of CMAM within the Indian health system (Burza et al., 2015). Building on such evidence, India has adopted a modified CMAM/IMAM approach across multiple states, including Assam, Bihar, Chandigarh, Chhattisgarh, Gujarat, Haryana, Jharkhand, Madhya Pradesh, Maharashtra, Odisha, Rajasthan, Telangana, Uttar Pradesh, and Meghalaya, in-line with national nutrition strategies in accordance with Poshan Abhiyaan (Ministry of Women and Child Development & Ministry of Health and Family Welfare, 2022).

In these states, frontline functionaries—Accredited Social Health Activists (ASHAs), auxiliary nurse midwives (ANMs), and AWWs—conduct active case-finding and screening using mid-upper arm circumference (MUAC) tapes and bilateral edema assessment, followed by referral or community-based management, depending on clinical status. Uncomplicated SAM cases are supported through locally produced, energy-dense therapeutic or supplementary foods, nutrition counseling, and periodic growth monitoring, while complicated cases are stabilized at NRCs before referral back to the community. This hybrid model reflects India's pragmatic adaptation of global CMAM principles, attempting to expand coverage while tackling safety, acceptability, and system capacity within the existing ICDS and public health delivery framework (Burza et al., 2015; Ministry of Health and Family Welfare, 2018; Ministry of Women and Child Development & Ministry of Health and Family Welfare, 2022).

2.3.8 The life-cycle model

The life-cycle model of malnutrition explains how nutritional deprivation at one stage of life contributes to adverse health, developmental, and socioeconomic outcomes in later stages, thereby perpetuating an intergenerational cycle of undernutrition (Gillespie & Flores, 2000; UNICEF, 2023). This perspective recognizes malnutrition as a cumulative biological and social process that begins before birth and continues across the lifespan (World Health Organisation, 2021). Global evidence demonstrates that the first 1000 days—from conception to age 2—is a critical window for physical growth, brain development, and long-term human capital formation (UNICEF, 2023). Nutritional deprivation during this period can lead to irreversible consequences for health, cognition, and productivity throughout the life course (Victora et al., 2021).

2.3.8.1 Key stages in the malnutrition cycle

Fetal stage (pregnancy)—Maternal undernutrition, anemia, and inadequate dietary intake during pregnancy increase the risk of intrauterine growth restriction (IUGR) and low birth weight. These early disadvantages are associated with impaired growth, reduced cognitive development, and elevated susceptibility to disease (World Health Organisation, 2021).

Infancy and early childhood—Poor IYCF practices, combined with infection and inadequate care, contribute to growth faltering and stunting. Stunted children are more likely to experience delayed cognitive development, poor school performance, and increased morbidity and mortality (UNICEF, 2023; Victora et al., 2021).

Adolescence—Adolescence represents a second critical period of rapid growth requiring increased nutritional intake. Undernourished adolescent girls who become pregnant face nutrient competition between maternal growth and fetal development, strengthening the intergenerational cycle of malnutrition (UNICEF, 2023; World Health Organisation, 2021).

Adulthood—Adults who experienced childhood undernutrition often have reduced physical capacity, lower productivity, and an increased risk of noncommunicable diseases such as diabetes and hypertension, notably in contexts undergoing a nutrition transition (Black et al., 2013; Victora et al., 2021).

Older age—In later life, cumulative nutritional disadvantage contributes to sarcopenia, functional decline, weakened immunity, and heightened vulnerability to chronic illness (World Health Organisation, 2021).

A growing body of empirical research supports the life-cycle model of malnutrition by demonstrating strong intergenerational and life-course linkages between maternal nutrition, birth outcomes, child growth, and adult health. Intergenerational transmission of undernutrition is a critical public health challenge in India, where maternal short stature, anemia, and poor nutritional status are strong predictors of low birth weight (LBW), child stunting, and mortality, independent of socioeconomic variables (Mamidi et al., 2011; Subramanian et al., 2009). Recent analyses of NFHS-5 data confirm that LBW is a key mediator in this pathway, significantly increasing the risk of subsequent childhood wasting and stunting (Khan et al., 2019; Meitei & Singh, 2024). Longitudinal research, particularly the Pune Maternal Nutrition Study, provides biological evidence for the "thin-fat" Indian phenotype, demonstrating that IUGR, followed by energy-dense diets, predisposes offspring to metabolic syndrome and noncommunicable diseases in adulthood (Fall et al., 2015; Yajnik & Deshmukh, 2008). This evidence of the double burden of malnutrition confirms the necessity of the life-cycle approach adopted in India's National Nutrition Strategy, which targets interventions at critical stages—preconception, pregnancy, and adolescence—to break the cycle of hardship (NITI Aayog, 2017).

2.3.8.2 Applications in India

India's nutrition strategy explicitly adopts a life-cycle approach through convergent programs targeting critical developmental windows. POSHAN Abhiyaan and the ICDS focus on the first 1000 days and early childhood (Ministry of Women and Child Development (MWCD), 2018), whereas initiatives, such as Pradhan Mantri Matru Vandana Yojana (PMMVY) and Anaemia Mukt Bharat, extend support to pregnant women and adolescents (Ministry of Health and Family Welfare, 2018). School-based interventions under PM POSHAN further ensure continuity into middle childhood, linking maternal health and child development within an integrated framework (Ministry of Health and Family Welfare, 2021).

Research confirms the necessity of this approach, as studies show that maternal undernutrition and adolescent anemia are strong predictors of child stunting and intergenerational disadvantage (Kim et al., 2017; Woode & Birner, 2021). However, the effectiveness of these interventions depends on tackling structural determinants, e.g., poverty, gender inequality, and sanitation. To break the cycle of malnutrition, India's policy framework emphasizes the combination of preventive and clinical strategies among generations to build sustained resilience (NITI Aayog, 2017).

2.3.9 Food system–based nutrition models

The food system–nutrition security models conceptualize childhood malnutrition as an outcome of interconnected processes involving food production, processing, distribution, food environments, dietary behavior, and supporting systems such as health, education, and social protection (Hammond & Dubé, 2012). This perspective emphasizes that improving nutrition requires transforming food systems to ensure access to multiple, safe, and affordable diets, rather than relying solely on supplementation (Hammond & Dubé, 2012; Ruel & Brouwer, 2024). Food systems, therefore, function as a central pathway linking agriculture, markets, and consumption patterns to nutrition security.

2.4 The HLPE Food Systems Framework

The HLPE Food Systems Framework, developed by the high-level panel of experts, conceptualizes food systems as the full set of activities from production, processing, distribution, preparation, and consumption of food, along with their social, economic, and environmental outcomes (High-Level Panel of Experts on Food Security and Nutrition, 2017). It emphasizes that nutrition outcomes depend not only on food availability but also on food environments, consumer behavior, and wider political, ecological, and economic drivers. The framework groups food systems into three interacting components: food supply chains, food environments, and consumer behavior (High Level Panel of Experts on Food Security and Nutrition, 2017). These operate inside broader drivers such as climate change, globalization, technological change, and governance, ultimately directing dietary quality and population nutrition.

A key contribution of the model is placing diet quality at the center of nutrition outcomes—including undernutrition, micronutrient deficiencies, and obesity—and endorsing nutrition-sensitive food systems that ensure access to safe and affordable different diets, especially for vulnerable groups (Global Panel on Agriculture and Food Systems for Nutrition, 2016; High Level Panel of Experts on Food Security and Nutrition, 2017). This perspective closely aligns with life-cycle approaches to nutrition by recognizing the importance of food environments in shaping eating habits across critical developmental stages.

The HLPE Food Systems Framework has been widely used to guide policy and research on sustainable nutrition interventions. It supports multisectoral strategies that integrate agriculture, public health, social protection, education, and environmental protection to address childhood malnutrition. By placing nutrition outcomes inside broader food-system dynamics the framework helps explain why interventions focused solely on food supplementation or clinical treatment may have limited long-term impact unless underlying food-system constraints are addressed (High Level Panel of Experts on Food Security and Nutrition, 2017).

In India the HLPE food-systems framework is reflected in a shift from calorie-based food security toward broader nutrition security through integrated agriculture, health, and social-protection programs. National initiatives such as the Public Distribution System (PDS), POSHAN Abhiyaan, ICDS, and the PM POSHAN school meal scheme together address food supply chains, food environments, and consumer behavior rather than treating malnutrition only as a clinical condition (Ministry of Health and Family Welfare, 2021). Agriculture policies increasingly promote nutrition-sensitive diversification, including millets, pulses, and biofortified crops, while Anganwadi and school feeding programs improve access and affordability of nutritious foods for women and children (FAO, 2019; Government of India, 2021). Behavior-change communication (BCC) under POSHAN Abhiyaan further influences eating, hygiene, and feeding habits, demonstrating how food environments and consumer actions jointly shape nutritional outcomes. This systems perspective explains why supplementation or therapeutic feeding alone cannot substantially reduce malnutrition unless livelihoods, sanitation, women's empowerment, and diet diversity improve simultaneously, leading

India to adopt multisectoral strategies aligned with the HLPE approach (HLPE, 2017; NITI Aayog, 2020).

2.5 The UNICEF Innocenti Framework

The UNICEF Innocenti Framework on Food Systems for Children and Adolescents (2019) embodies a critical paradigm shift from generic food security models to a child-centered approach, explicitly positioning children's diets as the central interface between broader food systems and health outcomes. Unlike classic models that focus primarily on agricultural production or household caloric availability, this system conceptualizes the "food environment" as a decisive factor, acknowledging that children's nutrition is determined by an intricate interaction of four distinct domains: food supply chains, external food environments (food availability, advertising, and pricing in the community), personalized food environments (household-level accessibility and affordability), and the behaviors of caregivers and children. This multilayered structure is key for addressing the changing "triple burden" of malnutrition—where persistent undernutrition coexists with micronutrient deficiencies and rapidly rising rates of childhood overweight—by mapping how macrolevel drivers such as urbanization, climate change, and commercial determinants trickle down to influence the daily nutritional decisions and physiological development of vulnerable young populations (UNICEF Office of Research-Innocenti, 2019).

Over the years, this system has deeply influenced India's national nutritional strategies, guiding the transition from calorie-centric welfare to "nutrition-sensitive" food systems. For instance, Mission Poshan 2.0 (Saksham Anganwadi and Poshan 2.0) adopts a systems-thinking approach to combat malnutrition by integrating the Supplementary Nutrition Programme (SNP) with Poshan Vatikas (nutri-gardens) to diversify the food available at the Anganwadi level (Ministry of Women and Child Development, 2021). Similarly the PM POSHAN (formerly midday meal) scheme strengthens the external food environment for school-aged children by mandating the inclusion of locally sourced vegetables and millets and by directly linking agricultural supply chains to child health outcomes (Ministry of Education, Government of India, 2021). The framework's emphasis on regulating unhealthy food environments is further operationalized through FSSAI's "Eat Right India" movement, which restricts the sale of high fat, sugar, and salt (HFSS) foods in school canteens to protect adolescents from the commercial determinants of health. By converging these sectors—agriculture, education, and food safety—India demonstrates how the Innocenti model can be applied in practice to bridge the gap between national food sovereignty and the specific nutritional rights of children (FSSAI, 2020; Ministry of Women and Child Development, 2022).

2.6 Farming Systems for Nutrition approach

The Farming Systems for Nutrition (FSN) approach, developed by the M. S. Swaminathan Research Foundation (MSSRF) (Swaminathan et al., 2012), integrates agriculture, nutrition, and livelihoods to address malnutrition through locally adapted farming systems. The FSN model is based on the premise that improving household-level production diversity, nutritional diversity, and nutrition awareness simultaneously is able to enhance nutrition security, particularly in rural and tribal communities that depend on smallholder agriculture. Unlike conventional agriculture strategies that focus primarily on yield and staple crop production, FSN emphasizes nutrition-sensitive agriculture by promoting the cultivation and consumption of nutrient-dense foods, including pulses, millets, fruits, vegetables, and small livestock.

The FSN framework links farm production systems directly to household diets through three pathways: food production for consumption, income generation, and women's empowerment. Through diversifying cropping systems and strengthening local food availability, FSN interventions seek to improve nutritional diversity and micronutrient intake among at-risk populations (Bhavani & Gopinath, 2017). Community participation, nutrition education, and use of indigenous foods are central components of the approach, rendering it especially relevant in resource-poor and ecologically fragile regions.

Empirical evidence from FSN pilot interventions in India (Bhavani & Gopinath, 2017; Pradhan et al., 2021) demonstrates improvements in nutritional variety, household food security, and consumption of nutrient-dense foods. Precisely the FSN pilots in Wardha (Maharashtra) and Koraput (Odisha) increased household nutritional diversity scores by 0.6–0.8 points over 3 years, with higher consumption of vegetables and animal sources. The endline surveys showed that 10%–15% of households achieved HDDS ≥ 9, corroborating the effectiveness of nutrition-sensitive agriculture in vulnerable areas (Pradhan et al., 2021). Studies conducted in rainfed and tribal regions show that including horticulture, backyard poultry, small livestock, and biofortified crops into farming systems can increase access to micronutrient-rich foods and strengthen resilience to seasonal food insecurity (Bhaskar et al., 2017). These findings show the potential of agriculture-based nutrition interventions to complement health-sector strategies to reduce childhood malnutrition.

The FSN approach matches closely with global food-systems thinking by emphasizing local resource endowments, crop diversification, and nutrition-sensitive agriculture (Bhavani et al., 2016; Nagarajan et al., 2014). It complements life-cycle nutrition interventions via addressing upstream determinants of malnutrition—specifically food availability and nutritional variety—at the household level (Nithya et al., 2017). As such, FSN provides a validated operational model for translating food-systems concepts for community-level action to improve maternal and child nutrition outcomes in developing contexts (Das et al., 2014).

2.7 Key interventions and evidence of food system models

2.7.1 Biofortification

A critical intervention within food-system strategies is biofortification, which addresses "hidden hunger" by breeding staple crops to increase their micronutrient density. In the Indian context, this strategy is fundamental for combating widespread anemia and zinc deficiency. The Indian Council of Agricultural Research (ICAR) has developed 152 biofortified varieties—rice (14), wheat (53), maize (24), millets (26), oilseeds (21), pulses (9), horticultural crops (19), and grain amaranth (5)—addressing micronutrient deficiencies such as Zn, Fe, vitamin A along with others (Press Information Bureau, 2025). Evidence from efficacy trials in Maharashtra demonstrates that the consumption of biofortified pearl millet significantly improves iron status and cognitive performance in adolescents, delivering a sustainable, cost-effective complement to supplementation programs (Finkelstein et al., 2019). Considering the need to scale up these biofortified varieties the ICAR—Central Tuber Crops Research Institute, Thiruvananthapuram, has developed an institutional intervention model, "Rainbow Diet Campaign" (Sivakumar et al., 2020). This program promotes the cultivation and consumption of biofortified tubers, specifically β-carotene-rich, orange-fleshed sweet potato (e.g., *Bhu Sona* and *Sree Kanaka*) and anthocyanin-rich, purple-fleshed varieties (*Bhu Krishna* and *Sree Neelima*). Implemented through "Nutriseed Villages" and school engagement programs in tribal belts such as Attapadi (Kerala) and Keonjhar (Odisha), the campaign has demonstrated that including these nutrient-dense tubers in local diets significantly increases vitamin A and antioxidant intake among at-risk populations (Nedunchezhiyan et al., 2024). This model validates biofortification as an expandable, cost-effective strategy when supported by strong institutional extension mechanisms.

2.7.2 Nutrition-sensitive agriculture and school feeding interventions

The interventions that explicitly link agricultural production to nutritional outcomes—termed nutrition-sensitive agriculture—are key for improving nutritional variety. In India the *FSN* approach, piloted in districts such as Wardha and Koraput, has shown that diversifying crop production to include pulses and millets, coupled with promoting "Poshan Vatikas" (nutri-gardens), leads to statistically considerable improvements in household nutritional diversity scores (Bird et al., 2019). Furthermore the PM POSHAN scheme (formerly the Mid-Day Meal Scheme) illustrates a home-grown school feeding model. By sourcing locally the program not only incentivizes smallholder production but also enhances the nutritional intake of school-aged children, acting as an important safety net against food insecurity.

2.7.3 Structural causes and the triple burden research

The triple burden research shows that structural food-system factors—including urbanization, market integration, and changing dietary patterns—strongly influence malnutrition outcomes. India is currently undergoing a "nutrition transition"—characterized by the simultaneous persistence of undernutrition and a rapid rise in obesity and noncommunicable diseases, known as the "triple burden of malnutrition." Studies by the Tata-Cornell Institute show that while India has achieved calorie sufficiency, the food system remains skewed toward staples, making nutrient-dense nonstaples (fruits, vegetables, eggs) unaffordable for many (Pingali et al., 2019). Consequently, panel data analyses suggest that transforming food systems to prioritize the cost and availability of diverse foods is critical to addressing these complex nutritional challenges (Sharma et al., 2020).

2.7.4 Multisectoral coordination

Although production-focused interventions are necessary, empirical evidence indicates that they are insufficient in isolation (Mejia et al., 2022). Effective food-system models require multisectoral coordination, which connects agriculture, health, and women's empowerment. The *POSHAN Abhiyaan* strategy demonstrates this by seeking to align agricultural availability with BCC and sanitation (NITI Aayog, 2023). Research indicates that agricultural interventions are most effective when they explicitly empower women—who are often the primary gatekeepers of household nutrition—improving their decision-making power and time allocation (Kadiyala et al., 2014). Thus the food systems–nutrition security model provides a comprehensive framework that supports public health approaches by addressing upstream structural determinants.

2.7.5 Behavior change and care practice models

2.7.5.1 Conceptual foundations of care and behavior in child nutrition

Research shows that childcare practice—specifically breastfeeding, complementary feeding, hygiene, and psychosocial care—are key determinants of nutritional status during the first 1000 days of life. Global evidence indicates that programs combining nutrition education with community health services significantly improve child growth outcomes (Bhutta et al., 2013; Engle et al., 1999). However, knowledge alone is often insufficient; caregiving is determined by a complex interplay between a caregiver's internal context (e.g., beliefs, self-efficacy) and external determinants, such as gender norms and family structure (UNICEF, 2020). Consequently, modern nutrition strategies have shifted from simple information dissemination to social and behavior change (SBC) models that address the gap between knowledge and practice by tackling the structural and psychological barriers to optimal care.

2.7.5.2 Care practices and household decision-making

Care is a multidimensional construct driven by psychological and communal factors, encompassing critical behaviors such as breastfeeding, hygiene, and psychosocial stimulation (Engle et al., 1999). These practices are strongly influenced by household power relations—specifically, women's autonomy in decision-making—which directly affects healthcare utilization and feeding outcomes (Bhutta et al., 2013). Furthermore deeply entrenched cultural principles and societal beliefs often shape caregiving norms, sometimes reinforcing traditional practices that unintentionally contribute to child undernutrition (Pelto et al., 2003).

2.7.5.3 The socioecological model in nutrition behavior change

To operationalize these concepts, practitioners frequently employ the socio-ecological model (SEM). This system conceptualizes behavior not as an isolated individual decision but as the result of layered influences ranging from the individual and interpersonal to community and policy levels (McLeroy et al., 1988). In the context of child nutrition the SEM highlights how intrahousehold decision-making power—particularly women's autonomy—and shared community beliefs shape feeding and health-seeking behaviors (Pelto et al., 2003). By placing the caregiver within these broader systems the model advocates interventions that extend beyond the mother to engage fathers, grandmothers, and community leaders, thereby fostering a supportive environment for sustainable behavior change.

2.7.5.4 Application in the Indian context

In India, these models are institutionalized through the ICDS and the POSHAN Abhiyaan (National Nutrition Mission). The strategy utilizes a "Jan Andolan" (People's Movement) approach to shift social norms around nutrition. Primary workers, including AWWs and ASHAs, leverage home visits and Village Health, Sanitation, and Nutrition Days (VHSNDs) to deliver interpersonal counseling (IPC) on IYCF. These communications are designed to be context-specific, addressing local cultural myths and strengthening positive practices through community-based events (Ministry of Women and Child Development, 2018). Programs such as Anaemia Mukt Bharat further integrate BCC to improve adherence to iron supplementation and dietary diversity.

2.7.5.5 Evidence of impact

Evaluations of these large-scale Indian interventions show the efficacy of integrating behavior change models into public health systems. Data from the NFHS and specific program assessments indicate that sustained exposure to BCC messages delivered by community health workers is associated with statistically significant improvements in early initiation of breastfeeding, exclusive breastfeeding rates, and complementary feeding diversity (International Institute for Population Sciences (IIPS) & ICF, 2021; Menon et al., 2018). These results indicate that when BCC strategies efficiently address the social and household determinants of care—rather than treating nutrition as a purely medical issue—they are a cost-effective means of improving maternal and child health outcomes throughout diverse demographic settings.

2.7.6 Equity-focused and gender-responsive models

Combating child malnutrition requires moving beyond simple food distribution and clinical treatment to tackling structural inequalities, gender relations, and social exclusion that limit access to care. Equity-focused and gender-responsive models emphasize that malnutrition is fundamentally determined by power relations within households, unequal access to resources, and system-wide barriers affecting marginalized populations (Bhutta et al., 2013; UNICEF, 2020). These approaches focus on identifying the underlying drivers of malnutrition, e.g., poverty and discrimination, and designing interventions that simultaneously improve nutrition outcomes and promote social fairness.

2.7.6.1 Gender-transformative frameworks

A central pillar of this strategy is the gender-transformative nutrition framework, which goes beyond gender-sensitive programming to actively change the social norms and institutional structures that maintain inequality. This approach operates across three dimensions: enhancing women's agency (decision-making power), improving relations (engaging men in caregiving), and reforming structures (addressing policy barriers, such as land ownership). Evidence consistently shows that when women are empowered, child feeding practices and nutritional diversity improve significantly, making gender equity a critical pathway for reducing malnutrition (Ruel et al., 2018).

2.7.6.2 Key operational models

To operationalize these concepts, practitioners employ models such as Integrated Community Case Management with Nutrition (iCCM + Nut) and the first 1000 days' approach. The iCCM + Nut improves equity by training community health workers to screen for and treat acute malnutrition alongside common childhood illnesses, thereby reducing the geographic and financial barriers that disproportionately affect poor households (Young et al., dat). Alongside this the first 1000 days model targets the critical window from conception to age 2, prioritizing the prevention of maternal anemia and the promotion of breastfeeding. This approach recognizes that maternal undernutrition is a main driver of low birth weight and intergenerational cycles of malnutrition (Black et al., 2013; Victora et al., 2021).

2.7.6.3 Applications in India

The Integrated Management of Neonatal and Childhood Illness (IMNCI) and the Home-Based Care for Young Child (HBYC) program are Indianized versions of the iCCM + Nut framework. While the IMNCI framework improves equity by training primary workers such as ASHAs and AWWs to screen and treat acute malnutrition alongside common illnesses, the HBYC initiative explicitly mandates home visits to ensure continued care, thereby reducing geographic and monetary barriers for poor rural households (Ministry of Health and Family Welfare, 2018). In addition, the first 1000 days model is institutionalized through POSHAN Abhiyaan and Anaemia Mukt Bharat, which target the critical window from conception to age 2. This approach prioritizes the prevention of maternal anemia and breastfeeding, recognizing that maternal undernutrition is a major cause of low birth weight and intergenerational cycles of malnutrition in India (Victora et al., 2021; NITI Aayog, 2023).

2.7.7 The "systems approach" model (2025–26 evolution)

2.7.7.1 Evolution and operational context

In recent global nutrition discourse the systems approach has evolved from a conceptual framework into an operational policy requirement. This shift acknowledges that malnutrition is not exclusively a health-sector issue but the result of interacting failures across five anchor systems: food, health, social protection, environment (WASH), and education (HLPE, 2020; UNICEF, 2020). The 2025–26 strategy emphasizes resilience and multisectoral governance, aligning nutrition action with the SDGs to address the "poly-crisis"—where climate change, conflict, and financial volatility simultaneously endanger global food and health security (Development Initiatives, 2024; FAO et al., 2023).

2.7.7.2 The five interlocking systems

Current thinking identifies five distinct systems that must function cooperatively to protect nutrition. The food system has shifted focus from simple calorie sufficiency to "nutrition security," emphasizing diet quality and regulating ultraprocessed foods (Global Panel on Agriculture and Food Systems for Nutrition, 2020). The health system integrates nutrition into primary care via antenatal support and anemia control (WHO, 2022). Simultaneously, Social Protection is moving toward "cash-plus" models that combine financial support with behavior change (Ruel & Alderman, 2013). These are underpinned by the WASH System, which reduces environmental enteric dysfunction caused by poor sanitation (Humphrey, 2009), and the Education System, which functions as a platform for adolescent nutrition and food literacy (Bundy et al., 2018).

2.7.7.3 Future directions: Resilience and equity

The latest evolution in systems thinking moves from merely "nutrition-sensitive" to "nutrition-smart" investment frameworks, which explicitly evaluate how sectoral investments influence diet quality (FAO et al., 2023). There is a heightened focus on data modernization, utilizing real-time administrative data to identify malnutrition hotspots more quickly than traditional surveys. Crucially, modern models place equity and gender at the center, addressing "time poverty" among women and extending interventions to adolescent girls to break the intergenerational cycle of malnutrition (UNICEF, 2020; Victora et al., 2021).

2.7.8 Application of the systems approach in India

2.7.8.1 Governance and convergence: The POSHAN model

India's nutrition strategy operationalizes these systems thinking mainly through POSHAN Abhiyaan (National Nutrition Mission), one of the world's largest multisectoral initiatives. Recognizing that malnutrition is multidetermined, the mission mandates "convergence" across critical ministries—Women and Child Development, Health, Education, Jal Shakti, and Agriculture (Government of India, 2018a, 2018b). This governance structure utilizes digital dashboards (Poshan Tracker) for immediate monitoring and emphasizes BCC (Jan Andolan), reflecting global best practices in coordinating action at the highest political levels (NITI Aayog, 2021).

2.7.8.2 *Programmatic integration across systems*

Implementation is visible across all five anchor systems. In health, programs such as *Anaemia Mukt Bharat* and IYCF counseling are integrated into primary care and Anganwadi services (Ministry of Health and Family Welfare, 2018). The food and social protection systems are linked through the PDS, *PM POSHAN* (school meals), and *PMMVY* (maternity benefits), which together address food security and maternal health (Drèze & Goyal, 2020). Furthermore the strategy integrates WASH through the *Swachh Bharat Mission* to reduce infection-related malnutrition and education through adolescent supplementation programs. Recent pushes for dietary diversification, such as the promotion of millets (Shree Anna), further demonstrate India's shift toward a climate-resilient, nutrition-smart food system (Government of India, 2023; UNICEF India, 2021).

2.8 Conclusion

Childhood malnutrition in India persists not because of a lack of knowledge or interventions, but because of the complex and interdependent nature of its determinants. This review demonstrates that malnutrition cannot be adequately understood or addressed through isolated, sector-specific approaches. Rather, it results from interacting failures across food systems, health services, caregiving practices, social protection, gender relations, environmental conditions, and governance structures, all of which operate across the life course and span generations. The evolution of nutritional thinking—from the UNICEF Conceptual Framework to life-cycle, food-systems, equity-focused, and contemporary systems approaches—reflects increasing recognition of these complications. Interventions are necessary to address immediate biological deficits; their population-level impact is constrained unless complemented by nutrition-sensitive and nutrition-smart strategies that address underlying and basic causes. Models such as the Lancet framework, CMAM/IMAM, and behavior change approaches demonstrate strong effectiveness when implemented with quality and coverage, yet their sustainability depends on supportive food environments, resilient health systems, effective social protection, and empowered caregivers—particularly women. Food system–based models, including the HLPE and UNICEF Innocenti frameworks, further underscore that diet quality, rather than caloric adequacy alone, must be central to nutrition policy in an era distinguished by the triple burden of malnutrition.

India's nutrition architecture, anchored in POSHAN Abhiyaan, ICDS, Anaemia Mukt Bharat, and allied sectoral missions, demonstrates a substantive shift toward multisectoral convergence and life-course programming. Nevertheless, persistent territorial disparities, micronutrient deficiencies, and increasing childhood overweight reveal ongoing gaps in last-mile delivery, nutritional diversity, gender equity, and system durability. The forthcoming 2025–2026 systems approach delivers a critical opportunity to strengthen governance coherence, incorporate real-time data systems, and embed equity and climate resilience into nutrition planning, thereby advancing from project-based interventions to adaptive, system-wide solutions.

To summarize, effectively confronting childhood malnutrition in India necessitates reframing nutrition as a development and governance challenge, rather than only a health or food issue. Future progress depends on institutionalizing systems thinking, aligning cross-sectoral investments with nutrition outcomes, and prioritizing the most at-risk populations through equity-focused and gender-responsive strategies. Through integrating biological, social, economic, and environmental dimensions across the life course, India can translate its major policy commitments into sustained nutritional gains and advance toward eliminating all forms of child malnutrition by 2030.

References

ASSOCHAM, EY. (2017). *Bridging the gap: Tapping the agriculture potential for optimum nutrition.* New Delhi: The Associated Chambers of Commerce and Industry of India (ASSOCHAM.

Bhaskar, A. V. V., Nithya, D. J., Raju, S., & Bhavani, R. V. (2017). Establishing integrated agriculture-nutrition programmes to diversify household food and diets in rural India. *Food Security, 9*(5), 981–999. https://doi.org/10.1007/s12571-017-0721-z.

Bhavani, R. V., & Gopinath, R. (2017). Farming systems for nutrition: An approach to leverage agriculture for nutritional outcomes. *Agricultural Research, 6*(3), 238–247. https://doi.org/10.1007/s40003-017-0261-1.

Bhavani, R. V., Jagarwal, N., Raju, S., et al. (2016). *Leveraging agriculture for nutrition in South Asia: Evidence from research 2012-2016 (LANSA working paper no. 25). Leveraging Agriculture for Nutrition in South Asia (LANSA) research programme.* https://www.lansa.ac.uk/publications/working-papers/

Bhutta, Z. A., Das, J. K., Rizvi, A., Gaffey, M. F., Walker, N., Horton, S., … MaternalChild Nutrition Study Group. (2013). Evidence-based interventions for improvement of maternal and child nutrition: What can be done and at what cost? *The Lancet, 382*(9890), 452–477. https://doi.org/10.1016/S0140-6736(13)60996-4.

Bird, F. A., Pradhan, A., Bhavani, R. V., & Dangour, A. D. (2019). Interventions in agriculture for nutrition outcomes: a systematic review focused on South Asia. (Special Issue: Leveraging agriculture for nutrition in South Asia.). Food Policy, 82, 39–49. https://doi.org/10.1016/j.foodpol.2018.10.015.

Black, R. E., Victora, C. G., Walker, S. P., Bhutta, Z. A., Christian, P., De Onis, M., Ezzati, M., Grantham-Mcgregor, S., Katz, J., Martorell, R., & Uauy, R. (2013). Maternal and child undernutrition and overweight in low-income and middle-income countries. *The Lancet, 382*(9890), 427–451. https://doi.org/10.1016/S0140-6736(13)60937-X.

Borooah, V. K. (2012). Social identity and educational attainment: The role of caste and religion in explaining differences between children in India. *Journal of Development Studies, 48*(7), 887–903. https://doi.org/10.1080/00220388.2011.621945.

Bundy, D. A. P., de Silva, N., Horton, S., Jamison, D. T., & Patton, G. C. (Eds.). (2018). *Re-imagining school feeding: A high-return investment in human capital and local economies.* World Bank https://openknowledge.worldbank.org/handle/10986/28926.

Burza, S., Mahajan, R., Marino, E., Sunyoto, T., Shandilya, C., Tabrez, M., Kumari, K., Mathew, P., Jha, A., Salse, N., & Mishra, K. N. (2015). Community-based management of severe acute malnutrition in India: New evidence from Bihar. *American Journal of Clinical Nutrition, 101*(4), 847–859. https://doi.org/10.3945/ajcn.114.093294.

Cleland, J.G., & Van Ginneken, J.K. (1988). Maternal education and child survival in developing countries: the search for pathways of influence. Social science & medicine (1982), 27(12), 1357–1368. https://doi.org/10.1016/0277-9536(88)90201-8

Collins, S., Sadler, K., Dent, N., Khara, T., Guerrero, S., Myatt, M., Saboya, M., & Walsh, A. (2006). Key issues in the success of community-based management of severe malnutrition. *Food and Nutrition Bulletin, 27*(3_suppl3), S49. https://doi.org/10.1177/15648265060273s304.

Dahir, H. M., Korse, A. H., & Mohamed, F. I. (2026). Water, sanitation, and hygiene and their association with child undernutrition: A hierarchical analysis of the 2020 Somaliland demographic health survey. *Frontiers in Public Health, 13*. https://doi.org/10.3389/fpubh.2025.1734101.

Das, J. K., Salam, R. A., Kumar, R., & Bhutta, Z. A. (2013). Micronutrient fortification of food and its impact on women and child health: A systematic review. *Annals of the New York Academy of Sciences, 1287*(1), 32–42. https://doi.org/10.1111/nyas.12056.

Das, P. K., Bhavani, R. V., & Swaminathan, M. S. (2014). A farming system model to leverage agriculture for nutritional outcomes. *Agricultural Research, 3*(3), 193–203. https://doi.org/10.1007/s40003-014-0119-5.

Development Initiatives. (2024). *Global nutrition report: The state of global nutrition*. https://globalnutritionreport.org/reports/2024-global-nutrition-report/

De Sanctis, V., Soliman, A., Alaaraj, N., Ahmed, S., Alyafei, F., & Hamed, N. (2021). Early and Long-term Consequences of Nutritional Stunting: From Childhood to Adulthood. *Acta biomedica : Atenei Parmensis, 92*(1), e2021168. https://doi.org/10.23750/abm.v92i1.11346.

Drèze, J., & Khera, R. (2020). Recent social security initiatives in India. *World Development, 136*, 105012. https://doi.org/10.1016/j.worlddev.2019.105012.

Engle, P. L., Menon, P., & Haddad, L. (1999). Care and nutrition: Concepts and measurement. *World Development, 27*(8), 1309–1337. https://doi.org/10.1016/S0305-750X(99)00059-5.

Fall, C. H. D., Sachdev, H. S., Osmond, C., Lakshmy, R., Biswas, S. D., Prabhakaran, D., & Tandon, N. (2015). Adult metabolic syndrome and impaired glucose tolerance are associated with different patterns of BMI gain during infancy and childhood: Evidence from the New Delhi Birth Cohort. *Diabetes Care, 38*(11), 2053–2061. https://doi.org/10.2337/dc15-0128.

FAO. (2019). Nutrition-sensitive agriculture and food systems in practice. Rome: Food and Agriculture Organization of the United Nations.

FAO, IFAD, UNICEF, WFP, and WHO. (2023). *The State of Food Security and Nutrition in the World 2023: Urbanization, agrifood systems transformation and healthy diets across the rural–urban continuum*. Rome: FAO.

FAO, IFAD, UNICEF, WFP and WHO. (2025). *The State of Food Security and Nutrition in the World 2025 – Addressing high food price inflation for food security and nutrition*. FAO.

FAO. (2016). *Influencing food environments for healthy diets*. Food and Agriculture Organisation of the United Nations.

FAO. (2017). *Nutrition-sensitive agriculture and food systems in practice: Options for intervention*. Food and Agriculture Organisation of the United Nations https://www.fao.org/3/a-i7848e.pdf.

Finkelstein, J. L., Fothergill, A., Johnson, C., Haas, J. D., Ghosh, S., Bhandari, N., O'Brien, K. O., & Scott, S. P. (2019). A 6-month randomised controlled efficacy trial of iron-biofortified pearl millet (ICTP 8203) in secondary school children in Maharashtra, India. *The Journal of Nutrition, 149*(2), 222–231. https://doi.org/10.1093/jn/nxy266.

Food Safety and Standards Authority of India. (2020). *Eat right India handbook*. Ministry of Health and Family Welfare https://eatrightindia.gov.in/eatright-toolkit.jsp.

Gillespie, S., & Flores, R. (2000). The life cycle of malnutrition (IFPRI 1999–2000 annual report essay). *International Food Policy Research Institute*.

Gillespie, S., Haddad, L., Mannar, V., Menon, P., & Nisbett, N. (2013). The politics of reducing malnutrition: Building commitment and accelerating progress. *The Lancet, 382*(9891), 552–569. https://doi.org/10.1016/S0140-6736(13)60842-1.

Global Panel on Agriculture and Food Systems for Nutrition. (2016). *Food systems and diets: Facing the challenges of the 21st century*. https://www.glopan.org/reports/food-systems-and-diets-facing-the-challenges-of-the-21st-century

Global Panel on Agriculture and Food Systems for Nutrition (2020). Future Food Systems: For people, our planet, and prosperity. Project Report. London School of Hygiene & Tropical Medicine. https://doi.org/10.17037/PUBS.04675674.

Government of India. (2018a). *Anaemia Mukt Bharat: Intensified national iron plus initiative operational guidelines*. Government of India https://anemiamuktbharat.info/wp-content/uploads/2019/09/AMB-Operational-Guidelines.pdf.

Government of India. (2018b). Home-Based Care for Young Child (HBYC): Operational guidelines. Government of India. https://nhm.gov.in/New_Updates_2018/NHM_Components/RMNCH_MH_Guidelines/HBYC-Guidelines.pdf

Government of India. (2021). Pradhan Mantri Poshan Shakti Nirman (PM POSHAN): Guidelines. Government of India. https://pmposhan.education.gov.in/guideline.html

Government of India, Ministry of Agriculture & Farmers' Welfare. (2023). International Year of Millets: India leading the way. Press Information Bureau, New Delhi, 18 March 2023.

Gupta, S., Borah, A., & Kochhar, E. (2025). *Understanding trends in dietary diversity in India: Moving towards sustainable consumption*. Council on Energy, Environment and Water.

Hammond, R. A., & Dubé, L. (2012). A systems science perspective and transdisciplinary models for food and nutrition security. *Proceedings of the National Academy of Sciences, 109*(31), 12356–12363. https://doi.org/10.1073/pnas.0913003109.

Hasan, M. dT., Magalhaes, R. J. S., Williams, G. M., & Mamun, A. A. (2016). The role of maternal education in the 15-year trajectory of malnutrition in children under 5 years of age in Bangladesh. *Maternal & Child Nutrition, 12*(4), 929–939. https://doi.org/10.1111/mcn.12178.

High Level Panel of Experts on Food Security and Nutrition. (2017). *Nutrition and food systems (HLPE report 12)*. Committee on World Food Security https://www.fao.org/3/i7846e/i7846e.pdf.

HLPE. (2020). *Food security and nutrition: building a global narrative towards 2030*. A report by the High Level Panel of Experts on Food Security and Nutrition of the Committee on World Food Security, Rome.

Humphrey, J. H. (2009). Child undernutrition, tropical enteropathy, toilets, and handwashing. *The Lancet*, 374(9694), 1032–1035. https://doi.org/10.1016/S0140-6736(09)60950-8.

International Institute for Population Sciences (IIPS) & ICF. (2021). *National Family Health Survey (NFHS-5), 2019-21: India*. IIPS https://dhsprogram.com/pubs/pdf/FR375/FR375.pdf.

Ji, N., Kumar, A., Joe, W., Kuriyan, R., Sethi, V., Finkelstein, J. L., & Mehta, S. (2024). Prevalence and correlates of double and triple burden of malnutrition among children and adolescents in India. *The Journal of Nutrition, 154*(10), 2932–2947. https://doi.org/10.1016/j.tjnut.2024.08.021.

Kadiyala, S., Harris, J., Headey, D., Yosef, S., & Gillespie, S. (2014). Agriculture and nutrition in India: Mapping evidence to pathways. *Annals of the New York Academy of Sciences, 1331*(1), 43–56. https://doi.org/10.1111/nyas.12477.

Khan, J., & Mohanty, S. K. (2024). Poverty induced inequality in nutrition among children born during 2010-2021 in India. *PloS one, 19*(11), e0313596. https://doi.org/10.1371/journal.pone.0313596.

Khan, J., Vesari, Y. B., & Pradhan, M. R. (2019). Low birth weight and its associated risk factors: Health facility-based case-control study. *Public Health, 171*, 54–62. https://doi.org/10.1016/j.puhe.2019.03.016.

Kim, R., Rajpal, S., Joe, W., Corsi, D. J., Sankar, R., Kumar, A., & Subramanian, S. V. (2017). Assessing the strength of association between stunting and wasting in India. *Maternal & Child Nutrition, 15*(1), e12693.

Kumar, A., & Joe, W. (2020). *Cost-benefit analyses of nutrition interventions in India's policy framework (IEG Working Paper No. 406).* Institute of Economic Growth https://iegindia.org/upload/profile_publication/doc-190820_174628wp406.pdf.

Macallan, D. (2009). Infection and malnutrition. *Medicine, 37*(10), 525–528. https://doi.org/10.1016/j.mpmed.2009.07.005.

Makwela, M. S., & Mashaba, R. G. (2025). Determinants of sub-optimal complementary feeding practices among caregivers of children aged 6–23 months in low-and middle-income countries: Scoping review. *Frontiers in Public Health, 13*. https://doi.org/10.3389/fpubh.2025.1655685.

Mamidi, R. S., Kulkarni, B., & Radhakrishna, K. V. (2011). Maternal short stature is associated with a high prevalence of stunting and underweight among children in India. *Public Health Nutrition, 14*(10), 1851–1856. https://doi.org/10.1017/S136898001100063X.

Mazumdar, S., & Roy, S. (2025). Gender inequality in nutritional status among Indian children: A systematic review and meta-analysis. *Ecology of Food and Nutrition, 64*(6), 373–394. https://doi.org/10.1080/03670244.2025.2602593.

McLeroy, K. R., Bibeau, D., Steckler, A., & Glanz, K. (1988). An ecological perspective on health promotion programs. *Health Education Quarterly, 15*(4), 351–377. https://doi.org/10.1177/109019818801500401.

Meitei, W. B., & Singh, L. (2024). Intergenerational transmission of poverty and stunting in India: Evidence from the National Family Health Survey (NFHS-5). *Child Indicators Research, 17*(1), 215–234. https://doi.org/10.1007/s12187-023-10085-3.

Mejia, L. A., Dary, O., & Bouis, H. (2022). Review of the impact pathways of biofortified foods and food products to reduce micronutrient deficiency. *Nutrients, 14*(6), 1204. https://doi.org/10.3390/nu14061204.

Menon, P., Nguyen, P. H., Saha, K. K., Khaled, A., Sanghvi, T., Baker, J., Afsana, K., Haque, R., & Ruel, M. T. (2018). Impacts of counselling and mass media on complementary feeding. *The Journal of Nutrition, 148*(5), 773–782.

Menon, P., Ruel, M. T., & Arimond, M. (2019). Social, biological, and programmatic factors linking adolescent pregnancy and early childhood undernutrition: A path analysis of India's 2016 National Family Health Survey. *The Lancet Child & Adolescent Health, 3*(11), 775–784. https://doi.org/10.1016/S2352-4642(19)30180-4.

Ministry of Education, Government of India. (2021). *Pradhan Mantri Poshan Shakti Nirman (PM POSHAN): Guidelines* https://pmposhan.education.gov.in.

Ministry of Health and Family Welfare. (2018). *Operational guidelines on facility-based management of children with severe acute malnutrition (SAM).* MoHFW.

Ministry of Health and Family Welfare. (2023). *Poshan Abhiyaan: Strategy and guidelines for addressing malnutrition in India.* MoHFW.

Ministry of Women and Child Development & Ministry of Health and Family Welfare. (2022). *Protocol for managing malnutrition in children.* Government of

India https://wcd.nic.in/sites/default/files/Protocol%20for%20Management%20of%20Malnutrition%20in%20Children.pdf.

Ministry of Women and Child Development (MWCD). (2018). *Administrative guidelines for implementation of POSHAN Abhiyaan*. Government of India https://wcd.nic.in/sites/default/files/Poshan_Abhiyaan_Administrative_Guidelines.pdf.

Ministry of Women and Child Development. (2021). *Mission Saksham Anganwadi and Poshan 2.0: Operational guidelines*. Government of India https://wcd.nic.in/sites/default/files/Poshan_2.0_Guidelines_Final.pdf.

Ministry of Women and Child Development. (2022). *Mission Saksham Anganwadi and Poshan 2.0: Operational guidelines*. Government of India https://wcd.nic.in/sites/default/files/Poshan_2.0_Guidelines_Final.pdf.

Monteiro, C. A., Cannon, G., Lawrence, M., Costa Louzada, M. L., & Pereira Machado, P. (2019). *Ultra-processed foods, diet quality, and health using the NOVA classification system*. FAO.

Mulyani, A. T., Khairinisa, M. A., Khatib, A., & Chaerunisaa, A. Y. (2025). Understanding Stunting: Impact, causes, and strategy to accelerate stunting reduction—A narrative review. *Nutrients, 17*(9). https://doi.org/10.3390/nu17091493.

Nagarajan, S., Bhavani, R. V., & Swaminathan, M. S. (2014). Operationalizing the concept of farming system for nutrition through the promotion of nutrition-sensitive agriculture. *Current Science, 107*(6), 959–964. http://www.currentscience.ac.in/Volumes/107/06/0959.pdf.

Nambiar, A., & Arunachalam, D. (2025). Child Food Deficiency in India: Socio-demographic and Regional Patterns. *Child Ind Res, 18*, 2131–2156. https://doi.org/10.1007/s12187-025-10246-6.

National Research Council (US) Subcommittee on Nutrition and Diarrheal Diseases Control. (1985). *Nutritional management of acute diarrhoea in infants and children*. National Academies Press https://www.ncbi.nlm.nih.gov/books/NBK219100/.

Nedunchezhiyan, M., Laxminarayana, K., Pati, K., & Byju, G. (2024). *Sustainable livelihoods through tuber crops-based agri-food systems (tribal sub-plan report)*. ICAR-Central Tuber Crops Research Institute.

Nguyen, P. H., Kachwaha, S., Tran, L. M., Sanghvi, T., Ghosh, S., Kulkarni, B., Beesabathuni, K., Menon, P., & Sethi, V. (2021). Maternal diets in India: Gaps, barriers, and opportunities. *Nutrients, 13*(10). https://doi.org/10.3390/nu13103534.

Nithya, D. J., Raju, S., Bhavani, R. V., Panda, A. K., Wagh, R. D., & Viswanathan, B. (2020). *Effect of farming systems for nutrition on nutritional intakes (working paper no. 2020-202)*. Madras School of Economics https://ideas.repec.org/p/mad/wpaper/2020-202.ht.

NITI Aayog. (2017). *National nutrition strategy*. Government of India https://niti.gov.in/writereaddata/files/document_publication/Nutrition_Strategy_Booklet.pdf.

NITI Aayog. (2019). *Transforming nutrition in India: POSHAN Abhiyaan first progress report*. Government of India https://www.niti.gov.in/sites/default/files/2020-02/POSHAN_Abhiyaan_first_progress_report_6_Feb_2019.pdf.

NITI Aayog (2020). Accelerating progress on nutrition in India: What will it take (Third progress report). Government of India. https://www.niti.gov.in/node/318.

NITI Aayog. (2021). Transforming nutrition in India: POSHAN Abhiyaan. New Delhi: NITI Aayog, Government of India.

NITI Aayog. (2023). *Transforming child nutrition: State-level approaches and practices for community-based comprehensive care and management of acute malnutrition*. Government of India https://www.niti.gov.in/sites/default/files/2023-12/CMAM-report-NITI-Aayog.pdf.

Paul, P., Saha, R., & Navaneetham, K. (2022). Is maternal autonomy associated with child nutritional status? Evidence from a cross-sectional study in India. *PLoS One, 17*(5), e0268126. https://doi.org/10.1371/journal.pone.0268126.

Pelto, G. H., Santos, I., & Gonçalves, H. (2003). Contextual constraints on the adoption of child feeding guidelines. *The Journal of Nutrition, 133*(9), 2963S–2968S.

Pingali, P., Aiyar, A., Abraham, M., & Rahman, A. (2019). Transforming Food Systems for a Rising India. Springer Nature. https://doi.org/10.1007/978-3-030-14409-8.

Pradhan, A., Raju, S., Nithya, D. J., Panda, A. K., Wagh, R. D., Maske, M. R., Bhavani, R. V., & Snapp, S. S. (2021). Farming System for Nutrition-a pathway to dietary diversity: Evidence from India. *PLoS One, 16*(3), e0248698. https://doi.org/10.1371/journal.pone.0248698.

Prasad, V. (2025). 50 years of a nation-wide child development programme in India. *BMJ Paediatrics Open, 9*(1), e003857. https://doi.org/10.1136/bmjpo-2025-003857.

Prentice, A. M. (2023). The triple burden of malnutrition in the era of globalisation. *Annals of Nutrition and Metabolism, 79*(Suppl. 1), 1–12. https://doi.org/10.1159/000529514.

Press Information Bureau. (2025, October 16). World Food Day 2025: Hand in hand for better foods and a better future [Press release]. Government of India. Retrieved from https://www.pib.gov.in/PressReleasePage.aspx?PRID=2179504&reg=48&lang=2.

Purwanti, E. D., Masitoh, S., & Ronoatmodjo, S. (2025). Association between basic immunization status and stunting in toddlers aged 12-59 months in Indonesia. *Journal of Preventive Medicine and Public Health, 58*(3), 298–306. https://doi.org/10.3961/jpmph.24.230.

Rachmadi, R. A., Ariani, Y., & Alatas, F. S. (2024). Impact of nutritional supplementation on environmental enteric dysfunction (EED) in children living in rural areas: A systematic review. *Arquivos de Gastroenterologia, 61*. https://doi.org/10.1590/S0004-2803.24612023-159.

Raghunathan, K., Headey, D., & Herforth, A. (2021). Affordability of nutritious diets in rural India. *Food Policy, 99*, 101982. https://doi.org/10.1016/j.foodpol.2020.101982.

Ruel, M. T., & Alderman, H. (2013). Nutrition-sensitive interventions and programmes: How can they help to accelerate progress in improving maternal and child nutrition? *The Lancet, 382*(9891), 536–551. https://doi.org/10.1016/S0140-6736(13)60843-0.

Ruel, M.T., & Brouwer, I.D. (2024). Diets and nutrition: The potential of a food systems approach. In Global food policy report 2024: Food systems for healthy diets and nutrition (pp. 18–24). International Food Policy Research Institute.

Ruel, M. T., Garrett, J., Yosef, S., & Olivier, M. (2017). Urbanisation, food security and nutrition. In S. dePee, D. Taren, & M. W. Bloem (Eds.), *Nutrition and health in a developing world* (pp. 661–691). Humana Press.

Ruel, M. T., Quisumbing, A. R., & Balagamwala, M. (2018). Nutrition-sensitive agriculture: What have we learned so far? *Global Food Security, 17*, 128–153. https://doi.org/10.1016/j.gfs.2018.01.002.

Sahoo, J., Mahajan, P. B., Paul, S., Bhatia, V., Patra, A. K., & Hembram, D. K. (2016). Operational assessment of ICDS scheme at grass root level in a rural area of Eastern India: Time to introspect. *Journal of Clinical and Diagnostic Research, 10*(12), LC28. https://doi.org/10.7860/JCDR/2016/23059.9041.

Sahoo, K., Sahoo, B., Choudhury, A. K., Sofi, N. Y., Kumar, R., & Bhadoria, A. S. (2015). Childhood obesity: Causes and consequences. *Journal of Family Medicine and Primary Care, 4*(2), 187–192. https://doi.org/10.4103/2249-4863.15462.

Saunders, J., & Smith, T. (2010). Malnutrition: Causes and consequences. *Clinical Medicine, 10*(6), 624–627. https://doi.org/10.7861/clinmedicine.10-6-624.

Sharma, S., Akhtar, F., Singh, R. K., & Mehra, S. (2020). Dietary intakes, patterns, and determinants of children under 5 years from marginalized communities in Odisha: A cross-sectional study. *Journal of Epidemiology and Global Health, 10*(4), 315–325. https://doi.org/10.2991/jegh.k.200515.002.

Sharn, A. R., Oliveros, E., Lai, S., Sánchez, C. P., Villa-Real Guno, M. J., & Rojas Montenegro, C. (2025). Multi-faceted nutritional interventions are imperative to the reduction of stunting among children in low- and middle-income countries. *Frontiers in Nutrition, 12*, 1479850. https://doi.org/10.3389/fnut.2025.1479850.

Shivakumar, N., Morrison, D. J., Hegde, S. G., Akbari, P., Nirmal Kumar, A., Athalye-Jape, G., Kar, B., Damodar, S., Kurpad, A. V., & Reeds, P. J. (2025). Is there dietary macronutrient malabsorption in children with environmental enteropathy? *European Journal of Clinical Nutrition, 79*, 181–194. https://doi.org/10.1038/s41430-024-01510-z.

Sinha, R., Dua, R., Bijalwan, V., Rohatgi, S., & Kumar, P. (2018). Determinants of stunting, wasting, and underweight in five high-burden pockets of four Indian states. *Indian Journal of Community Medicine, 43*(4), 279–283. https://doi.org/10.4103/ijcm.IJCM_151_18.

Sivakumar, P. S., Kesava Kumar, H., Immanuel, S., Sheela, M. N., Jayaprakas, C. A., Murugesan, P., Mohan, C., & Ravi, V. (2020). *Rainbow diet campaign: An extension strategy for scaling up biofortified tuber crop varieties*. ICAR-Central Tuber Crops Research Institute.

Smith, L. C., & Haddad, L. (2015). Reducing child undernutrition: Past drivers and priorities for the post-MDG era. *World Development, 68*, 180–204. https://doi.org/10.1016/j.worlddev.2014.11.014.

Soni, A., Fahey, N., Bhutta, Z. A., Li, W., Frazier, J. A., Simas, T. M., Nimbalkar, S. M., Allison, J. J., & Yount, K. M. (2021). Early childhood undernutrition, preadolescent physical growth, and cognitive achievement in India: A population-based cohort study. *PLoS Medicine, 18*(10), e1003838. https://doi.org/10.1371/journal.pmed.1003838.

Subramanian, S. V., Ackerson, L. K., Smith, G. D., & John, N. A. (2009). Association of maternal height with child mortality, anthropometric failure, and anemia in India. *JAMA, 301*(16), 1691–1701. https://doi.org/10.1001/jama.2009.548.

Swaminathan, M. S., Bhavani, R. V., & Rengalakshmi, R. (2012). Farming system for nutrition (FSN): An approach to leverage agriculture for nutritional outcomes. *Paper presented at the Leveraging Agriculture for Improving Nutrition and Health Conference*. M. S. Swaminathan Research Foundation https://www.fao.org/fileadmin/user_.

The Lancet. (2013). *Maternal and child nutrition: Executive summary of The Lancet Maternal and Child Nutrition Series*. The Lancet https://thousanddays.org/wp-content/uploads/Lancet-2013-Executive-summary.pdf.

UNICEF. (1990). *Strategy for improved nutrition of children and women in developing countries*. United Nations Children's Fund.

UNICEF. (2020). *Nutrition, for every child: UNICEF nutrition strategy 2020–2030*. United Nations Children's Fund https://www.unicef.org/reports/nutrition-strategy-2020-2030.

UNICEF. (2023). *Undernourished and overlooked: A global nutrition crisis in adolescent girls and women*. United Nations Children's Fund https://www.unicef.org/reports/undernourished-overlooked-nutrition-crisis-2023.

UNICEF India. (2021). *Everything about millets: POSHAN power*. New Delhi: UNICEF India.

UNICEF Office of Research–Innocenti. (2019). The state of the world's children 2019: Children, food and nutrition. New York: UNICEF.

Verma, D., & Singh, S. K. (2021). Knowledge, attitudes and practices regarding infant feeding among mothers of children with severe acute malnutrition in the rural areas of Northern India. *Pediatric Review: International Journal of Pediatric Research, 8*(3), 137–145. https://doi.org/10.17511/ijpr.2021.i03.03.

Victora, C. G., Bahl, R., Barros, A. J. D., França, G. V. A., Horton, S., Krasevec, J., Murch, S., Sankar, M. J., Walker, N., Rollins, N. C., Allen, K., Dharmage, S., Lodge, C., Peres, K. G.,

Bhandari, N., Chowdhury, R., Sinha, B., Taneja, S., Giugliani, E., … Richter, L. (2016). Breastfeeding in the 21st century: Epidemiology, mechanisms, and lifelong effect. *The Lancet., 387*(10017), 475–490. https://doi.org/10.1016/S0140-6736(15)01024-7.

Victora, C. G., Christian, P., Vidaletti, L. P., Gatica-Domínguez, G., Menon, P., & Black, R. E. (2021). Revisiting maternal and child undernutrition in LMICs. *The Lancet, 397*(10282), 1382–1399.

Wells, J. C. K., Marphatia, A. A., Amable, G., Siervo, M., Friis, H., Miranda, J. J., Haisma, H. H., & Raubenheimer, D. (2021). The future of human malnutrition: Rebalancing agency for better nutritional health. *Globalisation and health, 17*(1), 119. https://doi.org/10.1186/s12992-021-00767-4.

Woode, G., & Birner, R. (2021). How does governance impact malnutrition? A close look at factors associated with underweight in children under 5 years in Ghana. Journal of Nutrition & Food Sciences, 11, 822.

World Health Organisation. (2021). *Comprehensive implementation plan on maternal, infant and young child nutrition*. World Health Organisation https://www.who.int/publications/i/item/WHO-NMH-NHD-14.1.

World Health Organisation. (2022). *WHO recommendations on maternal health and nutrition services in antenatal care*. Geneva: World Health Organization.

World Health Organisation & United Nations Children's Fund (UNICEF). (2003). Global strategy for infant and young child feeding. Geneva: World Health Organisation.

World Health Organisation, World Food Programme, United Nations System Standing Committee on Nutrition, and United Nations Children's Fund (UNICEF). (2007). *Community-based management of severe acute malnutrition: A joint statement by the World Health Organization, the World Food Programme, the United Nations System Standing Committee on Nutrition and the United Nations Children's Fund*. Geneva: World Health Organization.

Yajnik, C. S., & Deshmukh, U. S. (2008). Maternal nutrition, intrauterine programming and consequential risks in the offspring. *Reviews in Endocrine and Metabolic Disorders, 9*(3), 203–211. https://doi.org/10.1007/s11154-008-9087-z.

Young, M., Wolfheim, C., Marsh, D. R., & Hammamy, D. (2012). World Health Organisation/UNICEF Joint Statement on integrated community case management. *American Journal of Tropical Medicine and Hygiene, 87*(5), 6–10.

Nutritional models of the Middle East

3

Arezoo Haghighian-Roudsari
Department of Community Nutrition, Faculty of Nutrition Sciences and Food Technology, National Nutrition and Food Technology Research Institute, Shahid Beheshti University of Medical Sciences, Tehran, Iran

3.1 Introduction

Food is what we eat and drink, and as food, it is usually composed of plants and animals and some minerals and chemicals that can provide nutrients and sustain life. The concept of food can be analyzed, and it is about what, when, and where; how; and with whom one consumes. Food can create different experiences for different people. On the one hand, as a basic need, it is a common right of all people on Earth. Despite the variety of views on food a wide range of methods, types of food, and tastes have been formed in relation to food, which creates various philosophical analyses. However, food is more than its ingredients and colors. Food is closely related to traditions, identities, and memories. The activities we do about food are wide, such as planting and producing food, buying, selling, and preparing and eating food. However, food is different from other things that we experience. Food is prepared not only for taste but also for eyes, nose, and even ears because we see it with our eyes, smell it with our nose, and hear the crisp sound of food with our ears. We also experience it as something we touch, taste, chew, swallow, and even feel in our bodies hours later. In addition, the experience of food is shaped by uncontrollable forces, unconscious motivations, and people's inclinations, all of which are influenced by social cues. Food experiences, the feeling of pleasure from eating or drinking, the beginning and end of eating are not completely under our control. In addition, the knowledge of taste and its origins is very wide. There are different tastes that, apart from the genetic origin, apparently exist in our minds. However, most people agree on the taste of food (sweet, salty, sour, or spicy), which means that taste is an objective property, found in food, not just in our minds (Kaplan, 2019).

3.2 The Middle East region

The term "Middle East" was first used in 1902 by an American named "Alfred Thayer Mahan" to describe the region between the Far and Near East. The term "Middle East" was used because it was viewed from the European continent, so it was neither the Near East nor the Far East. The definition of the Middle East in the 19th century was the area between the Arabian Peninsula, Mesopotamia, and Iran and Central Asia. Of course, what we know about the Middle East today is wider than the definitions

Nutritional Strategies, Predictive Models, and Sustainable Policies. DOI: https://doi.org/10.1016/B978-0-443-23671-6.00013-X

given by Mahan. There are many debates and misunderstandings about the countries that are in this region. What caused the lack of agreement in this regard is that the Middle East is mixed with political definitions. The countries of the Middle East, including Egypt, Jordan, Palestine, Lebanon, Syria, Yemen, Iran, Bahrain, Kuwait, Iraq, Oman, Qatar, Saudi Arabia, and the United Arab Emirates (UAE), have specific sociocultural, political, religious, and economic characteristics. Today, Islam is the dominant religion among at least 90% of the population of every country in the Middle East. The Middle East is home to numerous ethnic groups such as Arabs, Iranians (also known as "Persians"), Jews, Kurds, Berbers, Armenians, and Azeris. The Middle East has not been politically stable for more than a century and has experienced a lot of tension (Lewis, 1995). The Middle East region has different dimensions in eating habits and patterns because of cultural and geographical diversity and available food items.

3.3 Nutrition-related diseases in the Middle East

In the last half century the diet and nutritional status of humans have undergone major changes globally, and it seems that the diet change has increased more or less in different regions of the world. This concept, called the "nutritional transition," includes extensive changes in the overall structure and composition of the diet, changes such as a high-density diet, a reduction in complex carbohydrates, an increase in added sugar and other caloric sweeteners with processed foods. These changes can show their effects in body composition, health status as well as demographic changes.

In a large part of the world, including Latin American and Caribbean countries, Asian countries, and most African and Middle Eastern countries, the consumption of this food pattern is increasing. This eating behavior has caused diseases related to high-fat and low-fiber diets to become common in these populations. In addition, economic development among low-income populations has increased risk factors for chronic diseases. During the years of nutrition transition the Middle East region has experienced a new pattern of diseases. The reduction of communicable diseases and the increase of noncommunicable diseases (NCDs) such as cardiovascular diseases, cancer, diabetes, and chronic respiratory diseases are evident in this region as in other countries. NCDs are responsible for 70% of deaths in the world. Unhealthy eating, focusing on high intake of saturated and *trans* fatty acids, cholesterol, salt, and sugar, is one of the main causes of NCDs in the world, which are also considered main characteristics of nutrition transition.

Recent changes in diet and physical activity in low- and middle-income countries in Asia, Latin America, the Caribbean, Africa, and the Middle East have led to the emergence of an epidemic of overweight and obesity. The results of studies show that the highest levels of obesity (grade II and higher) are in the Middle East, Western Pacific, and Latin America, and in oil-exporting countries such as Kuwait and Saudi Arabia, more than a third of the adult population is overweight or obese (Semba & Bloem, 2002). According to the results of a systematic review and metaanalysis, obesity and overweight were determined as risk factors for many NCDs, including diabetes, various types of cancer, cardiovascular diseases, and high blood pressure. Moreover, the results of this study showed that the prevalence of overweight and obesity in the Middle East is 23.5%–62.1% and 14.5%–40.6%, respectively (Okati-Aliabad et al., 2022). The highest prevalence of obesity and overweight is reported in Kuwait and Syria. The cause of this high prevalence is considered to be recent changes in lifestyle, including the use of Arab diets (high-calorie and fatty foods such as fast foods), alcohol consumption, and reduced physical activity. On the other hand, some studies attribute the high prevalence of overweight and obesity in disadvantaged groups to the low quality of their diet (Batal et al., 2023).

3.4 Nutritional status in the Middle East countries

Macronutrients are present in larger amounts in food and are actually the main energy supplier of the body, whereas micronutrients exist in smaller amounts, such as milligrams or micrograms, in food, and they are more useful for maintaining the health of the body and helping to digest and absorb macronutrients. Micronutrients do not play a role in providing energy to the body. Therefore the importance of macronutrients is more in the field of energy supply for the body, and the importance of micronutrients is to help the body function to use macronutrients and carry out vital reactions in the body. Macronutrients include three main groups: carbohydrates, proteins, and fats. Micronutrients include two subgroups, vitamins and minerals. Each of these groups plays different roles in the body, and their presence is necessary for almost all body processes, and the lack of each of them in the body can cause complications for a person.

In the Middle East region a wide range of micronutrient deficiencies have been observed in recent decades, making it a major healthcare problem. Because of the wide spread of nutrition transition in the Middle East region and its major nutritional problems, the World Health Organization (WHO) has considered this region susceptible to conducting more comprehensive investigations and effective interventions and has divided the countries into

- *Advanced nutrition transition* countries, including Bahrain, Saudi Arabia, Kuwait, Oman, Qatar, and the UAE, with high rates of overweight and obesity and moderate prevalence of malnutrition and micronutrient deficiencies in some of the following population groups.
- *The countries in the initial transition of nutrition* include Egypt, Jordan, Lebanon, Iran, and Palestine, which are at medium levels in both areas of prevalence of overweight and obesity and malnutrition and lack of micronutrients.
- *Countries with significant malnutrition*, such as Iraq, Syria, Yemen, Palestine (Gaza Strip), have a high prevalence of acute and chronic malnutrition, widespread micronutrient deficiencies, and overweight, obesity, and malnutrition.

The micronutrients that have attracted the attention of the WHO are the lack/inadequate intake of calcium, iodine, iron, and zinc, as well as vitamin A, vitamin D, and folate, which in many countries of the region, especially in vulnerable groups such as children and women in fertility age, have been reported. More than a third of the population of this region suffers from iron deficiency or anemia (most of them are women) and are at risk of iodine deficiency disorders (Hwalla et al., 2017). The studies in the eastern Mediterranean region (EMR), where the Middle East countries are also part of this region, show low consumption of fruits and vegetables as the main sources of fiber, insufficient consumption of water, milk, and dairy products, high consumption of foods with high energy density from carbohydrate and fat sources, and at the same time, they have reported low amounts of nutrient intake such as calcium, iron, and zinc and vitamins A, D, C, and folate among children and adolescents. The concern of these dietary patterns is the increase in the prevalence of overweight and obesity, and it has caused the region to face the "triple burden of malnutrition" in children and adolescents, which is characterized by malnutrition with two spectra of overweight and obesity because of overeating and the continuation of stunting, underweight, and wasting because of malnutrition, as well as the high prevalence of micronutrient deficiency (Al-Jawaldeh et al., 2020).

3.5 The importance of dietary patterns

In the past, most of the analysis conducted by researchers in the field of nutrition epidemiology focused on the relationship between diseases and one or more nutrients or food. Despite being important the results of this type of analysis have limitations in understanding the impact of food-related factors on diseases. These restrictions fall into several categories: First, food is usually a combination of several nutrients that can affect each other and increase or decrease the effect of each other in this interaction, and it is very unlikely that each of these foods, is eaten alone. The "single nutrient" approach may be used more at the laboratory level. Second the effects of some nutrients are highly correlated with each other, such as sodium and potassium, which makes it difficult to study them independently. Third the cumulative effects of different nutrients in a dietary pattern are better detectable because the effect of a single nutrient may be difficult to distinguish. The relationship between food intake and disease incidence may differ from predictions based on the known effects of food components alone, as our knowledge of the myriad dimensions of foods, whether beneficial or harmful, is still limited. The study of dietary patterns is conducted to reduce these unforeseen effects and interactions that may exist between different components of a food and physical characteristics and unknown components (Hu, 2002). Dietary patterns study the amount, variety, or combination of different foods and beverages in a diet and the frequency of their consumption in the diet. A dietary pattern represents the totality of what people typically eat and drink, and parts of the pattern act synergistically to affect health. Healthy eating patterns can help reduce the risk of chronic diseases. There is now a global consensus that food and nutrition policies should be informed by evidence on dietary patterns. Assessment of dietary patterns is carried out using different approaches, of which two common types are "data-driven approaches" based on multivariate statistical techniques (e.g., principal component analysis, cluster analysis, and rank regression reduction) or models that are suggested by the researcher and according to "preliminary" dietary guidelines or recommendations (e.g., diet quality scores). Examining food patterns is used in many studies of nutrition science, including etiology research and compilation and updating of food guidelines. The study of changes and trends in the type and amount of food consumed by people in a certain period of time and in different societies can be traced in food patterns (McNaughton, 2020).

3.6 An overview of dietary pattern in the Middle East countries

A review of 47 years of changes in food items in the Middle East has shown that the access to energy and food items shows an increasing trend until the first decade of the 21st century. Available energy has increased by 42.2%, whereas the proportion of carbohydrates and fat in energy supply in this region has decreased by 5% for each macronutrient, whereas the proportion of protein remained constant. Cereals are the staple food consumed in the Middle East, and during this period, their proportion in energy supply has decreased. The consumption of fruits and vegetables in the Middle East showed an increase in all income groups during this period, and their proportion in energy supply increased; low-middle income countries were excluded from this increasing trend because their access to fruits and vegetables decreased during this period. Regarding the meat, eggs, fish, and legumes group, the availability in the Middle East has risen, and their proportion in daily energy supply showed an increase of 2.3%. Energy supply from milk and dairy products does not show much change, but per capita consumption of milk in the Middle East region is generally lower than the recommended value. The availability of vegetable oils in the 47-year period and their proportion in energy supply showed a very small increase in the Middle East. Moreover, the consumption of sugar and sweet drinks has grown significantly in the same period (Golzarand et al., 2012).

3.6.1 Egypt

Traditional foods in the Egyptian diet are grains, legumes, dark green leafy vegetables, fruits, cheese, oils, and white and red meat. The amount of food imports and the allocation of food subsidies to some high-calorie foods such as oil, bread, and sugar have caused the consumption of high-calorie foods to increase among the population. The development of urbanization and the reduction of physical activity and not having enough time have lowered the consumption of traditional foods (which take longer to prepare), and on the other hand, have increased the consumption of fast foods and prepared foods, drinks sweetened with sugar, and junk foods. The consequence of their higher prevalence is the increase in overweight and obesity statistics in this country, especially in the high socioeconomic status (SES) people who have the ability to buy all kinds of animal products, fruits and vegetables, and expensive foods.

The results of a study in Egyptian women aged 19–30 showed that the consumption of dietary sugars, Saturated Fatty acids (SFAs), and sodium exceeded the permissible limit, and the intake of vitamin D, folate, potassium, and iron was lower than the recommended amounts. The high prevalence of anemia in Egyptian women may be because of relatively low consumption of animal products rich in heme-type iron, high consumption of black tea, and foods containing phytate such as bread, which have a negative effect on the bioavailability of nonheme iron. High intake of total fats and SFAs is mainly because of high consumption of white cheese, especially feta cheese, which contains high amounts of sodium and SFA. The high share of sugar in carbohydrate intake is mainly from two sources of sugar and sugar-sweetened beverages. Moreover, high sodium intake was observed in more than 93% of the studied population (Brouzes et al., 2020).

The results of a study on Egyptian children aged 6 months to 18 years showed that a high percentage of the studied population (86 and 83) received insufficient amounts of calcium and vitamins A and C. Among children of different ages the prevalence of insufficient intake of calcium and iron in adolescents between 12 and 18 years old was higher than in other groups. Inadequate intake of iron and vitamin C was observed in about one third of the studied children. Inadequate intake of vitamin A was present in 83% of children, which was higher in the first 2 years of life. The prevalence of zinc deficiency among children aged 6–60 months (43.8%) and adolescents (49.4%) also had a high percentage (Saleh et al., 2023).

The results of another study among 18–40-year-old university students in Egypt showed that in men, the contribution of plant-based food in providing daily energy intake is greater than in women, and snacks in girls have a greater contribution to supplying daily calories, which is because of their desire to consume sweet and fatty foods such as cookies, candies, and sweet drinks. On the other hand, animal proteins have a more prominent place in women's snacks than men, and it seems that they get more iron in this way. About 35%, 40%, and 25% of the daily fat intake of students comes from vegetable foods, animal products, and snacks, respectively (Saraya et al., 2021).

The prevalence of malnutrition in the elderly population of Egypt is about 30%, which is slightly higher in women than in men. Malnutrition is also more common in the elderly who do not consume one serving per day of dairy products, meat, fish, and poultry (Mahfouz et al., 2013).

3.6.2 *Jordan*

Jordan is a middle-income country in the Middle East region that has experienced nutrition transition and, as a result, malnutrition and NCDs at a high speed in recent years. In Jordan, nutrition-related problems such as stunting and wasting in school-aged children have attracted the attention of decision-makers. Stunting and wasting happen in many cases because of lack of protein or lack of energy and protein as well as micronutrients. Stunting is more common, especially in the underdeveloped regions of Jordan, and is caused by long-term poor nutritional status. Moreover, the lack of vitamins A and E in these children can be factors for the occurrence of stunting and wasting. However, in recent years, the prevalence of short stature is decreasing. Another nutritional problem is anemia, which can be caused by insufficient access to iron sources such as animal proteins, but generally, anemia is a multifactorial complication (Khatib & Sa, 2009).

Bread is the staple food in the Lebanese diet, so in 2002, this country decided to fortify bread with iron, folate, vitamins B and A, and zinc. Considering that the average daily intake of bread in the Lebanese diet was about 270 g, fortification is an effective solution to reduce the lack of micronutrients. In 2010 a survey showed that there were positive changes in the intake of micronutrients, especially iron, in children, but this change was not major among women, and the prevalence of folate deficiency and insufficiency was reported as 13.6% and 82.9%, respectively (Serdula et al., 2014).

Eating during the transition period of entering the university, there may be changes that affect people's eating patterns. In Lebanon, because of the presence of about 300,000 students in university centers, food pattern is very important because the formation of food patterns in this era can be a basis for people's eating habits in the future. The results of a study in Lebanon identified three types of food patterns among students: The first component, "snacking pattern," represented a high consumption of western and Arabic desserts, ice cream, juice, mayonnaise, soft drinks, junk food, pastries, ka'ak, canned fruit, fresh juice, cakes, cookies, biscuits, yellow cheeses, processed meats, chocolate, falafel, and white bread. The second component, "healthy" dietary pattern, included bulgur, freekeh and oats, dried fruits, fish, canned fish, milk, honey, nuts, fresh fruits, eggs, breakfast cereals, herbal drinks, red meat, maftool, brown bread, green leafy vegetables, starchy vegetables, and other vegetables. The third component was defined as "accessible" dietary pattern with high intake of olives, olive and vegetable oil, green-leafy vegetables, starchy vegetables and other vegetables, tea, legumes, falafel, pickles, sugar, white bread, yogurt, tahini, coffee, labaneh, and junk food (Sbaih et al., 2020).

The prevalence of anemia in children aged 6–59 months is one of the public health concerns in Jordan. The evidence shows that with the start of complementary feeding, half of the children aged 6–23 months experience low dietary diversity, which can be a major contributing factor to iron deficiency anemia (IDA). The intake of vitamin A in children under 5 years old and women of reproductive age is not reported within the normal range. In children under 5 years of age, a relatively high prevalence of vitamin D deficiency and inadequate intake among women have been observed. The most important nutritional problems are the low consumption of fruits and vegetables among different age groups in Jordan, the increase in the consumption of soft drinks, the insufficient consumption of dairy products in teenagers, the high consumption of sweet drinks, sweets and chocolates, cakes and cookies, fried potatoes and potato chips, and high salt consumption. These patterns of improper food consumption are a warning for the prevalence of the Western diet, which can lead to an increase in the burden of obesity with a lack of micronutrients and an increase in the incidence of NCDs in adolescence and adulthood (Al-Awwad et al., 2021).

Considering the increase in the global prevalence of metabolic syndrome (MetS), which is characterized by insulin resistance, hypertension, dyslipidemia, and obesity, examining the characteristics of food patterns in this group can be useful in planning prevention at the policy-making level. In Lebanon the results of a study in this group showed that there is a significant difference in energy intake, the share of energy supply from carbohydrates and fat, and the intake of some macro- and micronutrients. Moreover, the intake of saturated and *trans* fatty acids and some micronutrients such as phosphorus and B-vitamins is higher. The possible reason for the increased intake of saturated and *trans* fatty acids as well as phosphorus is the high intake of animal proteins and, in relation to group B vitamins, because of the high intake of carbohydrates. Because of the high consumption of fast food in this population, the amount of sodium intake was higher than usual (Tayyem et al., 2020).

3.6.3 Palestine

About 5.5 million Palestinians live in the Middle East region, which in the last three decades has faced a lot of demographic, economic, political, and social changes. Such changes had a great impact on their physical and mental health. Some of these Palestinians have shifted their diets because of migration to other countries. However, during the covid epidemic, changes in the food pattern were also made in Palestine, including more consumption of fried food, snacks, and coffee among the population. With a population of about 1.4 million people the Gaza Strip is one of the areas with inhabitants with low purchasing power because of economic restrictions and low-income levels, and a large part of the population (about 69%) lacks food security, although international institutions have allocated food aid to a large population of the Gaza Strip.

In the last decade the micronutrient status of women and preschool children showed a wide deficiency of micronutrients such as iron, zinc, vitamins A, B12, E, and D in the Gaza Strip, especially among pregnant women and preschool children. Iron and vitamin E deficiencies affect one-third of pregnant women, whereas deficiencies in vitamin A and B12 are observed in about half of them. In addition, approximately 70% suffer from zinc deficiency, and almost all pregnant women show signs of vitamin D deficiency. Recent surveys also indicate the continuation of shortages in this region. The prevalence of anemia and deficiency of iron, zinc, and folate in pregnant women was observed to be about 43%, 39%, 85%, and 10%, respectively, in the third trimester of pregnancy. The results published in 2020 indicate the growth of this statistic for vitamin A, B12, and D to 51%, 78.6%, and 69%, respectively, in the third trimester of pregnancy. In children aged 6–59 months the prevalence of anemia and deficiency of zinc, vitamins D, and A was about 31%, 71%, 62.5%, and 35.3%, respectively (Horino et al., 2020). The continuation of this shortage trend can be because of social political instability and low access to food resources because of various conflicts. The most important groups at risk are children and pregnant women who need national and international solutions.

The study of nutritional behaviors and food choices in adolescents showed that the area of residence and the lifestyle of its people can have different patterns of eating behaviors. In Palestine, people who live in the West Bank follow healthier food choices compared to Gaza. Adolescents in the West Bank consume fruits, sweets, soft drinks, meat, and chicken, but in Gaza, where there is a high population density and less access to food, the consumption of these foods is lower. This finding is also confirmed in the adult population of the West Bank, which shows a significant increase in the consumption of industrial foods such as cakes, fruit juices, and sweet drinks. Meanwhile, compared to boys, girls have healthier food choices, in which the consumption of more fruits and vegetables is evident, and the consumption of soft drinks and milk is higher in boys than in girls (Al Sabbah et al., 2007). In Gaza, one of the most important reasons for the high prevalence of anemia is that almost half of the population consumes red meat three or more times a week, and a quarter of people consume red meat once or twice a week, mainly because of food aid from related organizations. Investigating the nutritional status of pregnant women in the Gaza Strip, using the data of the 98-item food frequency questionnaire, elucidated 2 prominent types of food patterns: (1) Asian pattern, in which the consumption of whole grains, potatoes, legumes, fish, low-fat dairy products, vegetables, fruits, vegetable oils olives, and nuts is high; and (2) the Western pattern, which is characterized by high consumption of grains, red meat, fast foods, eggs, high-fat dairy products, hydrogenated oils, salt, sugar, sweets, and soft drinks. Analysis showed that women who follow the Asian model may have a lower prevalence of premature birth, Low Birth Weight (LBW), and congenital anomalies, whereas premature birth may be more frequent in the followers of the Western model (El Bilbeisi et al., 2020).

3.6.4 Lebanon

In Lebanon, which is a small country in the Middle East region, two dietary patterns were identified among children aged 2–5, which are somehow related to the increasing prevalence of obesity in Lebanese children in the last decade. The first pattern is entitled "Fast Food and Sweets," which is very similar to the Western food pattern and has a lot of carbohydrates, fats, and sugars; and includes fast food and sweets, sweet drinks, salty snacks, and the "traditional Lebanese" pattern characterized by high intake of bread and cereals, dairy products, fruits and vegetables, and traditional Lebanese mixed foods (Nasreddine et al., 2019).

In school-aged children, almost half of energy was provided by carbohydrates, whereas 12% of children had protein intakes below the recommended amount, but their intake of fat and sugar exceeded the recommended amount, and they obtained more from foods such as sweets, sweetened beverages and desserts and than from cereals and mixed foods. A high percentage of children aged 4–13 are deficient in micronutrients such as vitamin D, calcium, and vitamin A (Nasreddine et al., 2022). Of course the food sources of important micronutrients, such as iron, zinc, calcium, and vitamins D and A, and folate, are different in different ages of childhood, from infant formula and cereals in toddlers to meat and fish, cow's milk, and even sweet drinks in preschool children (Chokor et al., 2024).

Since overweight and obesity in childhood are the basis of obesity in adolescence and adulthood, studies on the relationship between food patterns in children and adolescents, and the occurrence of obesity in Lebanon have also been conducted. Surveys in adolescents have shown that in this age group, the common patterns include the "Western pattern" and the "traditional Lebanese pattern." The Western food pattern includes all kinds of fast food and sweet drinks, all kinds of sauces, red meat, and eggs. Like the traditional Lebanese pattern in children, in this age group, the traditional pattern includes vegetables, fruits, bread, rice, beans, pasta, and plant oils (Naja et al., 2015). According to other studies conducted in Lebanon, similar findings of common dietary patterns have been identified in adults, which shows that the prevalence of a dietary pattern in childhood can continue into adulthood and make it more difficult to modify the diet in adulthood.

However, the food pattern identified in pregnant women is slightly different from other age groups in Lebanon. The components of these patterns can be categorized into three patterns: "Western," "mixed," and "neo-Mediterranean" patterns. In the Western dietary model, a high frequency of fast-food consumption combined with low intake of fruits, vegetables, and protein sources can be observed. Following this pattern during pregnancy often leads to excessive energy intake from carbohydrates and fats, along with higher than recommended levels of sodium and inadequate intake of essential micronutrients such as magnesium, folate, and iodine, which can negatively affect maternal and fetal health. On the opposite point the mixed diet includes vegetables, fruits, and seeds, and some Lebanese street food, where again, the energy intake from this model is high from the source of carbohydrates, but the intake of zinc, iron, and iodine also promotes the quality of the diet. The "neo-Mediterranean" food pattern, whose structure is similar to the high-protein pattern, is mainly followed by women living in the urban area with a higher level of education or employed and includes eggs, milk and dairy products, lean meat, which contain significant amounts of calcium, vitamins A and D, folate, and magnesium in the diet (Papazian et al., 2022). However, among the foods consumed in Lebanon, traditional foods and Arabic sweets are good sources of fiber intake, 23% and 30%, respectively. Nonetheless, this food category is poor in vitamins A, D, E, and C (Hoteit et al., 2024).

3.6.5 Syria

The most obvious feature of the diet in Syria is the consumption of grains, especially bread, at the rate of 18.4%–22% in the daily calorie supply. Meat, poultry, and fish have a contribution of 18%–21% in providing daily calories, although the consumption of fish among adolescents is low, whereas potato chips (5%) and chocolate (5%) have a significant share in providing daily calories in adolescents (Al-Jawaldeh et al., 2020).

The results of a study on children aged 6–12 in Syria showed that bread consumption was the most frequent and was reported by 86% among children. Moreover, they had a great desire to consume rice, chips, and popcorn daily. From the group of vegetables, tomatoes (44%); and from the group of fruits, apples (30%), oranges (26%), and bananas (21%) were consumed more than other fruits. From the dairy group the consumption of yogurt (62%) and cheese (50%) was more than the consumption of milk (38%). In the group of meat and protein, 38% of children mainly consume eggs daily, whereas they consume peas (10% in the form of falafel and 6% in the form of hummus) and red meat (7%). The oils used were mainly olives and olive oil, but the consumption of sugar was the most important problem in the diet of these children in the form of sugar with tea or in the form of simple biscuits, biscuits with chocolate, and chocolate, 52%, 44%, and 33% of which were consumed. However, the consumption of important food groups in the growth and development of children did not match the recommended amounts (Jaghasi et al., 2012).

Syria is a country that produced most of its food because of the prosperity of agriculture, and the occupation of the majority of people is therefore agriculture. But in recent years, Syria, like many countries in the world, has undergone a nutritional and epidemiological transition, which has caused a rapid change in people's lifestyle. The type of employment has changed from agriculture to office work and more use of computers, resulting in a decrease in physical activity. Among adolescents, these conditions have increased the level of sedentary behavior, especially in urban areas such as Damascus. There is a significant difference in the eating habits of adolescent boys and girls in Syria. Skipping a meal (The omission or lack of consumption of one or more of the traditional main meals) such as breakfast is more common among girls than boys, which is probably due to a greater desire to go on a diet, reduce calorie intake, body image, and obesity concern. The consumption of vegetables, milk and dairy products, red meat, and soft drinks showed a significant difference between girls and boys so that the consumption of fast food and soft drinks was more prevalent among boys. Considering the high prevalence of overweight and obesity as risk factors for NCDs, low consumption of vegetables and fruits can be a warning (Musaiger & Kalam, 2014).

Five dietary patterns have been identified among Syrian adults aged 40–65 years. The characteristic of dietary pattern 1 is foods with protein, saturated fat, and high calories that are based on animal consumption and the highest level of energy intake, protein, and vitamins A, D, and B12. Dietary pattern 2 is a traditional pattern and consists of traditional Syrian foods, which are based on starch and contain a high amount of carbohydrates and sugar intake and vitamin K (probably because of the high content of vegetables); whereas pattern 3 includes foods that are high in fat, carbohydrates, and saturated fat. In pattern 4, there are traditional Syrian foods with monounsaturated and polyunsaturated fatty acids (MUFA and PUFA) and folic acid, which are based on many vegetables. Lastly, pattern 5 is related to the consumption of fast food with high energy and sodium content (Atasi et al., 2022).

Pregnant women need more energy and micronutrients because of physiological changes during pregnancy. Therefore studying the food pattern and food security of this group is particularly important. According to studies, 73% of Syrian pregnant women suffer from food insecurity, and this high number is probably because of the war, economic crises in the country, the COVID-19 pandemic, and the impact of the war between Russia and Ukraine, which has reduced access to food sources. The number of meals in Syrian pregnant women is 2.4, which is contrary to the recommendation of UNICEF (three meals a day for pregnant women) and, in turn, can reduce the intake of necessary micronutrients (Zabad et al., 2024).

3.6.6 Yemen

Civil wars in recent years have turned Yemen into one of the poorest Arab countries and caused Yemenis to experience a humanitarian crisis. The consequences of this war are severe food insecurity and mental problems and malnutrition, especially in children. Of course, in the last three decades, this country has undergone both an epidemiological transition and changes in their eating habits. A comparison of studies conducted in Yemen shows that the prevalence of overweight and obesity in this country has increased in recent years, which is a sign of the double burden of malnutrition. The prevalence of obesity and overweight was 10.3% and 20.3%, respectively, and the prevalence of underweight was 21.2%, which is probably because of the popularization of the modern lifestyle, which is characterized by low physical activity and high consumption of cheap foods with high calorie density. Urbanization is one of the factors that increase people's access to food sources, especially with the origin of carbohydrates and sugars, and the choice of easy foods also increases because of the busy life in the city (Ibrahim Sr et al., 2023).

The high prevalence of malnutrition among Yemeni children has also attracted the attention of researchers and policymakers. The prevalence of stunting and wasting in Yemeni children is 42.5% and 7.9%, respectively. More than half of the children living in the mountainous areas of Yemen suffer from stunting, whereas the prevalence of short stature in the areas at sea level is 8%. Moreover, there is a big difference between the prevalence of stunting in urban areas (28%) compared to rural areas (46%). Unsanitary drinking water is one of the most important problems in children's nutrition and a risk factor for increasing their mortality. This statistic shows the close relationship with protein consumption, so 65% of children in their families who did not consume protein during the last week were stunted, but if they consumed protein daily during the last week, this statistic reaches less than 30% (De Souza, 2017). Anemia has been observed among 38% of Yemeni adolescents, which can indicate the continuation of micronutrient malnutrition in children until adolescence.

About 80% of the population of Yemen is below the national poverty line, and this has caused many public health problems for the people of this country. Improper health conditions, lack of many micronutrients, and limited access to drinking water are the most important factors in the spread of infectious diseases among people, especially malnourished children. Anemia because of iron deficiency or parasite contamination has also been reported among children between 31.7% and 49% (Al-Halani et al., 2023).

Nutrition status of women of reproductive age is one of the most important factors predicting the spread of disease or mortality among pregnant women and even their children. They investigated the nutritional status of Yemeni women aged 15–49 through their common patterns. Two types of food patterns were identified: The first one includes different types of cereals, oil, honey, sugar, and dairy products; and the second food pattern includes honey, sugar, dairy, oil, and legumes. The relationship between these two types of food patterns with mid-upper arm circumference (MUAC) showed that in women who followed the first food pattern, MUAC was larger than the second group of food patterns (Al Mansoob & Masood, 2019).

The results of a metaanalysis showed that the intake of energy, protein, carbohydrate, and fat in adults of the EMR, of which Yemen is one of the countries, was more than recommended. High sodium intake also causes a constant decrease in calcium and potassium (Doggui et al., 2021).

Vitamin D is one of the micronutrients whose deficiency is very common in different sex and age groups. A study among Yemeni women also showed a wide deficiency of this vitamin. Hypovitaminosis D was reported in 2.87% of women and severe vitamin D deficiency in 4.4% of them. These results emphasize the necessity of implementing interventions aimed at increasing serum vitamin D levels (Alwabr & Al-Wadhaf, 2020).

3.6.7 Iran

Adolescence is an important period in life, in which the style of food choices has changes that can continue until adulthood. During the nutrition transition the quality of the diet of Iranian adolescences has also decreased, which is because of the increase in the consumption of fast food, soft drinks, and salty snacks and the decrease in the consumption of fruits and vegetables. Dietary patterns of Iranian adolescences have been identified in four main dietary patterns: "prudent," "fast food," "animal fat," and "Mediterranean." A prudent diet included high intake of dried fruits, legumes, raw vegetables, walnuts, fruits, fresh fruit juices, pickles, nuts, cooked vegetables, and potatoes. Fast food diet was described with frequent consumption of junk food, carbonated soft drinks, sausages, hamburgers, sweets and biscuits, and chocolate. An animal fat diet is characterized by a low amount of low-fat dairy products as well as a high consumption of whole dairy products and animal fat. In the Mediterranean diet, hydrogenated vegetable oil is consumed in small amounts and nonhydrogenated vegetable oil, fish, raw vegetables, and olive oil in larger amounts (Kafeshani et al., 2015).

A study of women aged 20–50 in Iran showed that older women, with university education, bigger house, higher household income, shorter stay in Tehran, more physical activity, and history of high blood pressure, most likely had a healthy pattern. On the other hand, younger women of Turk ethnicity, who consume a lot of sweets and fat in their eating habits or currently smoke, follow an unhealthy eating pattern. Healthy food pattern includes vegetables, low-fat dairy products, yogurt drinks, chicken, olives, nuts, natural fruit juice, potatoes, coffee, and garlic; and the unhealthy food pattern consists of processed meats, mayonnaise, soft drinks, sweets, refined grains, snacks, industrial fruit juices, red meat, nuts, hydrogenated fats, butter, French fries, high-fat dairy products, eggs, organ meats, and sugars (Rezazadeh et al., 2010).

The study of the common food pattern in Iranian adults identified two types of "regular" meal pattern in 60% of adults and "irregular" meal pattern in 40% of them, which were named based on their major eating habits. In the regular food pattern, three meals are consumed in a day, and 48% of people receive these three meals regularly, and 98% and 81% of them eat breakfast and lunch, respectively (Saneei et al., 2016).

Iran, like other countries in the world, has an increasing trend in the number of its elderly population. The nutritional issues of the elderly not paying attention to the quality and quantity of their food can be related to the occurrence of various diseases in this age group. Common breads (as staple food consumed in Iran) in Iranian culture are Berberi, Sangak, and Lavash, which are also consumed by the elderly, but one of the problems of these breads, despite the good content of fiber (in Barbari and

Sangak bread), is the high amount of salt. In the case of Lavash bread, because of its high glycemic load, there is a risk of increasing blood sugar in these people. Rice and beans are among the most consumed food items among Iranians, including the elderly (Mirrafiei & Shab-Bidar, 2023).

In the study of the dietary pattern of the Iranian elderly over 60 years old, four main dietary patterns were identified in this population: (1) a "healthy" pattern characterized by more consumption of vegetables, tomatoes and tomato sauce, vegetable oil, olives, and fruits; (2) an "unhealthy" pattern, including red meat, fast food, snacks, sugar, honey and jam, soft drinks, and high-fat dairy products; (3) a "traditional" pattern characterized by consumption of whole grains, hydrogenated oil and animal fat, beans, salt, and pickles; and (4) a "high-protein" pattern, which is characterized by the consumption of chicken and poultry, fish, grains, and organ meats (Abdollahi et al., 2015). Another study on the dietary patterns of people over 18 years of age in Iran identified three dietary patterns: "healthy" dietary pattern (more consumption of chicken; low-fat and high-fat dairy products; cabbage; yellow and dark green vegetables; other vegetables; legumes; whole grains; fish; olives; and fruits); "western" dietary pattern (high consumption of red and processed meat, organ meats, margarine, flavorings, desserts, soft drinks, snacks, nuts, and sweets); and "traditional" dietary pattern (higher consumption of eggs, tea, water, fruit juice, refined grains, nuts, pickles, hydrogenated fats, sugar, salt, and spices) (Falahi, 2013).

What can be understood from the comparison of the patterns identified in these two studies is the similarity in the healthy and traditional patterns, and the unhealthy and Western patterns have almost the same characteristics in the two studies. What is evident in some studies of food patterns in Iran is the difference in food patterns explored in the same age groups, which can be because of the differences in food culture and geographical features of these regions, which determine the level of access to different food, items and knowledge and skills to cook these food items.

The study of Iranian diet quality in seven provinces showed that calcium intake in 80% of the population is less than the recommended amount. Moreover, the amount of iron intake is 40%–70% less than the recommended standard. These amounts satisfy one-half and one-third of calcium and iron requirements (Valaei et al., 2017). The results of the study on the intake of some micronutrients in adults aged 20–50 years showed that the average intake of zinc, copper, and magnesium was higher than the average needs of people, and the intake of calcium and phosphorus was less than their required amount. Moreover, the intake of sodium in these people was higher than the allowed amount (Babaali et al., 2020). Eating less than the recommended amount of calcium and phosphorus has been confirmed in another study (Jafari Giv et al., 2018).

3.6.8 Bahrain

Traditional foods in Bahrain are one of its cultural and historical manifestations. Fifty-two food items and drinks have been identified in this country, which are consumed according to different occasions and ceremonies. Some of them are consumed in all seasons of the year, such as *harees, momowash, sambosa, halwa, assidah*, and *legaimaat*; and others, such as *madquq bisr, mattaai, khabees, gurs al-taabi*, and *khubez zinjibari*, are consumed in family celebrations or special holidays. The most important cooking methods are boiling and frying (Alalwan et al., 2017). The food consumption pattern in Bahrain has two aspects: high consumption of foods harmful to health and low consumption of healthy foods. Accordingly the consumption of fruits and vegetables, milk, nuts, whole grains, and seafood is less than the recommended amounts. The consumption of red meat, processed meats, sweet drinks, and soft drinks in Bahrain is higher than the recommended value.

In Bahraini students the average energy intake was somewhat close to the recommended values, whereas the protein intake and sugar consumption in them were higher than the recommended amounts, which was because of the high consumption of sweets, snacks, and sweet drinks. On the other hand the consumption of milk, fruits, and vegetables was less than the recommended amounts (Gharib & Rasheed, 2011).

Studies of eating habits in Bahraini teenagers indicate the increasing prevalence of unhealthy eating habits, which has provided concerns for health planners. For example, 62.8% of teenage girls skip breakfast, which is more compared to boys. Despite the omission of breakfast, lunch, and dinner, most of the students consume and provide their daily energy needs from these two meals. A high percentage of students eat snacks. The consumption of chicken and fast food is high among students, but fish is consumed in small quantities (Musaiger et al., 2011). Similar findings have been reported in the eating habits of university students. Wide advertisements about energy drinks have made the consumption of this type of drink popular among Bahraini youth in recent years, and they consume it for reasons such as reducing fatigue, maintaining alertness, and increasing academic performance.

One of the most important nutritional problems in Bahrain is the lack of micronutrients such as iron and vitamin D, so 41.4% of adults are reported to be vitamin D deficient. Anemia in pregnant women and its prevention and treatment are one of the top priority actions of the health system. In Bahrain the prevalence of anemia among pregnant women in 2014 was about 19.8%, but surveys in 2020 showed that its prevalence reached 28.8%, which is classified as mild-to-moderate anemia. Types of anemia were also identified, which were IDA, vitamin B12 deficiency, and hemoglobinopathy in 39%, 30.8%, and 16% of cases, respectively (Almohri et al., 2023). The diet of the elderly is often deficient in several nutrients, including protein, vitamins A and C, folic acid, calcium, and iron. Energy and nutrient intakes of older Bahrainis, such as iron and calcium, were lower than the United States' recommended daily allowance. In the elderly, calcium absorption and the total energy intake decrease, and therefore, the need for calcium in the elderly increases. Iron intake in Bahraini elderly meets 77% of men's needs and 63% of women's needs (Obaid Musaiger, 2004).

3.6.9 Kuwait

Before the oil discovery, Kuwait had limited food resources. Available foods included rice, dates, seafood, camel milk, sheep, goat meat, and their by-products. Meat indicated wealth and was consumed weekly or monthly by the general public. Arabic coffee and milk were the main drinks, whereas sweet tea was reserved for special occasions. Kuwait's economic growth is evident through increased Gross Domestic

Product (GDP) per capita, overall GDP, and population growth. However, this growth led to greater reliance on imported food, which now constitutes 85% of the market. Traditional foods have given way to Western-style fast food because of increased availability and reduced prices (thanks to government subsidies). The results of the energy intake survey of Kuwaitis showed that half of Kuwaiti children and one-third of adults receive energy in excess of their needs and between 70% and 100% more protein and carbohydrates than they need. Like many countries undergoing nutrition transition, Kuwait has intakes of many micronutrients, such as vitamin D, vitamin E, calcium, and n-3 and n-6 fatty acids, that are lower than the recommended amounts. Despite the general deficiency of many vitamins and minerals the intake level of adults is better than that of children. (Zaghloul et al., 2013).

Food culture, access and ability to prepare food, hot and dry climate of Kuwait have caused changes in the eating habits of Kuwaiti people. These eating habits can be the reason for the high prevalence of NCDs in Kuwait (72%). The most important of these habits include eating time, number of meals per day, skipping meals, and prolonged hunger. Kuwaiti people consume 4.4 meals per day on average. Dinner time, which is directly related to the occurrence of insulin resistance, is after 10 p.m. in the majority of Kuwaiti adults. Skipping breakfast in Kuwaiti adolescents and its relationship with the incidence of overweight and obesity in adolescents who eat breakfast less than five times a week have been reported. Skipping breakfast (29%) and dinner (about 10%) is also seen in this population, whereas skipping breakfast and long hours of fasting are common among women (Alkhulaifi et al., 2023).

Three types of dominant dietary patterns were identified in Kuwaiti adults at risk of heart disease, which are fast-food dietary pattern, a refined-grains/poultry dietary pattern, and a vegetable-rich dietary pattern. People who had a fast-food diet had a higher body mass index and waist circumference and elevated blood pressure. Followers of this dietary pattern consume a lot of French fries and sugar-sweetened beverages. For people who had a grain/poultry diet including refined grains and poultry, along with other aspects of the traditional Kuwaiti diet such as dates, vegetables, and fish, the incidence of increased glucose levels is mostly because of insulin resistance. Vegetable-rich dietary pattern, including vegetables, is mostly consumed as an ingredient of mixed dishes, stews, soups, or salads and showed relationship with reduced dyslipidemia (Al-Lahou et al., 2020). Fast food and refined grains/poultry dietary patterns are more popular among the young generation of Kuwait, so about a third of teenagers consume fast food more than three times a week, and 60% of them consume sweets and sweetened drinks more than three times a week. Meanwhile, more than two-thirds of Kuwaiti adolescents do not consume dairy products, fruits, and vegetables on a daily basis (Allafi et al., 2014). The prevalence of these types of dietary patterns among adolescents and adults emphasizes the need for behavioral change interventions and national policies in the field of food and nutrition in Kuwait.

3.6.10 Saudi Arabia

The nutrition transition and the economic growth of Saudi Arabia during the last decades have raised concerns about dietary patterns and the resulting risks in the incidence of NCDs. Access to food in terms of quantity, quality, and variety has increased in Saudi Arabia, and food items such as sugar, meat, various oils, organs meat, eggs, and other foods are more available than in the past, increasing the demand for food consumption, and overeating has become at different age groups. The people of Saudi Arabia use the basic ingredients to prepare food: Fava beans, wheat, rice, yogurt, dates, and chicken are staple foods for all Saudis. The variety of food traditions in different regions, the difference in access to food sources, and the weather have been effective in the formation of dietary patterns in Saudi Arabia. Wheat is the most consumed grain in the diet of Saudi people, providing 41% of their energy and 40% of their protein intake. Rice is the main food in Saudi Arabia, which can be consumed up to two times a day. The proportion of carbohydrates providing energy needed by Saudis has decreased in the last few years, but the proportion of fat and protein providing energy shows a gradual increase. The consumption of milk and eggs has also increased in recent years, and the consumption of fruits and vegetables has decreased, which may be because of their price increase, especially during holidays and occasions such as Ramadan (Adam et al., 2014).

Young adults between the ages of 15 and 24 exhibited a notable trend characterized by elevated consumption levels of sugar-sweetened beverages, processed meat, and other similar food items, alongside a limited intake of fruits and vegetables. These detrimental dietary patterns emerge at an even earlier stage in school-aged children. In comparison to the dietary guideline recommendations the consumption levels of fruits, vegetables, dairy products, and nuts are notably deficient, with less than 45% of individuals in the Saudi Arabia adhering to the recommended intake of fish. Conversely, there exists a marked prevalence of excessive consumption of processed meat and sugar-sweetened beverages in contrast to the established guidelines (Moradi-Lakeh et al., 2017). Approximately 28.5% of adolescents reported frequent consumption of fast food, exceeding two times per week, with a higher prevalence among male adolescents than female ones. Adolescents from households with the highest monthly income demonstrated a notably elevated rate of fast-food intake when contrasted with those from lower income families. The regularity of fast-food consumption was linked to poorer dietary quality, alongside increased consumption of carbohydrates and free sugars among adolescents (Mumena et al., 2022). University students generally follow the pattern of convenient snacks and fast food, except for students who have a higher income level or are more active and tend to have healthier snacks.

In Saudi adults aged 35–65, five dietary patterns were obtained: "sweet and starch" pattern, "dates and coffee" pattern, "healthy" pattern, "traditional" pattern, and "protein" pattern. In cereals, bread, bakery products, beans, rice, pasta, and cooked foods were identified. The pattern of dates and coffee included, as expected, the consumption of dates and coffee; the healthy pattern represented the consumption of fruits, vegetables, and seafood; the traditional pattern consisted mostly of traditional foods of Saudi Arabia, including meat and chicken, fat, oil, and fruits; and the pattern of protein included the consumption of eggs and dairy products (Bawazeer et al., 2021). Elderly people in Saudi Arabia tend to have a higher intake of fruits and vegetables while consuming fewer processed foods. The inclination toward a more nutritious diet among the elderly may be attributed to various factors, including increased longevity associated with healthy eating habits, interactions with healthcare professionals among older adults in comparison to their younger counterparts, and a higher level of compliance with dietary recommendations among older individuals driven by their perceived susceptibility to illness and mortality (Moradi-Lakeh et al., 2017).

Iron and vitamin D are two important micronutrients in children's growth and health, and in Saudi children who have a normal body mass index, iron and vitamin D show a deficiency of 20% and 78%, respectively (Al-Hussaini et al., 2022). The study of Saudi children shows that their intake of calcium, potassium, and phosphorus is less than the recommended amount, but two-thirds of them get vitamin B12 and more than half of them get enough vitamin C and phosphorus, with a very low intake of magnesium and vitamin E (Kutbi, 2021). The prevalence of vitamin B2 deficiency in Saudi adults is reported to be about 37%, but still in this age group, vitamin B12 deficiency is common and folate deficiency is less common (Aljaadi et al., 2023). Examining the status of vitamin D in Saudi women aged 19–40 showed that the deficiency of this vitamin is very common among women, so 79.1% of them are severely deficient in vitamin D and about 21% are at an insufficient level (Al-Mogbel, 2012). The prevalence of vitamin D deficiency among all age groups is 81% (Al-Daghri, 2018).

3.6.11 United Arab Emirates

In recent years, the UAE has faced changes such as population growth, urbanization development, and economic developments, which have also been accompanied by nutrition transition in the Middle East region. Advertisements, smart food marketing, increased access to various food sources and drinks have caused changes in the food pattern of Emiratis, which gradually have negative effects on health and increase the incidence of many NCDs in them. This pattern has caused changes in the trend of overweight and obesity among Emiratis, especially in children. The prevalence of overweight, obesity, stunting, and wasting among 0–4-year-old Emirati children is reported as 5%, 3%, 10%, and 6%, respectively. The prevalence of some micronutrient deficiencies that are effective in children's growth, such as calcium, zinc, folate, and vitamins A and D, has also been observed. Despite the children consuming enough protein the intake of fruits and vegetables was at the lowest level. Sugar-sweetened beverages and sweets from the same period of starting complementary feeding, i.e., from 6 to 12 months, provide 5% of the energy intake of children, which reaches 17% in children 3–4 years old (Nassreddine et al., 2022). This trend is also seen in older children and adolescents (6–18 years old), and studies show that a significant proportion of the daily energy intake of girls aged 9–13 years comes from sweets and sugar-sweetened drinks and saturated fats. Although the intake of calcium and vitamins A, D, and E was less than the average of their needs, and the consumption of milk and dairy products and vegetables was also very low in most of them (Ali et al., 2013). Part of micronutrient deficiencies is related to insufficient intake, and another part can be related to socioeconomic conditions or, in the case of vitamin D, lack of sunshine exposure. Prevalence of anemia has been reported in different age groups, which can be because of low intake of iron-containing foods, consumption of foods with low nutritional value. Unhealthy dietary patterns have become increasingly prevalent among adolescent individuals. The literature highlights trends such as skipping breakfast and reduced intake of fruits and dairy products, as well as elevated consumption of fast food and sweetened beverages or energy drinks. Gender disparities are evident, with females exhibiting a higher likelihood of engaging in unhealthy eating behaviors compared to their male counterparts, barring energy drink consumption. A significant proportion of Emirati female adolescents display a complete absence of dairy consumption, a concerning trend given the rising incidence of vitamin D insufficiency in the Gulf region. Despite the region's abundant sunshine, females face an elevated susceptibility to osteoporosis and compromised bone development, thereby impeding their optimal growth potential.

3.6.12 Qatar

The nutritional paradox observed in the Arab countries manifests through the presence of two distinct categories of nutritional issues currently being encountered by these nations. These issues encompass challenges associated with nutrient deficiencies such as anemia and growth retardation, alongside those arising from rapid transformations in lifestyle and dietary patterns, leading to NCDs. Qatar, positioned at an advanced stage of nutrition transition, exhibits a significant proportion of its population grappling with overweight and obesity, complemented by certain demographic subgroups experiencing undernourishment and deficiencies in essential micronutrients. Despite the escalating preference for fast food, traditional culinary preparations, either homemade or procured from eateries and markets, continue to constitute a substantial portion of the dietary habits prevalent among the Qatari community (ElObeid et al., 2015). Qatar has a population of Qatari nationals and a large number of non-Qatari residents. The mean quantity of food purchased by households in Qatar exceeded that of non-Qatari households; nevertheless, the distribution of food purchases across different categories was comparable between the two groups. The average daily energy intake per individual was nearly two times higher in Qatari households compared to non-Qatari households. Food items included in the subsidy program for Qatari citizens contributed to 41% of the total daily energy consumption. Nutrient density levels surpassed the recommended values for proteins (29.2 g), fats (39.2 g), sodium (3.3 mg), and vitamin C (32.5 mg). Conversely, calcium (227 mg), vitamin A (302.3 μg), fiber (2.0 g), and carbohydrates (132.6 g) fell below the recommended nutrient energy density levels. The food basket composition in Qatar primarily consists of fruit and vegetables, representing around 30% of the total, followed by animal products at 29% and cereals at 21%. The Qatari diet is characterized by a high consumption of meat products, sugar, and sodium, while being deficient in calcium and fiber. Excessive intake of free sugars poses a threat to the nutritional value of diets, as they provide substantial energy without essential nutrients. Overconsumption of high-energy foods contributes to weight gain and various NCDs and associated morbidity and mortality (Al-Thani et al., 2017).

In the last decade the prevalence rates of overweight and obesity were 18.5% and 19.1%, respectively. Among males the prevalence of obesity was significantly higher at 25.3% compared to females at 12.6%, whereas overweight prevalence among females was significantly higher at 21.0% than among males at 16.3%. When obesity and overweight rates were combined, they were significantly higher among males at 25.6% than in females at 23.7%. The analysis of the students' eating habits revealed that the frequency of consuming fruits, milk, and energy drinks per week was significantly higher among males than females, whereas the intake of sweets, French fries, and cake/doughnuts was higher among females than males (Daradkeh et al., 2015).

In the university students aged 18 and older, four distinct dietary patterns, namely, "fast food," "healthy diet," "traditional diet," and "protein shake," were explored. Those who closely followed the "fast food" pattern were characterized as "juvenile and hectic," predominantly male, preuniversity students who perceive themselves as too occupied to consume healthy meals and tend to skip breakfast. Individuals adhering to the "traditional diet" pattern were more "traditionalist and sedentary," regularly eating breakfast and dinner, and showing reluctance toward vegetarianism or dietary restrictions. Students embracing the "healthy diet" pattern were perceived as "salubrious and resolute," prioritizing regular consumption of nutritious meals such as breakfast and lunch while being more inclined toward supplement intake. Lastly, those following the "protein shake" pattern demonstrated an "active and self-controlled," engaging in vigorous physical activity at higher rates (Cheema et al., 2023).

The prevalence of anemia in 12-month-old infants was 23.5%; iron deficiency was 9.2%; and IDA was 7.8%. The WHO has identified iron deficiency among adolescents as one of the most important issues in the health system. The prevalence of iron deficiency among Qatari adolescents aged 10–19 years was 26.4%.

3.6.13 Oman

Oman has experienced significant economic growth over the past decades, and at the same time, a decrease in some indicators of malnutrition such as short stature, weight loss and underweight in young children and malnutrition in nonpregnant women have also been reported. But in-line with the increase in global overweight and obesity, 73.4% of women in Oman are overweight or obese, and the lack of many micronutrients is also common among women. According to a nutritional assessment of Oman in 2004, Omani women and children suffer from high prevalence of iron deficiency and moderate prevalence of vitamin A deficiency. On average, about 23.8% of Omani children suffer from anemia, which was less prevalent in children from wealthy families. A rate of 10.2% of children had iron deficiency, and 1.6% had IDA. The prevalence of vitamin A deficiency in children is 9.5%, and its percentage is higher in infants aged 6–12 months than in other children. The percentage of children who had insufficient vitamin D was 53.8, but overall, the prevalence of vitamin D deficiency was reported as 10.6. The prevalence of stunting, wasting, and underweight in children was 11.4%, 9.3%, and 11.2%, respectively. On the other hand, overweight and obesity, with a prevalence of 4.2%, were more common in children aged 6–23 months than in older children. Pregnant women had higher anemia than nonpregnant women (29.3% vs. 27.8%). The prevalence of various micronutrient deficiencies in nonpregnant women was reported as 24.8% for iron deficiency (ID), 13.3% for ID-Anaemia, 16.2% for vitamin D deficiency, 41.5% for vitamin D insufficiency, 11.6% for folate deficiency, 8.9% and for vitamin B_{12} deficiency, 8.9% was reported. The prevalence of overweight and obesity in nonpregnant women increased with age, from 25.7% in women aged 15–19 to 88% in women aged 45–49 (Petry et al., 2020).

The rate of overweight and obesity among school children in Oman has increased in recent years, which is related to the increase in the consumption of high-energy fast foods and carbonated drinks, skipping breakfast and regular meals, insufficient consumption of fruits, vegetables, fish, and sedentary lifestyle (Al-Saadi et al., 2020). The majority of adolescents adhere to the recommendations of food guide pyramids by consuming regular meals based on the specified daily and weekly serving sizes. Many adolescents of both genders believed in the importance of consuming diverse foods to achieve a well-rounded and nourishing diet. A nutritious diet is defined as one that incorporates a higher quantity of fruits and vegetables while limiting fat intake. Conversely a considerable number of adolescents reported consuming daily snacks and fried foods as being a leading contributor to obesity because of their high energy and fat content. Male adolescents reported high intake of red meat and saturated fat and moderate intake of fruits and vegetables. Both genders showed a positive trend in daily fruit and vegetable consumption. The study also highlighted a common unhealthy habit of skipping breakfast, with 32% of Omani adolescents admitting to this practice. Omani females tend to consume fast food more frequently than males (63.3% vs. 50.2%) (Kilani et al., 2013).

The change in the food style of Arab countries such as Oman, such as receiving high energy from foods with high energy density, has caused an increase in the prevalence of overweight and obesity in the elderly population. On the other hand, in this age group, there is not enough information about the relationship between food intake and the occurrence of various diseases, the benefits of consuming food groups such as fruits and vegetables, and the harms of sweets, salt, and fat. Per capita consumption of salt in Oman is high, at 11.5 g/day, and a high rate (6.38%) of the prevalence of hypertension has also been reported in this country. About 40% of the consumption of milk and dairy products in elderly is from the high-fat dairy group. Strategies such as nutrition education and strategies to provide micronutrients in the elderly population of Oman seem necessary (Al Riyami et al., 2010).

3.6.14 Iraq

Iraq is one of the countries in the Arab world that involves the consumption of nutrients either in insufficient amounts or in excess. Following the 2003 conflict in Iraq, many Iraqis faced challenges in accessing vital healthcare services because of ongoing security limitations. Stunting and overweight are prevalent in Iraq in the amount of 22% and 7.7%, respectively. Dietary habits and lifestyle have been changed in Iraq, with a choice for energy-dense foods, sugar-sweetened beverages, and processed foods, which contribute to increased overweight and obesity across all age groups in Iraq. Assessment of dietary patterns among overweight adult individuals classified into class I, II, and III reveals a strong correlation between the levels of obesity and dietary behaviors. The dietary habits have significant effects on obesity, in the amount of 42%, with the consumption of foods rich in saturated fats and sugars and low consumption of fruits and vegetables.

The study of lactating women showed that they do not consume enough protein and healthy fats, iron, zinc, vitamin C, pantothenic acid, folate, vitamin C, vitamin A, vitamin D, zinc, iodine, potassium, and linoleic acid. Lactating women living in urban areas have a better nutritional status than rural women, which is because of greater access to diverse and nutrient-rich food sources; ease of food preparation in supermarkets and markets that supply fresh vegetables, dairy, and protein; and transportation networks. On the other hand, breastfeeding mothers who have higher education, higher income, and higher SES have a higher level of nutritional status (Shabib et al., 2024).

In recent years the prevalence of anemia has decreased from moderate to mild, which is because of various reasons such as deficiency of iron, vitamin B12, and folate (5%, 30%, and 19%, respectively) (Sabeeh et al., 2022). The prevalence of IDA in Iraqi children is 20%, which is higher in children aged 9–23 months and residents of rural areas. A lower level of vitamin D is usually seen in children suffering from iron deficiency (Al-Zuhairy et al., 2022).

The survey of 65–74-year-old Iraqi people also indicates insufficient intake of many micronutrients, and the prevalence of these deficiencies was the highest for vitamin B12 (59.2%). The proportion of intake of many food items was lower than the average recommended daily intake, which was 98.4%, 97.3%, 96.7% for milk, vegetables, fruits, and 95.1%, 70.7%, 59.3% for fish and seafood, meat and poultry, legumes, and 57.6% and 88% for eggs and cereals, respectively (AlSharbaty, 2013). Anemia is a common health problem among pregnant women, which has a lot to do with being a housewife, living in rural areas, multiple births, and low education of women. In general, about 91% had IDA, and in the majority of those women, it was related to drinking tea with breakfast or after meals, low consumption of meat and low consumption of vegetables fresh and dried fruits (Abdul-Fatah et al., 2018).

3.7 The policies of different countries in the Middle East for better nutrition

The general goal of developing food and nutrition policies is to develop nutrition-sensitive policies that help establish healthy nutrition and food security and promote health in society. A wide range of policies can be formulated in this direction, from the production of healthy food in the agriculture sector to the import and supply of food. Based on these policies the quality and quantity of available food, the ability to buy healthy food, people's food choices, and the amount of macro- and micronutrients intake will increase. The output of these strategies can reduce various dimensions of the triple burden of malnutrition, from improving the growth of children and adolescents and preventing malnutrition to reducing the prevalence of micronutrient deficiency and preventing the occurrence of overweight and obesity in society. In this section the most important strategies that have been developed and implemented in recent years are presented (Leppäniemi et al., 2023).

3.7.1 National nutrition strategy or action plan

Following the formulation of the WHO strategy on nutrition for EMR (2020–2030) in October 2019, a commitment was made in the countries of the region to improve the nutritional status of different age groups (World Health Organization, Regional Office for the Eastern Mediterranean, 2019b). By August 2022, all countries in the Middle East region had developed a national nutrition strategy or action plan. In these programs, countries emphasize the centrality of nutrition in formulating appropriate strategies for each demographic group.

3.7.2 Plan for obesity prevention

In the EMR, which also includes the countries of the Middle East, obesity prevention strategies 2019–23 presented with various topics such as food supply, food trade, public education campaigns, food labeling, and food reformulation to produce healthy products. All countries in the Middle East, except Iraq and the UAE, follow a plan to prevent obesity (Al-Jawaldeh et al., 2020; World Health Organization, Regional Office for the Eastern Mediterranean, 2019a). The development of the "Nutrition-Friendly School" framework by the WHO provided a basis for the formation of a healthier food environment for society, especially for children and adolescents (World Health Organization, 2021). This framework provides recommendations to countries regarding the marketing and supply of food and beverages, especially those containing sugar, salt, saturated, and *trans* fats. Among the countries of the Middle East, Egypt, Iran, and Saudi Arabia have enacted laws to achieve this goal.

3.7.3 Code of marketing of breast milk substitutes

The production and marketing of breast milk substitutes (BMSs) by baby food industry producers can have negative effects on the health of the child, the mother, and the economic status of the family. Therefore the World Health Assembly (WHA) approved the International Code of Marketing of Breast Milk Substitutes in 1981 and later updated it based on changes in marketing methods and new scientific information. This code includes all products that are considered BMSs in the market (Becker et al., 2022). Among the countries of the Middle East region, Bahrain, Kuwait, Lebanon, Yemen, Saudi Arabia, and the UAE have fully established ample laws and measures; Syria's measures provide the majority of the code provisions; and the countries of Jordan, Iran, Iraq, Palestine, Oman, and Egypt have laws for some of these codes. Only Qatar is currently studying the matter (Leppäniemi et al., 2023).

3.7.4 Food-based dietary guidelines

Food-based dietary guidelines (FBDG) provide recommendations based on food groups and nutritional principles with the aim of preventing malnutrition and other diseases and improving health by considering a sustainable diet. These guidelines are in accordance with the food culture of each country and their local food patterns

(Cámara et al., 2021). FBDG has been developed in many Middle Eastern countries such as Bahrain, UAE, Saudi Arabia, Oman, Kuwait, Qatar, Jordan, Lebanon, Iran, Palestine, and Syria. Some recommendations are general in all of the FBDGs, such as recommendations on obesity prevention, but some countries have included recommendations based on their country's situation, such as prevalent diseases or specific demographic groups or their concern. For example, there are dietary recommendations for heart diseases and diabetes in the FBDG of Lebanon, Iran, Oman, and Qatar. Regarding specific groups, such as pregnant and lactating mothers, Lebanon, Oman, and Jordan have recommendations for specific concern, such as Saudi Arabia for nutrition labels and Iran, Lebanon, Oman, and Qatar for preventing micronutrient deficiencies (Leppäniemi et al., 2023).

3.7.5 Policy to limit sugar/fatty acids/salt consumption

The WHO has introduced the policy of reducing the consumption of salt, sugar, and *trans* fat as one of the most cost-effective intervention policies to reduce NCDs. Several policy statements have been issued regarding the reduction of sugar, fat, and salt consumption, and the implementation of these policies can gradually reduce sugar, salt, and fat in the diet and help to decrease the prevalence of NCDs. Among the countries in the Middle East, Bahrain, Oman, Qatar, Saudi Arabia, Kuwait, the UAE, Jordan, Iran, Palestine have established policies to reduce the consumption of trans fatty acids. The mentioned countries, along with Iraq and Egypt, also formulate and implement policies to reduce salt/sodium consumption. However, Lebanon and Syria currently do not have policies to reduce sugar and salt/sodium (Leppäniemi et al., 2023).

3.7.6 Sugar-sweetened beverages tax

A tax on sugar-sweetened beverages is one of the financial policies to improve community nutrition. The revenues obtained from this tax should be invested for low-income households or treatment of diseases. In the meantime, food-producing industries also have some resistance to this taxation because price increases may have a negative effect on their sales. Often these rates are very low and have little effect on consumption. One of the proposed solutions is to increase the current tax rate, which in some Middle Eastern countries, such as Saudi Arabia, Qatar, and the UAE, have imposed an indirect tax of 50%–100% on this group of drinks (Popkin & Ng, 2021). According to the findings of a metaanalysis, with a 10% increase in the price of sugar-sweetened beverages, consumption decreases by 10% (Teng et al., 2019). This tax has been implemented in the high-income countries of the Middle East, namely Bahrain, Kuwait, Oman, Qatar, Saudi Arabia, and the UAE s, and some low-middle income countries, such as Egypt, Iran, and Palestine. The percentage of tax on soft drinks and energy drinks in 2016 was set at 50 and 100, respectively, in the countries of the Persian Gulf Cooperation Council (GCC), and in the next stages, Saudi Arabia, UAE, and Bahrain in 2017 and Oman and Qatar in 2019 and Kuwait in 2020 implemented this policy (Leppäniemi et al., 2023).

3.7.7 Policy to reduce the impact of marketing of food to children

Marketing of food and beverages can influence children's food choices and can gradually change their preferences. WHO's efforts to adopt the proper approach to marketing began in 2004, and in 2010, the WHA, Food and Beverage Marketing Rules, and asked the countries to formulate and implement laws related to marketing based on their own priorities. The 2018 WHO's report shows the limited implementation of these rules in the EMR, which are mostly focused on local television and radio marketing (Al-Jawaldeh & Jabbour, 2022). Bahrain, Kuwait, Oman, Qatar, Saudi Arabia, the UAE, Jordan, Lebanon, Iran, and Egypt have developed this policy (Leppäniemi et al., 2023).

3.7.8 Front-of-pack labeling

To achieve a healthy diet and with the aim of preventing NCDs, the WHO proposed another policy to the governments as front-of-pack (FOP) nutrition labels. Because of the simplicity, graphicness, and attention grabbing of the labels, it can help the consumer to understand the quality of the food he/she chooses. There are different formats for FOP such as stars, traffic lights, stop signs (Jones et al., 2019). FOP has been implemented in the Middle East region in the countries of Saudi Arabia, the UAE, and Iran. As the first country in 2017, Iran made it mandatory to include a traffic light labeling on packaged food products so that 80% of the country's food products have this label. After that, Saudi Arabia implemented it voluntarily, in 2018, and the UAE implemented this labeling in 2022 (Leppäniemi et al., 2023).

3.7.9 Salt iodization

Iodine insufficiency has a detrimental impact on human well-being and overall quality of life. A supplementary source of iodine is essential for most individuals because of its relatively limited presence in dietary sources. The act of iodizing salt involves fortifying it with iodine for human consumption, proving to be a successful approach in enhancing iodine consumption on a societal scale. All salt intended for households and food production purposes must undergo iodine fortification as a secure and efficient method in the prevention and management of iodine deficiency ailments among populations residing in both stable and crisis environments (Doggui et al., 2020). In 1991 the WHO asked different countries to implement the salt iodization program. Currently, this program is implemented in all countries of the Middle East.

3.7.10 Flour fortification

Staple foods are the best vehicles of fortification with vitamins and minerals because they are accessible for a large population. Every year, millions of tons of wheat around the world are milled, and flour is used in the preparation of various foods, from baking bread to the confectionery industry, and many households use it. Micronutrients, such as iron, folate, and group B vitamins, can be used to fortify flour, and the deficiency identified in each country determines which of these micronutrients should be used for fortification. About 34.1% of food industries around the world fortified flour with iron and folic acid in 2016 (World Health Organization, 2009). Flour fortification has been implemented in all the countries of the Middle East in the form of voluntary and mandatory regulations. Iron and folic acid were the top micronutrients used in the wheat flour fortification, but vitamins B, A, D, and zinc were used for fortification to a lesser extent (Leppäniemi et al., 2023).

3.7.11 Micronutrient supplementation

Supplementing with micronutrients in special population groups such as children and pregnant women is one of the ways to combat micronutrient deficiency. In this short-term solution, micronutrients are distributed among vulnerable groups in the form of tablets, powders, or pills. Despite the fact that this method is useful in combating acute and chronic deficiency of micronutrients, it is not justified in large populations and in the long term. Extensive investment, participation of the private and public sectors, as well as the need for continuous monitoring, are some of the things that should be considered in micronutrients supplementation (Pritwani & Mathur, 2015). Considering the prevalence of various micronutrient deficiencies in the Middle East region, supplementing with micronutrients can be a suitable solution to prevent higher prevalence and treat some deficiencies.

3.7.12 Food and nutrition literacy promotion

Promoting food and nutrition literacy is important to choose healthy food, food preparation, eating behaviors, and dietary quality via elevated vegetables and fruits and reduced processed foods among children and adolescents, specifically. In addition, a lack of food skills has been demonstrated to be connected with an increased consumption of highly processed foods. Furthermore, inadequate food literacy has worsened food insecurity by hindering appropriate food utilization. Although research on the relationship between nutrition outcomes and food and nutrition literacy is still evolving, the interventions based on food and nutrition literacy in the Middle East and North Africa (MENA) region hold significant promise. The countries in the MENA region should initiate measures to enhance the food literacy and nutrition literacy of individuals in the area. Nutrition education, as well as food and nutrition programs and policies, are crucial in creating a supportive environment for promoting healthy dietary habits and eliciting a response from the food system. Introducing nutrition and food education in childcare and school environments is just one of several steps that can be taken to progress toward the achievement of the sustainable development goals by the year 2030 (Mohsen et al., 2022).

3.8 Outlook of strategies that should be considered in future research

Despite all the strategies that are carried out to improve the nutritional status in age groups, cooperation between different countries in the region and achieving effective solutions are recommended. In this regard the proposed areas are as follows:

- Considering local and cultural foods of different countries in updating food composition tables
- Conducting national studies and preparing evidence about food consumption patterns and food intakes of different age groups using validated and standardized methods
- Developing programs to assess the amount of salt, sugar, and *trans* fat in various food sources
- Capacity building of nutritionists and their evidence-based education to design and conduct appropriate education for different population groups
- Designing educational programs on nutrition suitable for different age groups of the society, considering the SES of the target groups
- Paying attention to the social determinants of health in conducting nutritional interventions in each country

References

Abdollahi, S., Zeinali, F., Azam, K., Toupchian, O., & Djafarian, K. (2015). Identifying major dietary patterns among the elderly in Tehran health homes. *Jundishapur Journal of Health Sciences, 7*(4), e30395.

Abdul-Fatah, B. N., Murshid, R. M., & Ahmed, T. E. (2018). Assessment of iron deficiency anemia (IDA) and dietary pattern among pregnant women in Baghdad city, Iraq. *Journal of Pharmaceutical Sciences and Research, 10*(9), 2279–2284.

Adam, A., Osama, S., & Muhammad, K. I. (2014). Nutrition and food consumption patterns in the Kingdom of Saudi Arabia. *Pakistan Journal of Nutrition, 13*(4), 181.

Alalwan, T. A., Mandeel, Q. A., & Al-Sarhani, L. (2017). Traditional plant-based foods and beverages in Bahrain. *Journal of Ethnic Foods, 4*(4), 274–283.

Al-Awwad, N. J., Ayoub, J., Barham, R., Sarhan, W., Al-Holy, M., Abughoush, M., Al-Hourani, H., Olaimat, A., & Al-Jawaldeh, A. (2021). Review of the nutrition situation in Jordan: Trends and way forward. *Nutrients, 14*(1), 135.

Al-Daghri, N. M. (2018). Vitamin D in Saudi Arabia: Prevalence, distribution and disease associations. *The Journal of Steroid Biochemistry and Molecular Biology, 175*, 102–107.

Al-Halani, A. A., Edrees, W. H., Alrahabi, L. M., Thabit, J. M., Al-Bahloul, S., Al-washali, F. A., Al-Qhali, R. M., Morshed, M. M., Al-Hossainy, A. S., Al-Maflhi, E. A., & Al-Sufi, N. H. (2023). Prevalence of intestinal parasites, malnutrition, anemia and their risk factors among orphaned children in Sana'a city, Yemen. *Universal Journal of Pharmaceutical Research., 8*(2), 32–39.

Al-Hussaini, A. A., Alshehry, Z., AlDehaimi, A., & Bashir, M. S. (2022). Vitamin D and iron deficiencies among Saudi children and adolescents: A persistent problem in the 21st century. *Saudi Journal of Gastroenterology, 28*(2), 157–164.

Ali, H. I., Ng, S. W., Zaghloul, S., Harrison, G. G., Qazaq, H. S., El Sadig, M., & Yeatts, K. (2013). High proportion of 6 to 18-year-old children and adolescents in the United

Arab Emirates are not meeting dietary recommendations. *Nutrition Research, 33*(6), 447–456.

Aljaadi, A. M., Alsunaid, F. F., Abdulrahim, M., Almehmadi, N. H., & Alzaben, A. S. (2023). The status of B vitamin in Saudi Adults: A review. *Current Research in Nutrition and Food Science Journal, 11*(3), 894–909.

Al-Jawaldeh, A., & Jabbour, J. (2022). Marketing of food and beverages to children in the eastern mediterranean region: A situational analysis of the regulatory framework. *Frontiers in Nutrition, 9*, 868937.

Al-Jawaldeh, A., Taktouk, M., & Nasreddine, L. (2020). Food consumption patterns and nutrient intakes of children and adolescents in the Eastern Mediterranean Region: A call for policy action. *Nutrients, 12*(11), 3345.

Alkhulaifi, F., Al-Hooti, S., Al-Zenki, S., AlOmirah, H., & Darkoh, C. (2023). Dietary habits, meal timing, and meal frequency in Kuwaiti adults: Analysis of the Kuwait National Nutrition Surveillance data. *Nutrients, 15*(21), 4537.

Allafi, A., Al-Haifi, A. R., Al-Fayez, M. A., Al-Athari, B. I., Al-Ajmi, F. A., Al-Hazzaa, H. M., Musaiger, A. O., & Ahmed, F. (2014). Physical activity, sedentary behaviours and dietary habits among Kuwaiti adolescents: Gender differences. *Public Health Nutrition, 17*(9), 2045–2052.

Al-Lahou, B., Ausman, L. M., Peñalvo, J. L., Huggins, G. S., Al-Hooti, S., Al-Zenki, S., & Zhang, F. F. (2020). Dietary patterns associated with the prevalence of cardiovascular disease risk factors in Kuwaiti adults. *Journal of the Academy of Nutrition and Dietetics, 120*(3), 424–436.

Al Mansoob, M. A. K., & Masood, M. S. A. (2019). The impact of food consumption pattern on women's health at Sana'a Governorate, Yemen. *Global Journal of Nutrition & Food Science, 2*(2), 2019.

Al-Mogbel, E. S. (2012). Vitamin D status among adult Saudi females visiting primary health care clinics. *International Journal of Health Sciences, 6*(2), 116.

Almohri, M., Al Salehi, S., Al Ghawi, A., Husain, E., & Al Fardan, M. (2023). Prevalence of anemia, and associated risk factors among pregnant women attending primary healthcare centers in the Kingdom of Bahrain. *Bahrain Medical Bulletin, 45*(3), 1581–1587.

Al Riyami, A., Al Hadabi, S., Aty, A., Al Kharusi, H., Morsi, M., & Jaju, S. (2010). Nutrition knowledge, beliefs and dietary habits among elderly people in Nizwa, Oman: Implications for policy. *EMHJ-Eastern Mediterranean Health Journal, 16*(8), 859–867.

Al-Saadi, L. S., Ali, A., Waly, M. I., & Al-Zuhaibi, K. (2020). Impact of dietary patterns and nutritional status on the academic performance of Omani school students. *Journal of Pharmacy and Nutrition Sciences, 10*(3), 74–87.

Al Sabbah, H., Vereecken, C., Kolsteren, P., Abdeen, Z., & Maes, L. (2007). Food habits and physical activity patterns among Palestinian adolescents: Findings from the national study of Palestinian schoolchildren (HBSC-WBG2004). *Public Health Nutrition, 10*(7), 739–746.

AlSharbaty, S. S. (2013). Dietary assessment and food intake in elderly individuals attending public health centers in urban areas of Baghdad city in Iraq. *Journal of the Faculty of Medicine Baghdad, 55*(3), 224–229.

Al-Thani, M., Al-Thani, A.-A., Al-Mahdi, N., Al-Kareem, H., Barakat, D., Al-Chetachi, W., Tawfik, A., & Akram, H. (2017). An overview of food patterns and diet quality in Qatar: Findings from the National Household Income Expenditure Survey. *Cureus, 9*(5), e1249.

Alwabr, G. M., & Al-Wadhaf, A. Y. (2020). Risk factors and prevalence of vitamin D deficiency among Yemeni women attending Al-Zahrawi Medical Center in Sana'a City. *MicroMedicine, 8*(1), 12–21.

Al-Zuhairy, S. H., Darweesh, M. A., Othman, M. A-M., & Noor, A. (2022). Vitamin D deficiency in young children with iron deficiency in Misan province, Iraq. *Journal of Medicine and Life, 15*(3), 387.

Atasi, M., Kammar-García, A., Almendra-Pegueros, R., & Navarro-Cruz, A. R. (2022). Dietary patterns and their association with metabolic syndrome and their components in middle-class adults from Damascus, Syria: A cross-sectional study. *Journal of Nutrition and Metabolism, 2022*, 5621701.

Babaali, E., Rahmdel, S., Berizi, E., Akhlaghi, M., Götz, F., & Mazloomi, S. M. (2020). Dietary intakes of zinc, copper, magnesium, calcium, phosphorus, and sodium by the general adult population aged 20–50 years in Shiraz, Iran: A total diet study approach. *Nutrients, 12*(11), 3370.

Batal, M., Deaconu, A., & Steinhouse, L. (2023). The nutrition transition and the double burden of malnutrition. In *Nutritional health: Strategies for disease prevention* (pp. 33–44). Springer.

Bawazeer, N. M., Al-Qahtani, S. J., & Alzaben, A. S. (2021). The association between dietary patterns and socio-demographic and lifestyle characteristics: A sample of Saudi Arabia. *Current Research in Nutrition and Food Science Journal, 9*(3), 1046–1057.

Becker, G. E., Zambrano, P., Ching, C., Cashin, J., Burns, A., Policarpo, E., Datu-Sanguyo, J., & Mathisen, R. (2022). Global evidence of persistent violations of the international code of marketing of breast-milk substitutes: A systematic scoping review. *Maternal & Child Nutrition, 18*, e13335.

Brouzes, C. M., Darcel, N., Tomé, D., Dao, M. C., Bourdet-Sicard, R., Holmes, B. A., & Lluch, A. (2020). Urban Egyptian women aged 19–30 years display nutrition transition-like dietary patterns, with high energy and sodium intakes, and insufficient iron, vitamin D, and folate intakes. *Current Developments in Nutrition, 4*(2), nZz143.

Cámara, M., Giner, R. M., González-Fandos, E., López-García, E., Mañes, J., Portillo, M. P., Rafecas, M., Domínguez, L., & Martínez, J. A. (2021). Food-based dietary guidelines around the world: A comparative analysis to update AESAN scientific committee dietary recommendations. *Nutrients, 13*(9), 3131.

Cheema, S., Maisonneuve, P., Abraham, A., Chaabna, K., Yousuf, W., Mushannen, T., Ibrahim, H., Tom, A., Lowenfels, A. B., & Mamtani, R. (2023). Dietary patterns and associated lifestyle factors among university students in Qatar. *Journal of American College Health, 71*(9), 2795–2803.

Chokor, F. A. Z., Hwalla, N., Naja, F., & Nasreddine, L. (2024). Food sources of fiber and micronutrients of concern among infants and young children in Lebanon: A national cross-sectional study. *BMC Pediatrics, 24*(1), 57.

Daradkeh, G., Muhannadi, A., Chandra, P., Fadlalla, A., & Hajr, M. (2015). Dietary habits and intakes associated with obesity and overweight among adolescents in the state of Qatar. *Journal of Nutritional Disorders & Therapy, S1*, 005.

De Souza, L. R. (2017). Correlates of child undernutrition in Yemen. *Bandung, 4*(1), 1–27.

Doggui, R., Al-Jawaldeh, H., & Al-Jawaldeh, A. (2020). Trend of iodine status in the eastern mediterranean region and impact of the universal salt iodization programs: A narrative review. *Biological Trace Element Research, 198*(2), 390–402.

Doggui, R., Al-Jawaldeh, H., El Ati, J., Barham, R., Nasreddine, L., Alqaoud, N., Aguenaou, H., El Ammari, L., Jabbour, J., & Al-Jawaldeh, A. (2021). Meta-analysis and systematic review of micro- and macro-nutrient intakes and trajectories of macro-nutrient supply in the Eastern Mediterranean Region. *Nutrients, 13*(5), 1515.

El Bilbeisi, A., El Afifi, A., Baloushah, S., Alblbeisi, A., Albelbeisi, A., & Taleb, M. (2020). Maternal dietary patterns during early pregnancy and their association with pregnancy outcome among obese women in Gaza Strip, Palestine: A prospective cohort study. *Austin Journal of Nutrition and Food Sciences, 8*(1), 1138.

ElObeid, T., Phoboo, S., & Magdad, Z. (2015). Proximate and mineral composition of indigenous Qatari dishes: Comparative study with similar Middle Eastern dishes. *Journal of Food Chemistry and Nutrition, 3*(1), 27–34.

Falahi, E. (2013). Identification of dietary patterns among Iranian adults. *Yafteh, 14*(5), 29–39.

Gharib, N., & Rasheed, P. (2011). Energy and macronutrient intake and dietary pattern among school children in Bahrain: A cross-sectional study. *Nutrition Journal, 10*, 1–12.

Golzarand, M., Mirmiran, P., Jessri, M., Toolabi, K., Mojarrad, M., & Azizi, F. (2012). Dietary trends in the Middle East and North Africa: An ecological study (1961 to 2007). *Public Health Nutrition, 15*(10), 1835–1844.

Horino, M., Bahar, L., Al-Jadba, G., Habash, R., Akihiro, S., & We st, K. P., Jr (2020). Dietary inadequacy, micronutrient deficiencies, and approaches to preventing poor nutrition in the Gaza Strip. *Food and Nutrition Bulletin, 41*(4), 503–511.

Hoteit, M., Zoghbi, E., Rady, A., Shankiti, I., Sacre, Y., Hanna-Wakim, L., Mahfouz, R., Ibrahim, C., & Al-Jawaldeh, A. (2024). The dietary fiber and micronutrient composition of traditional foods from Lebanon and their contribution to dietary adequacy: A call for action. *PLoS One, 19*(10), e0312429.

Hu, F. B. (2002). Dietary pattern analysis: A new direction in nutritional epidemiology. *Current Opinion in Lipidology, 13*(1), 3–9.

Hwalla, N., Al Dhaheri, A. S., Radwan, H., Alfawaz, H. A., Fouda, M. A., Al-Daghri, N. M., Zaghloul, S., & Blumberg, J. B. (2017). The prevalence of micronutrient deficiencies and inadequacies in the Middle East and approaches to interventions. *Nutrients, 9*(3), 229.

Ibrahim Sr, A. I. M., Bourkhime, H., Benmaamar, S., El Harch, I., Otmani, N., Mohammed, S., Benazzouz, B., & El Rhazi, K. (2023). The double burden of obesity and underweight in Yemeni Adults. *Cureus, 15*(12), e50829.

Jafari Giv, Z., Avan, A., Hamidi, F., Tayefi, M., Khayyatzadeh, S. S., Javandoost, A., Nematy, M., Ferns, G. A., & Mobarhan, M. G. (2018). Nutrients intake, and serum calcium and phosphorus levels: An evidence-based study. *Journal of Clinical Laboratory Analysis, 32*(2), e22235.

Jaghasi, I., Hatahet, W., & Dashash, M. (2012). Dietary patterns and oral health in schoolchildren from Damascus, Syrian Arab Republic. *Eastern Mediterranean Health Journal, 18*(4), 358–364.

Jones, A., Neal, B., Reeve, B., Mhurchu, C. N., & Thow, A. M. (2019). Front-of-pack nutrition labelling to promote healthier diets: Current practice and opportunities to strengthen regulation worldwide. *BMJ Global Health, 4*(6), e001882.

Kafeshani, O., Sarrafzadegan, N., Nouri, F., & Mohammadifard, N. (2015). Major dietary patterns in Iranian adolescents: Isfahan healthy heart program, Iran. *ARYA Atherosclerosis, 11*(Suppl 1), 61.

Kaplan, D. M. (2019). *Food philosophy: An introduction*. Columbia University Press.

Khatib, D., & Sa, H. (2009). Micronutrient deficiencies among children may be endemic in underprivileged areas in Jordan. *Jordan Medical Journal, 43*(4), 324–332.

Kilani, H., Al-Hazzaa, H., Waly, M. I., & Musaiger, A. (2013). Lifestyle habits: Diet, physical activity and sleep duration among Omani adolescents. *Sultan Qaboos University Medical Journal, 13*(4), 510.

Kutbi, H. A. (2021). Nutrient intake and gender differences among Saudi children. *Journal of Nutritional Science, 10*, e99.

Leppäniemi, H., Ibrahim, E., Abbass, M. M., Borghi, E., Flores-Urrutia, M. C., Dominguez Muriel, E., Gatica-Domínguez, G., Kumapley, R., Hammerich, A., &

Al-Jawaldeh, A. (2023). Nutrition profile for countries of the Eastern Mediterranean region with different income levels: An analytical review. *Children, 10*(2), 236.

Lewis, B. (1995). *The Middle East: A brief history of the last 2,000 years*. Simon and Schuster.

Mahfouz, E., Mohammed, E., & Abd El-Rhman, T. (2013). Assessment of nutritional status of elderly populations in rural Minia, Egypt. *Journal of Aging Research & Clinical Practice, 2*(3), 300–302.

McNaughton, S. A. (2020). Dietary patterns. In B. P. Marriott, D. F. Birt, & V. A. Stallings (Eds.), *Present knowledge in nutrition* (11th edition) (pp. 235–248). Academic Press.

Mirrafiei, A., & Shab-Bidar, S. (2023). Traditional dietary patterns in the elderly: Iranian aspect. In *Ancient and traditional foods, plants, herbs and spices used in the Middle East* (pp. 71–81). CRC Press.

Mohsen, H., Sacre, Y., Hanna-Wakim, L., & Hoteit, M. (2022). Nutrition and food literacy in the MENA region: A review to inform nutrition research and policy makers. *International Journal of Environmental Research and Public Health, 19*(16), 10190.

Moradi-Lakeh, M., El Bcheraoui, C., Afshin, A., Daoud, F., AlMazroa, M. A., Al Saeedi, M., Basulaiman, M., Memish, Z. A., Al Rabeeah, A. A., & Mokdad, A. H. (2017). Diet in Saudi Arabia: Findings from a nationally representative survey. *Public Health Nutrition, 20*(6), 1075–1081.

Mumena, W. A., Ateek, A. A., Alamri, R. K., Alobaid, S. A., Alshallali, S. H., Afifi, S. Y., Aljohani, G. A., & Kutbi, H. A. (2022). Fast-food consumption, dietary quality, and dietary intake of adolescents in Saudi Arabia. *International Journal of Environmental Research and Public Health, 19*(22), 15083.

Musaiger, A., Bader, Z., Al-Roomi, K., & D'Souza, R. (2011). Dietary and lifestyle habits amongst adolescents in Bahrain. *Food & Nutrition Research, 55*(1), 7122.

Musaiger, A. O., & Kalam, F. (2014). Dietary habits and lifestyle among adolescents in Damascus, Syria. *Annals of Agricultural and Environmental Medicine, 21*(2), 416–419.

Naja, F., Hwalla, N., Itani, L., Karam, S., Sibai, A. M., & Nasreddine, L. A. (2015). Western dietary pattern is associated with overweight and obesity in a national sample of Lebanese adolescents (13–19 years): A cross-sectional study. *British Journal of Nutrition, 114*(11), 1909–1919.

Nasreddine, L., Hwalla, N., Al Zahraa Chokor, F., Naja, F., O'Neill, L., & Jomaa, L. (2022). Food and nutrient intake of school-aged children in Lebanon and their adherence to dietary guidelines and recommendations. *BMC Public Health, 22*(1), 922.

Nasreddine, L., Shatila, H., Itani, L., Hwalla, N., Jomaa, L., & Naja, F. (2019). A traditional dietary pattern is associated with lower odds of overweight and obesity among preschool children in Lebanon: A cross-sectional study. *European Journal of Nutrition, 58*, 91–102.

Nassreddine, L. M., Naja, F. A., Hwalla, N. C., Ali, H. I., Mohamad, M. N., Fatima Al Zahraa, S. C., Chehade, L. N., O'Neill, L. M., Kharroubi, S. A., Ayesh, W. H., Kassis, A. N., Cheikh Ismail, L. I., & Al Dhaheri, A. S. (2022). Total usual nutrient intakes and nutritional status of United Arab Emirates children (<4 years): Findings from the Feeding Infants and Toddlers Study (FITS) 2021. *Current Developments in Nutrition, 6*(5), nZac080.

Obaid Musaiger, A. (2004). Health status, lifestyle and nutrient intake of home resident elderly in Bahrain. *Nutrition and Health, 17*(4), 285–295.

Okati-Aliabad, H., Ansari-Moghaddam, A., Kargar, S., & Jabbari, N. (2022). Prevalence of obesity and overweight among adults in the middle east countries from 2000 to 2020: A systematic review and meta-analysis. *Journal of Obesity, 2022*, 8074837.

Papazian, T., Salameh, P., Abi Tayeh, G., Kesrouani, A., Aoun, C., Abou Diwan, M., & Khabbaz, L. R. (2022). Dietary patterns and birth outcomes of healthy Lebanese pregnant women. *Frontiers in Nutrition, 9*, 977288.

Petry, N., Al-Maamary, S. A., Woodruff, B. A., Alghannami, S., Al-Shammakhi, S. M., Al-Ghammari, I. K., Tyler, V., Rohner, F., & Wirth, J. P. (2020). National prevalence of micronutrient deficiencies, anaemia, genetic blood disorders and over- and undernutrition in Omani women of reproductive age and preschool children. *Sultan Qaboos University Medical Journal, 20*(2), e151.

Popkin, B. M., & Ng, S. W. (2021). Sugar-sweetened beverage taxes: Lessons to date and the future of taxation. *PLoS Medicine, 18*(1), e1003412.

Pritwani, R., & Mathur, P. (2015). Strategies to combat micronutrient deficiencies: A review. *International Journal of Health Sciences and Research, 5*(2), 362–373.

Rezazadeh, A., Rashidkhani, B., & Omidvar, N. (2010). Association of major dietary patterns with socioeconomic and lifestyle factors of adult women living in Tehran, Iran. *Nutrition, 26*(3), 337–341.

Sabeeh, H. K., Ali, S. H., & Al-Jawaldeh, A. (2022). Iraq is moving forward to achieve global targets in nutrition. *Children, 9*(2), 215.

Saleh, S. M., El-Sayed, H. H., Mostafa, A. E., & El Gezery, H. M. (2023). Micronutrients intake among a group of Egyptian children in different demographic areas of Egypt. *Bulletin of the National Nutrition Institute of the Arab Republic of Egypt, 61*(1), 62–86.

Saneei, P., Esmaillzadeh, A., Keshteli, A. H., Feizi, A., Feinle-Bisset, C., & Adibi, P. (2016). Patterns of dietary habits in relation to obesity in Iranian adults. *European Journal of Nutrition, 55*, 713–728.

Saraya, M. A., Soliman, I., & El-Shorbagy, G. A. (2021). Dietary pattern of some egyptian university youth. *Zagazig Journal of Agricultural Research, 48*(4), 1033–1041.

Sbaih, R. A., Hourani, H. A., Khader, Y., Khawaja, N., Hyassat, D., & Ajlouni, K. (2020). *Dietary Patterns of University Students in Jordan: A Cross-Sectional Study* https://doi.org/10.21203/rs.3.rs-53972/v1.

Semba, R. D., & Bloem, M. W. (2002). *Nutrition and health in developing countries*. Taylor & Francis.

Serdula, M., Nichols, E., Aburto, N., Masa'd, H., Obaid, B., Wirth, J., Tarawneh, M., Barham, R., Hijawi, B., & Sullivan, K. M.Jordan Fortification Working Group. (2014). Micronutrient status in Jordan: 2002 and 2010. *European Journal of Clinical Nutrition, 68*(10), 1124–1128.

Shabib, M. A., Ahmed, J. T., & Alshawi, R. (2024). Food consumption pattern among lactating mothers during 2023 in Babil governorate, Iraq. *European Journal of Modern Medicine and Practice, 4*(5), 566–578.

Tayyem, R., Al-Qawasmeh, R., & Khawaja, N. (2020). Dietary patterns and nutrients associated with metabolic syndrome: Preliminary findings from Jordanian case-control study. *Nutrition & Food Science, 50*(2), 253–268.

Teng, A. M., Jones, A. C., Mizdrak, A., Signal, L., Genç, M., & Wilson, N. (2019). Impact of sugar-sweetened beverage taxes on purchases and dietary intake: Systematic review and meta-analysis. *Obesity Reviews, 20*(9), 1187–1204.

Valaei, S., Rashidi, A., Haghighian Roudsari, A., Houshyarrad, A., Abadi, A., Abdollahi, M., & Bonab, A. M. (2017). Evaluation of Iranian household's diet in terms of calcium and iron density in the seven provinces of Iran. *Journal of Nutrition and Food Security, 2*(2), 157–163.

World Health Organization. (2021). Nutrition action in schools: A review of evidence related to the nutrition-friendly schools initiative. World Health Organization. Retrieved October 8, 2020, from https://www.who.int/nutrition/topics/nutrition_friendly_schools_initiative/en/.

World Health Organization, Regional Office for the Eastern Mediterranean. (2019a). *Regional framework for action on obesity prevention 2019–2023*. World Health Organization.

World Health Organization, Regional Office for the Eastern Mediterranean. (2019b). *Strategy on nutrition for the Eastern Mediterranean region 2020–2030*. World Health Organization, Regional Office for the Eastern Mediterranean Retrieved July 12, 2022, from https://apps.who.int/iris/bitstream/handle/10665/330059/9789290222996-eng.pdf?sequence=1 .

World Health Organization. (2009). *Recommendations on wheat and maize flour fortification meeting report: Interim consensus statement*. World Health Organization http://www.who.int/nutrition/publications/micronutrients/wheat_maize_fort.pdf.

Zabad, K., Alnesr, A., Alkadah, H., Alchikha, M., Mohammad, K., & Abbassi, H. Food insecurity among Syrian pregnant women: A cross-sectional study. https://doi.org/10.21203/rs.3.rs-3793039/v1.

Zaghloul, S., Al-Hooti, S. N., Al-Hamad, N., Al-Zenki, S., Alomirah, H., Alayan, I., Al-Attar, H., Al-Othman, A., Al-Shami, E., Al-Somaie, M., & Jackson, R. T. (2013). Evidence for nutrition transition in Kuwait: Over-consumption of macronutrients and obesity. *Public Health Nutrition, 16*(4), 596–607.

Current nutritional status in South America: Challenges, strategies, and policies

4

A. Gomez-Zavaglia[a,*], *A.D. Carboni*[a], *M.V. Salinas*[a], *F.A. Silva*[b], *M.W.S. Barbosa*[b], *M.C. Puppo*[a] *and M. Magnani*[b,*]
[a]Center for Research and Development in Food Science and Technology (CIDCA, CCT-CONICET, La Plata), La Plata, Argentina, [b]Laboratory of Microbial Process in Foods, Department of Food Engineering, Federal University of Paraíba, João Pessoa, Brazil
*Corresponding Authors.

4.1 Introduction

4.1.1 General aspects of South American countries

South America is composed of 12 countries, including Argentina, Bolivia, Brazil, Chile, Colombia, Ecuador, Guyana, Paraguay, Peru, Surinam, Uruguay, and Venezuela, and a total size of ca. 17.8 million km^2, representing 41.4% of the American continent. South America has 423 million inhabitants (5.2% of the global population), nearly half of whom live in Brazil, followed by Argentina, with has ca. 45 million inhabitants (Avezum et al., 2009; Sposob, 2024). The South American subcontinent has a wide range of geographical differences in terms of climates, ranging from humid tropical conditions near the equator to cold, dry climates in the southernmost regions. The dominant climates include tropical (hot and rainy year-round), temperate (moderate temperatures with differentiated seasons), cold (freezing conditions in the far south), arid/desert (hot and dry with little rainfall), and high-altitude (cool temperatures at higher elevations, especially in the Andes). Such geographical diversity, along with significant cultural differences and availability of local food products, are the main factors determining the nutritional status and dietary patterns of South American population. General aspects of South America subcontinent and location of Brazil and Argentina are presented in Fig. 4.1.

This chapter is focused on the two largest countries in the subcontinent, Brazil and Argentina. In recent decades the traditional diets of South American countries, which were based on minimally processed foods, have been replaced by diets with a higher content of industrialized products, often rich in salt, saturated fats, and simple sugars (Hernández-Ruiz et al., 2022). This shift has led to an increase in both overnutrition and undernutrition, which can coexist, indicating an early stage of nutritional transition (De La & Sánchez, 2016; Romaguera et al., 2007) and is referred to as the "double burden of malnutrition" by Hernández-Ruiz et al. (2022). Consequently, there has been a rise in the prevalence of overweight, obesity, and other

Nutritional Strategies, Predictive Models, and Sustainable Policies. DOI: https://doi.org/10.1016/B978-0-443-23671-6.00009-8

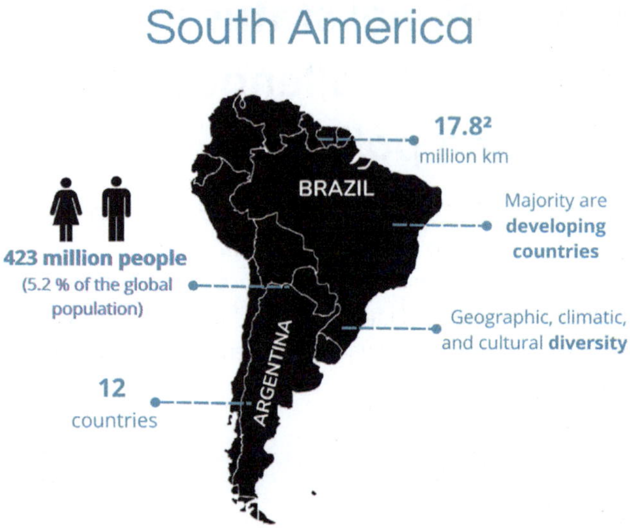

Figure 4.1 General characteristics of South America.

nutrition-related health issues (Malik et al., 2020; Rivera et al., 2004). Different factors can cause this situation, including socioeconomic aspects and consuming behaviors. Hernández-Ruiz et al. (2022) identified the increased availability and accessibility of unhealthy industrialized products for the South American population as one of the main drivers of the rise in nutrition-related diseases. According to some authors, low-income populations tend to replace their traditional food products with others that are more energy-dense and with a high content of sugars, fat, or sodium (World Health Organization & Food and Agriculture Organization, 2003). In addition, the behavior of people toward new or nontraditional food products is strongly influenced by advertisement and marketing. The lack of time to prepare and consume healthy meals also impacts the diet populational patterns. Higher rates of urbanization may also explain some of the weight gain observed in the South American population, as it affects the amount of physical effort or activity individuals exert, and their stress levels (Avezum et al., 2009). These factors together have led to increased consumption of ready-to-eat products, which are generally high in saturated and *trans* fats, sodium, and simple sugars.

Different national and international organizations, along with local governments in South American countries have undertaken efforts to address the diet-related challenges affecting the subcontinent. Such strategies include school feeding programs, food fortification policies, and food cards, which have achieved different degrees of success. However, it is worth mentioning that solving such issues is extremely complex because of the intricate socioeconomic and cultural circumstances. Apart from Brazilian and Argentinian-specific problems, global issues such as pandemics, financial crises, and climate change have put potential advancements in nutrition at risk. Therefore specific strategies and sustainable policies that take into account the particularities of each country are required. This chapter aims to outline the situation in Brazil and Argentina regarding this issue, focusing on three main pillars: the description of the current nutritional status, the policies implemented by both countries to address the problem, including achievements and challenges, and, finally, a critical discussion with educational suggestions, directly addressed to consumers.

4.2 Nutritional status in Argentina and Brazil

4.2.1 General overview of nutritional status

The nutritional status of the Argentinian population is a complex issue determined by different factors, including cultural habits, territory components, changing economic status, public policies, food safety, and security issues. Despite the vast land resources and favorable climatic conditions for agriculture and livestock production, undernutrition persists in certain vulnerable regions of the territory (Zonta et al., 2022). At the same time, many diseases linked to overnutrition or insufficient intake of nutrient-dense foods remain highly prevalent, with some of these conditions strongly associated with cultural habits. One of the most representative examples is the paradox of being a major producer of legumes and having low consumption because of dietary lifestyles. Another cultural practice very common among Argentinians is the high intake of simple sugars, often used to sweeten infusions, industrial dairy products (e.g., yogurts and dairy desserts), and juices. This habit strongly contributes to nutritional imbalances at the population level. Associated with this issue is the lack of variety in children's diets, even though families have access to a wide range of foods, school environments, or other cultural factors often result in a limited intake of certain nutritious foods. For instance, despite the availability, many children do not consume vegetables and legumes, which are often replaced with industrialized products high in saturated fats and salt. This combination of factors may lead to malnutrition caused by deficiencies in different minerals and vitamins. This form of malnutrition is not directly linked to a low-income, but rather to poor dietary choices resulting from a lack of education and consciousness about nutrition importance. On the other hand, chronic malnutrition associated with unbalanced diets resulting from restricted access to food products affects approximately 7.1% of children under the age of 5, leading to individuals with low height for age (Argentinian Ministry of Health, 2019; Food and Agriculture Organization (FAO) et al., 2024). Both cases are clear examples of deficiencies related to undernutrition, leading to widespread micronutrient deficiencies (Le Coq et al., 2022), including iron deficiency anemia, which affects more than 15% of children under 5 years old, as well as zinc and vitamin A deficiencies among the vulnerable population (Argentinian Ministry of Health, 2019; FAO, 2022).

Regarding health-related conditions associated with overnutrition, it should be stated that nearly 40% of adults are overweight at a worldwide level. This problem affects over 60% of the Argentinian adult population and 41% of children and adolescents. Obesity, a risk factor for noncommunicable diseases (NCD) (e.g., cardiovascular diseases, type 2 diabetes, metabolic disorders -hyperlipidemia-, and certain types of cancer) (Popkin, 2015), represents a public health problem affecting all socioeconomic classes, with women being more likely than men to be obese (Argentinian Ministry of Health, 2019). Overweight and obesity are directly related to low physical activity and the consumption of industrialized products high in saturated fats, simple sugars, and sodium, which account for 28% of the average daily caloric intake (PAHO, 2020) and contribute to more than 70% of deaths (PAHO, 2021a; Piñeiro, 2023). In addition, according to Argentina's 2019 National Nutrition Survey, less than 40% of the population reported consuming fruit and vegetables at least once a day, thus not covering the recommended fruit and vegetable intake (Argentinian Ministry of Health, 2019).

The nutritional status of the Brazilian population reflects the deep-rooted social and regional inequalities that have historically characterized the country (Medina et al., 2019). Although certain population groups continue to suffer from food insecurity and malnutrition, others face issues related to overweight and NCDs associated with inadequate dietary habits (Malta et al., 2024). In the north and northeast regions, high rates of malnutrition persist, particularly among children, pregnant women, and Indigenous communities. These groups experience exacerbated vulnerabilities because of poverty, food insecurity, lack of access to basic services, and inadequate diets (Canella et al., 2020). In addition to the more visible forms of malnutrition, Brazil faces widespread nutritional inadequacies, with insufficient intake of fiber, vitamins, and minerals common across diverse population groups (Verly Junior et al., 2021).

Brazil showed recent progress in partial reversal of food insecurity, with severe food insecurity dropping by 85% in 2023 and 14.7 million people no longer facing hunger, mainly because of the impact of public policies and social programs focused on hunger alleviation (Ministério do Desenvolvimento e Assistência Social, Família e Combate à Fome, 2024). However, moderate and mild food insecurity, characterized by poor dietary quality, still affects millions of Brazilians, producing less visible but equally harmful consequences (Santos et al., 2021). This situation was significantly worsened by the COVID-19 pandemic, which heightened food insecurity across the country between 2020 and 2022. Many families lost their income, encountered physical barriers to food access, and were forced to adopt lower quality dietary habits. Returning to prepandemic levels of food security remains a substantial challenge, requiring structural and sustained interventions (Penssan, 2022).

Conversely, according to data from the Brazilian telephone survey Vigitel 2006–23, more than half of the adult population is overweight, with a notable and continuous increase among young people (Ministério da Saúde. Secretaria de Vigilância em Saúde e Ambiente. Departamento de Análise Epidemiológica e Vigilância de Doenças Não Transmissíveis, 2023). Brazil's ongoing nutritional transition reveals a dietary pattern increasingly centered on unhealthy ultraprocessed products, which are rich in sugar, sodium, and fats (Fox et al., 2019). This dietary trend encourages automatic, high-calorie, and nutrient-poor consumption, contributing to a phenomenon known as the double burden of malnutrition, which, as previously mentioned is characterized by the coexistence of undernutrition and obesity (Kroker-Lobos et al., 2022; Malta et al., 2024).

The ultraprocessed foods, engineered to be hyperpalatable and long-lasting, have increasingly dominated the food market and compromised the overall nutritional quality of the Brazilian diet. The NOVA, a system for classifying foods based on the extent and purpose of industrial processing, groups foods as unprocessed or minimally processed foods (group 1), processed culinary ingredients (group 2), processed foods (group 3), and ultraprocessed food products (group 4). This system was developed by Brazilian researchers concerned with the changes in food processing worldwide and is already recognized and applied in several countries. Ultraprocessed foods are defined as industrial formulations usually containing many ingredients, including sugar, fats, salt, additives, and substances not commonly used in culinary preparations (Monteiro et al., 2016). However, despite being widespread, the term ultraprocessed is often mistakenly used to encompass all types of processed food. In this context, awareness campaigns and regulatory policies, such as front-of-package labeling and restrictions on child-targeted advertising, have become increasingly urgent. Furthermore, these findings reinforce the need for comprehensive public policies aimed at improving the food environment, promoting nutritional education, and ensuring the human right to adequate food, as established by Law No. 11.346, which created the National Food and Nutrition Security System (SISAN) (Institui o Sistema de Segurança Alimentar e Nutricional (SISAN), 2006).

4.2.2 Micronutrient deficiencies and excesses: A comparative perspective

4.2.2.1 Micronutrient inadequacies and deficiencies

Micronutrient inadequacies and deficiencies remain a significant public health concern in South American countries directly impacting the population's growth, development, and overall quality of life (Argentinian Ministry of Health, 2019; Verly Junior et al., 2021). Although micronutrient deficiencies are often associated with food scarcity and undernutrition, it is important to note that overweight and obesity can also coexist with vitamin and mineral imbalances (Chapela et al., 2024). Despite the fortification and supplementation policies implemented in Argentina and Brazil to address nutrients such as iron, folic acid, and iodine, other forms of nutritional deficiencies have notably increased. These are particularly prevalent among the elderly, women, and urban populations, reflecting a dietary pattern increasingly reliant on ultraprocessed foods with low nutritional value. The *Dietary Guidelines for the Brazilian Population* and the *Food Guidelines for Argentinian Population* emphasize the importance of diets based on fresh and minimally processed foods, such as vegetables, fruits, and legumes as a key strategy to prevent such nutritional deficiencies (Argentinian Ministry of Health, 2020a; Ministério da Saúde, 2014; Monteiro et al., 2016). However, unequal access to these food options hinders the adoption of balanced and adequate eating practices.

The most prominent nutritional deficiencies currently observed in both Argentina and Brazil are presented below, with emphasis on emerging deficiencies and their implications for public health.

4.2.2.1.1 Vitamin D

Vitamin D is critical for bones, muscles, immune system, and neurological health, as well as for calcium absorption. The recommended daily allowance (RDA) for vitamin D is 10–20 μg/day (Cavagnari et al., 2021; National Institutes of Health (NIH), 2024a). Its deficiency has been associated with an increased risk of osteopenia, sarcopenia, infections, autoimmune diseases, and depression (Kaur et al., 2025). According to the ELANS (Latin American Nutrition and Health Study) survey, vitamin D intake in the Latin American population is primarily derived from milk, fish, eggs, and meat (Leme et al., 2021).

Vitamin D deficiency and inadequacy are currently among Brazil's most prevalent nutritional issues, particularly affecting older adults, women, individuals with limited sun exposure, and residents of urban areas (Monge-Rojas et al., 2024). Although Brazil is a tropical country, factors such as urbanization, sedentary lifestyles, and the widespread use of sunscreen significantly reduce cutaneous synthesis of vitamin D. In addition, the Brazilian diet is typically low in dietary sources of this nutrient, such as fatty fish, eggs, and mushrooms (Benedik, 2022). There is currently no national policy for universal vitamin D supplementation, contributing to this deficiency's growing and largely unaddressed prevalence.

The daily intake of vitamin D is around 3.2–3.8 μg/day in Argentinian adults (women and men) (Cavagnari et al., 2021), and among children under 2 years old, approximately 40% presented a mild deficiency of vitamin D (Argentinian Ministry of Health, 2007).

4.2.2.1.2 Calcium

Calcium is essential for the formation and maintenance of bones and teeth, as well as for muscle contraction and neuromuscular function. The RDA for calcium rounds between 1000 and 1300 mg/day for adults (National Institutes of Health (NIH), 2024b).

Deficiency of this mineral has become increasingly common among adolescents and older adults, contributing to a heightened risk of osteoporosis and fractures. One of the primary factors behind this deficiency is the reduced consumption of milk and dairy products, which are often replaced by ultraprocessed beverages with low nutritional value. The lack of alternative calcium-rich sources and insufficient nutritional guidance exacerbates the issue among individuals with lactose intolerance or specific dietary restrictions (Martini et al., 2013).

Studies carried out in Argentinian population showed that calcium recommendations are generally not covered. Cavagnari et al. (2021) evaluated more than 1200 adults, finding that the media of calcium daily intake was 703 mg for women and 831 mg for men. These authors observed that calcium intake was less close to the recommended value in adolescents and adults over 50 years of age. Besides, they showed an inversely proportional relationship between calcium intake and body mass index (BMI) in women. Negro et al. (2020) evaluated calcium intake in university students and determined that less than 10% met the RDA of 1000 mg calcium/day. Other study made by Cormick et al. (2014) showed that calcium intake among pregnant women was approximately 660 mg/day.

In Brazil, Verly Junior's, (2021) study on calcium intake, based on data from the National Health Survey (PNS), highlights that the average intake of this mineral is significantly below the established daily recommendations. In 2008–09 the average calcium intake was 470.1 and 447.2 mg/day for male and female adolescents, respectively. By 2017–18 these values dropped to 457.1 mg/day for males and 406.6 mg/day for females. For adults the intake was 483.7 mg/day for men and 429.4 mg/day for women in 2008–09, and in 2017–18, it was 472.7 mg/day for men and 429.3 mg/day for women. Among the elderly the intake was 469.3 mg/day for men and 451.3 mg/day for women in 2008–09, dropping to 446.3 mg/day for men and 429.3 mg/day for women in 2017–18. These findings demonstrate that in all analyzed age groups the average calcium intake remains well below the recommended daily intake (RDI), especially among lower income populations. This underscores the urgency for public policies focused on nutritional education and increasing access to calcium-fortified foods, especially in regions of greater socioeconomic vulnerability.

4.2.2.1.3 B-Complex vitamins

B-complex vitamins, particularly B12, B6, and folic acid, play essential roles in energy metabolism, neurological function, DNA synthesis, and red blood cell formation. Vitamin B12 deficiency is especially common among older adults (because of impaired absorption), vegetarians, and individuals undergoing long-term treatment with medications such as metformin and proton pump inhibitors. This deficiency can lead to megaloblastic anemia, muscle weakness, neurological disturbances, and cognitive decline (Choudhury et al., 2023; Pardo-Cabello et al., 2023).

Folic acid (also known as vitamin B9 or folate) is a critical nutrient for the perinatal period, as it is directly linked to neural tube defects (a group of congenital malformations) in newborns, and lifelong disabilities or death (Martinez et al., 2023a; Rodrigues et al., 2023). RDA for folate round between 65 and 600 μg/day being the lower values for children and the highest for pregnant women (National Institutes of Health (NIH), 2022). Inadequate intake of folate-rich foods, such as leafy greens and legumes, is a leading cause of this issue, disproportionately affecting vulnerable populations (Santos et al., 2021). Besides, wet cooking of foods can lead to a reduction in the amount of this folic acid (Scott et al., 2000). These deficiencies can be reversed through food fortification programs (Castillo-Lancellotti et al., 2013).

Folate deficiency, although partially mitigated by flour fortification programs, remains a significant concern. Folate supplementation is advised in those women who are going through the pregnancy period to prevent problems in fetal development. According to a study carried out in public hospitals of Argentina from 2004 to 2006, with more than 6000 women in the perinatal period, only 52.5% of them adequately adhered to a folate supplementation regimen, consisting of 350 mg/day of folic acid (Karolinski et al., 2009). In contrast, according to a national survey conducted in 2007 in Argentina, only 22.9% of the pregnant women evaluated reported taking a folic acid supplement the day before the survey (Argentinian Ministry of Health, 2007).

Although the Brazilian government has implemented folic acid fortification policies, the deficiency remains a public health issue, especially in geographically isolated regions. Raising awareness about the importance of this nutrient, particularly among pregnant women, continues to be a challenge. Although food fortification with folic acid has proven to be effective, sustained efforts are needed to ensure that all women of reproductive age have access to this essential nutrient (Magalhães et al., 2023). The implementation of comprehensive nutritional education programs should be prioritized to reduce the prevalence of neural tube defects.

4.2.2.1.4 Iron and iodine

Iron RDA rounds between 7 and 27 mg/day for adults, being the lowest recommended values for children and male population, and the highest for pregnant women (National Institutes of Health (NIH), 2024c). Although iron and iodine nutrients are covered by relatively well-structured public health policies in Brazil, deficiencies in both nutrients persist in certain regions and among specific social groups. Iron deficiency anemia primarily affects children and women of reproductive age. It is exacerbated by low heme iron and vitamin C intake and the excessive consumption of ultraprocessed foods (Levi et al., 2019). Despite being a major producer of iron-rich foods such as meat, Brazil continues to experience a high prevalence of iron deficiency anemia, particularly in economically disadvantaged regions (Magalhães et al., 2023). The fortification of wheat and corn flour with iron is an important strategy, but it is insufficient to solve the problem.

In Argentina, dietary iron-deficiency anemia remains a significant public health concern, particularly among children under 5 years old and pregnant women (WHO, 2022). According to a survey carried out in Argentina in 2007 the average intake of iron among children was 7.42–10.48 mg/day, whereas for adult women this value was of 12.43 mg/day (Argentinian Ministry of Health, 2007). Despite the Argentinian diet typically including substantial meat consumption, dietary imbalances remain because of food choices that lead to the intake of highly industrialized food products and refined grains, whereas fruits, vegetables, and legumes (which are essential components that enhance iron absorption and help prevent deficiency) are consumed in insufficient amounts. In consequence, promoting balanced diets and nutritional education, emphasizing iron-rich foods and combinations that improve iron absorption, is crucial for reducing the prevalence of iron-deficiency anemia among high-risk groups.

Iodine is a nutrient that is generally found in seawater and in the soils of coastal areas. It is primarily present in saltwater fish and seafood, such as clams, sardines, lobsters, and oysters, which are the richest sources, containing between 300 and 3000 μg/kg of meat (National Institutes of Health (NIH), 2024d). Areas located far from coastal regions, such as plateaus, mountains, and flatlands distant from the sea, are more prone to iodine deficiency-related health issues, including endemic goiter and cretinism. Foods grown in these soils contain little to no iodine, and livestock raised on pasture in these areas may also suffer from iodine deficiency (Scaramella, 2020). RDA for iodine is between 90 and 250 μg/day (Argentinian Ministry of Health, 2025; National Institutes of Health (NIH), 2024d).

Iodine deficiency, while significantly reduced following the implementation of salt iodization policies, still exists in some parts of Brazil, especially in inland regions far from coastal areas, where consumption of iodine-rich foods such as fish and seafood is limited. Although the country has adopted effective salt fortification measures, the ongoing lack of access to fresh foods and iodized salt in certain areas contributes to this nutritional deficiency (Araújo et al., 2021). Nutritional education and the sustained implementation of fortification policies are essential to eliminate iodine deficiency nationwide (Fisberg et al., 2024; Kroker-Lobos et al., 2022). To fully eradicate this deficiency, it is critical to ensure that all regions of the country have access to iodine-rich foods and benefit from comprehensive nutrition education programs (Araújo et al., 2021). In Argentina the region close to Mendoza (34.5869° S and 68.1431° W) has reported iodine deficiency problems in the past. Other parts of the country showed the nonexistence of iodine deficiency (Rodríguez et al., 2013).

4.2.2.2 *Excess intake of critical nutrients*

Hernández-Ruiz et al. (2022) mentioned that although great advances have been made in several countries in alleviating the burden of undernutrition and micronutrient deficiencies, the health conditions associated with excess nutrition are still not adequately addressed.

Brazil is facing the growing challenge of excessive intake of critical nutrients such as sugars, fats, and sodium, particularly in the context of accelerated nutritional transition and increasing urbanization. These nutrients, which are present in large quantities in most ultraprocessed foods, are directly associated with the rising prevalence of obesity, type 2 diabetes, hypertension, dyslipidemia, and other NCDs (Louzada, 2022). Although the *Dietary Guidelines for the Brazilian Population* and the *Food Guidelines for Argentinian Population* recommend reducing the consumption of ultraprocessed foods and promoting fresh and minimally processed foods, changing dietary habits remains a persistent challenge. To ensure access to healthy food options for the population, comprehensive nutrition education strategies and regulatory measures targeting the food industry are required (Magalhães et al., 2023).

Data on the consumption of some of the nutrients that are present in excess in the diets of both the Argentinian and the Brazilian populations are presented in detail below.

4.2.2.2.1 Sugars

Excessive sugar consumption is one of the main contributors to the rise in obesity and NCDs in Brazil and Argentina. The high intake of sugar-sweetened beverages and highly industrialized products has significantly contributed to the increasing prevalence of conditions such as type 2 diabetes and hypertension. The World Health Organization (WHO) recommends that free sugars account for less than 10% of total daily caloric intake, with an ideal target of below 5%. However, the Brazilian dietary pattern far exceeds these recommendations, particularly among children, adolescents, and young adults (PAHO, 2019).

Despite WHO recommendations to reduce sugar intake, especially added sugars, the Brazilian dietary reality remains marked by high consumption of this nutrient, which exacerbates the prevalence of obesity and metabolic diseases (Ramos & Meneses, 2021). Although scientific evidence regarding the harms of sugar consumption is increasingly robust, the food industry strongly influences on advertising and eating behaviors, particularly among children (Ferreira et al., 2021). Public policies promoting clear front-of-package labeling, restricting marketing aimed at children, and taxing sugar-sweetened beverages may be effective strategies to reduce sugar intake. In addition, public initiatives strengthening nutrition education are essential to promote long-term improvements in the population's eating habits (Fisberg et al., 2024; Magalhães et al., 2023).

Total sugar consumption in the Argentinian population is twice the maximum amount recommended by the WHO, and significantly higher than in many other countries (Argentinian Ministry of Health, 2019; Fisberg et al., 2018; WHO, 2015). The mean added sugar intake in Argentina in 2019 was estimated at 91.4 g/day. Part of this sugar derives from the high consumption of sweetened beverages and candies, with more than 35% of the population reporting that they consume sugary drinks at least once a day and sweets twice a week or more (Argentinian Ministry of Health, 2019). Zapata et al. (2022) evaluated the diet of Argentinian women, finding that free sugars accounted for 18% of the total energy intake. Socioeconomic factors play a role in the consumption of sweetened beverages, as lower levels of education and health insurance were associated with higher consumption of this type of products (Argentinian Ministry of Health, 2019).

4.2.2.2.2 Fats

High consumption of saturated fats, particularly those found in ultraprocessed products, is a significant risk factor for cardiovascular disease and obesity in Brazil (Izar et al., 2021). The Brazilian diet has increasingly deviated from international recommendations regarding healthy fat intake, favoring foods rich in saturated fats, such as fast food and unhealthy industrialized products. This dietary pattern has contributed to the growing burden of NCDs, including hypertension and heart disease (WHO, 2023a).

As mentioned before, candies are highly consumed by the Argentinian population, which not only explains the high intake of sugar but also of fats. A study carried out on Argentinian women of 20–49 years old showed that saturated fats accounted for 11% of the total energy intake, whereas *trans* fats represented 1% of the total energy intake (Zapata et al., 2022).

Raising awareness about the importance of choosing healthy fat sources, such as vegetable oils, and reducing saturated fat intake are essential steps toward improving the population's nutritional status and lowering the prevalence of diet-related chronic diseases (Santos et al., 2021). Promoting healthy alternatives and regulating the food industry to limit saturated fats are critical strategies for mitigating the impact of poor dietary habits on public health.

4.2.2.2.3 Sodium

Excessive sodium intake represents a serious public health concern in Brazil, primarily because of the high levels of salt found in most of the ultraprocessed and ready-to-eat foods. The WHO recommends a maximum daily intake of 2 g of sodium (equivalent to 5 g of salt). However, the average sodium consumption in Brazil significantly exceeds this limit, particularly among adults (Ministério da Saúde. Secretaria de Atenção Primária à Saúde. Departamento de Promoção da Saúde, 2022a).

In recent years in Argentina, and as mentioned above, there has been an evident change in the food consumption patterns, contributing to a more processed food intake than observed in previous patterns (FAO et al., 2017; PAHO, 2015; WHO, 2004). This type of food tends to have a high sodium content, which has led the Argentinian population to an average sodium consumption of 7.8 g/person/day (Argentinian Ministry of Health, 2019).

High sodium intake is strongly associated with an increased prevalence of hypertension and other related diseases, including cardiovascular disease, stroke, and coronary heart disease (He et al., 2002; Verly Junior et al., 2021). Reducing salt consumption remains a key priority in Brazilian public health policies, yet public acceptance and adopting healthier eating habits continue to pose considerable challenges (PAHO, 2021b). Promoting the consumption of fresh, unprocessed foods with minimal added salt should be a central strategy to address this issue. Moreover, regulating the food industry, specifically aimed at reducing the salt content of processed foods, is an urgent measure needed to reverse the current trend (Kroker-Lobos et al., 2022).

4.2.2.2.4 Energy intake

Excessive caloric intake, when combined with a sedentary lifestyle and the consumption of ultraprocessed foods, has contributed significantly to the rise in obesity in Brazil (Ministério da Saúde, 2014). The combination of calorie-dense diets and low levels of physical activity has played a key role in the increasing incidence of metabolic disorders, such as type 2 diabetes and hypertension (Sanches et al., 2024). Public policies that promote physical activity and encourage the consumption of fresh, unprocessed foods are essential for reversing this trend. Promoting physical education in schools and implementing programs that support physical activity among adults and the elderly can significantly contribute to reducing the burden of weight-related diseases (Institui o Sistema de Segurança Alimentar e Nutricional (SISAN), 2006; Magalhães et al., 2023; Santos et al., 2021).

In Argentina, highly processed unhealthy foods represent an important part of the energy intake in children and adolescents diets (Zapata et al., 2022). Moreover, energy intake from industrialized products has increased at the expense of fresh and homemade foods. Changes in food patterns obey a mixture of social, economic, environmental, and demographic factors that determine the general food habits of the population, including affordability, food production models, availability, marketing, and forms of commercialization that have probably generated obesogenic environments (Argentinian Ministry of Health, 2019).

The recommended and actual intake of each nutrient by the Argentinian and Brazilian populations are shown in Table 4.1.

4.3 Policies and strategies for enhancing nutritional status

4.3.1 Argentina

Several policies have been implemented in Argentina with different degrees of success to address the nutritional challenges outlined in the previous section. Such actions aim

Table 4.1 Recommended and actual intake of different critical nutrients by the population of Argentina and Brazil.

Nutrient	Recommended intake	Actual intake		References
		Argentina	Brazil	
Vitamin D (μg/day)	10–20	3.2–3.8	1.3–2.0	National Institutes of Health (NIH) (2024a), Cavagnari et al. (2021), Instituto Brasileiro de Geografia e Estatística (IBGE) (2020)
Calcium (mg/day)	1000–1200	660–830	399–473	National Institutes of Health (NIH) (2024b), Cavagnari et al. (2021), Instituto Brasileiro de Geografia e Estatística (IBGE) (2020)
Iron (mg/day)	6–27	7.4–15.8	8.7–12.7	Argentinian Ministry of Health (2025), National Institutes of Health (NIH) (2024c), Cavagnari et al. (2021), Argentinian Ministry of Health (2007), Instituto Brasileiro de Geografia e Estatística (IBGE) (2020)

(*continued on next page*)

Sugars (% of total energy intake)	≤5–10	16.4	8.3–12.3	WHO (2023b), Argentinian Ministry of Health (2019), WHO (2015), Instituto Brasileiro de Geografia e Estatística (IBGE) (2020)
Fat (% of total energy intake)	≤30	31	28.4–29.6	WHO (2023a), Argentinian Ministry of Health (2007), Instituto Brasileiro de Geografia e Estatística (IBGE) (2020)
Trans fat (% of total energy intake)	≤1	1	0.6–0.9	WHO (2023a), Zapata et al. (2022), Instituto Brasileiro de Geografia e Estatística (IBGE) (2020)
Sodium (g/day)	≤2	7.8	2.4–2.9	Argentinian Ministry of Health (2019), Instituto Brasileiro de Geografia e Estatística (IBGE) (2020)

at combating malnutrition, reducing overweight, obesity and high blood pressure, and promoting healthy eating habits adapted to the socioeconomic and cultural context. The main strategies adopted include the incorporation of micronutrients in different food products or ingredients, the regulation of *trans* fats and the presentation of nutritional information through the incorporation of warning labels on the front-of-package labeling of packaged foods and nonalcoholic beverages.

4.3.1.1 Strategies for increasing critical nutrients in food products

The incorporation of proteins, amino acids, vitamins, minerals, or/and essential fatty acids in food is regulated in Chapter XVII of the Argentinian Alimentarius Code (AAC) (ANMAT, 2025). These foods are referred to as **fortified** or **enriched**.

Fortified foods are those in which a naturally present nutrient is added in a higher amount. A food is considered fortified with fat-soluble vitamins and/or minerals if a serving provides between 20% and 50% of the RDI of these nutrients, or between 20% and 100% for water-soluble vitamins (ANMAT, 2025, Art. 1363). When proteins are used to fortify food products, they must meet specific requirements: the protein content must be at least twice that of the nonfortified version, with no less than 20% w/w of the product; the ratio of the caloric value of protein to the total caloric value of the product must be at least 0.2; and the biological value of the protein and its true digestibility must exceed 60% and 80%, respectively. In addition, these products may also be enriched with vitamins and/or minerals, provided that the previously established requirements align with these criteria (ANMAT, 2025, Art. 1364).

In turn, **enriched foods** are those to which essential nutrients have been added to compensate for nutritional deficiencies leading to population deficiency. These products should meet the following requirements: first, it must be established that the deficiencies cannot be corrected through ordinary foods; second the relevant health authority must identify the deficiencies, the affected population groups, and the extent of the deficiencies (whether provincial, regional, or national) based on epidemiological data; and third the health authority must determine the necessary additions, their concentrations, the type of food to be enriched, labeling requirements, distribution characteristics, and the overall scope of the measure (ANMAT, 2025, Art. 1369).

Although both fortified and enriched foods have added nutrients, the purpose of these additions is different. In the first case a naturally occurring nutrient in the food is voluntarily added to meet specific nutritional needs of the healthy population and improve the nutritional profile of the product for sale. In contrast, in enriched foods, nutrients are added to a food product that does not naturally contain them on a mandatory basis and to solve a nutritional deficiency of the population that results in collective deficiency diseases. As these deficiencies affect the population as a whole, enriched foods are typically selected based on their accessibility, low cost, and widespread consumption. In this context, in Argentina two ingredients need to be enriched: salt and wheat flour.

Salt enriched with **iodine** (Law No. 17259, 08.05.67): In Argentina, in 1952, the government of the province of Mendoza (34.5869° S and 68.1431° W) sanctioned provincial Law No. 2112, which established the mandatory fortification of salt with iodine, making this province the first area in the entire American continent to have a law to combat goiter. Thanks to salt iodine fortification a 93% decrease in goiter was observed between 1941 and 1968 (Scaramella, 2020). This law was the basis for the subsequent enactment of National Law No. 17259, which establishes that salt for human or animal consumption must be fortified with iodine (potassium iodate). The same treatment must be applied to sodium-free or modified salts with a lower sodium content, which are recommended for the prevention of arterial hypertension (Law No. 24786, 04.04.1997). This law was regulated considering that in large areas of Argentina there is endemic goiter, which is a disease caused by iodine deficiency in the diet, frequent in areas where the amount of iodine in soil and water is low.

Fortification of wheat flour **with iron and B vitamins** (Law No. 25630, 23.08.2002): This law aimed at preventing anemia and neural tube defects (e.g., anencephaly and spina bifida) and mandates that wheat flour intended for human consumption and sold on the domestic market must be fortified with iron (as ferrous sulfate) and B vitamins, including folic acid (B9), thiamine (B1), riboflavin (B2), and niacin (B3), in appropriate proportions. Studies have shown that fortifying wheat flour with iron has had a positive impact on reducing anemia prevalence (Field et al., 2020; González, 2020; Martorell et al., 2015), although some research has failed to confirm significant improvements, possibly because of the type of iron used and its low bioavailability (Sadighi et al., 2019).

In Buenos Aires (Argentina), 1 year after implementing Law 25630, the prevalence of anemia in children under 2 years old decreased from 55% to 39% as a result of the synergistic effect of providing micronutrient-fortified foods and the regulation of the enrichment law (Varea et al., 2011). In this regard, Hurrell et al. (2010) reported that the greatest impact of wheat flour fortification with iron can be observed during the first year of implementing the strategy. These authors found that only 9 out of 78 studied programs (including those in Argentina, Chile, and Uruguay) were considered likely to have a significant positive impact on iron status if coverage were optimized. Recently, Mapelli et al. (2021) evaluated the iron content in fortified wheat flour and its derivatives, and the contribution of these to the recommendations for children aged 6 months to 7 years ($n = 120$) attending the public health system in La Plata, Buenos Aires, Argentina. They found that most of the studied ingredients and/or commercial foods met the iron amount established by the law, except for small baguettes and grated bread. Furthermore, they reported that the foods covered a low percentage of the RDI for children aged 6 months to 1 year (7%), whereas the coverage was higher for older children: 81% in the 1–3 years group and 45% in children over 4 years old.

Currently, there is a cultural trend to reduce wheat flour consumption, which could lead to deficiencies in iron and B group vitamins that should be monitored and considered. Attention can also be paid to people with celiac disease, considering that, in general, these individuals cannot access to fortified flours.

4.3.1.2 Strategies for reducing critical nutrients in food products

Considering the increase in hypertension and pathologies related to it, there is a trend to reduce salt and sodium consumption. According to data summarized by

Innova Market Insights (2024), globally 22% of consumers look for low salt food products. Argentina has implemented measures to decrease sodium consumption as a strategy to prevent high blood pressure and reduce the risk of cardiovascular diseases (Ferrante et al., 2015). In 2010 the Ministry of Health launched the "less salt, more life," a program aiming to reduce sodium consumption both by stimulating the decrease of the sodium content in processed foods and by educating the community to decrease sodium consumption (FAO, 2014). In 2013 the National Law No. 26905 to reduce sodium consumption in the population was passed, establishing clear goals for food products. These measures include health warnings on packaging, actions in the food service sector, communication strategies, and the development of an evaluation and monitoring plan.

Trans fats found in food products can be generated through both biological and industrial processes. The first group results from the partial biohydrogenation process carried out by microorganisms in the rumen and are naturally present in the meat, milk, and dairy products of ruminant animals. These fats include vaccenic acid (C18:1 *trans*-11) and the conjugated linoleic acid (CLA) isomers (C18:2 *cis*-9 and C18:2 *trans*-11) and would have a positive effect on health (e.g., reducing the risk of diabetes and preventing cardiovascular and cerebrovascular diseases) although their use is recommended with caution (Badawy et al., 2023; Pipoyan et al., 2021). The second group of *trans* fats is produced by partial hydrogenation of vegetable and marine oils and is found in the fats used in baked goods, margarines, shakes, sweet doughs, puff pastry, cookies, crackers, snacks, filling creams for sweet cookies and wafers, cereal bars, confectionery coatings, and other similar products (Allemandi et al., 2014). Consumption of industrial *trans* fats increases the risk of coronary disorders, insulin resistance, and obesity (Mozaffarian et al., 2006).

As the nutritional information on food labels typically does not mention the origin of *trans* fats, the general recommendation is to reduce their consumption, regardless of the origin (Pipoyan et al., 2021). The WHO recommends that adults and children reduce the intake of *trans* fatty acids to less than 1% of the total energy intake and recommends replacing them with healthier fats and oils in the food supply (WHO, 2023a). This goal should be achieved by developing, monitoring, and enforcing effective policies. Therefore a legal limit of up to 2 g of *trans* fat per 100 g of fat in all foods was established, along with a ban on the use of partially hydrogenated oils (PHOs). Since 2018, when the WHO first recommended the global elimination of industrially produced *trans* fats, mandatory *trans* fat limits have been implemented, covering 54.7% of the global population as of 2023 (WHO, 2025).

In the 1990s Argentina had the fourth-highest rate of cardiovascular mortality in the Americas (PAHO, 1990), which was directly related to the consumption patterns of industrialized products high in *trans* fats. In 2000 Tavella et al. (2000) made a survey about the consumption of total fat, saturated fat, and *trans* fatty acid content (e.g., elaidic acid) in 46 food items, confirming that the Argentinian investigated products (margarines, butter, oils—sunflower, corn, and mixed—mayonnaises, crackers, cookies, sliced bread, french fries, and cheetos) had higher *trans* fat content compared to those reported in other parts of the world.

To address this serious nutritional issue and promote a healthy lifestyle, in 2007, the Pan American Health Organization (PAHO)/WHO convened public health authorities, representatives from the food industry, and oil companies from across the Americas to form a working group, which ultimately signed the Rio de Janeiro Declaration: "The Americas free of *trans* fats" (PAHO, 2008). This group was tasked with evaluating the impact of *trans* fats on nutrition and health and discussing practical strategies for their gradual elimination from food products. Naturally, Argentinian specialists were part of this initiative, which was committed to working at the national level to promote different actions aimed at eliminating industrially produced *trans* fats. As a result of the work of that Intersectoral Commission, in 2008, the Argentinian Ministry of Health established an Interinstitutional Commission, including the Ministry of agriculture, livestock, and fisheries, ANMAT (National Administration of Medicines, Food, and Medical Technology), the Ministry of Social Development, the academic sector, and the main Chambers of the Food Industry in the country, to start working on the recommendations issued by PAHO/WHO, under the national group "Argentina: Free of *trans* fats," aimed at reducing the consumption of these fats through different channels.

First, communication efforts were directed at informing consumers about the negative health effects of *trans* fats. In addition, the industry was provided with information and tools to help comply with regulations and improve product quality. Furthermore the group worked on amending the AAC, leading to the introduction of Article 155 tris in 2010. This article underwent modifications until 2023 to align with the WHO's 2025 goal of globally eliminating *trans* fats. Initially, Article 155 tris established that "The content of industrially produced *trans* fatty acids in foods must not exceed 2% of the total fats in vegetable oils and margarines intended for direct consumption, and 5% of the total fats in other foods, including those used as ingredients and raw materials. These limits do not apply to fats from ruminants, including dairy fat" (joint resolution SCS and SAByDR No. 3/2021). The regulation provided a transition period with a deadline of January 2022 for ingredients and raw materials. Nevertheless, the limits for vegetable oils, margarines, and foods were already in effect since December 2014. In 2021, a new modification was made to Article 155 tris of the AAC, reducing the maximum limit of industrially produced *trans* fatty acids to 2% of the total fats in all foods, including ingredients and raw materials. Furthermore, on May 19, 2023, through Joint Resolution No. 16/2023 between the Secretariat of agriculture, livestock, and fisheries of the Ministry of economy and the Secretary of Health Quality of the Ministry of Health, Article 155 tris of the AAC was replaced to implement new limits on the content of industrially produced *trans* fatty acids to no more than 2% of the total fats in foods, including those used as ingredients and raw materials, excluding fats from ruminants. A transition period of 2 years was established for foods and 3 years for ingredients and raw materials. In addition, the use of PHOs and fats in the food industry was prohibited, with a transition period of 4 years from the enactment of the regulation (May 20, 2023). These measures position Argentina as a leader in the elimination of industrial *trans* fats, aligning with international recommendations to improve public health.

Argentina has the "*Trans* fat content reduction control and surveillance program" within the framework of the comprehensive inspection plan carried out by the INAL

(National Food Institute), under the ANMAT, which conducts chemical analysis of samples or evaluates labeling in relation to the ingredient list of food products marketed in Argentina, both domestic and imported, that use fats and/or vegetable oils in their production. The evaluation is carried out by checking if the labels correspond to the *trans* fat values declared in the nutritional information table and if they comply with the regulations for food labeling and advertising. The products monitored include margarines and oils, snacks and prefried foods, cereal bars, breakfast cereals, cookies, packaged baked goods, and sweets. The program has shown a high level of compliance with the law, as in 2014, 73% (n = 249) of the products met the established *trans* fat limits. This percentage improved in the years 2015, 2018, and 2019, with compliance rates of 93% (n = 390), 96% (n = 476), and 92% (n = 198), respectively. In the 2023 survey, it was found that 88% (n = 43) of the products complied with the maximum *trans* fat limit set by the current legislation. Noncompliance was observed in the categories of oils and fats and spreadable products (INAL, 2023).

4.3.2 Brazil

To improve the population's nutritional status, it is essential to combine policies and programs of various sectors to promote access to adequate food (Amorim et al., 2022). Similar to Argentina the main strategies adopted in Brazil include the incorporation of micronutrients in different food products or ingredients and the implementation of the front-of-package labeling of packaged foods. In addition, Brazil also has a significant number of public policies focused on promoting an adequate and healthier diet.

4.3.2.1 *Strategies for increasing critical nutrients in food products*

Food fortification plays a crucial role in public health policies aimed at combating micronutrient deficiencies. It has long been utilized as a strategic approach in various countries to address micronutrient deficiencies and has significantly contributed to reducing diseases linked to this issue (Steluti et al., 2017). Food fortification involves adding one or more nutrients to foods in amounts regulated by each country's health authority (WHO, 2006). In Brazil the National Agency for Sanitary Vigilance (ANVISA) establishes that every 100 g or 100 mL of a ready-to-consume product must provide at least 30% or 15% of the RDI of a given nutrient (Agência Nacional de Vigilância Sanitária (ANVISA), 1998). Brazil has adopted universal food fortification strategies aimed at preventing specific nutrient deficiencies. The main strategies include the mandatory fortification of wheat and corn flour with iron and folic acid and the adding iodine to salt (Ministério da Saúde. Secretaria de Atenção Primária à Saúde. Departamento de Promoção da Saúde, 2022b).

Universal salt iodization has been widely adopted in over 120 countries, significantly reducing the prevalence of iodine deficiency disorders (IDD) worldwide (WHO, 2014). Salt iodization has been mandatory in Brazil since the 1950s (Law No. 1.944/15.08.1953) to prevent IDD, including goiter and cretinism (Santos et al., 2011). In 2003 the Resolution of the Collegiate Board (RDC) No. 130 established iodine content between 20 and 60 mg/ kg of salt (Ministério da Saúde. Agência Nacional de Vigilância Sanitária (ANVISA), 2003a). Because of evidence of excessive iodine intake the regulation was updated in 2022 (RDC No. 604), which currently mandates iodine levels between 15 and 45 mg/kg (Ministério da Saúde. Agência Nacional de Vigilância Sanitária (ANVISA), 2022a). Salt is an ideal vehicle for iodine fortification because of its universal use in food preparation and regular consumption in small amounts (Santos et al., 2011). Furthermore, iodine deficiency control relies on systematic monitoring of nutritional status, regulation of salt production, and periodic legislative updates to ensure the effectiveness of the iodization policy (Nimer et al., 2009).

The mandatory fortification of wheat and corn flour with iron and folic acid was introduced in Brazil in 2002 and officially implemented in 2004. The regulation, updated by ANVISA in 2022 (RDC No. 604), requires that every 100 g of flour contain 4.0 mg of iron and 140 μg of folic acid (Ministério da Saúde. Agência Nacional de Vigilância Sanitária (ANVISA), 2022a). This policy aims to prevent iron deficiency anemia and neural tube defects by using flour as a widely consumed food vehicle to improve the population's micronutrient intake (Ministério da Saúde. Secretaria de Atenção Primária à Saúde. Departamento de Promoção da Saúde, 2022b).

Research on flour fortification in Brazil remains limited, with few studies evaluating the fortified products' impact on iron and folic acid intake. Santos et al. (2015) estimated iron intake based on folic acid data and assessed Brazil's flour fortification program, revealing that iron absorption from fortified flour is low (around 0.2 mg/day) for both men and women. This result is attributed to the use of electrolytic iron, which has low bioavailability, and the fact that actual flour consumption in Brazil was lower than expected when the policy was designed. However, increasing flour consumption is not advisable because of high obesity rates, making it more effective to use a form of iron with higher absorption. Another issue identified is noncompliance by food manufacturers, highlighting the need for stricter control of the industry's compliance with regulations (Santos et al., 2015).

Vieira et al. (2017) analyzed iron intake before and after mandatory fortification, noting a significant reduction in deficiency prevalence, except among women of reproductive age. Before fortification, primary iron sources were natural sources of this nutrient, whereas postfortification, bread, and cookies became key contributors. Similarly, Steluti et al. (2017) evaluated the impact of 10 years of folic acid fortification in the São Paulo population, finding a low plasma folate deficiency rate (1.76%). However, inadequate folate intake remained more prevalent in women. Processed wheat-based foods were the primary folate sources, especially among younger populations. In addition, despite the lack of biochemical data comparing folate levels pre- and postfortification on a national scale, a review analyzing nearly 50 Brazilian studies found that folate concentrations increased by 57% in children and adolescents and nearly doubled in adults after fortification. However, it is important to note that the review included studies that used varying methodologies to measure folate concentration (Britto et al., 2014).

Although the intake of wheat and corn flour fortified with iron and folic acid has been rising, it is essential that public policies related to this fortification are adequately regulated and closely monitored to ensure that nutrient levels remain safe and do not pose health risks to children, either in the short or long term (Salvatte et al., 2023).

4.3.2.2 Strategies for reducing critical nutrients in food products

Brazil played a leading role among Mercosur (southern common market) countries in implementing mandatory nutritional labeling and proposing reforming food labeling regulations to include the mandatory declaration of industrially produced *trans* fats (Moreno & von Atzingen, 2022). The Brazilian regulations RDC No. 359 and RDC No. 360, published by ANVISA in 2003, established rules for mandatory nutritional labeling, including the declaration of *trans* fat content per portion in packaged foods. According to RDC No. 360, foods containing 0.2 g or less of *trans* fats per serving may be labeled as "does not contain *trans* fats" or "zero *trans*" (Ministério da Saúde. Agência Nacional de Vigilância Sanitária (ANVISA), 2003b, 2003c).

In parallel with labeling regulations, Brazil promoted initiatives to reduce industrial *trans* fats through voluntary reformulation agreements between the Ministry of Health and the Brazilian Association of Food Industries (ABIA), including a technical cooperation established in 2007 that created the healthy eating forum to support the reduction of *trans* fats, sugar, and salt in processed foods (Block & Herrera, 2014; Moreno & von Atzingen, 2022). Although these initiatives encouraged the food industry to replace PHOs with alternatives such as palm oil or polyunsaturated fats, they primarily involved ABIA-affiliated companies, leaving out many smaller producers, who often continued to produce foods high in *trans* fats and/or saturated fats (ANVISA, 2019).

Despite the evidence of a reduction in *trans* fats over time, as a result of mandatory labeling since 2003 and voluntary reformulations by the industry, *trans* fats have remained present in many processed foods and continued to be widely consumed in Brazil (ANVISA, 2019; Aued-Pimentel & Kus-Yamashita, 2021; Dias et al., 2018a). A significant portion of Brazilian food products labeled as "low *trans*" showed labeling inconsistencies, and some products labeled "zero *trans*" still contained levels above legal limits (Pinto et al., 2016; Sobral et al., 2024). A market analysis evaluating around 600 products sold in São Paulo between 2005 and 2018 revealed discrepancies between declared and actual *trans* fats content, with about 30% of samples exceeding the 2 g/100g fat limit (Aued-Pimentel & Kus-Yamashita, 2021).

In response to increasing concerns about the health risks associated with industrial *trans* fats, Brazil implemented RDC No. 332/2019, consolidated by RDC No. 632/2022, progressively restricting the use of industrial *trans* fats in food products (Ministério da Saúde. Agência Nacional de Vigilância Sanitária (ANVISA), 2019, 2022b; Moreno & von Atzingen, 2022). The regulation was implemented in three phases: initially limiting *trans* fats in refined oils to 2 g per 100 g of fat by July 2021, extending this limit to all food products until January 2023, and ultimately banning the production, import, use, and sale of artificially hydrogenated oils from January 1, 2023. These actions align with WHO's global recommendation to eliminate *trans* fats by 2023 (Aued-Pimentel & Kus-Yamashita, 2021). Nevertheless, ongoing inconsistencies in label information highlight the limitations of current monitoring and enforcement mechanisms (Sobral et al., 2024). To effectively eliminate

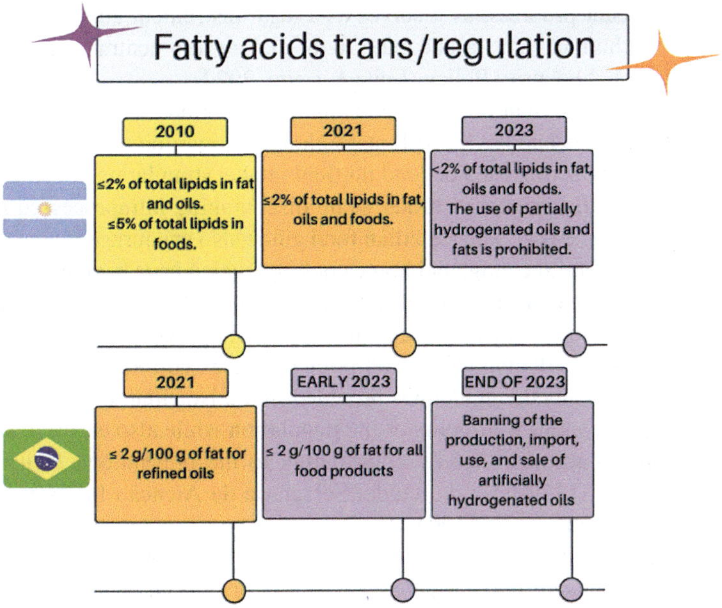

Figure 4.2 Timeline of the regulation of *trans* fats in Argentina and Brazil.

trans fats, Brazil must strengthen regulatory controls, ensure that replacements are safe for consumption, and promote consumer education (Moreno & von Atzingen, 2022) (Fig. 4.2).

4.3.2.3 *Other strategies for improving nutritional status in Brazilian population*

Public policies promoting healthy eating include initiatives encouraging and empowering individuals to make informed food choices through public campaigns and educational materials aligned with local food cultures (Santos et al., 2021).

Several programs and policies focused on food and nutrition have been implemented over the years in Brazil. The National Policy of Food and Nutrition (Política Nacional de Alimentação e Nutrição—PNAN) was created in 1999, with its most recent edition published in 2013 (Ministério da Saúde. Secretaria de Atenção à Saúde. Departamento de Atenção Básica, 2013). At the federal level the PNAN's actions are formalized in national plans and other official planning instruments, demonstrating the growing relevance of food and nutrition on the public agenda and in national policy. Since 2003 the debate and actions on Food and Nutrition Security have advanced in Brazil, resulting in the creation of the SISAN in 2006 and the inclusion of the Human Right to Adequate Food in the Federal Constitution in 2010 (Santos et al. 2021).Brazil also has a specific law in the field of food security and the right to food, the Organic Law on Food and Nutritional Security (LOSAN), established by Law 11.346/2006, which represents significant progress, as it serves as a legal instrument aimed at promoting and ensuring the human right to adequate food, making it a central objective of the Food and Nutritional Security Policy (Leite & Leite, 2022).

Furthermore the Brazilian food guide is another important strategy for promoting healthier food practices and has gained international recognition (Santos et al., 2021). It stands out for considering food beyond nutrient intake, stimulating the consumption of fresh and minimally processed foods while discouraging ultraprocessed products (Ministério da Saúde, 2014). The Brazilian food guide also encourages behaviors such as meal planning, mindful eating, and home cooking, which have been linked to better diet quality and lower consumption of ultraprocessed foods. Research suggests that these practices are associated with a higher intake of fruits, vegetables, legumes, whole grains, and nuts while reducing the consumption of processed foods and added sugars (Gabe et al., 2023). Thus the guidelines provided in the Brazilian food guide support both the health and overall well-being of the population while also ensuring sufficient intake of essential nutrients, thereby contributing to the prevention of vitamin and mineral deficiencies (Ministério da Saúde. Secretaria de Atenção Primária à Saúde. Departamento de Promoção da Saúde, 2022b).

Another important public policy is the Brazilian school food program (Programa Nacional de Alimentação Escolar—PNAE), which originated in the 1930s decade (Amorim et al., 2022). Over the years the program has evolved from an assistance-based approach to food supplementation to a reference model for promoting healthy eating, particularly after legislative improvements in 2009 (Boklis-Berer et al., 2021; Ministério da Educação. Fundo Nacional de Desenvolvimento da Educação, 2009). The program has gained international recognition and inspired similar initiatives, such as the Food for Peace Program by USAID (United States Agency for International Development), the Food Program for Development (focused on populations in poverty and school-age children), and the Program Food World by the FAO/UN (United Nations for Food and Agriculture) (Martinez et al., 2023b).

Since 2009 the PNAE has ensured the offer of unprocessed and minimally processed foods and restricted the purchase of ultraprocessed foods (Ministério da Educação. Fundo Nacional de Desenvolvimento da Educação, 2009). Recent legislative updates in 2020 further strengthened these regulations by increasing the required portions of fruits and vegetables while imposing stricter limits on ultraprocessed food offerings. The guidelines also provide recommendations for meal composition, setting limits on added sugars, total fat, saturated fat, *trans* fat, and sodium (Ministério da Educação. Fundo Nacional de Desenvolvimento da Educação, 2020). The consumption of school meals provided by the PNAE has been associated with healthier dietary habits, improved diet quality, and lower obesity rates among students (Boklis-Berer et al., 2021; Locatelli et al., 2018). These findings reinforce the public health significance of a well-structured school feeding program as a strategy for obesity prevention and the reduction of chronic diseases associated with poor nutrition (Boklis-Berer et al., 2021).

In addition, PNAE is recognized as a key program supporting food and nutritional security, primarily because of its universal scope, the requirement that at least 30% of food purchases come from family farming, its strong focus on food and nutrition education, and the strict regulation of the nutritional quality of the meals provided

(Dias et al., 2018b). Amorim et al. (2022) identified a positive correlation between food insecurity and school meal consumption, with food-insecure children having a higher frequency of regular consumption of school meals. This finding highlights the crucial role of school meals, particularly in socially vulnerable areas, where they often serve as a primary food source for students facing food insecurity. The PNAE benefits more than 40 million students (Ministério da Educação. Fundo Nacional de Desenvolvimento da Educação, 2025) and is crucial in shaping eating habits and influencing nutritional status, especially in vulnerable communities where food insecurity is prevalent (Boklis-Berer et al., 2021).

Brazil also has National Micronutrient Supplementation Programs designed according to the country's specific health needs, focusing on the most common and significant nutritional issues. The main initiatives include the NutriSUS program, which fortifies children's food with powdered micronutrients, the national iron supplementation program (PNSF), and the national vitamin A supplementation program (PNSVA). All three are part of the country's preventive supplementation strategy to combat nutritional deficiencies (Ministério da Saúde. Secretaria de Atenção Primária à Saúde. Departamento de Promoção da Saúde, 2022b).

Shifts in the dietary habits of the Brazilian population, marked by increased consumption of ultraprocessed foods and reduced intake of fresh foods, have contributed to a rise in micronutrient deficiencies despite a decline in overall malnutrition (Dias et al., 2018b). Organizing the care flow for children's micronutrient supplementation within primary health care is crucial to ensure effective and nonoverlapping coverage. In addition, strategies to prevent and manage micronutrient deficiencies should be integrated into broader food and nutrition policies, encompassing surveillance, health promotion, and preventive measures. These efforts must also stimulate collaboration across sectors to effectively address the challenges posed by malnutrition (Brazil, 2022a).

4.3.3 Front nutrition labeling in Brazil and Argentina

In Brazil the "Healthy Eating Promotion Law" No. 27642 was enacted in 2021 and further regulated on March 22, 2022 (Decree 151/2022). The objective of this law was to ensure the right to health and proper nutrition by requiring warning labels on nonalcoholic food and beverages, indicating critical nutrients such as sugars, total fats, saturated fats, sodium, and calories, as well as the presence of caffeine and sweeteners. It also aimed to provide consumers with clearer, more visible, precise, and nonmisleading nutritional information to help them make informed food choices. In addition, the law sought to promote the prevention of malnutrition and reduce the prevalence of NCDs.

In South America, Republic of Ecuador and Bolivia were the first countries to implement traffic light-type warning labels in 2014 and 2017, respectively. Since 2016, Chile, Uruguay, and Peru have incorporated black octagon-shaped warning labels (Marichal, 2022). In Argentina the Ministry of Health concluded that black octagons are the most effective front labeling system for consumers to identify critical nutrients, as they provide better visibility, attention, and clear, quick, and easy-to-understand information (Argentinian Ministry of Health, 2020a, 2020b).

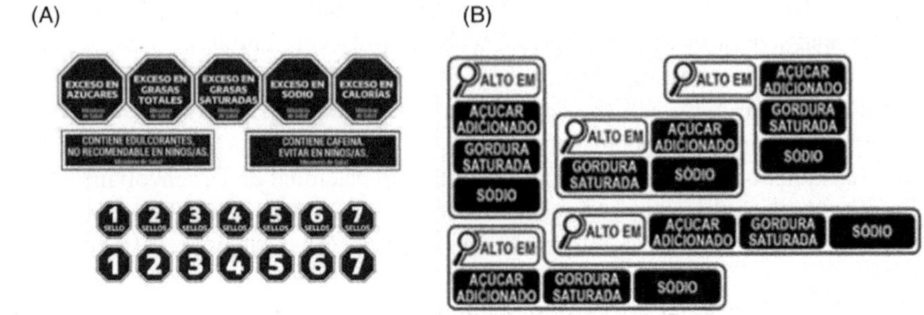

Figure 4.3 Warning labels implemented by the front nutrition labeling laws in Argentina (A) and Brazil (B).

In Brazil the regulation was created in 2020 through RDC No. 429/2020 and Normative Instruction No. 75/2020 and gradually implemented from 2022 to 2025. These regulations introduced an innovative warning label design on the front of food packaging, featuring a black magnifying glass icon accompanied by the phrase "high in" to alert consumers about excessive amounts of added sugars, sodium, and saturated fats (Ministério da Saúde. Agência Nacional de Vigilância Sanitária (ANVISA), 2020). Nevertheless, ANVISA excluded *trans* fat from this labeling system, given that a regulatory initiative was already underway to eliminate its presence from food products (Moreno & von Atzingen, 2022; Santos et al., 2021).

The selection of the magnifying glass symbol distinguishes Brazil from other Latin American countries, such as Chile and Argentina, which have adopted the black octagon model (Fig. 4.3). Nevertheless, research indicates that both formats enhance label readability and support healthier consumer decision-making (Alcântara et al., 2025). Evidence suggests that many Brazilian consumers, particularly those with limited health knowledge, experience difficulties interpreting traditional nutritional labels, limiting their effectiveness as public health tools. Thus implementing this new system using warning labels emerges as a regulatory instrument designed to minimize informational asymmetries, helping to reduce the consumption of products containing high levels of nutrients associated with NCDs (Sousa et al., 2023).

Fig. 4.3 A shows the warning labels implemented in Argentina. These are black octagons with white letters inside, including the text "**EXCESS IN**" followed by **SUGARS, TOTAL FATS, SATURATED FATS, CALORIES, or SODIUM,** one for each nutrient in excess. If the product contains sweeteners and caffeine, it shall be warned with black rectangles, with the text "**CONTAINS SWEETENERS, NOT RECOMMENDED FOR CHILDREN**" and "CONTAINS CAFFEINE, AVOID IN CHILDREN," respectively (Official Bulletin of the Argentinian Republic, 2021). Small packages, such as candies, contain microlabels (Fig. 4.3B) with a number indicating the amount of critical nutrients, calories, sweeteners, and/or caffeine in the product. However, because of their small size, they do not fit on the package itself, but the full information can be found on the box or bag in which these units are packaged (Table 4.2). Figure 4.3B shows the warning labels adopted by Brazil. These

Table 4.2 Current limits established by the laws of front nutritional labeling for critical nutrients in Argentina and Brazil.

Critical nutrient	Argentina	Brazil
Added sugars	≥10% of the food calories	≥15 g/100 g of solid and semisolid foods and ≥7.5 g/100 mL of liquid foods
Total fats	≥30% of the food calories	–
Saturated fats	≥10% of the food calories	≥6 g/100 g of solid and semisolid foods and ≥3 g/100 mL of liquid foods
Sodium	Foods: ≥1 mg/kcal or 300 mg/100 (g or mL of food), regardless of the energetic content[a] Nonalcoholic beverages: >40 mg sodium/100 mL	≥600 mg /100 g of solid and semisolid foods and ≥300 g /100 mL of liquid foods
Calories	Foods: at least one of the warning labels, and provide ≥275 kcal/100 g product. Nonalcoholic beverages: at least one warning label and provide ≥25 kcal/100 mL product	–
Sweeteners	If the list of ingredients contains it	
Caffeine	If the list of ingredients contains it	

[a] The condition that is met first determines that the food exceeds the maximum established values for sodium.

are a rectangle featuring a black magnifying glass icon and the phrase "**EXCESS IN**" accompanied by "**ADDED SUGAR**", "**SATURED FAT**", and/or "**SODIUM**". The warning labels are optional for certain products, including foods in packaging with a main display panel smaller than 35 cm^2, foods packaged at the point of sale upon consumer request, and foods prepared, portioned, and sold within the same establishment [Brasil, 2020b].

Argentina sets the maximum values at which products must display a front-of-package label, using the nutritional profile system (NPS) as a tool (Table 4.2). The NPS proposed by the PAHO/WHO is the only system based on nutrient recommendations with international standards and is the one that best aligns with the recommendations of the Argentinian Food Guidelines, which, by Resolution 693/2019, is the standard for establishing food policies (Tiscornia et al., 2020). Therefore, by implementing front labeling based on the PAHO/WHO nutrient profile system, national food sovereignty is not at risk, because both documents (Argentinian Food Guidelines and the PAHO/WHO Nutrient Profile Model) are based on the same recommendations.

Complementary policies include the ban on advertising, promotion, and sponsorship of packaged foods and nonalcoholic beverages that carry at least one warning label. In this sense, any product containing one or more warning labels is not allowed to advertise through children's characters, cartoons, animals, celebrities, or athletes, in addition, these products cannot be associated with the provision of gifts, prizes, or any type of accessory. Besides, educational institutions (schools and kindergartens) are prohibited from offering, selling, advertising, promoting, or sponsoring packaged foods that contain at least one warning label or precautionary statement, as a measure to promote nutritional education among children and their families. Furthermore, food products with warning labels are not allowed to display positive health claims (Official Bulletin of the Argentinian Republic, 2021).

4.3.4 Critical discussion about front nutritional labeling implementation

In Argentina the healthy eating promotion law was implemented in two stages. The first stage required compliance by August 20, 2022, for large companies and by February 20, 2023, for small and medium-sized enterprises (SMEs), during which intermediate threshold values were established. The second stage introduced more restrictive measures, with deadlines set for May 20, 2023, for large companies and November 20, 2023, for SMEs (Brizuela et al., 2022).

As a result of the law's implementation, products such as cheese and yogurt began carrying warning labels, as they naturally contain saturated fats and lactose, respectively. This also meant they could no longer be promoted with nutritionally positive claims, such as being fortified with minerals or vitamins or containing added probiotics, because of the presence of warning labels. In response to these concerns the law was amended in December 2024 to differentiate between naturally occurring and added nutrients. Now, labels only warn about added nutrients, and foods with warning labels can still highlight other positive qualities, as long as they are not related to the excess nutrients declared. In addition, advertising regulations were adjusted to improve the law's clarity and predictability (ANMAT, 2024).

In Brazil the law regarding nutritional labeling of packaged foods had an implementation deadline by October 9, 2022, for new food products launched to the market after the regulation was approved; by October 9, 2023, for food products already on the market prior to its approval; by October 9, 2024, for food products from small-scale producers; and by October 9, 2025, for nonalcoholic beverages in returnable packaging (Ministério da Saúde. Agência Nacional de Vigilância Sanitária (ANVISA), 2020).

One limitation of front-of-package labeling is that it only applies only to packaged foods, excluding products such as pastries and other artisanal foods. In addition, products classified as dietary supplements or foods for medical purposes are not subjected to the law. The same happens with alcoholic beverages because they are exempted from the regulation. Therefore consumer education campaigns are essential to complement the labeling system.

Front labeling is another public health strategy implemented by several countries and is expected to help reduce healthcare costs (Cecchini et al., 2010). It has been recommended as a policy to protect the right to health, as it helps guide consumers in choosing healthier foods, encourages the food industry to reformulate products to be healthier, and supports the design of public policies for healthy eating. One of the main drivers of its implementation is the rising prevalence of diet-related NCDs. In addition, cultural aspects and the interplay between businesses, the state, and consumers should be considered (Tobón, 2021).

Recent studies have explored the impact of nutritional labeling and front-of-package warnings on consumer behavior. A study carried out by UNICEF/FIC Argentina (2024) evaluated the knowledge of the Argentinian population about the front nutritional labeling. This research established that 94% of the evaluated individuals agreed with the front labeling. Besides the study showed a positive effect on the purchasing intention of consumers before and after the implementation of the law, being the "excess sugars" label the one with the greatest influence on the purchase decision (UNICEF/FIC, 2024). Castagna et al. (2024) analyzed how labeling influenced the food purchasing decisions of adults with type 2 diabetes in Buenos Aires in 2023. Their findings suggest that warning labels affect purchasing behavior, encouraging consumers to choose products with lower sugar and sodium content. Similarly, Malzoni and Sechi (2024) examined the impact of front labeling on packaged food purchases in Argentina ($n = 1150$). However, their study presents a potential bias, as 97% of respondents were university-educated women (aged 25–34), and more than 90% were already familiar with (98.5%) and understood (94.1%) the warning labels. Further studies on the impact of implementing front-of-package nutrition labels are needed. On one hand, it will be interesting to assess the long-term effects of the law after a significant amount of time has passed, because it is important to consider whether consumers may become habituated to the presence of the labels. On the other hand, it may be relevant to assess whether the law affects consumers' purchasing choices, considering that a large majority of certain available products (e.g., cookies, snacks, and candies) would likely have warning labels.

Alcântara et al. (2025) investigated Brazilian consumers' behavior toward products displaying the magnifying glass warning and observed a positive impact on food choices in three of the four product categories assessed. However, the study also revealed that established brands and appealing nutritional claims exert considerable influence on purchasing decisions, partially undermining the intended effects of the labeling. These findings underscore the need for an integrated regulatory approach that combines labeling with nutrition education initiatives and stricter controls on marketing practices.

4.4 Conclusion

The nutritional landscape in Brazil and Argentina presents a complex scenario, marked by the coexistence of malnutrition and a rising prevalence of diet-related NCDs. This combination contributes to the persistence of undernutrition alongside an increase in metabolic disorders linked to unhealthy diets, which are characterized by high consumption of foods rich in saturated fats, salt, and simple sugars. In addition, cultural habits, such as high intake of sweetened products and low consumption of nutritionally valuable foods (e.g., legumes, vegetables, and fruits), further exacerbate the situation.

Public policies implemented by Brazil and Argentina, such as front-of-package nutritional labeling and educational campaigns, have proven to be important steps in addressing these issues. However, the effectiveness of these policies should be continuously reviewed and reassessed to enhance their efficiency.

Despite these challenges, Brazil and Argentina have significant potential to improve the nutritional status of their populations. Integrating nutrition policies that emphasize food education and the promotion of diets based on fresh and locally sourced foods can also contribute to sustainable food production. Moreover, regional cooperation and the establishment of partnerships between governments, international organizations, and civil society can play a crucial role in addressing nutritional issues comprehensively and effectively.

In conclusion, although nutrition-related policies face significant challenges regarding public health and the overall nutritional status, the strategies already in place pave the way for improvement. A multisectoral approach, focusing on sustainability, nutritional education, and the promotion of healthier, more accessible food products, is key to advancing public health and food security in the region.

Acknowledgments

This project has received funding from the Argentinean Agency for the Promotion of Science and Technology (ANPCyT) (Project PICT2020/0482). V.S., M.C.P., and A.G.-Z. are members of the CONICET Research Career; A.C. is a CONICET postdoctoral fellow.

Glosary

AAC	Argentinian Alimentarius Code
ABIA	Brazilian Association of Food Industries
ANMAT	National Administration of Medicines, Food, and Medical Technology (Argentina)
ANVISA	National Agency for Sanitary Vigilance (Brazil)
ELANS	Latin American Nutrition and Health Study
FAO	Food and Agriculture Organization
IDD	iodine deficiency disorders
INAL	National Food Institute (Argentina)
NCDs	noncommunicable diseases
NPS	nutritional profile system
PAHO	Pan American Health Organization
RDI	recommended daily intake
RDC	Resolution of the Collegiate Board (Brazil)
SISAN	National Food and Nutrition Security System (Brazil)
SMEs	small and medium-sized enterprises
WHO	World Health Organization

References

Agência Nacional de Vigilância Sanitária (ANVISA). (1998). *Resolução da Diretoria Colegiada—RDC n° 31, de 13 de janeiro de 1998. Regulamento Técnico para Fixação de*

Identidade e Qualidade de Alimentos Adicionados de Nutrientes Essenciais. Diário Oficial da União.

Alcântara, M., Martins, I. B. A., Ares, G., & Deliza, R. (2025). Relative effect of warning labels on food choice: Case study with four product categories after the implementation of the Brazilian regulation. *Food Quality and Preference, 124*, 105359. doi:10.1016/j.foodqual.2024.105359.

Allemandi, L., Tiscornia, V., Clemente, A., Castronuovo, L., Schoj, V., & Samman, N. (2014). *Análisis de los niveles de grasas trans en los alimentos industrializados en Argentina.* Fundación Interaméricana del Corazón http://www.ficargentina.org/wp-content/uploads/2017/11/informe_grasas_trans_02_10_2014-1.Pdf.

Amorim, A. L. B., Dalio Dos Santos, R., Ribeiro Junior, J. R. S., Canella, D. S., & Bandoni, D. H. (2022). The contribution of school meals to food security among households with children and adolescents in Brazil. *Nutrition, 93*, 111502. doi:10.1016/j.nut.2021.111502.

ANMAT. (2024). Official Gazette of the Argentine Republic (Law 27.642, Disposition 11362/2024). Retrieved May 12, 2025, from https://www.boletinoficial.gob.ar/detalleAviso/primera/318798/20241226.

ANMAT. (2025). *Argentinian food code (Law 18.284)*. National Administration of Drugs, Food and Medical Technology Retrieved March 12, 2025, from https://www.argentina.gob.ar/codigoalimentario .

ANVISA. (2019). Relatório de análise de impacto regulatório sobre ácidos graxos trans em alimentos. Agência Nacional de Vigilância Sanitária. Retrieved April 12, 2025, from https://www.gov.br/anvisa/pt-br/assuntos/regulamentacao/air/analises-de-impacto-regulatorio/2019/25351-906891_2017-15-acidos-graxos-trans-em-alimentos.pdf.

Araújo, D., Carrillo, B., & Sampaio, B. (2021). The long-run economic consequences of iodine supplementation. *Journal of Health Economics, 79*, 102490. doi:10.1016/j.jhealeco.2021.102490.

Argentinian Ministry of Health. (2007). *First national survey on nutrition and health (SNSN&H)*. Retrieved May 6, 2025, from https://www.extensioncbc.com.ar/wp-content/uploads/ENNyS-2007.pdf.

Argentinian Ministry of Health. (2019). *Second national survey on nutrition and health (SNSN&H)*. Retrieved March 17, 2025, from https://bancos.salud.gob.ar/.

Argentinian Ministry of Health. (2020a). *Food guidelines for Argentina's population.* Retrieved May 12, 2025, from https://www.argentina.gob.ar/sites/default/files/bancos/2020-08/guias-alimentarias-para-la-poblacion-argentina_manual-de-aplicacion_0.pdf.

Argentinian Ministry of Health. (2020b). *Front-of-package nutritional labeling.* Retrieved March 17, 2025, from https://www.fagran.org.ar/wp-content/uploads/2020/08/MINSAL-Investigacio%CC%81n-Etiquetado-Frontal-de-Alimentos.pdf.

Argentinian Ministry of Health. (2025). *National administration of laboratories and institutes of health. Iodine, nutrition, and health.* Retrieved May 12, 2025, from https://www.argentina.gob.ar/salud/anlis/cnin/yodo-nutricion-y-salud.

Aued-Pimentel, S., & Kus-Yamashita, M. M. M. (2021). Analysis of the fat profile of industrialized food in Brazil with emphasis on trans-fatty acids. *Journal of Food Composition and Analysis, 97*, 103799. doi:10.1016/j.jfca.2020.103799.

Avezum, Á, Braga, J., Santos, Í., Guimarães, H. P., Marin-Neto, J. A., & Piegas, L. S. (2009). Cardiovascular disease in South America: Current status and opportunities for prevention. *Heart, 95*(18), 1475–1482. doi:10.1136/hrt.2008.156331.

Badawy, S., Liu, Y., Guo, M., Liu, Z., Xie, C., Marawan, M. A., Ares, I., Lopez-Torres, B., Martínez, M., Maximiliano, J. E., Martínez-Larrañaga, M. R., Wang, X., Anadón, A., &

Martínez, M. A. (2023). Conjugated linoleic acid (CLA) as a functional food: Is it beneficial or not? *Food Research International, 172*. doi:10.1016/j.foodres.2023.113158.

Benedik, E. (2022). Sources of vitamin D for humans. *International Journal for Vitamin and Nutrition Research, 92*(2), 118–125. doi:10.1024/0300-9831/a000733.

Block, J. M., & Herrera, M. L. (2014). Trans fats replacement solutions in South America. In *Trans fats replacement solutions* (pp. 313–336). Elsevier Inc. doi:10.1016/B978-0-9830791-5-6.50019-8.

Boklis-Berer, M., Rauber, F., Azeredo, C. M., Levy, R. B., & da Costa Louzada, M. L. (2021). The adherence to school meals is associated with a lower occurrence of obesity among Brazilian adolescents. *Preventive Medicine, 150*. doi:10.1016/j.ypmed.2021.106709.

Britto, J. C., Cançado, R., & Guerra-Shinohara, E. M. (2014). Concentrations of blood folate in Brazilian studies prior to and after fortification of wheat and cornmeal (maize flour) with folic acid: A review. *Revista Brasileira de Hematologia e Hemoterapia, 36*(4), 275–286. doi:10.1016/j.bjhh.2014.03.018.

Brizuela, G., Cova, C., Monzón, J., & Varona, P. (2022). *2.22. Ley 27642 de Promoción de la Alimentación Saludable—Recomendaciones de políticas de fomento a la reformulación de alimentos*. Recuperado 02 de abril de 2023, from https://www.argentina.gob.ar/sites/default/files/2021/03/35_-_ley_de_promocion_de_alimentacion_saludable_-_arg._productiva.pdf.

Canella, D. S., Duran, A. C., & Claro, R. M. (2020). Malnutrition in all its forms and social inequalities in Brazil. *Public Health Nutrition, 23*(1), S29. http://journals.cambridge.org/PHN. doi:10.1017/S136898001900274X.

Castagna, C., Castagna, J., Di Maio, M., Maddaloni, M. J., Concilio, C., & Marcandrés, M. (2024). Influencia del rotulado nutricional y etiquetado frontal en la compra de productos alimenticios por parte de adultos con diabetes tipo 2. *Revista Nutrición Investiga, 24*, 1–10. https://escuelanutricion.fmed.uba.ar/revistani/24anco.html.

Castillo-Lancellotti, C., Tur, J. A., & Uauy, R. (2013). Impact of folic acid fortification of flour on neural tube defects: A systematic review. *Public Health Nutrition, 16*(5), 901–911. doi:10.1017/S1368980012003576.

Cavagnari, B. M., Favieri, A., Zonis, L., Guajardo, V., Gerardi, A., Fisberg, M., & Kovalskys, I. (2021). Inadecuación de micronutrientes en adolescentes y adultos argentinos de población urbana. Resultados del Estudio Latinoamericano de Nutrición y Salud (ELANS). *Actualización en Nutrición, 22*(3). doi:10.48061/san.2021.22.3.71.

Cecchini, M., Sassi, F., Lauer, J. A., & Lee, Y. Y. (2010). Abordar las dietas poco saludables, la inactividad física y la obesidad: Efectos en la salud y rentabilidad. *The Lancet, 376*(9754), 1775–1784. doi:10.1016/S0140-6736(10)61514-0.

Chapela, S. P., Martinuzzi, A. L. N., Llobera, N. D., Ceriani, F., Gonzalez, V., Montalvan, M., Verde, L., & Frias-Toral, E. (2024). Obesity and micronutrients deficit, when and how to suplement. *Food and Agricultural Immunology, 35*(1). doi:10.1080/09540105.2024.2381725.

Choudhury, A., Jena, A., Jearth, V., Dutta, A. K., Makharia, G., Dutta, U., Goenka, M., Kochhar, R., & Sharma, V. (2023). Vitamin B12 deficiency and use of proton pump inhibitors: A systematic review and meta-analysis. *Expert Review of Gastroenterology and Hepatology, 17*(5), 479–487. doi:10.1080/17474124.2023.2204229.

Cormick, G., Zhang, N. N., Andrade, S. P., Quiroga, M. J., Di Marco, I., Porta, A., Althabe, F., & Belizán, J. M. (2014). Gaps between calcium recommendations to prevent pre-eclampsia and current intakes in one hospital in Argentina. *BMC Research Notes, 7*(1). doi:10.1186/1756-0500-7-920.

De La, E. E., & Sánchez, C. (2016). La transición nutricional. Abordaje desde de las políticas públicas en América Latina. *Opcion, 32*(11), 379–402. http://produccioncientificaluz.org/index.php/opcion/article/download/21955/21691.

Dias, F. S. L., Lima, M. F., De Velasco, P. C., Salles-Costa, R., De Carvalho Sardinha, F. L., & Carmo, M. D. G. T. D. (2018a). Were policies in Brazil effective to reducing trans fat from industrial origin in foods? *Revista de Saúde Pública, 52*, 34. doi:10.11606/s1518-8787.2018052000292.

Dias, P. C., Henriques, P., Ferreira, D. M., Barbosa, R. M. S., Soares, D. S. B., Luquez, T. M. S., Feijão, M. D., & Burlandy, L. (2018b). Desafios da intersetorialidade nas políticas públicas: O dilema entre asuplementação nutricional e a promoção da alimentação saudável em escolas. *Cadernos de Saúde Pública, 34*(12), e00035218. doi:10.1590/0102-311X00035218FA.

FAO, OMS, & OPS. (2017). *Panorama de la Seguridad Alimentaria y Nutricional. Sistemas alimentarios sostenibles para poner fin al hambre y la malnutrición.* https://iris.paho.org/handle/10665.2/33680

FAO. (2014). *Governments adopt Rome declaration on nutrition and framework for action.* Food and Agriculture Organization of the United Nations https://www.fao.org/about/meetings/icn2/news/news-detail/en/c/251870/.

FAO. (2022). *The state of food security and nutrition in the world.* FAO https://www.fao.org/.

Ferrante, D., Gautero, M. E., Carles, M., Elorza, C., Duymovich, C., Konfino, J., Laspiur, S., & Koakof, M. (2015). Iniciativa Menos sal, más vida: Estrategia para la reducción de la ingesta de sodio en Argentina. *Revista Argentina de Salud Pública, 6*(22), 35–39.

Ferreira, M. M. C., Matos, Y. S., & Carvalho, L. M. F. (2021). Evidências científicas sobre a influência da publicidade no desenvolvimento do hábito alimentar infantil. *Research, Society and Development, 10*(15), e100101522381. doi:10.33448/rsd-v10i15.22381.

Field, M. S., Mithra, P., Estevez, D., & Peña-Rosas, J. P. (2020). Wheat flour fortification with iron for reducing anaemia and improving iron status in populations. *Cochrane Database of Systematic Reviews, 2020*(7). doi:10.1002/14651858.CD011302.pub2.

Fisberg, M., Batista, L. D., Previdelli, A. N., Ferrari, G., & Fisberg, R. M. (2024). Exploring diet and nutrient insufficiencies across age groups: Insights from a population-based study of Brazilian adults. *Nutrients, 16*(5). doi:10.3390/nu16050750.

Fisberg, M., Kovalskys, I., Gómez, G., Rigotti, A., Sanabria, L., García, M., Torres, R., Herrera-Cuenca, M., Zimberg, I., Koletzko, B., Pratt, M., Aznar, L., Guajardo, V., Fisberg, R., Sales, C., & Previdelli, Á. (2018). Total and added sugar intake: Assessment in eight Latin American countries. *Nutrients, 10*(4), 389. doi:10.3390/nu10040389.

Food and Agriculture Organization (FAO), International Fund for Agricultural Development, World Health Organization, World Food Programme, & United Nations Children's Fund. (2024). *The state of food security and nutrition in the world 2024: Financing to end hunger, food insecurity, and malnutrition in all its forms.* Retrieved March 17, 2025, from doi: 10.4060/cd1254es.

Fox, A., Feng, W., & Asal, V. (2019). What is driving global obesity trends? Globalization or "modernization"? *Globalization and Health, 15*(1). doi:10.1186/s12992-019-0457-y.

Gabe, K. T., Dos Santos Costa, C., Dos Santos, F. S., Souza, T. N., & Jaime, P. C. (2023). Is the adherence to the food practices recommended by the dietary guidelines for the Brazilian population associated with diet quality? *Appetite, 190*. doi:10.1016/j.appet.2023.107011.

González, H. F. (2020). Deficiencia de hierro, la injusta herencia. *Archivos Argentinos de Pediatría, 118*(3), 156–158.

He, F. J., & MacGregor, G. A. (2002). Effect of modest salt reduction on blood pressure: A meta-analysis of randomized trials. Implications for public health. *Journal of Human Hypertension, 16*, 761–770. doi:10.1038/sj.jhh.1001459.

Hernández-Ruiz, Á., Madrigal, C., Soto-Méndez, M. J., & Gil, Á. (2022). Challenges and perspectives of the double burden of malnutrition in Latin America. *Clinica e Investigacion en Arteriosclerosis, 34*, S3. doi:10.1016/j.arteri.2021.11.005.

Hurrell, R., Ranum, P., Pee, S., Biebinger, R., Hulthen, L., Johnson, Q., & Lynch, S. (2010). Revised recommendations for iron fortification of wheat flour and an evaluation of the expected impact of current national wheat flour fortification programs. *Food and Nutrition Bulletin, 31*(1_suppl1), S7. doi:10.1177/15648265100311s102.

INAL. (2023)*Programa Federal de Vigilancia del Contenido de Grasas Trans en Alimentos. Plan Integral de Fiscalización Año 2023*. National Food Institute. Retrieved May 12, 2025, from https://www.argentina.gob.ar/sites/default/files/informe_grasas.pdf.

Innova Market Insights. (2024). *Sodium reduction trends, global market overview*. Retrieved May 12, 2025, from https://www.innovamarketinsights.com/trends/sodium-reduction-trends/.

Institui o Sistema de Segurança Alimentar e Nutricional (SISAN). (2006). *Lei n° 11.346, de 15 de setembro de 2006. Institui o Sistema de Segurança Alimentar e Nutricional—SISAN*. Diário Oficial da União.

Instituto Brasileiro de Geografia e Estatística (IBGE). (2020). *Instituto Brasileiro de Geografia e Estatística. Pesquisa de orçamentos familiares 2017-2018: Análise do consumo alimentar pessoal no Brasil*. IBGE Retrieved May 14, 2025, from https://biblioteca.ibge.gov.br/visualizacao/livros/liv101742.pdf .

Izar, D. O. M. C., Lottenberg, A. M., Giraldez, V. Z. R., Santos, R. D. D., Machado, R. M., Bertolami, A., Assad, M. H. V., Saraiva, J. F. K., Faludi, A. A., Moreira, A. S. B., Geloneze, B., Magnoni, C. D., Scherr, C., Amaral, C. K., De Araújo, D. B., Cintra, D. E. C., Nakandakare, E. R., Fonseca, F. A. H., Mota, I. C. P., ... Machado, V. A. (2021). Posicionamento sobre o Consumo de Gorduras e Saúde Cardiovascular–2021. *Arquivos Brasileiros de Cardiologia, 116*(1), 160–212. doi:10.36660/abc.20201340.

Karolinski, A., Micone, P., Mercer, R., Gibbons, L., Althabe, F., Belizán, J. M., Messina, A., Lapidus, A., Correa, A., Taddeo, C., Lambruschini, R., Bertin, M., Dibiase, L., Varela, D. M., & Laterra, C. (2009). Evidence-based maternal and perinatal healthcare practices in public hospitals in Argentina. *International Journal of Gynecology and Obstetrics, 105*(2), 118–122. Www.elsevier.com/locate/ijgo. doi:10.1016/j.ijgo.2009.01.003.

Kaur, J., Khare, S., Sizar, O., & Givler, A. (2025). Vitamin D deficiency. *StatPearls*. StatPearls Publishing https://www.ncbi.nlm.nih.gov/books/NBK532266/.

Kroker-Lobos, M. F., Mazariegos, M., Guamuch, M., & Ramirez-Zea, M. (2022). Ultraprocessed products as food fortification alternatives: A critical appraisal from Latin America. *Nutrients, 14*(7), 1413. doi:10.3390/nu14071413.

Le Coq, J.-F., Grisa, C., Guéneau, S., & Niederle, P. (2022). *Public policies and food systems in Latin America* éditions Quae. doi:10.35690/978-2-7592-3536-0.

Leite, M. L. S., & Leite, J. F. (2022). (In)segurança alimentar e agricultura familiar: Políticas públicas como estratégia de superação da fome. *Revista Katálysis, 25*(3), 528–538. doi:10.1590/1982-0259.2022.e86341.

Leme, A. C. B., Fisberg, R. M., de Mello, A. V., Sales, C. H., Ferrari, G., Haines, J., Rigotti, A., Gómez, G., Kovalskys, I., Sanabria, L. Y. C., Herrera-Cuenca, M., Garcia, M. C. Y., Pareja, R. G., & Fisberg, M. (2021). Food sources of shortfall nutrients among Latin Americans: Results from the Latin American study of health and nutrition (ELANS). *International Journal of Environmental Research and Public Health, 18*(9). doi:10.3390/ijerph18094967.

Levi, M., Simonetti, M., Marconi, E., Brignoli, O., Cancian, M., Masotti, A., Pegoraro, V., Heiman, F., Cricelli, C., & Lapi, F. (2019). Gender differences in determinants of

iron-deficiency anemia: A population-based study conducted in four European countries. *Annals of Hematology, 98*(7), 1573–1582. doi:10.1007/s00277-019-03707-w.
Locatelli, N. T., Canella, D. S., & Bandoni, D. H. (2018). Positive influence of school meals on food consumption in Brazil. *Nutrition, 53*, 140–144. doi:10.1016/j.nut.2018.02.011.
Louzada, D. C. M. L., Costa, C. D. S., Souza, T. N., Da Cruz, G. L., Levy, R. B., & Monteiro, C. A. (2021). Impacto do consumo de alimentos ultraprocessados na saúde de crianças, adolescentes e adultos: Revisão de escopo. *Cadernos de Saúde Pública, 37*(Suppl 1). doi:10.1590/0102-311x00323020.
Magalhães, N. V., Waitzberg, D. L., Lopes, N. C., Vicedomini, A. C. C., Prudêncio, A. P. A., Jacob-Filho, W., Busse, A. L., Ferdinando, D., Alves, T. P., Pereira, R. M. R., Torrinhas, R. S., & Belarmino, G. (2023). High prevalence of energy and nutrients inadequacy among Brazilian older adults. *Nutrients, 15*(14). doi:10.3390/nu15143246.
Malik, V. S., Willet, W. C., & Hu, F. B. (2020). Nearly a decade on—Trends, risk factors and policy implications in global obesity. *Nature Reviews Endocrinology, 16*(11), 615–616. doi:10.1038/s41574-020-00411-y.
Malpeli, A., Varea, A., Vargas, V., Fritz Heck, H., Fasano, V., Asens, D., & Martins, E. (2021). Contribución de la harina de trigo enriquecida y derivados a los requerimientos de hierro en niños de 6 meses a 7 años. *Archivos Argentinos de Pediatría, 119*(5), 304–309. doi:10.5546/aap.2021.eng.304.
Malta, D. C., Gomes, C. S., Felisbino-Mendes, M. S., Veloso, G. A., Machado, I. E., Cardoso, L. O., Azeredo, R. T., Jaime, P. C., Vasconcelos, L. L. C., Naghavi, M., & Ribeiro, A. L. P. (2024). Undernutrition, and overweight and obesity: The two faces of malnutrition in Brazil, analysis of the global burden of disease, 1990 to 2019. *Public Health, 229*, 176–184. doi:10.1016/j.puhe.2023.12.037.
Malzoni, D., & Secchi, C. M. (2024). Impact of front-of-package labeling on the purchase patterns of packaged foods in Argentina. *Actualización en Nutrición, 25*. doi:10.48061/SAN.2024.25.3.137.
Martinez, H., Benavides-Lara, A., Arynchyna-Smith, A., Ghotme, K. A., Arabi, M., & Arynchyn, A. (2023a). Global strategies for the prevention of neural tube defects through the improvement of folate status in women of reproductive age. *Child's Nervous System, 39*(7), 1719–1736. doi:10.1007/s00381-023-05913-4.
Martinez, P., De Lourdes Saturnino Gomes, M., & Marini, F. S. (2023b). Public policies strengthen the relationship between family farming and food security in Brazilian schools—A case study of Paraíba state. *Heliyon, 9*(10), e20482. doi:10.1016/j.heliyon.2023.e20482.
Martini, L. A., Verly, E., Marchioni, D. M. L., & Fisberg, R. M. (2013). Prevalence and correlates of calcium and vitamin D status adequacy in adolescents, adults, and elderly from the health survey-São Paulo. *Nutrition, 29*(6), 845–850. doi:10.1016/j.nut.2012.12.009.
Martorell, R., Ascencio, M., Tacsan, L., Alfaro, T., Young, M. F., Addo, O. Y., Dary, O., & Flores-Ayala, R. (2015). Effectiveness evaluation of the food fortification program of Costa Rica: Impact on anemia prevalence and hemoglobin concentrations in women and children. *American Journal of Clinical Nutrition, 101*(1), 210–217. doi:10.3945/ajcn.114.097709.
Medina, L. P. B., Barros, M. B. A., da Silva Sousa, N. F., Bastos, T. F., Lima, M. G., & Szwarcwald, C. L. (2019). Desigualdades sociais no perfil de consumo de alimentos da população brasileira: Pesquisa Nacional de Saúde, 2013. *Revista Brasileira de Epidemiologia, 22*(suppl 2). doi:10.1590/1980-549720190011.supl.2.
Ministério da Educação. Fundo Nacional de Desenvolvimento da Educação. (2009). *Resolução/CD/FNDE n° 38, de 16 de julho de 2009. Dispõe sobre o atendimento da alimentação escolar aos alunos da educação básica no Programa Nacional*

de Alimentação Escolar—PNAE. https://www.gov.br/fnde/pt-br/acesso-a-informacao/legislacao/resolucoes/2009/resolucao-cd-fnde-no-38-de-16-de-julho-de-2009

Ministério da Educação. Fundo Nacional de Desenvolvimento da Educação. (2020). *Resolução/CD/FNDE n° 6, de 8 de maio de 2020. Dispõe sobre o atendimento da alimentação escolar aos alunos da educação básica no âmbito do Programa Nacional de Alimentação Escolar—PNAE.* https://www.gov.br/fnde/pt-br/acesso-a-informacao/legislacao/resolucoes/2020/resolucao-no-6-de-08-de-maio-de-2020/view

Ministério da Educação. Fundo Nacional de Desenvolvimento da Educação. (2025). *PNAE—Programa Nacional de Alimentação Escolar.* Retrieved April 12, 2025, from https://www.gov.br/fnde/pt-br/acesso-a-informacao/acoes-e-programas/programas/pnae.

Ministério da Saúde. (2014). *Guia alimentar para a população brasileira: Promovendo a alimentação saudável.* Retrieved April 12, 2025, from https://bvsms.saude.gov.br/bvs/publicacoes/guia_alimentar_populacao_brasileira_2ed.pdf.

Ministério da Saúde. Agência Nacional de Vigilância Sanitária (ANVISA). (2003a). *RDC n° 130, de 26 de maio de 2003. Dispõe sobre o teor de iodo que deve conter o sal destinado ao consumo humano.* Diário Oficial da União.

Ministério da Saúde. Agência Nacional de Vigilância Sanitária (ANVISA). (2003b). *RDC n° 359, de 23 de dezembro de 2003. Aprova o Regulamento Técnico de Porções de Alimentos Embalados para Fins de Rotulagem Nutricional.* Diário Oficial da União.

Ministério da Saúde. Agência Nacional de Vigilância Sanitária (ANVISA). (2003c). *RDC n° 360, de 23 de dezembro de 2003. Aprova o Regulamento Técnico sobre Rotulagem Nutricional de Alimentos Embalados, tornando obrigatória a rotulagem nutricional.* Diário Oficial da União.

Ministério da Saúde. Agência Nacional de Vigilância Sanitária (ANVISA). (2019). *RDC n° 332, de 23 de dezembro de 2019. Define os requisitos para uso de gorduras trans industriais em alimentos.* Diário Oficial da União.

Ministério da Saúde. Agência Nacional de Vigilância Sanitária (ANVISA). (2020).*RDC n° 429, de 08 de outubro de 2020. Dispõe sobre a rotulagem nutricional dos alimentos embalados.* Diário Oficial da União.

Ministério da Saúde. Agência Nacional de Vigilância Sanitária (ANVISA). (2022b). *RDC n° 632, de 24 de março de 2022. Dispõe sobre a restrição de uso de gorduras trans industriais em alimentos.* Diário Oficial da União.

Ministério da Saúde. Agência Nacional de Vigilância Sanitária (ANVISA). (2022c). *RDC n° 604, de 10 de fevereiro de 2022. Dispõe sobre o enriquecimento obrigatório do sal com iodo e das farinhas de trigo e de milho com ferro e ácido fólico destinados ao consumo humano.* Diário Oficial da União.

Ministério da Saúde. Secretaria de Atenção à Saúde. Departamento de Atenção Básica. (2013). *Política Nacional de Alimentação e Nutrição.* Retrieved April 12, 2025, from https://bvsms.saude.gov.br/bvs/publicacoes/politica_nacional_alimentacao_nutricao.pdf.

Ministério da Saúde. Secretaria de Atenção Primária à Saúde. Departamento de Promoção da Saúde. (2022a). *Policy brief: Redução do sódio em alimentos processados e ultraprocessados no Brasil.* Retrieved April 12, 2025, from https://bvsms.saude.gov.br/bvs/publicacoes/policy_brief_sodio_alimentos_processados.pdf.

Ministério da Saúde. Secretaria de Atenção Primária à Saúde. Departamento de Promoção da Saúde. (2022b).*Caderno dos programas nacionais de suplementação de micronutrientes.* Retrieved April 12, 2025, from https://bvsms.saude.gov.br/bvs/publicacoes/caderno_programas_nacionais_suplementacao_micronutrientes.pdf

Ministério da Saúde. Secretaria de Vigilância em Saúde e Ambiente. Departamento de Análise Epidemiológica e Vigilância de Doenças Não Transmissíveis. (2023). *Vigitel Brasil 2023:*

Vigilância de fatores de risco e proteção para doenças crônicas por inquérito telefônico: Estimativas sobre frequência e distribuição sociodemográfica de fatores de risco e proteção para doenças crônicas nas capitais dos 26 estados brasileiros e no Distrito Federal em 2023. https://bvsms.saude.gov.br/bvs/publicacoes/vigitel_brasil_2023.pdf

Ministério do Desenvolvimento e Assistência Social, Família e Combate à Fome. (2024). *Insegurança alimentar severa cai 85% no Brasil em 2023, conforme dados extraídos de Relatório da ONU sobre a Insegurança Alimentar Mundial (SOFI 2024).* Retrieved April 12, 2025, from https://www.gov.br/mds/pt-br/noticias-e-conteudos/desenvolvimento-social/noticias-desenvolvimento-social/mapa-da-fome-da-onu-inseguranca-alimentar-severa-cai-85-no-brasil-em-2023.

Monge-Rojas, R., Vargas-Quesada, R., Previdelli, A. N., Kovalskys, I., Herrera-Cuenca, M., Cortés, L. Y., García, M. C. Y., Liria-Domínguez, R., Rigotti, A., Fisberg, R. M., Ferrari, G., Fisberg, M., & Gómez, G. (2024). A landscape of micronutrient dietary intake by 15- to 65-years-old urban population in 8 Latin American countries: Results from the Latin American study of health and nutrition. *Food and Nutrition Bulletin, 45*(2), S11. doi:10.1177/03795721231215267.

Monteiro, C. A., Cannon, G., Levy, R., Moubarac, J. C., Jaime, P., Martins, A. P., & Parra, D. (2016). NOVA. The star shines bright. *World Nutrition, 7*(1–3), 28–38. https://worldnutritionjournal.org/index.php/wn/article/view/5.

Moreno, L. P. Z., & von Atzingen, M. C. B. C. (2022). Rotulagem de ácidos graxos trans: Revisão sobre Brasil e Estados Unidos. *Vita et Sanitas, 16*(2), 16–32.

Mozaffarian, D., Katan, M. B., Ascherio, A., Stampfer, M. J., & Willett, W. C. (2006). Trans fatty acids and cardiovascular disease. *New England Journal of Medicine, 354*(15), 1601–1613. doi:10.1056/NEJMra054035.

National Institutes of Health (NIH). (2022). *Folate—Health professional fact sheet.* U.S. Department of Health & Human Services Retrieved May 12, 2025, from https://ods.od.nih.gov/factsheets/Folate-HealthProfessional/ .

National Institutes of Health (NIH). (2024a). *Vitamin D—Health professional fact sheet.* U.S. Department of Health & Human Services Retrieved May 12, 2025, from https://ods.od.nih.gov/factsheets/VitaminD-HealthProfessional/ .

National Institutes of Health (NIH). (2024b). *Calcium—Health professional fact sheet.* U.S. Department of Health & Human Services Retrieved May 12, 2025, from https://ods.od.nih.gov/factsheets/Calcium-HealthProfessional/ .

National Institutes of Health (NIH). (2024c). *Iron—Health professional fact sheet.* U.S. Department of Health & Human Services Retrieved May 12, 2025, from https://ods.od.nih.gov/factsheets/Iron-HealthProfessional/ .

National Institutes of Health (NIH). (2024d). *Iodine—Health professional fact sheet.* U.S. Department of Health & Human Services Retrieved May 12, 2025, from https://ods.od.nih.gov/factsheets/Iodine-Consumer/ .

Negro, E., Hochstrasser, A., Vega Joubert, M., & Rosa Williner, M. (2020). Ingesta de calcio en jóvenes estudiantes de Licenciatura en Nutrición de Santa Fe (Argentina). *Nutrición Clínica y Dietética Hospitalaria, 40*(3). doi:10.12873/403williner.

Nimer, M., Ansaloni, J. A., & Silva, M. E. (2009). *Iodization of salt: The control of iodine deficiency disorders in Brazil comprehensive handbook of iodine* (pp. 1203–1212). Elsevier Inc. doi:10.1016/B978-0-12-374135-6.00124-2.

Official Bulletin of the Argentinian Republic. (2021). *Promotion of healthy eating—Law 27,642.* https://www.boletinoficial.gob.ar/detalleAviso/primera/252728/20211112

PAHO. (1990). Health conditions in the Americas. *Scientific Publication N° 524.* OPS.

PAHO. (2008). *Trans-fat free Americas: Declaration of Rio de Janeiro 2008*. Retrieved March 17, 2025, from https://www.paho.org/es/documentos/americas-libres-grasas-trans-declaracion-rio-janeiro-2008.

PAHO. (2015). *Alimentos y bebidas ultraprocesados en América Latina: Tendencias, efecto sobre la obesidad e implicaciones para las políticas públicas*. http://iris.paho.org/xmlui/bitstream/handle/123456789/7698/9789275318645_esp.pdf

PAHO. (2019). *Alimentação saudável*. Pan American Health Organization. Retrieved April 12, 2025, from https://www.paho.org/pt/topicos/alimentacao-saudavel.

PAHO. (2020). *Consumption of ultra-processed food and drink products in Latin America*. Pan American Health Organization https://www.paho.org/.

PAHO. (2021a). *Noncommunicable diseases in the Americas*. Pan American Health Organization https://www.paho.org/.

PAHO. (2021b). *OPAS lança novas metas para reduzir consumo de sal na população e prevenir doenças cardiovasculares*. Retrieved April 12, 2025, from https://www.paho.org/pt/noticias/28-10-2021-opas-lanca-novas-metas-para-reduzir-consumo-sal-na-populacao-e-prevenir-doenças

Pardo-Cabello, A. J., Manzano-Gamero, V., & Puche-Cañas, E. (2023). Vitamin B12: For more than just the treatment of megaloblastic anemia? *Revista Clínica Española (English Edition), 223*(2), 114–119. doi:10.1016/j.rceng.2022.11.004.

Penssan. (2022). *Rede Brasileira de Pesquisa em Soberania e Segurança Alimentar e Nutricional. Inquérito Nacional sobre Insegurança Alimentar no contexto da pandemia da COVID-19 no Brasil*. Retrieved April 12, 2025, from https://pesquisassan.net.br/2o-inquerito-nacional-sobre-inseguranca-alimentar-no-contexto-da-pandemia-da-covid-19-no-brasil/.

Piñeiro, V. (2023). *La seguridad alimentaria y el comercio agroalimentario en América Latina y el Caribe*. International Food Policy Research Institute. doi:10.4060/cc8592es.

Pinto, A. L. D., Miranda, T. L. S., Ferraz, V. P., Athayde, D. D., & Salum, A. (2016). Determinação e verificação de como a gordura trans é notificada nos rótulos de alimentos, em especial naqueles expressos "0% gordura trans". *Brazilian Journal of Food Technology, 19*. http://www.scielo.br/pdf/bjft/v19/1981-6723-bjft-1981-67234315.pdf. doi:10.1590/1981-6723.4315.

Pipoyan, D., Stepanyan, S., Stepanyan, S., Beglaryan, M., Costantini, L., Molinari, R., & Merendino, N. (2021). The effect of trans fatty acids on human health: Regulation and consumption patterns. *Foods, 10*(10), 2452. doi:10.3390/foods10102452.

Popkin, B. M. (2015). Nutrition transition and the global diabetes epidemic. *Current Diabetes Reports, 15*(9). doi:10.1007/s11892-015-0631-4.

Ramos, V. P., & Meneses, C. O. R. (2021). Efeitos do consumo excessivo de açúcar sobre o desempenho cognitivo: Uma revisão de literatura/Effects of excessive sugar consumption on cognitive performance: A literature review. *Brazilian Journal of Health Review, 4*(6), 24931–24951. doi:10.34119/bjhrv4n6-106.

Rivera, J. A., Barquera, S., González-Cossío, T., Olaiz, G., & Sepúlveda, J. (2004). Nutrition transition in Mexico and in other Latin American countries. *Nutrition Reviews, 62*(7 Pt 2), S149–S157. doi:10.1111/j.1753-4887.2004.tb00086.x.

Rodrigues, V. B., da Silva, E. N., dos Santos, A. M., & Santos, L. M. P. (2023). Prevented cases of neural tube defects and cost savings after folic acid fortification of flour in Brazil. *PLoS ONE, 18*(2). doi:10.1371/journal.pone.0281077.

Rodríguez, F., Mendez, V., Lutzky, C., Ilera, V., Zunino, A., Junco, M., … Gauna, A. (2013). Evaluación de yodurias en embarazadas eutiroideas residentes en Buenos Aires. *Revista Argentina de Endocrinología y Metabolismo, 50*(16), 64.

Romaguera, D., Samman, N., Farfán, N., Lobo, M., Pons, A., & Tur, J. (2007). Nutritional status of the Andean population of Puna and Quebrada of Humahuaca, Jujuy, Argentina. *Public Health Nutrition, 11*(6), 606–615. doi:10.1017/s1368980007001061.

Sadighi, J., Nedjat, S., & Rostami, R. (2019). Systematic review and meta-analysis of the effect of iron-fortified flour on iron status of populations worldwide. *Public Health Nutrition, 22*(18), 3465–3484. doi:10.1017/s1368980019002179.

Salvatte, K., Farias, D. R., Normando, P., Berti, T. L., de Castro, I. R. R., & Kac, G. (2023). High serum folate concentration, vitamin B12 deficiency, and Anthropometric Nutritional Status in Brazilian children aged 6–59 months: Data from the Brazilian National Survey of Child Nutrition. *Journal of Nutrition, 153*(7), 2094–2104. doi:10.1016/j.tjnut.2023.05.020.

Sanches, M. H. F., Gripp, M. S. D. M., Caetano, R. B., & Lopes, T. P. (2024). Obesidade em adultos: Visão geral do tratamento. *Brazilian Journal of Implantology and Health Sciences, 6*(10), 1500–1520. doi:10.36557/2674-8169.2024v6n10p1500-1520.

Santos, Q., Nilson, E. A., Verly Junior, E., & Sichieri, R. (2015). An evaluation of the effectiveness of the flour iron fortification programme in Brazil. *Public Health Nutrition, 18*(9), 1670–1674. doi:10.1017/S1368980014002055.

Santos, S. M., Mazon, E. M. A., & Freitas, V. P. S. (2011). Teores de iodo em sal fortificado para o consumo humano. *Revista do Instituto Adolfo Lutz, 70*(3), 349–353. doi:10.53393/rial.2011.v70.32543.

Santos, S. M. C., Ramos, F. P., Medeiros, M. A. T., Mata, M. M., & Vasconcelos, F. A. G. (2021). Avanços e desafios nos 20 anos da Política Nacional de Alimentação e Nutrição. *Cadernos de Saúde Pública, 37*(Suppl 1), e00150220. doi:10.1590/0102-311X00150220.

Scaramella, J. C. (2020). *Contenido de yodo en sal de mesa y variación del mismo durante el proceso de cocción (Dissertation for the degree of Degree in Bromatology).* National University of Cuyo.

Scott, J., Rébeillé, F., & Fletcher, J. (2000). Folic acid and folates: The feasibility for nutritional enhancement in plant foods. *Journal of the Science of Food and Agriculture, 80*(7), 795–824. doi:10.1002/(SICI)1097-0010(20000515)80:7⟨795::AID-JSFA599⟩3.0.CO;2-K.

Sobral, C. T. C., Gomes, A. S., Da Conceição, C. W., Da Silva Cavichioli, B. N. B., Sá, A. B., De Sousa Barroso, A., & Da Silva Júnior, A. Q. (2024). Avaliação do teor de ácidos graxos trans em margarinas após a RDC 632/2022. *Brazilian Journal of Health Review, 7*(9), e75588. doi:10.34119/bjhrv7n9-319.

Sousa, I. C., Mucinhato, R. M. D., Prates, C. B., Zanin, L. M., da Cunha, D. T., Capriles, V. D., de Rosso, V. V., & Stedefeldt, E. (2023). Do Brazilian consumers intend to use food labels to make healthy food choices? An assessment before the front-of-package labelling policy. *Food Research International, 172.* doi:10.1016/j.foodres.2023.113107.

Sposob, G. (2024). *South America. Enciclopedia Concepto.* Retrieved March 17, 2025, from https://concepto.de/america-del-sur/.

Steluti, J., Selhub, J., Paul, L., Reginaldo, C., Fisberg, R. M., & Marchioni, D. M. L. (2017). An overview of folate status in a population-based study from São Paulo, Brazil and the potential impact of 10 years of national folic acid fortification policy. *European Journal of Clinical Nutrition, 71*(10), 1173–1178. doi:10.1038/ejcn.2017.60.

Tavella, M., Peterson, G., Espeche, M., Cavallero, E., Cipolla, L., Perego, L., & Caballero, B. (2000). Trans fatty acid content of a selection of foods in Argentina. *Food Chemistry, 69*(2), 209–213. doi:10.1016/s0308-8146(99)00257-5.

Tiscornia, M. V., Costronuovo, L., Guarnieri, L., Martins, E., & Allemandi, L. (2020). Evaluación de los sistemas de perfiles nutricionales para la definición de una política de etiquetado frontal en Argentina. *Revista Argentina de Salud Pública, 12*, 17. https://rasp.msal.gov.ar/index.php/rasp/article/view/117.

Tobón, L. M. S. (2021). Etiquetado nutricional frontal y su impacto en la salud pública. Consideraciones bioéticas. *Revista de Nutrición Clínica y Metabolismo, 4*(3), 26–34. doi:10.35454/rncm.v4n3.214.

UNICEF/FIC Argentina. (2024). *Valoración de los efectos de la Ley de Promoción de Alimentación Saludable*. UNICEF/FIC Argentina https://www.unicef.org/argentina/informes/valoracion-de-los-efectos-de-la-ley-de-promocion-de-alimentacion-saludable.

Varea, A., Malpeli, A., Etchegoyen, G., Vojkovic, M., Disalvo, L., Apezteguía, M., Pereyras, S., Pattín, J., Ortale, S., Carmuega, E., & González, H. F. (2011). Short-term evaluation of the impact of a food program on the micronutrient nutritional status of Argentinean children under the age of six. *Biological Trace Element Research, 143*(3), 1337–1348. doi:10.1007/s12011-011-8978-0.

Verly Junior, E., Marchioni, D. M., Araujo, M. C., De Carli, E., de Oliveira, D. C. R. S., Yokoo, E. M., Sichieri, R., & Pereira, R. A. (2021). Evolution of energy and nutrient intake in Brazil between 2008–2009 and 2017–2018. *Revista de Saude Publica, 55*(1). doi:10.11606/S1518-8787.2021055003343.

Vieira, D. A. D. S., Steluti, J., Verly-Jr, E., Marchioni, D. M., & Fisberg, R. M. (2017). Brazilians' experiences with iron fortification: Evidence of effectiveness for reducing inadequate iron intakes with fortified flour policy. *Public Health Nutrition, 20*(2), 363–370. doi:10.1017/S1368980016001981.

WHO. (2006). *Guidelines on food fortification with micronutrients*. World Health Organization.

WHO. (2014). *Guideline: Fortification of food-grade salt with iodine for the prevention and control of iodine deficiency disorders*. World Health Organization.

(2015). *Guideline: Sugars intake for adults and children* (p. 49). World Health Organization.

(2022). *Anaemia* (p. 10). World Health Organization. https://www.who.int/health-topics/anaemia.

WHO. (2023a). *Saturated fatty acid and trans-fatty acid intake for adults and children: WHO guideline*. World Health Organization.

WHO. (2023b). *Reducing free sugars intake in adults to reduce the risk of noncommunicable diseases*. World Health Organization Retrieved May 12, 2025, from https://www.who.int/tools/elena/interventions/free-sugars-adults-ncds .

World Health Organization & Food and Agriculture Organization. (2003). *Diet, nutrition and the prevention of chronic diseases: Report of the joint WHO/FAO expert consultation (WHO Technical Report Series, No. 916)*. World Health Organization Retrieved March 17, 2025, from https://www.who.int/dietphysicalactivity/publications/trs916/summary/en/ .

World Health Organization (WHO). Global database on the Implementation of Nutrition Action (GINA). TFA Country Score Card. Retrieved February 25, 2025, from https://extranet.who.int/nutrition/gina/en/scorecard/TF.

Zapata, M. E., Cediel, G., Arrieta, E., Rovirosa, A., Carmuega, E., & Monteiro, C. A. (2023). Ultra-processed foods consumption and diet quality among preschool children and women of reproductive age from Argentina. *Public Health Nutrition, 26*(11), 2304–2313. doi:10.1017/s1368980022002543.

Zonta, M. L., Servián, A., Panisse, G., Oyhenart, E. E., & Navone, G. T. (2022). Nutritional status, intestinal parasitic infections, and socio-environmental conditions in Mbyá-guaraní children: The current situation in communities in central Misiones, Argentina. *American Journal of Human Biology., 34*(7). http://onlinelibrary.wiley.com/journal/10.1002/(ISSN)1520-6300. doi:10.1002/ajhb.23749.

Nutritional status across different age groups in Southeast Asia

5

Sharmin Zaman Emon[a] *and Dam Sao Mai*[b]
[a]Centre for Advanced Research in Sciences (CARS), University of Dhaka, Dhaka, Bangladesh, [b]Institute of Food technology and Biotechnology, Industrial University of Ho Chi Minh City, Ho Chi Minh City, Vietnam

5.1 Introduction

Southeast Asia (SEA), an area recognized for its unique cultures, weather, and socioeconomic conditions, provides a complicated picture of nutritional status across age groups. The association of traditional diets, economic transformations, and public health initiatives has a considerable impact on the nutritional health of people in this region. Understanding these variances is crucial for combating malnutrition in three forms: undernutrition, overnutrition, and micronutrient deficiencies.

SEA consists of eleven countries: Brunei, Burma (Myanmar), Cambodia, Timor-Leste, Indonesia, Laos, Malaysia, the Philippines, Singapore, Thailand, and Vietnam. SEA has a total population of 697 million, with diverse food habits shaped by cultural history and agricultural techniques (Worldometer, 2024). Urbanization, farming, and food exchange have a significant impact on the region's nutritional environment. Traditional cuisines such as rice, fish, and vegetables are rapidly changing because of urbanization and the introduction of manufactured foods. This dietary adaptability, combined with socioeconomic inequality, has increased the burden of malnutrition, with undernutrition and obesity coexisting in communities and even households (Gaupholm et al., 2023).

For better understanding the nutritional status of these countries, intricate interplay between cultural, economic, and environmental factors is also important. The dual burden of malnutrition—characterized by the coexistence of undernutrition and obesity—is particularly pronounced in SEA. For instance, whereas rural areas grapple with issues such as stunting and wasting, urban regions face rising rates of obesity and noncommunicable diseases (NCDs). These challenges are further exacerbated by gender disparities, socioeconomic inequalities, and limited access to healthcare and education. Children, women of reproductive age, and the elderly are particularly vulnerable to these nutritional challenges, which have far-reaching implications for individual well-being and socioeconomic development.

The role of policy interventions, such as school meal programs, food fortification, and public health campaigns, is pivotal in mitigating these issues. In addition, international organizations, such as WHO, UNICEF, and FAO, have been instrumental in supporting regional efforts to combat malnutrition (United Nations Children's Fund (UNICEF), 2024; World Health Organization, 2023). However, achieving sustainable progress requires a holistic approach that integrates traditional practices with

Nutritional Strategies, Predictive Models, and Sustainable Policies. DOI: https://doi.org/10.1016/B978-0-443-23671-6.00002-5

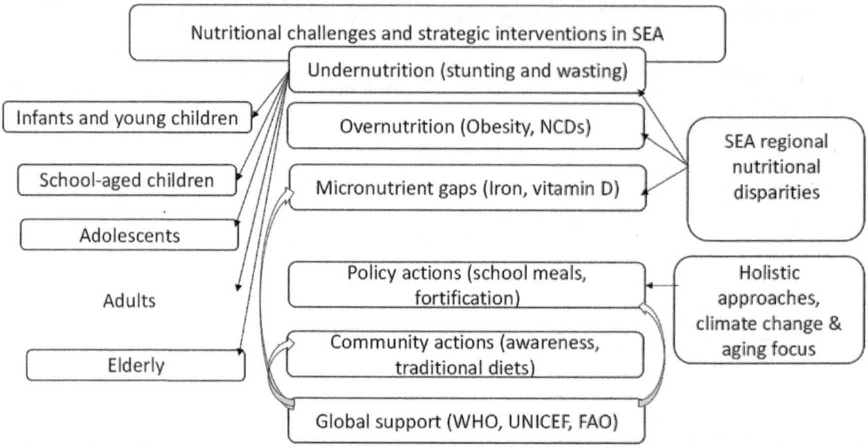

Figure 5.1 Outline of nutritional challenges and interventions in SEA. *NCDs*, Noncommunicable diseases; *SEA*, Southeast Asia.

modern solutions, emphasizing local context and inclusivity. For example, community-based initiatives that leverage traditional diets can be aligned with modern nutritional standards to improve dietary diversity and nutritional outcomes.

Furthermore, climate change and fast urbanization have a significant impact on food security and nutrition in SEA. Climate-induced disruptions in agriculture jeopardize the availability and cost of healthful foods, whereas urbanization promotes processed and convenience foods over traditional, nutrient-dense diets. This emphasizes the need for resilient food systems and policies that address the unique difficulties of SEA's fast changing population and environmental situation.

The nutritional status of SEA communities necessitates a comprehensive approach that takes into account cultural, economic, and environmental factors. To address the region's unique nutritional concerns, governments, communities, and international organizations must work together to ensure fair access to nutritious foods, promote healthy lifestyles, and create sustainable development. This chapter lays the groundwork for investigating the individual nutritional issues and strategic responses across different age groups in SEA. Fig. 5.1 shows the outline of this chapter.

5.2 Nutritional status of infants and young children

For humans the first 1000 days are critical for both physical and cognitive development. Significant progress has been achieved in SEA toward improving infants' nutrition through breastfeeding promotion and vitamin supplementation. However, in terms of undernutrition, micronutrient deficiencies, and exclusive breastfeeding, the nutritional health of newborns and young children throughout SEA exhibits significant disparities between undernutrition in some nations and growing obesity in others.

1. **Cambodia**: Cambodia is one of the least developed countries in SEA, facing substantial socioeconomic issues such as high poverty rates and inadequate access to healthcare and clean water, especially in rural areas. Stunting affects approximately 32% of children under the age of 5, with wasting affecting 10%. Micronutrient deficits, such as vitamin A and iron, are common. Exclusive breastfeeding rates are at 65% (United Nations Children's Fund (UNICEF), 2024). Chronic poverty, combined with food insecurity and insufficient maternal nutrition during pregnancy, contributes to chronically high rates of malnutrition. Furthermore, restricted access to diverse meals and fortified foods increases the prevalence of micronutrient deficits. On the other hand, traditional breastfeeding habits are widely promoted and reinforced by public health initiatives, which contributes to the relatively high incidence of exclusive breastfeeding. These initiatives highlight the importance of culturally embedded methods in tackling nutrition-related issues.
2. **Laos**: Laos shares many socioeconomic challenges with neighboring Cambodia, including widespread poverty and an underdeveloped healthcare infrastructure. Stunting rates remain alarmingly high at 33.4%, with wasting at 9% (FAO, 2022). Iron deficiency anemia is widespread. Exclusive breastfeeding is practiced by 55% of mothers (World Health Organization, 2023). Food insecurity, caused by low agricultural output and unequal access to resources, is a major factor in malnutrition. The country's reliance on staple foods like rice, along with limited dietary diversity, exacerbates micronutrient inadequacies, especially iron insufficiency. Furthermore, cultural norms greatly favor nursing, laying a good basis for child nutrition. However, maternal workload, sometimes combined with hunger among mothers, creates hurdles to good breastfeeding practices. Addressing these difficulties needs integrated initiatives to boost agricultural productivity, expand healthcare services, and provide targeted nutritional education to communities.
3. **Myanmar**: Myanmar is facing serious socioeconomic issues caused by political instability, which has disrupted key services and worsened poverty. Malnutrition is widespread, with 26.7% of children stunted and 7.4% wasting. Vitamin A supplementation coverage is below recommended levels. The rate of exclusive breastfeeding is 51% (United Nations Children's Fund (UNICEF), 2024). Limited access to healthcare, along with persistent violence and relocation, severely hinders attempts to combat hunger. Conflict-related displacement and food shortages have resulted in widespread malnutrition, particularly in vulnerable groups. Fortified foods are not widely known or accessible, causing deficits in critical nutrients such as vitamin A and iron. Furthermore, urbanization and a lack of education about the benefits of exclusive breastfeeding are leading to a decrease in breastfeeding practices, particularly in metropolitan areas. Malnutrition prevention efforts in Myanmar must include improving healthcare access, providing fortified foods, and boosting educational programs to promote exclusive breastfeeding and better dietary practices.
4. **Vietnam**: Vietnam is a fast-developing country with significant economic growth. However, rising income inequality in urban and rural areas has resulted in discrepancies in healthcare access and nutritional outcomes. Although stunting is down to 19.6%, rural areas continue to encounter issues. Iron and zinc deficiencies persist. Exclusive breastfeeding rates are relatively low, at 45% (World Bank, 2023). Undernutrition is primarily prevalent in rural and ethnic minority areas, where healthcare infrastructure and access to resources are scarce. Furthermore the dietary trend toward processed foods in cities has failed to address the requirement for diversified and nutrient-dense diets, worsening iron and zinc deficiencies. On the other side, urbanization and workplace rules that do not fully support mother leave and breastfeeding have contributed to a drop in breastfeeding rates. To solve these issues, Vietnam must focus on strengthening healthcare facilities in rural regions, increasing dietary

diversity, and enacting policies that support breastfeeding, particularly among working women in metropolitan centers.

5. **Thailand**: Thailand is an upper-middle-income country experiencing rapid urbanization and economic growth. Despite its advancements, significant disparities exist, particularly affecting marginalized and rural populations. Stunting is low at 10.5%, but obesity is on the rise. Micronutrient deficiencies are present in marginalized populations. Exclusive breastfeeding rates are 23% (United Nations Children's Fund (UNICEF), 2024). Although stunting rates are reduced in general, undernutrition persists in marginalized communities and rural areas with inadequate access to healthcare and nutritional foods. Low-income families and migrant workers are more likely to suffer from deficiencies because of a lack of dietary diversity and limited availability to fortified foods. The low percentage of exclusive breastfeeding can be attributed to the widespread use of formula feeding, aggressive marketing by formula producers, and limited maternity leave rules, which prevent working mothers from breastfeeding. To address these obstacles, focused interventions are required, such as support for vulnerable communities, public health campaigns to promote breastfeeding, and policies to increase parental leave and control formula marketing practices.
6. **Malaysia**: Malaysia is a high-income country with large differences between cities and rural areas. Health disparities are more severe in indigenous groups, which have limited access to healthcare and dietary resources. In Malaysia, urban obesity rates are rising, indicating a shift in dietary and lifestyle habits. At the same time, indigenous and rural groups continue to be concerned about undernutrition. Exclusive breastfeeding is uncommon, with only 41% of newborns receiving only breast milk (World Health Organization, 2023). Undernutrition disproportionately affects indigenous and rural groups because of limited access to healthcare facilities, adequate food, and clean water. Urban dietary habits are frequently nutritionally imbalanced, with greater intake of processed and high-calorie meals contributing to micronutrient deficits despite rising wages. Furthermore the rate of exclusive breastfeeding has decreased, owing to urbanization, an increase in the number of working mothers, and a greater reliance on formula feeding as a substitute. To address these challenges, efforts should be focused on reducing health disparities by improving access to healthcare for marginalized populations, promoting balanced dietary habits across all income levels, and implementing supportive policies for breastfeeding mothers, including workplace accommodations and public health campaigns.
7. **Singapore**: As a high-income country, Singapore has an excellent healthcare system and strong government-led health initiatives. However, urban living problems and socioeconomic gaps among immigrant and low-income populations continue to pose health risks. Rising childhood obesity in Singapore has become a serious public health concern, highlighting the influence of urban lifestyle choices. Despite the country's high adherence to vitamin supplementation programs, exclusive breastfeeding rates remain low at 31% (Singapore Ministry of Health, 2023). Undernutrition is rare in Singapore because of strong government health programs and extensive access to nutritious meals. Deficiencies are primarily concentrated among immigrants and low-income populations, who may encounter challenges to getting diversified and nutrient-dense meals. The low percentage of exclusive breastfeeding is caused by workplace stress, short maternity leave for some working mothers, and a preference for formula feeding in metropolitan families. To overcome these difficulties, Singapore must focus on combating obesity through public health campaigns, supporting exclusive breastfeeding through workplace policies and education, and ensuring that marginalized people have equitable access to nutritious meals and healthcare facilities.
8. **Indonesia**: Indonesia is a lower-middle-income country with extensive rural and isolated areas. Significant wealth disparity and limited infrastructure contribute to gaps in healthcare

and nutritional access for the general population. Food insecurity is a big problem in rural and isolated places where agricultural productivity is low and access to affordable healthy food is scarce. In Indonesia, stunting affects 24.4% of children under the age of 5, whereas 7.1% experience wasting, highlighting persistent nutritional challenges. Widespread micronutrient deficiencies, particularly in iodine and iron, further exacerbate health issues. Exclusive breastfeeding rates stand at 55%, indicating moderate adherence to recommended practices (FAO, 2022). The absence of effective food fortification programs and limited access to healthcare services, particularly in rural regions, contribute to widespread deficits in important elements such as iodine and iron. Otherwise, cultural views, insufficient support networks for breastfeeding women, and a lack of public knowledge on the benefits of exclusive breastfeeding all contribute to low rates. To address these difficulties, Indonesia must increase food security initiatives, extend healthcare and fortification programs in rural regions, and undertake targeted education and support programs to encourage breastfeeding patterns.

9. **Philippines**: As a middle-income country the Philippines experiences major gaps in healthcare and nutrition, notably between urban and rural, underprivileged areas. Furthermore, economic inequality and inadequate infrastructure accentuate the discrepancies. In the Philippines, 28.7% of children under the age of 5 are stunted, and 6.1% are wasting, highlighting the ongoing burden of malnutrition. Exclusive breastfeeding rates stand at 49%, indicating moderate adherence to recommended feeding methods. Severe iron insufficiency is common, particularly in rural regions with inadequate access to nutritious diets (United Nations Children's Fund (UNICEF), 2024). Food instability, poverty, and a lack of access to healthcare and clean water in remote areas all contribute to stunting and waste. Severe iron deficiency is also frequent, particularly in rural areas, where there is little access to iron-rich or fortified foods. On the other hand, breastfeeding rates are influenced by a lack of maternal education, aggressive formula marketing, and insufficient workplace policies to encourage breastfeeding moms. Efforts to resolve these issues should include improving access to healthcare and fortified foods in remote regions, developing better public health campaigns to promote breastfeeding, and enacting legislation that supports working women' exclusive breastfeeding habits.
10. **Brunei**: Brunei is a high-income country with universal healthcare and a solid economic base. Childhood obesity and micronutrient deficiencies are rising public health concerns in Brunei, highlighting the influence of modern lifestyle choices. Exclusive breastfeeding rates are moderate, at 46% (World Health Organization, 2023). However, increased obesity and nutritional changes connected with urbanization pose considerable public health risks. Although undernutrition is uncommon, it occurs in underprivileged populations with inadequate access to resources and healthcare. Changing dietary patterns, such as eating less vegetables and relying more on processed foods, contribute to vitamin shortages. Breastfeeding rates are hampered by an increasing reliance on formula feeding in urbanized homes, as well as a lack of general education about the long-term benefits of exclusive breastfeeding. To address these concerns, Brunei should prioritize public health measures that promote balanced meals, encourage exclusive breastfeeding through workplace policies and community education, and target underserved communities for fair access to healthcare and nutritional resources.
11. **Timor-Leste**: Timor-Leste is one of the region's poorest countries, with minimal infrastructure, widespread poverty, and inadequate healthcare facilities. In Timor-Leste, 47.1% of children under the age of 5 suffer from stunting, making it one of the highest rates in SEA. Wasting is also high, affecting 11% of children. Despite the limitations, exclusive breastfeeding rates remain reasonably high at 61%

(United Nations Children's Fund (UNICEF), 2024). Severe food insecurity, combined with insufficient maternal nutrition during pregnancy and early childrearing, contributes to the high frequency of stunting and wasting. Diets frequently lack variation, relying largely on staple foods and consuming insufficient amounts of critical vitamins and minerals. Although breastfeeding rates are quite high, they are not completely ideal because of maternal malnutrition and a lack of healthcare support for breastfeeding mothers. To address these concerns, Timor-Leste must prioritize improving food security, strengthening healthcare infrastructure, and establishing community-based nutritional initiatives that promote mother and child health. In addition, tailored interventions to improve dietary diversity and provide nutritional education are critical for long-term progress.

The nutritional quality of infants and young children in SEA is influenced by a variety of circumstances, emphasizing the importance of the first 1000 days in shaping lifetime health. In addition, maternal nutrition has a major impact on birth outcomes, emphasizing the importance of addressing maternal anemia and malnutrition. Furthermore, although exclusive breastfeeding is necessary, it encounters challenges including cultural norms, aggressive formula marketing, and limited workplace support. Micronutrient supplementation and food fortification initiatives, which target vitamin A, zinc, and iron deficits, have proven beneficial but need to be scaled up. Furthermore, hygiene and sanitation improvements are critical for lowering malnutrition-related illnesses, especially in conflict-affected areas where food security and healthcare access are compromised. In this regard, cultural traditions serve a dual purpose, with some promoting nutrition and others impeding progress. Emerging issues, such as overnutrition from processed meals, necessitate balanced treatments. Strengthening data systems, evaluating progress, and addressing the cognitive effects of malnutrition can all help to steer more complete and effective nutritional interventions.

5.3 Nutritional challenges in school-aged children

School-aged children face unique nutritional challenges that impact their learning and long-term health. Malnutrition, micronutrient deficiencies, and dietary habits are the three categories divided in the case of school-aged children's nutritional challenges. SEA countries face diverse nutritional challenges among school-aged children, ranging from persistent undernutrition to rising trends of overnutrition, exacerbated by micronutrient deficiencies and shifting dietary habits.

1. **Cambodia**: Malnutrition affects rural children, with 22% underweight (World Bank, 2023). Vitamin A and iron deficiencies are rampant. Diets are primarily rice-based, lacking protein and diversity (FAO, 2022). Heavy reliance on rice as the staple food, leading to a lack of dietary diversity. Moreover, limited access to nutrient-rich foods such as fruits, vegetables, and protein sources because of poverty also increases malnutrition. Moreover, poor maternal nutrition and inadequate breastfeeding practices contribute to childhood malnutrition.
2. **Laos**: Stunting (33%) and wasting (9%) extend into school-aged children. Iron-deficiency anemia is widespread, exacerbated by limited access to fortified foods. Traditional diets dominate, with low fruit and vegetable intake (UNICEF, 2021). In remote areas, poor access to fortified foods and healthcare services exacerbated malnutrition. But traditional diets are

low in fruits, vegetables, and protein. Poor sanitation and lack of awareness about balanced diets contribute to iron-deficiency anemia and stunting.

3. **Myanmar**: Myanmar faces food nutrition challenges marked by rural undernutrition, urban obesity, micronutrient deficiencies, poor dietary diversity, and economic disparities. In Myanmar, malnutrition among school-aged children remains a critical issue, especially in rural areas, where poverty limits access to nutritious food. Chronic undernutrition leads to stunted growth, whereas in urban areas, rising obesity linked to processed food consumption and sedentary lifestyles presents a contrasting challenge. Micronutrient deficiencies, particularly iodine, iron, and vitamin A, persist, adversely affecting cognitive and physical development. Poor dietary habits are widespread, driven by economic constraints, lack of nutrition education, and reliance on staple foods like rice, which lacks essential nutrients. Addressing these issues requires holistic interventions, including school-based feeding programs and awareness campaigns for improved dietary practices (World Health Organization, 2023).
4. **Vietnam**: Vietnam has made progress in reducing poverty, yet socioeconomic disparities persist, impacting children's nutrition. In rural areas, malnutrition remains prevalent because of limited access to diverse foods and healthcare. Urbanization has led to increased consumption of processed foods, contributing to rising obesity rates among school-aged children in cities. Micronutrient deficiencies, particularly in iron, vitamin A, and zinc, affect growth and cognitive development, especially in underprivileged communities. Dietary habits often lack diversity, with a heavy reliance on rice and limited protein and vegetable intake. Addressing these challenges requires targeted programs promoting nutrition education, affordable food access, and balanced school meal initiatives (World Bank, 2023).
5. **Thailand**: Thailand, a middle-income country, faces diverse nutritional challenges among school-aged children influenced by socioeconomic disparities. Rising obesity affects 10% of school-aged children, whereas undernutrition persists in underserved regions. Sugar-rich snacks and beverages dominate dietary habits (United Nations Children's Fund (UNICEF), 2024). In rural areas, malnutrition and stunted growth remain significant because of poverty and limited access to nutritious foods. Conversely, urbanization and economic growth have led to increasing obesity rates in cities, driven by sedentary lifestyles and rising consumption of processed and fast foods. Micronutrient deficiencies, particularly in iron and iodine, persist, impacting cognitive and physical development. Dietary habits often lack diversity, with overreliance on rice and insufficient fruits and vegetables. Comprehensive strategies, including school meal programs and nutrition education, are vital for addressing these challenges.
6. **Malaysia**: Malaysia, a rapidly developing upper-middle-income country, experiences dual nutritional challenges among school-aged children. In rural areas, malnutrition and stunting persist because of poverty and limited access to nutrient-rich foods. Urbanization and economic growth have led to rising obesity rates in urban children, driven by sedentary lifestyles and increased consumption of processed foods and sugary beverages. Micronutrient deficiencies, particularly in iron, iodine, and vitamin D, remain common, affecting overall growth and development. Dietary habits often lack balance, with high carbohydrate intake dominating over protein and vegetables. Addressing these issues requires school-based programs, public awareness, and policies to promote healthy eating habits. Overweight and obesity affect 15% of children in this country. Iron and vitamin D deficiencies are also common. Urban dietary habits lean toward processed and calorie-dense foods (World Health Organization, 2023).
7. **Singapore**: Singapore, a high-income nation, has largely overcome issues of severe malnutrition but faces emerging nutritional challenges in school-aged children. Urban lifestyles

and economic affluence have contributed to rising childhood obesity up to 14%, driven by sedentary habits and consumption of processed and fast foods. Despite widespread food availability, micronutrient deficiencies, including vitamin D and calcium, persist because of limited sun exposure and dietary patterns. Poor eating habits, such as skipping meals and overreliance on convenience foods, exacerbate these issues. Singapore's efforts to combat these challenges include school-based nutrition programs, health education campaigns, and policies promoting balanced diets and active lifestyles for children. Government programs encourage healthy eating, but high consumption of sugary drinks and fast food remains an issue (Singapore Ministry of Health, 2023).

8. **Indonesia**: In Indonesia, malnutrition among school-aged children remains a significant concern, with stunting and underweight rates influenced by socioeconomic disparities. Many children from low-income families face limited access to nutritious food, resulting in micronutrient deficiencies such as anemia because of inadequate iron intake. Conversely, urban areas witness a rise in obesity because of poor dietary habits, including high consumption of processed foods. Economic inequality exacerbates these issues, as rural and impoverished communities struggle with food insecurity, whereas wealthier urban populations adopt unhealthy diets. Addressing these challenges requires targeted interventions to improve nutrition education, access to affordable healthy food, and public health initiatives (FAO, 2022).
9. **Philippines**: In the Philippines, malnutrition remains a pressing issue among school-aged children in rural areas, around 28%, with high rates of stunting and wasting linked to poverty and food insecurity. Children in low-income households often lack access to diverse and nutritious food, leading to micronutrient deficiencies such as vitamin A deficiency and anemia. Simultaneously, urbanization and economic disparity contribute to unhealthy dietary habits, with processed and sugary foods becoming more common, increasing the risk of obesity. Socioeconomic inequalities exacerbate these challenges, as rural and impoverished areas face inadequate health and nutrition services, whereas urban centers struggle with the dual burden of undernutrition and overnutrition (United Nations Children's Fund (UNICEF), 2024).
10. **Brunei**: Brunei faces fewer nutritional concerns among school-aged children than neighboring countries, but rising issues require attention. Although malnutrition is uncommon because of Brunei's high income and strong social assistance programs, micronutrient deficiencies such as vitamin D inadequacy are documented, owing to lifestyle circumstances that limit sun exposure. Urbanization and prosperity have altered dietary habits, resulting in increasing intake of processed and high-calorie foods, which contribute to childhood obesity. Socioeconomic stability ensures universal food access, but sedentary lifestyles and changing eating patterns pose health hazards, stressing the need for targeted nutrition education and lifestyle interventions (World Health Organization, 2023).
11. **Timor-Leste**: Timor-Leste experiences major nutritional issues among school-aged children, with high rates of malnutrition, including stunting and wasting, and 37% of children being underweight, which are mostly caused by poverty and food insecurity. Many families struggle to obtain a varied and nutritious diet, resulting in widespread micronutrient shortages, particularly in vitamin A, iron, and iodine. Dietary habits are determined by the scarcity of fresh produce and reliance on staple foods such as rice and maize, which are deficient in critical nutrients. Socioeconomic restrictions, combined with insufficient healthcare and education systems, intensify the problem. Addressing these concerns needs coordinated efforts to increase food security, nutrition education, and access to fortified foods and healthcare (United Nations Children's Fund (UNICEF), 2024).

School-aged children in SEA countries suffer a variety of nutritional difficulties that affect their growth, cognitive development, and long-term health. Malnutrition and micronutrient shortages, such as iron and iodine, impair scholastic performance and mental focus, whereas "hidden hunger" exacerbates developmental difficulties even with adequate calorie intake. Urban-rural differences, on the other hand, show undernutrition in rural areas and increased obesity in urban settings, indicating a double burden of malnutrition. Otherwise, aggressive marketing of unhealthy foods and sedentary lifestyles contribute to poor eating habits and obesity, which are exacerbated by low physical activity and increasing screen time. Cultural views, peer influence, and gender-specific difficulties, such as anemia in females, all have an impact on eating patterns. Furthermore, climate change and food system disturbances limit access to nutritional foods, whereas body image issues, driven by social media, contribute to poor eating habits. Addressing these challenges through school food programs, integrated nutrition education, regular health screenings, and targeted legislation can promote healthier generations and reduce the long-term risk of noncommunicable illnesses.

5.4 Adolescents and emerging nutritional risks

Adolescents in SEA are particularly vulnerable to nutritional imbalances because of rapid growth and lifestyle changes. Here, social media and cultural shifts are also influencing this group in case of eating style. Undernutrition and anemia, obesity, and body image issues are the main concerns in the case of adolescents influenced by socioeconomic disparities, urbanization, and cultural perceptions. Below is a detailed country-wise analysis:

1. **Cambodia**: In Cambodia, adolescents face dual nutritional challenges influenced by socioeconomic disparities. Undernutrition and anemia remain prevalent among rural and low-income communities, with 45% of girls because of poor dietary diversity, where limited access to nutritious foods and healthcare services perpetuates poor health outcomes. Conversely, urban areas are witnessing a rise in obesity among wealthier adolescents because of increasing consumption of processed foods and sedentary lifestyles. Body image issues are also emerging, influenced by globalized media and cultural pressures, affecting mental health and dietary behaviors. Addressing these risks requires multisectoral approaches, including improving food security, nutrition education, healthcare access, and awareness campaigns to foster balanced dietary habits and positive body image (World Bank, 2023).
2. **Laos**: In Laos, adolescents face nutritional challenges closely tied to socioeconomic conditions. Undernutrition and anemia are prevalent with nearly 38% of adolescent girls, especially in rural areas, where poverty limits access to diverse, nutrient-rich foods and health services. Adolescents often depend on rice-heavy diets lacking essential vitamins and minerals, impacting growth and cognitive development. In urban centers, rising incomes and globalization are driving increased consumption of processed foods, leading to obesity among wealthier adolescents. Body image issues are also emerging because of media influences, creating psychological stress and unhealthy dietary behaviors. Addressing these challenges requires initiatives in nutrition education, equitable food access, and mental health awareness (FAO, 2022).

3. **Myanmar**: In Myanmar, adolescents face a spectrum of nutritional risks shaped by socioeconomic disparities and ongoing political instability. Undernutrition and anemia are widespread in rural and conflict-affected areas, with anemia nearly 38% of adolescent girls, where poverty and limited healthcare access hinder the availability of nutritious food and iron supplements. In urban centers, economic growth has led to dietary shifts, with increased consumption of processed foods contributing to rising obesity rates among wealthier adolescents. Body image issues, influenced by globalized media, are also becoming a concern, particularly in urban youth, impacting mental health and eating behaviors. Comprehensive strategies are needed to promote balanced nutrition and mental well-being (World Health Organization, 2023).
4. **Vietnam**: In Vietnam, adolescents experience diverse nutritional challenges linked to the country's socioeconomic landscape. Undernutrition and anemia are more prevalent in rural areas, affecting 29% of adolescents, where poverty and limited access to health services restrict the availability of nutrient-rich foods. In contrast, urbanization and economic growth have introduced issues like obesity, as increased income leads to higher consumption of fast food and sugary beverages. Body image concerns are rising among urban youth, influenced by social media and modern beauty standards, leading to unhealthy eating behaviors. Addressing these challenges requires targeted nutrition education, equitable food access, and programs promoting balanced lifestyles and self-esteem (World Bank, 2023).
5. **Thailand**: In Thailand, socioeconomic disparities significantly impact adolescent nutrition. Undernutrition and anemia are prevalent among adolescents in low-income families, often linked to limited access to nutrient-rich foods and inadequate healthcare. Conversely, obesity is rising (15%) among urban adolescents from higher socioeconomic groups because of sedentary lifestyles and consumption of calorie-dense, processed foods. In addition, body image issues are becoming widespread, fueled by social media and cultural beauty standards, disproportionately affecting middle and upper-class adolescents. These nutritional risks highlight the need for targeted interventions addressing both undernutrition and obesity while promoting healthy body image across diverse socioeconomic contexts in Thailand.
6. **Malaysia**: In Malaysia, socioeconomic status plays a crucial role in shaping adolescent nutritional risks. Undernutrition and anemia (25%) are more prevalent among adolescents from lower income families, often because of limited access to balanced diets and healthcare services. In contrast, obesity is on the rise among adolescents (17%) in higher income urban households, driven by sedentary lifestyles and the consumption of fast food. Body image issues are also increasing, particularly among urban adolescents, influenced by societal beauty standards and exposure to social media. Addressing these challenges requires policies that promote equitable access to nutrition, healthcare, and education on healthy lifestyles across all socioeconomic groups (World Health Organization, 2023).
7. **Singapore**: In Singapore, socioeconomic status influences adolescent nutritional risks in complex ways. Undernutrition and anemia are rare but can affect adolescents in lower income households because of financial constraints limiting access to diverse, nutrient-rich foods. Obesity is a growing concern, particularly among middle-income groups (around 14%), linked to sedentary lifestyles and the availability of calorie-dense convenience foods. Body image issues are prevalent across all socioeconomic levels, exacerbated by cultural and social media pressures promoting unattainable beauty standards. Singapore's well-established healthcare and educational systems offer opportunities for targeted interventions to address these risks, focusing on promoting balanced diets, active lifestyles, and positive body image (Singapore Ministry of Health, 2023).

8. **Indonesia**: In Indonesia, socioeconomic disparities significantly affect adolescent nutritional risks. Undernutrition and anemia (35%) are more prevalent among adolescents from low-income rural areas, where access to nutrient-dense foods and healthcare is limited. In contrast, urban adolescents from higher income families face rising obesity rates because of sedentary lifestyles and increased consumption of processed and fast foods. Body image issues are also becoming prominent, driven by cultural ideals and social media influence, particularly affecting middle and upper-class adolescents. Addressing these challenges requires targeted policies to reduce nutritional disparities, promote balanced diets, and foster healthy body image perceptions across all socioeconomic groups in Indonesia (FAO, 2022).
9. **Philippines**: In the Philippines, socioeconomic status significantly influences adolescent nutritional challenges. Undernutrition and anemia (37%) remain widespread among adolescents in low-income communities, driven by poverty, limited access to nutritious food, and inadequate healthcare. Meanwhile, obesity is emerging in urban areas among higher income groups, often linked to sedentary lifestyles and the growing popularity of processed and fast foods. Body image issues are prevalent across socioeconomic strata, exacerbated by cultural beauty standards and social media pressures. Addressing these risks requires multifaceted interventions, including food security programs for disadvantaged communities, education on balanced diets, and awareness campaigns promoting healthy body image among Filipino adolescents (United Nations Children's Fund (UNICEF), 2024).
10. **Brunei**: In Brunei, adolescent nutritional risks are influenced by socioeconomic status, though the effects are less pronounced because of the country's wealth and accessible healthcare system. Undernutrition and anemia are relatively rare but may affect lower income families or those in rural areas with limited access to diverse diets. Obesity, however, is rising among adolescents in urban areas and higher income groups, driven by sedentary lifestyles and the availability of fast food. Body image issues are also growing, influenced by societal standards and social media. Effective interventions in Brunei should focus on promoting balanced diets, active lifestyles, and fostering positive body image attitudes (World Health Organization, 2023).
11. **Timor-Leste**: In Timor-Leste, socioeconomic challenges deeply affect adolescent nutritional risks. Undernutrition and anemia are widespread, with 50% of girls being anemic, especially in low-income rural areas, where poverty and limited access to diverse, nutrient-rich foods persist. These conditions are compounded by inadequate healthcare and education about nutrition. Obesity is less common but emerging among adolescents in urban settings with greater exposure to processed foods and sedentary lifestyles. Body image issues are gradually becoming a concern, influenced by global media and societal shifts, though less prevalent than in neighboring countries. Addressing these challenges requires improved food security, healthcare access, and nutrition education across all socioeconomic levels (UNICEF, 2021).

Adolescents in SEA countries face unique nutritional challenges because of rapid physical and cognitive growth, requiring increased intake of protein, calcium, iron, and vitamins. Gender-specific issues, such as iron-deficiency anemia in girls and body image pressures, exacerbate nutritional disparities. Otherwise, dietary transitions toward processed and fast foods contribute to micronutrient deficiencies and rising obesity rates, whereas social media and societal beauty standards fuel body image issues and disordered eating patterns. In contrast, poor nutrition affects mental health, linking unhealthy diets to anxiety, depression, and reduced academic performance. Sedentary lifestyles and substance use further compromise nutritional health, particularly in urban settings. Socioeconomic inequalities limit access to nutritious food and healthcare, particularly in rural and conflict-affected areas. Addressing these risks requires school-based nutrition programs, empowerment initiatives, and policies promoting healthy eating. In addition, climate change and food security challenges demand targeted interventions to ensure adolescents have equitable access to affordable, nutritious food.

5.5 Adult nutrition: Balancing undernutrition and overnutrition

Among adults, nutritional status varies widely across socioeconomic strata, as do underweight and rising adults and micronutrient gaps. SEA presents a dual burden of undernutrition and overnutrition among adults, influenced by economic transitions, dietary changes, and lifestyle factors.

1. **Cambodia**: In Cambodia, adult nutrition reflects stark socioeconomic disparities. Undernutrition and underweight issues are prevalent among low-income rural populations, driven by poverty, food insecurity, and limited access to healthcare and diverse diets. Micronutrient deficiencies, such as iron and vitamin A, are widespread, exacerbating health risks. Meanwhile, overnutrition is emerging in urban areas among higher income groups, with rising rates of obesity linked to sedentary lifestyles and increased consumption of processed foods. Addressing these challenges requires a dual approach: ensuring equitable access to nutrient-rich foods and healthcare while promoting education on balanced diets and healthy lifestyles across all socioeconomic groups in Cambodia (World Bank, 2023).
2. **Laos**: In Laos, socioeconomic disparities significantly influence adult nutrition. Undernutrition and underweight are prevalent in low-income rural areas, where food insecurity, limited healthcare, and poor dietary diversity hinder nutritional outcomes. Micronutrient deficiencies, including iron, iodine, and vitamin A, remain critical concerns, particularly among economically disadvantaged groups. Conversely, overnutrition is emerging in urban areas as higher income populations adopt diets high in processed foods and lead sedentary lifestyles, contributing to obesity. Bridging these nutritional gaps requires targeted interventions, such as improving access to diverse diets, strengthening healthcare systems, and raising awareness about balanced nutrition to address the dual burdens of under- and overnutrition (FAO, 2022).
3. **Myanmar**: In Myanmar, adult nutrition is deeply affected by socioeconomic status and regional disparities. Undernutrition and underweight are prevalent among low-income populations, especially in rural and conflict-affected areas, where poverty and food insecurity limit access to diverse and sufficient diets. Micronutrient deficiencies, such as iron, iodine, and vitamin A, are widespread, exacerbating health challenges for economically disadvantaged groups. In urban areas, higher income adults are experiencing rising rates of overnutrition and obesity because of increased consumption of processed foods and sedentary lifestyles. Addressing these challenges requires a multifaceted approach, including improving food security, healthcare access, and nutrition education across socioeconomic groups (World Health Organization, 2023).
4. **Vietnam**: In Vietnam, adult nutrition reflects a dual burden influenced by socioeconomic disparities. Undernutrition and underweight remain concerns in low-income rural areas, where limited access to diverse foods and healthcare services perpetuates malnutrition. Micronutrient deficiencies, particularly in iron, iodine, and vitamin A, are prevalent among disadvantaged populations, affecting productivity and health. Meanwhile, urbanization

and economic growth have led to rising rates of overnutrition and obesity (18%) among higher income groups, fueled by sedentary lifestyles and processed food consumption. Tackling these challenges requires targeted interventions, including food security programs, healthcare improvements, and public education on balanced diets and active lifestyles across all socioeconomic levels (World Bank, 2023).

5. **Thailand**: In Thailand, adult nutrition faces challenges shaped by socioeconomic status. Undernutrition and underweight persist in rural and low-income areas, where poverty limits access to balanced diets and healthcare services. Micronutrient deficiencies, such as iron, iodine, and zinc, are common in these groups, affecting overall health and productivity. On the other hand, overnutrition is a growing concern in urban and higher income populations, with rising obesity (around 22%) rates driven by sedentary lifestyles and the widespread availability of calorie-dense processed foods. Addressing these issues requires targeted strategies, including improving food security, enhancing healthcare access, and promoting nutritional education for all socioeconomic groups in Thailand (United Nations Children's Fund (UNICEF), 2024).
6. **Malaysia**: In Malaysia, adult nutrition reflects a dual burden influenced by socioeconomic status. Undernutrition and underweight are prevalent among lower income groups, particularly in rural areas, where access to diverse diets and healthcare is limited. Micronutrient deficiencies, including iron, calcium, and vitamin D, are widespread in these populations, impacting overall health and well-being. Conversely, overnutrition is on the rise among urban and higher income groups, with obesity in adults being 30%, which is fueled by sedentary lifestyles and increased consumption of processed foods. Bridging these gaps requires holistic strategies, including food security programs, nutrition education, and policies promoting balanced diets and active lifestyles for all socioeconomic levels (World Health Organization, 2023).
7. **Singapore**: In Singapore, adult nutrition challenges are influenced by socioeconomic status, though the country's advanced infrastructure mitigates disparities. Undernutrition and underweight are rare but can affect low-income groups, particularly the elderly or those with limited access to balanced diets. Micronutrient gaps, such as vitamin D and calcium deficiencies, are present across all socioeconomic levels because of dietary habits and urban lifestyles. Overnutrition and obesity are more common, around 25%, with chronic diseases on the rise among higher income groups, driven by sedentary lifestyles and convenience food consumption. Singapore addresses these issues through robust public health policies, education on balanced diets, and programs promoting active lifestyles and food accessibility for all (Singapore Ministry of Health, 2023).
8. **Indonesia**: In Indonesia, adult nutrition reflects stark socioeconomic inequalities. Undernutrition and underweight (10%) are prevalent in low-income rural areas, where poverty limits access to diverse diets and healthcare services. Micronutrient gaps, including deficiencies in iron, vitamin A, and zinc, are common, particularly among economically disadvantaged populations, leading to long-term health challenges. Conversely, overnutrition and obesity (28%) are rising among urban and higher income groups, driven by increasing consumption of processed foods and sedentary lifestyles. Addressing these dual burdens requires tailored strategies, such as improving food security, enhancing healthcare access, and promoting nutritional education to bridge the gaps across diverse socioeconomic contexts in Indonesia (FAO, 2022).
9. **Philippines**: In the Philippines, adult nutrition is heavily influenced by socioeconomic disparities. Undernutrition and underweight are prevalent among low-income groups, particularly in rural areas, where poverty and limited access to diverse diets and healthcare persist. Micronutrient deficiencies, such as iron, iodine, and vitamin A, are widespread, affecting productivity and overall health. Meanwhile, overnutrition and obesity (24%) are emerging

challenges in urban and higher income populations, driven by increased consumption of processed foods and sedentary lifestyles. Bridging these gaps requires comprehensive interventions, including food security programs, better healthcare access, and education on balanced diets to address undernutrition and overnutrition across socioeconomic strata (United Nations Children's Fund (UNICEF), 2024).

10. **Brunei**: In Brunei, adult nutrition challenges are less pronounced compared to regional neighbors, but socioeconomic disparities still play a role. Undernutrition and underweight are rare because of the nation's strong economic foundation and widespread access to healthcare. However, micronutrient gaps, such as vitamin D and calcium deficiencies, can affect lower income groups with limited dietary diversity. Overnutrition is a growing issue, particularly among higher income adults, driven by sedentary lifestyles and consumption of processed and calorie-dense foods. Addressing these concerns requires promoting balanced diets, public health campaigns on nutrition education, and initiatives to encourage active lifestyles across all socioeconomic levels in Brunei (World Health Organization, 2023).
11. **Timor-Leste**: In Timor-Leste, adult nutrition is significantly impacted by socioeconomic challenges. Undernutrition and underweight (20%) are prevalent, particularly among low-income and rural populations, where poverty, food insecurity, and limited healthcare access hinder proper dietary intake. Micronutrient deficiencies, such as iron, iodine, and vitamin A, are widespread, contributing to health issues and reduced productivity. Overnutrition and obesity remain minimal but are emerging in urban areas with increased access to processed foods. Addressing these nutritional disparities requires targeted efforts to improve food security, enhance healthcare infrastructure, and implement educational programs promoting balanced diets and awareness of nutritional needs across socioeconomic levels (United Nations Children's Fund (UNICEF), 2024).

Adult nutrition in SEA is marked by the dual challenges of undernutrition and overnutrition, shaped by socioeconomic disparities. Low-income groups face food insecurity, leading to undernutrition, whereas urbanization and processed food consumption drive obesity in higher income populations. In cities, workplace environments and sedentary lifestyles exacerbate these trends, alongside persistent micronutrient deficiencies, particularly in iron, calcium, and vitamin D. Moreover, traditional diets are increasingly replaced by calorie-dense, nutrient-poor foods, contributing to the rising burden of NCDs such as diabetes and hypertension. Mental health issues, stress, and cultural pressures further influence eating behaviors, whereas gender-specific challenges, such as maternal nutrition, remain critical. Moreover, age-specific nutritional needs, particularly for older adults, highlight gaps in dietary diversity. In addition, climate change and food system disruptions worsen access to nutrient-rich foods. Addressing these issues requires policy interventions, technology-driven solutions, workplace wellness programs, and improved monitoring systems to promote balanced diets and healthier lifestyles across all socioeconomic groups.

5.6 Nutritional concerns for the elderly

The aging population in SEA presents a new set of nutritional challenges, such as undernutrition, obesity-related NCDs and micronutrient needs. These are compounded by age-related declines in nutrient absorption and dietary quality.

1. **Cambodia**: In Cambodia, elderly nutrition is shaped by socioeconomic disparities. Undernutrition is prevalent among low-income older adults, especially in rural areas, where poverty and limited access to diverse diets and healthcare services contribute to inadequate calorie and nutrient intake. Conversely, obesity-related NCDs, such as diabetes and hypertension, are rising among wealthier urban populations because of sedentary lifestyles and processed food consumption. Micronutrient deficiencies, particularly in calcium, vitamin D, and iron, are widespread, affecting bone health and overall well-being. Addressing these challenges requires targeted interventions, including improved healthcare access, nutrition education, and programs to support balanced diets for all socioeconomic groups (World Bank, 2023).
2. **Laos**: In Laos, elderly nutrition is strongly influenced by socioeconomic status. Undernutrition is prevalent among low-income populations, particularly in rural areas, where limited access to diverse and nutrient-rich foods exacerbates issues such as muscle wasting and frailty. Micronutrient deficiencies, including calcium, vitamin D, and iron, are common, further impacting bone health and immunity. In urban areas, higher income groups face rising rates of obesity-related NCDs, such as diabetes and hypertension, driven by sedentary lifestyles and unhealthy diets. Addressing these disparities requires comprehensive strategies, including food security programs, healthcare access, and nutrition education tailored to the needs of the elderly (FAO, 2022).
3. **Myanmar**: In Myanmar, socioeconomic disparities significantly impact elderly nutrition. Undernutrition is prevalent among low-income and rural populations, where food insecurity and limited healthcare access contribute to insufficient calorie and nutrient intake, leading to frailty and poor health outcomes. Micronutrient deficiencies, such as calcium, vitamin D, and iron, are widespread, exacerbating issues such as bone fragility and anemia. Among wealthier urban groups, obesity-related NCDs, including diabetes and cardiovascular diseases, are increasing because of sedentary lifestyles and dietary shifts toward processed foods. Addressing these challenges requires improving healthcare access, food security, and education on balanced diets for elderly individuals across all socioeconomic levels (World Health Organization, 2023).
4. **Vietnam**: In Vietnam, elderly nutrition is closely linked to socioeconomic status. Undernutrition remains a concern for low-income groups around 18%, particularly in rural areas, where limited access to diverse diets and healthcare results in insufficient calorie and protein intake, leading to frailty and health decline. Micronutrient deficiencies, such as calcium, vitamin D, and iron, are widespread, impacting bone health and immunity. In urban areas and among higher income groups, obesity-related NCDs, including diabetes and hypertension, are rising because of dietary changes and sedentary lifestyles. Addressing these challenges requires tailored interventions, including improved healthcare, nutrition education, and access to balanced diets (World Bank, 2023).
5. **Thailand**: In Thailand, elderly nutrition reflects socioeconomic disparities. Undernutrition is prevalent among low-income and rural populations, where poverty limits access to diverse, nutrient-rich diets, leading to frailty and increased health risks. Micronutrient deficiencies, such as calcium, vitamin D, and iron, are widespread across disadvantaged groups, contributing to bone fragility and anemia. In contrast, higher income urban populations face rising rates of obesity-related NCDs, such as diabetes and hypertension, because of sedentary lifestyles and increased consumption of processed foods. Addressing these challenges requires targeted efforts to improve food security, healthcare access, and education on balanced diets for all elderly individuals (United Nations Children's Fund (UNICEF), 2024).

6. **Malaysia**: In Malaysia, elderly nutrition is influenced by socioeconomic disparities. Undernutrition is more common among low-income and rural populations, where limited access to diverse diets and healthcare leads to inadequate intake of calories and nutrients, causing frailty and poor health outcomes. Micronutrient deficiencies, including calcium, vitamin D, and iron, are prevalent, affecting bone health and immunity. In urban and higher income groups, obesity-related (15%) NCDs, such as diabetes, cardiovascular diseases, and hypertension, are rising because of sedentary lifestyles and processed food consumption. Addressing these concerns requires inclusive policies to improve healthcare access, nutrition education, and balanced diets across all socioeconomic levels (World Health Organization, 2023).
7. **Singapore**: In Singapore, elderly nutrition challenges vary with socioeconomic status, though the country's robust healthcare system mitigates some disparities. Undernutrition is uncommon but can affect lower income seniors who face limited access to diverse diets and nutritional support, leading to frailty. Micronutrient deficiencies, including calcium, vitamin D, and iron, are observed across all groups, exacerbated by dietary patterns and reduced physical activity. Higher income elderly populations are more prone to obesity-related NCDs, such as diabetes (30%) and hypertension, because of sedentary lifestyles and high-calorie diets. Addressing these concerns requires integrated healthcare programs, education on balanced diets, and accessible nutrition support for all (Singapore Ministry of Health, 2023).
8. **Indonesia**: In Indonesia, elderly nutrition reflects significant socioeconomic disparities. Undernutrition is prevalent among low-income and rural populations, driven by poverty, food insecurity, and limited access to healthcare, leading to frailty and reduced quality of life. Micronutrient deficiencies, particularly in calcium, vitamin D, and iron, are widespread, further compromising bone health and immunity. In contrast, obesity-related NCDs, such as diabetes and hypertension, are rising in urban and wealthier populations because of sedentary lifestyles and increased consumption of processed foods. Addressing these issues requires targeted interventions to enhance healthcare, promote balanced diets, and improve food security across socioeconomic levels (FAO, 2022).
9. **Philippines**: In the Philippines, elderly nutrition is shaped by socioeconomic inequalities. Undernutrition is widespread among low-income and rural populations, where limited access to diverse diets and healthcare leads to insufficient calorie and nutrient intake, causing frailty and health deterioration. Micronutrient deficiencies, including calcium, vitamin D, and iron, are common, further exacerbating health risks. Conversely, obesity-related NCDs, such as diabetes and hypertension, are rising among urban and higher income elderly populations because of sedentary lifestyles and high-calorie diets. Tackling these challenges requires improved healthcare access, food security programs, and education on balanced diets tailored to the needs of all socioeconomic groups (United Nations Children's Fund (UNICEF), 2024).
10. **Brunei**: In Brunei, elderly nutrition concerns are influenced by socioeconomic status, though the country's wealth and healthcare infrastructure help mitigate disparities. Undernutrition is relatively rare but can affect lower income individuals who face barriers to accessing diverse diets and proper nutritional care. Micronutrient deficiencies, including calcium and vitamin D, are common across all socioeconomic levels, impacting bone health and immunity. Obesity-related NCDs, such as diabetes and hypertension, are prevalent among higher income groups because of sedentary lifestyles and consumption of calorie-dense foods. Addressing these issues requires comprehensive public health campaigns, healthcare accessibility, and education promoting balanced diets and active lifestyles (World Health Organization, 2023).

11. **Timor-Leste**: In Timor-Leste, elderly nutrition is heavily influenced by socioeconomic challenges. Undernutrition is a significant concern, particularly in low-income rural areas where poverty and food insecurity limit access to sufficient calories and nutrients, leading to frailty and poor health. Micronutrient deficiencies, including iron, calcium, and vitamin D, are widespread, further compromising bone health and immunity. Obesity-related NCDs are minimal but may emerge with urbanization and dietary shifts. Addressing these challenges requires focused interventions, such as enhancing food security, improving healthcare access, and educating communities about balanced diets to support healthy aging across all socioeconomic levels (United Nations Children's Fund (UNICEF), 2024).

Nutritional concerns for the elderly in SEA are shaped by physiological changes, such as reduced appetite, slower metabolism, and impaired nutrient absorption, leading to increased risks of micronutrient deficiencies, particularly in calcium, vitamin D, and vitamin B12. Moreover, age-related chronic diseases such as diabetes, hypertension, and arthritis necessitate tailored dietary approaches, whereas adequate protein intake is essential to prevent muscle loss and maintain functionality. In contrast, cognitive health is impacted by deficiencies in omega-3s, antioxidants, and B vitamins, highlighting the need for brain-supportive diets. Barriers such as limited income, social isolation, and oral health issues, including tooth loss, affect food choices. Hydration is often neglected because of reduced thirst perception. Cultural diets offer nutritional benefits but must be adapted to modern needs. Food safety, accessibility, and counseling are critical, alongside community meal programs and gender-specific strategies. Climate change, economic transitions, and the judicious use of supplements further influence elderly nutrition, requiring comprehensive, targeted interventions.

5.7 Regional initiatives and policy interventions

Governments and organizations in SEA are working to address these nutritional disparities through various initiatives, such as school feeding programs, public awareness campaigns, fortification programs, and collaborative efforts. SEA countries have implemented various initiatives to address nutritional challenges, with programs tailored to local needs, often supported by international organizations.

1. **Cambodia**: The *World Food Programme* supports school feeding programs, providing fortified rice to combat undernutrition. Public campaigns promote dietary diversity, whereas fortification programs address vitamin A and iodine deficiencies (WFP, 2023).
2. **Laos**: School meals supported by *UNICEF* and *FAO* focus on reducing stunting and improving micronutrient intake. Public awareness campaigns emphasize balanced diets, and salt iodization programs are implemented nationally (FAO, 2022).
3. **Myanmar**: School feeding initiatives led by *WFP* and *Save the Children* target malnutrition. Fortification programs for rice and flour address micronutrient gaps, whereas national campaigns promote healthy eating (World Health Organization, 2023).
4. **Vietnam**: The government partners with *UNICEF* and *FAO* to support school meals and promote breastfeeding. Fortification programs focus on iron and zinc, whereas campaigns raise awareness of obesity risks (World Bank, 2023).

Table 5.1 Ongoing national and international initiatives to improve the nutritional status in SEA countries.

Countries	Initiatives and policy interventions	Focus area
Cambodia	–World Food Programme supports school feeding programs with fortified rice –Public campaigns promoting dietary diversity –Fortification programs addressing vitamin A and iodine deficiencies –National programs improving access to safe drinking water and sanitation facilities	Combating undernutrition, improving hygiene, and reducing waterborne diseases
Laos	–School meals supported by UNICEF and FAO –National salt iodization programs –Public campaigns emphasizing balanced diets –Efforts to expand rural access to safe drinking water and sanitation	Reducing stunting, improving micronutrient intake, and hygiene standards
Myanmar	–School feeding programs by WFP and Save the Children –Rice and flour fortification programs –National campaigns on healthy eating –Infrastructure projects for clean water supply and sanitation facilities	Addressing malnutrition, micronutrient gaps, and waterborne illnesses
Vietnam	–School meal programs with UNICEF and FAO –Fortification initiatives focusing on iron and zinc –Awareness campaigns on obesity risks –Initiatives to improve access to clean drinking water and sanitation facilities	Promoting child nutrition, addressing obesity, and improving hygiene

(continued on next page)

Thailand	–Mandatory fortification of salt with iodine –School lunch program for balanced meals –Campaigns promoting active lifestyles and addressing obesity –Programs to ensure urban and rural water supply access and sanitation facilities	Tackling malnutrition, lifestyle diseases, and hygiene challenges
Malaysia	–Targeted school feeding programs for underprivileged children –Fortification efforts for vitamin D and iron –"Eat Right Malaysia" campaign addressing undernutrition and obesity –National efforts to provide clean water and sanitation in underserved areas	Balancing undernutrition, overnutrition, and improving public health infrastructure
Singapore	–Healthier Choice Symbol campaigns for healthy eating –Mandatory fortification programs for vitamin D and calcium –School initiatives promoting balanced diets –Advanced water sanitation and recycling technologies ensuring universal access to clean drinking water	Encouraging healthier dietary practices and leading in water management
Indonesia	–Government-WFP partnership for fortified school meals –Public campaigns on dietary diversity –Salt iodization programs –Clean water access and sanitation facility improvements, especially in rural areas	Improving dietary quality, combating deficiencies, and hygiene

(continued on next page)

Table 5.1 Ongoing national and international initiatives to improve the nutritional status in SEA countries—cont'd

Countries	Initiatives and policy interventions	Focus area
Philippines	–DepEd's school-based feeding program –"Pinggang Pinoy" campaign promoting balanced diets –Fortification programs for rice and oil –WASH programs focusing on schools and communities	Addressing undernutrition, promoting balanced diets, and improving hygiene
Brunei	–Health programs promoting balanced school diets –Fortification initiatives for calcium and vitamin D –Awareness campaigns addressing obesity –Comprehensive sanitation infrastructure and safe water access programs	Addressing obesity, improving nutrition, and ensuring hygiene
Timor-Leste	–WFP and FAO collaboration on school feeding programs –National salt iodization programs –Public campaigns promoting dietary diversity –Programs improving rural access to safe drinking water and sanitation	Tackling severe undernutrition, deficiencies, and hygiene challenges

SEA, Southeast Asia; *WASH*, water, sanitation, and hygiene.

5. **Thailand**: The *School Lunch Program* provides balanced meals to reduce malnutrition. Fortification of salt with iodine is mandatory, whereas public campaigns address rising obesity and promote active lifestyles (United Nations Children's Fund (UNICEF), 2024).
6. **Malaysia**: School feeding programs target underprivileged children, and fortification efforts include vitamin D and iron. National campaigns, such as "Eat Right Malaysia," address obesity and undernutrition (World Health Organization, 2023).
7. **Singapore**: The *Health Promotion Board* implements campaigns like "Healthier Choice Symbol" to encourage healthy eating. Fortification programs for vitamin D and calcium are mandatory. School initiatives promote balanced diets (Singapore Ministry of Health, 2023).
8. **Indonesia**: The government partners with *WFP* for school meals, focusing on fortified foods. Public campaigns promote dietary diversity, and salt iodization programs combat deficiencies (FAO, 2022).
9. **Philippines**: *DepEd's School-Based Feeding Program* addresses undernutrition, whereas campaigns like "Pinggang Pinoy" promote balanced diets. Fortification programs for rice and oil combat micronutrient deficiencies (United Nations Children's Fund (UNICEF), 2024).
10. **Brunei**: Health programs promote balanced diets in schools, and fortification efforts ensure calcium and vitamin D supplementation. Awareness campaigns address rising obesity (World Health Organization, 2023).
11. **Timor-Leste**: *WFP* and *FAO* collaborate on school feeding programs to address severe undernutrition. Salt iodization programs are widespread, and public campaigns emphasize the importance of diverse diets (United Nations Children's Fund (UNICEF), 2024).

Ongoing national and international initiatives to improve the nutritional status in SEA countries are given in Table 5.1.

5.8 Conclusion: Toward a holistic approach

Addressing nutritional challenges in SEA requires a multifaceted approach that considers cultural diversity, economic conditions, and demographic transitions. By leveraging traditional dietary practices and integrating modern nutritional science, the region can combat both undernutrition and the rising prevalence of overnutrition. Governments must prioritize policies that ensure equitable access to nutritious foods, foster public-private partnerships, and invest in education campaigns to promote healthy eating habits.

The involvement of international organizations, such as WHO and UNICEF, is critical for guiding national governments in developing evidence-based strategies. Initiatives such as fortifying staple foods and improving maternal and child health programs have shown potential but require expansion and sustained funding to maximize their impact.

Research plays a vital role in addressing emerging issues, such as the dietary impacts of climate change and the nutritional needs of rapidly aging populations. Scholars and policymakers should collaborate to monitor and evaluate the effectiveness of interventions, ensuring they are adaptive and inclusive.

In conclusion, SEA has the potential to transform its nutritional landscape through concerted efforts that combine traditional knowledge, scientific advancements, and comprehensive policy frameworks. A sustained commitment from all stakeholders—governments, communities, and international partners—is essential to achieving nutrition security and fostering healthier generations.

References

FAO. (2022). *Regional nutrition overview*. Food and Agriculture Organization Retrieved from https://openknowledge.fao.org/server/api/core/bitstreams/8452ccd1-96eb-45bf-90ec-a4864f5a757e/content.

Gaupholm, J., Papadopoulos, A., Asif, A., Dodd, W., & Little, M. (2023). The influence of food environments on dietary behaviour and nutrition in Southeast Asia: A systematic scoping review. *Nutrition and Health, 29*(2), 231–253. https://pubmed.ncbi.nlm.nih.gov/35850565/.

Singapore Ministry of Health. (2023). *Childhood nutrition in Singapore*. Singapore Ministry of Health Retrieved from https://corp.nhg.com.sg/Media%20Releases/NEW%20SINGAPORE%20STANDARD%20TO%20GUIDE%20NUTRITION%20AND%20FOOD%20SERVICES%20FOR%20INFANTS%20AND%20CHILDREN_31%20May%202023_FINAL.pdf.

UNICEF. (2021). *Southeast Asia Regional Report on maternal nutrition and complementary feeding. UNICEF East Asia and Pacific Region*. UNICEF Retrieved from https://www.unicef.org/eap/media/9466/file/Maternal%20Nutrition%20and%20Complementary%20Feeding%20Regional%20Report.pdf.

United Nations Children's Fund (UNICEF). (2024). *The state of the world's children 2024: Nutrition*. UNICEF Retrieved from https://www.unicef.org/reports/state-of-worlds-children/2024.

WFP. (2023). *School* feeding programs *in Southeast Asia*. WFP Retrieved from https://www.wfp.org/stories/how-school-meals-transform-futures-children-and-communities-cambodia.

World Bank. (2023). *Nutrition data Southeast Asia*. World Bank Retrieved from https://www.worldbank.org/en/topic/nutrition/overview.

World Health Organization. (2023). *Nutrition challenges in Southeast Asia: Stunting, wasting, and obesity trends*. WHO Regional Office for South-East Asia Retrieved from https://iris.who.int/bitstream/handle/10665/380407/SEA-NCD-112-eng.pdf?sequence=1.

Worldometer. (2024). Population of South-Eastern Asia (2025). Worldometer-World Population. https://www.worldometers.info/world-population/south-eastern-asia-population/

6 Nutrition study of young children in Bangladesh: Scope of improvement

Md. Latiful Bari[a] *and Sabina Yeasmin*[b]
[a]Center for Advanced Research in Sciences, University of Dhaka, Dhaka, Bangladesh, [b]Department of Genetic Engineering and Biotechnology, University of Dhaka, Dhaka, Bangladesh

6.1 Introduction

Nutrition and food are among the most basic human requirements, and children's nutritional condition can be used as a health indicator of a country's progress. Undernutrition is defined by a lack of vital nutrients such as proteins, vitamins, and minerals, which can result in stunting (impaired growth and development), wasting (rapid weight loss), and micronutrient deficiencies such as iron, iodine, or vitamin A. Overnutrition, on the other hand, refers to an excessive intake of calories, which frequently results in obesity and other health problems such as diabetes, cardiovascular disease, and certain malignancies. The word "malnutrition" has been used to encompass all types of undernutrition (wasting, stunting, and underweight), insufficient vitamin and mineral intake, obesity, and the resulting noncommunicable diseases (NCDs) associated with diet. Acute childhood malnutrition is associated with a higher risk of dying from childhood infections such as diarrhea, pneumonia, and malaria, as well as a variety of psychological issues (World Health Organization (WHO), 2024b). In the 1990s 60% of Bangladeshi children were stunted, 52% were underweight, and 21% were wasting (NIPORT, 1997). However, various intervention approaches and policies were developed and implemented across the country to enhance children's nutritional status. The most current Demographic and Health Survey (BDHS) statistics revealed that 23.6% of children were stunted, 22.3% were underweight, and 11% were wasting (NIPORT, 2023). Despite significant economic progress and poverty reduction, child food poverty remains a significant challenge in Bangladesh, with recent reports indicating that two out of every three children under the age of 5 are affected (UNICEF, 2024). This situation is exacerbated by inadequate dietary diversity; one in five children consumes only one or two food groups daily, leading to severe nutritional deficiencies (UNICEF, 2024). Despite this, millions of parents and families are failing to provide the nutritious and diverse foods that young children require to attain their full potential as a result of child food insecurity. Child food poverty, according to UNICEF, is defined as children's inability to access and consume a nutritious and diverse diet during their early childhood. Child food poverty affects all children, but it is especially harmful

Nutritional Strategies, Predictive Models, and Sustainable Policies. DOI: https://doi.org/10.1016/B978-0-443-23671-6.00016-5

in early childhood, when insufficient dietary intake of essential nutrients can have the greatest impact on child survival, physical growth, and cognitive development, trapping children and their families in a cycle of poverty and deprivation. Growing disparities, conflict, and climatic problems, along with growing food prices, an oversupply of unhealthy foods, destructive food marketing methods, and poor child feeding practices, are causing millions of children to become food insecure.

Furthermore, maternal nutrition inadequacies are significant in both children under 5 years old and nonpregnant and nonlactating (NPNL) women of reproductive age in Bangladesh. Common deficiencies include iron, folic acid, calcium, vitamin A, and iodine. Around 40%–50% of pregnant women are anemic because of poor dietary intake, frequent pregnancies, and parasitic infections. Vitamin D and zinc deficiencies are highly prevalent in NPNL women in Bangladesh. Iodine, folate, iron deficiency, and anemia prevalence are also persistent among women of reproductive age warrants urgent attention of the policymakers. However, maternal malnutrition requires a multisectoral response, coordinated efforts in health, agriculture, education, and social protection. To address maternal malnutrition effectively a combination of health, nutritional, social, and policy-based intervention strategies is required. In addition, strong leadership and community engagement are crucial to ensuring long-term success and breaking the cycle of malnutrition in mothers and their children. In Bangladesh, undernutrition is still a major problem, but overweight and obesity are increasingly growing issues; 10% of unmarried women aged 15–19 and 16% of married women are overweight or obese (NIPORT, 2023). In 2019 38% of adolescent girls had started having children by the age of 19 (Bangladesh Bureau of Statistics (BBS), 2019). Adolescent underweight is on the rise, whereas adolescent pregnancy rates remain high. Adolescent pregnancy is related with a 50% greater risk of stillbirths and neonatal fatalities, as well as an increased risk of low-birth weight (LBW) (23% in Bangladesh) (National Nutrition Service (NNS) et al., 2017), premature birth, asphyxia, and maternal mortality (Bhutta et al., 2013).

Poor sanitation and hygiene, which cause diarrhea and other infectious disorders, lead to child malnutrition. Gender inequality in decision-making over household production and consumption also contributes to the consequent poor nutritional condition of mothers and young children. Undernutrition is compounded by a lack of dietary diversity, with grains accounting for 70% of the diet, and insufficient protein and micronutrient consumption (Magnani et al., 2015). Almost two-thirds of children aged 6 months to 2 years do not receive the nutritional diversity necessary for optimal growth and development. In addition, breastfeeding practices, though improving, remain inconsistent, with many infants not exclusively breastfed during the critical early months of life. Thus insufficient infant and young child feeding (IYCF) practices contribute to the high prevalence of malnutrition. Furthermore, vitamin deficiencies remain an issue in Bangladesh. The national salt iodization policy has been effective in lowering iodine shortage, with 76% of households using iodized salt. However, deficiencies in vitamins A, B12, zinc, and folate, as well as maternal and child anemia, remain a problem. Preschool children are projected to have a 21% vitamin A deficit, 45% zinc insufficiency, and 51% anemia (Bangladesh Bureau of Statistics (BBS), 2019).

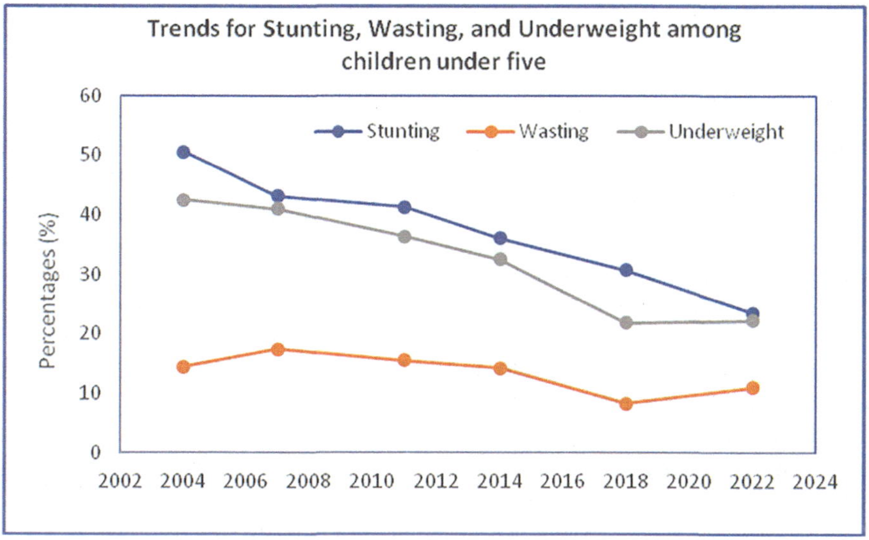

Figure 6.1 Trends of stunting, wasting, and underweight in Bangladesh (2004–22).

6.2 Nutritional status of young children in Bangladesh

6.2.1 *Prevalence of malnutrition*

Child nutrition in Bangladesh remains a pressing concern, with significant portions of the population affected by malnutrition. According to recent reports, approximately 23.6% of children under 5 years old are stunted, and 9% are severely stunted, reflecting chronic undernutrition. Wasting, a marker of acute malnutrition, affects about 11% of children in this age group (NIPORT, 2022). The nutritional landscape for children under 5 in Bangladesh has undergone substantial changes over the past decade. The trends for stunting, wasting, and underweight reveal both progress and persistent challenges in addressing different dimensions of malnutrition.

Stunting: The prevalence of stunting has decreased significantly from 50.6% in 2004 to 23.6% in 2022 (Fig. 6.1). This decline reflects improvements in maternal and child healthcare services, increased access to nutrition education, and community-based programs promoting dietary diversity. However, regional disparities remain, with rural and marginalized populations facing higher rates. Although the sharp reduction in stunting is encouraging, the prevalence still exceeds the World Health Organization (WHO)'s thresholds for public health concern in some regions. Long-term interventions aimed at improving maternal nutrition, antenatal care (ANC), and sanitation are vital for sustaining this trend.

Wasting: Wasting rates have reduced more gradually, from 14.5% in 2004 to 11.0% in 2022. This slower progress indicates that acute malnutrition is harder to address because of recurring factors such as food insecurity, natural disasters, and disease outbreaks. Wasting is still a critical public health issue requiring urgent intervention.

The relatively slower decline in wasting highlights the urgent need for responsive measures such as ready-to-use therapeutic foods (RUTFs) and better integration of emergency response mechanisms into routine healthcare.

Underweight: The proportion of underweight children has fallen from 42.5% in 2004 to 22.3% in 2022. This improvement suggests that a combination of enhanced food security and targeted nutrition programs has positively influenced weight-for-age metrics in children. The improvements in underweight prevalence reflect gains in addressing general malnutrition. Scaling up food fortification and maternal education programs can accelerate this progress.

Micronutrient deficiencies: Micronutrient deficiencies are widespread among Bangladeshi children under the age of 5, and the situation has not improved considerably during the last decade (2011–21). Bangladesh completed its first National Micronutrient Survey (NMS) in 2011–12, followed by a second in 2019–20. The prevalence of important micronutrients, such as vitamin A, iron, zinc, vitamin D, and iodine, was calculated among children under the age of 5, school-aged children, and NPNL women. Overall vitamin A deficiency (mild to severe) was recorded as 50.9% (95% CI: 46.3%–55.5%), where mild vitamin A deficiency was recorded as 43.7% and moderate vitamin A deficiency was recorded as 7.2% and no severe deficiency was observed in the NMS 2019–20. Mild vitamin A deficiency reduced 12.6% and moderate vitamin A deficiency reduced 12.8% compared to 2011–12 NMS. Overall vitamin D deficiency was recorded as 21.9% (95% CI: 18.8%–25.5%) in 2019–20 NMS, which was 39.6% in 2011–12 NMS, indicating 18% reduction of vitamin D deficiency in children under 5 years.

Fig. 2 Comparison of micronutrient deficiency in children under 5 years in the national micronutrient survey 2011–12 and 2019–20.

Zinc deficiency in children under 5 years in NMS 2011–12 was recorded as 44.6%, and these values in NMS 2019–20 survey was recorded as 31.0%, revealed a 13.6% reduction. On the contrary, iron deficiency increased by 4.4% (from 10.7% in 2011–12 NMS to 15.1% in 2019–20 NMS) among children under 5 years. The national prevalence of iodine deficiency was not reported in 2011–12 NMS; however, the 2019–20 NMS reported an overall of 19.7% (95% CI: 17.2%–22.1%), with 11.7% mild, 6.8% moderate, and 1.2% severe iodine deficiency. Furthermore the overall prevalence of anemia in 2011–12 NMS was recorded as 33.1% and reduced 12.0%–21.1% (95% CI: 18.6%–23.9%), with mild 14.0%, moderate 6.7%, and severe only 0.4% in NMS 2019–20 survey.

6.2.2 Overnutrition

Overnutrition, characterized by excess energy intake leading to overweight and obesity, is an emerging public health concern in Bangladesh. Traditionally associated with high-income countries the rise in overnutrition among children in Bangladesh reflects a shift in dietary habits, urbanization, and lifestyle changes, particularly in urban areas. The prevalence of overweight/obesity among children under 5 years was recorded as 0.7% in 2000, which increases to 2.1% in 2022 [World Health Organization (WHO), 2024a]. An increasing trend was observed, whereas undernutrition remains a major challenge in

Bangladesh; rates of overweight and obesity among children are increasing, especially in urban and affluent populations. The Bangladesh Demographic and Health Survey (BDHS, 2023) indicates a growing double burden of malnutrition, where overnutrition coexists with undernutrition. Parents and caregivers often do not recognize obesity as a problem and think that overweight children may be perceived as healthier; as a result, children are more likely to become overweight adults, perpetuating a cycle of intergenerational overnutrition. Overweight children may experience low self-esteem, bullying, and body image issues. Furthermore, hormonal imbalances associated with obesity can lead to early puberty and may increase risk of NCDs, including Type 2 diabetes, hypertension, cardiovascular diseases, and fatty liver disease in later life, which will increase healthcare costs for families and the health system to manage obesity-related conditions.

6.3 Determinants of malnutrition

Malnutrition in Bangladesh is a multifaceted issue influenced by a combination of economic, social, cultural, environmental, and healthcare-related factors. The immediate causes of child undernutrition can be categorized into two primary factors, including inadequate dietary intake and disease or illness, both of which directly affect a child's nutritional status. The underlying causes of child undernutrition have been linked to a number of factors, including food insecurity in the home, poor feeding and care practices, an unpleasant home environment, and insufficient or nonexistent access to health care. The basic causes of undernutrition are rooted in systemic and structural factors that impact the availability and access to resources necessary for adequate nutrition. All these factors contribute to persistent undernutrition among children in Bangladesh. The following are some of the key factors contributing to child malnutrition in Bangladesh (Table 6.1).

6.3.1 Dietary diversity and illness

Dietary diversity is the variety of foods or food groups ingested over a specific period, usually a day or week. It is a key indicator of diet quality and nutritional adequacy. A diverse diet ensures a broad intake of essential macronutrients (carbohydrates, proteins, and fats) and micronutrients (vitamins and minerals), which are critical for health and development. Child nutrition and feeding practices are pivotal in shaping the physical, cognitive, and emotional development of children, particularly during the first 1000 days of life (from conception to the child's second birthday). Inadequate nutrition during this vital period can cause permanent damage, such as stunting, decreased brain development, and diminished immunity. Minimum dietary diversity (MDD) is consuming foods from five or more of the following eight food groups: (1) breast milk; (2) grains, white or pale starchy roots, tubers, and plantains; (3) legumes, nuts, and seeds; (4) dairy items (fresh, bottled, and powdered milk; newborn formula; yogurt; cheese); (5) meat, fish, poultry, and organ meats; (6) eggs; (7) vitamin A-rich fruits and vegetables; and (8) other fruits and vegetables. However, heavy reliance on staple foods

Table 6.1 Key factors contributing to child malnutrition in Bangladesh.

Sl. no.	Major factors	Subfactors
1	**Socioeconomic factors**	**Poverty:** Nearly 18.7% of the population lives below the poverty line (World Bank, 2022), limiting access to diverse and nutritious foods. Families often prioritize calorie-dense staples like rice over more expensive nutrient-rich foods such as fruits, vegetables, and proteins **Education:** Mothers are the primary caregivers for their children, and the quality of care they provide is strongly dependent on their knowledge of nutrition and health-related topics. Maternal education is strongly associated with better child nutrition outcomes (Banu et al., 2023). **Employment:** Limited employment opportunities reduce purchasing power, affecting food security and dietary quality
2	**Food security and dietary patterns**	**Food insecurity:** Seasonal food shortages, natural disasters, and climate variability impact food production and availability. Households often face chronic or acute food insecurity, particularly in rural and disaster-prone areas **Dietary monotony:** Heavy reliance on staple foods like rice contributes to energy sufficiency but lacks essential micronutrients. Low intake of protein, fruits, and vegetables results in widespread micronutrient deficiencies
3	**Healthcare and nutrition services**	**Limited access to healthcare:** Many people in rural and remote areas lack access to quality healthcare facilities for preventive and curative nutrition services **Inadequate antenatal and childcare services:** Low coverage of maternal and child health programs reduces opportunities for early detection and treatment of malnutrition **Insufficient micronutrient supplementation:** Limited distribution and poor compliance with programs for iron, folic acid, and vitamin A supplementation

(*continued on next page*)

Table 6.1 Key factors contributing to child malnutrition in Bangladesh—cont'd

Sl. no.	Major factors	Subfactors
4	**Gender inequality and social norms**	**Early marriage and pregnancy:** High rates of adolescent pregnancies lead to young mothers who are biologically unprepared for the nutritional demands of pregnancy and lactation **Gender disparities in food allocation:** In many households, women and girls eat last and often consume smaller portions, leading to undernutrition **Low female education and empowerment:** Lack of education and decision-making power among women limits their ability to prioritize their health and nutrition
5	**Cultural and behavioral factors**	**Food taboos and myths:** Cultural beliefs often restrict the consumption of certain nutritious foods during pregnancy and lactation **Inadequate knowledge:** Poor awareness about proper dietary practices and the importance of nutrition during pregnancy, lactation, and early childhood **Suboptimal infant and young child feeding practices:** High rates of delayed breastfeeding initiation, inadequate exclusive breastfeeding, and poor complementary feeding practices
6	**Environmental and climatic factors**	**Natural disasters:** Frequent floods, cyclones, and droughts disrupt food production, supply chains, and healthcare access, exacerbating malnutrition **Climate change:** Rising temperatures and changing rainfall patterns affect agricultural yields and food security
7	**Policy and governance issues**	**Weak implementation of programs:** Nutrition-specific and nutrition-sensitive programs often face implementation challenges, including lack of coordination and inadequate funding **Limited safety nets:** Social safety net programs often fail to cover the most vulnerable populations effectively **Insufficient monitoring:** Poor data collection and monitoring mechanisms hinder the ability to track malnutrition trends and the effectiveness of interventions

(*continued on next page*)

Table 6.1 Key factors contributing to child malnutrition in Bangladesh—cont'd

Sl. no.	Major factors	Subfactors
8	**Disease and health-related factors**	**High disease burden:** Infections such as diarrhea, respiratory illnesses, and parasitic infections increase nutrient requirements and reduce absorption **Poor sanitation and hygiene:** Lack of access to clean water and proper sanitation contributes to frequent illnesses, perpetuating the cycle of malnutrition **Low immunization rates:** Inadequate vaccination coverage exposes children to preventable diseases that exacerbate malnutrition

like rice contributes to energy sufficiency but lacks essential micronutrients. Low intake of protein, fruits, and vegetables results in widespread micronutrient deficiencies. The major challenges in feeding diverse diet to children include limit access to diverse and nutrient-rich foods, lack knowledge of mother or caregivers on optimal feeding practices, including the importance of dietary diversity and hygienic preparation of complementary foods. Furthermore, misconceptions about food during illness and postpartum periods often restrict nutrient intake for mothers and children. Animal proteins, nutritional diversity, and foods high in micronutrients are recognized as essential elements of a healthy diet for children.

6.3.1.1 Breastfeeding

Exclusive breastfeeding (EBF) for the first 6 months of life is a key recommendation by the WHO. However, in Bangladesh, while breastfeeding initiation rates are high, EBF rates drop significantly before the 6-month mark. Only 62% of infants are exclusively breastfed for the first 6 months. Breastfeeding significantly improves immunity, reduces infant mortality, and supports healthy growth and development. A mixed-methods study also found considerable gaps in breastfeeding behaviors among Bangladeshi mothers, primarily because of a lack of understanding about why medically prescribed breastfeeding practices are helpful, the costs of not doing them, and how to practice them. Interactions between health providers to promote and support optimal breastfeeding are exceedingly low (Haider et al., 2010). During the first 6 months of infancy, there is often confusion over EBF techniques in which other liquids are also offered. Misconceptions regarding breastfeeding, supplemental feeding, and dietary diversity contribute to poor nutrition practices.

6.3.1.2 Complementary feeding

After 6 months of EBF, supplemental feeding is advised; however, in Bangladesh, only around 34% of children aged 6–23 months receive the MDD required for healthy growth. Optimal infant feeding practices are crucial for promoting healthy growth and improving nutritional outcomes in infants. Key components of these practices include appropriate portion sizes, regular feeding frequency, the inclusion of micronutrient-rich foods, and active encouragement during feeding. A study published in the Journal of Health, Population and Nutrition emphasizes that adhering to these feeding recommendations—such as proper portion sizes, consistent feeding schedules, offering nutrient-dense foods, and encouraging infants to eat—significantly contributes to better growth during infancy and early childhood (Saha et al., 2008). According to a Dhaka-based study (Jesmin et al., 2011), approximately 26% of mothers give their children complementary food less than four times a day, which can have a negative impact on a child's nutritional status. Undernutrition is most common in children older than 7 months, and the primary cause of malnutrition is inadequate supplemental food given following EBF (Ahmed et al., 2012). Poor feeding habits include insufficient frequency and reliance on nutrient-deficient staple meals, which frequently lack vital vitamins and minerals such as iron and vitamin A. Furthermore the growing reliance on processed and packaged meals that are thought to be healthier or more convenient exacerbates nutrient deficiencies in children.

6.3.2 *Disease/Illness*

In Bangladesh, children under 5 years old face significant health challenges, with common illnesses including fever, cough, diarrhea, and acute respiratory infections (ARIs) (Islam et al., 2024). Common ailments include respiratory infections, diarrhea, malnutrition, and vaccine-preventable diseases such as measles and whooping cough. ARIs, particularly pneumonia, remain a leading cause of mortality in this age group (World Health Organization (WHO), 2023). ARIs and diarrheal diseases are leading causes of mortality among children under 5 years old. ARI accounts for approximately 25% of deaths in this age group (Islam et al., 2022), whereas diarrheal diseases contribute to about 13% of under-5 child deaths (Ahmed et al., 2018). These statistics highlight the significant impact of ARI and diarrheal diseases on child mortality in Bangladesh. In addition, malnutrition, including stunting, wasting, and micronutrient deficiencies, affects a substantial proportion of children, weakening their immunity and making them more susceptible to infections, with approximately 24% of Bangladeshi children under 5 experiencing stunted growth (World Bank, 2022). Furthermore, floods and other natural disasters increase the risk of waterborne diseases, further threatening child health. Although government programs and international initiatives have improved vaccination coverage and healthcare access, significant disparities remain, particularly in rural and impoverished communities. Addressing these challenges requires comprehensive strategies focusing on improving nutrition, enhancing access to clean water and sanitation, and strengthening healthcare services to reduce the burden of disease among young children in Bangladesh.

6.4 Maternal malnutrition

Poor maternal nutrition during pregnancy is typically associated with LBW and developmental delays in offspring. Poor maternal nutrition, which is widespread in Bangladesh, particularly among adolescent girls, plays a crucial role in perpetuating a cycle of hunger and poverty. Malnourished adolescent females are more likely to become malnourished mothers, which can have consequences ranging from the intrauterine development period to the health and nutritional status of birth outcomes (Ahmed et al., 2012). Maternal health, both during pregnancy and EBF, as well as while caring for a child, is a good predictor of pregnancy outcomes and a child's nutritional status.

6.4.1 Nutritional status of mothers

In Bangladesh, severe and moderate acute undernutrition were significantly impacted by maternal nutrition status. A increased risk of wasting, LBW, and acute undernutrition in children was linked to low maternal nutrition levels (Rahman et al., 2009). Numerous studies have demonstrated that a mother's nutritional status can impact the size of her fetus at birth (Rahman et al., 2009). A 2008 study found that the prevalence of child undernutrition decreased with the quality of maternal care (Das & Hossain, 2008). According to the Bangladesh NMS; 2019–20, 42.4% of NPNL women are zinc deficient, 29% are folate deficient, and 28.9% of NPNL women suffer from anemia. Furthermore, 8% of women aged 15–19 who are single and 4% of women who have ever been married are underweight (BMI < 18.5). In Bangladesh, undernutrition is still a major problem, but overweight and obesity are increasingly growing issues; 10% of unmarried women aged 15–19 and 16% of married women are overweight or obese (NIPORT, 2021). According to the Bangladesh Bureau of Statistics (BBS) (2019), 38% of teenage girls had started having children before the age of 19. A worrying trend is the rising incidence of underweight among adolescents coupled with high and ongoing rates of adolescent pregnancies. Teenage pregnancy is linked to a 50% higher chance of stillbirths and neonatal fatalities, as well as a higher chance of LBW (23% in Bangladesh), premature birth, asphyxia, and maternal death (Bhutta et al., 2013).

Fig. 3 Micronutrient deficiency and anemia among NPNL women in Bangladesh in NMS 2019–20. *NMS*, National Micronutrient Survey; *NPNL*, nonpregnant and nonlactating.

Limited access to nutritious food, early marriage and early pregnancies results in higher nutritional demands on young mothers. Seasonal food shortages and reliance on staple crops like rice, which lack essential nutrients. Poor awareness of dietary needs during pregnancy, inadequate access to prenatal care and supplementation, are the contributing factors of maternal malnutrition. All of these factors contributed to the consequences of LBW and stunting, increased neonatal mortality and morbidity, and long-term cognitive and physical impairments.

6.4.2 Health and well-being of caregivers

The nutritional status and general development of a kid are significantly impacted by the health and wellbeing of caregivers, especially mothers. Research indicates that caregivers in good physical and mental health are better equipped to provide consistent, responsive, and nurturing care, which directly influences feeding practices and dietary quality for children (World Health Organization (WHO), 2020). Maternal mental health, such as the presence of depression or anxiety, has been linked to suboptimal breastfeeding and inadequate complementary feeding, which can lead to malnutrition (Black et al., 2013). Antepartum depression symptoms were shown to predict infant stunting, whereas postpartum depression symptoms were linked to LBW and impaired motor development in newborns (Nasreen et al., 2010, 2013). In addition, children's birth order and birth interval are also associated with undernutrition, and short birth intervals can affect health outcomes, put more pressure on caregivers, and influence children's nutritional condition. There is proof that a birth interval of more than 24 months lowers the prevalence of stunting in Bangladesh's rural areas as well as wasting and stunting in urban children (Khan & Raza, 2013). Furthermore, caregivers with better nutritional health are more likely to model healthy eating behaviors and make informed food choices for their children (Walker et al., 2011). Addressing caregiver well-being through health interventions, social support, and education can, therefore, play a critical role in improving child nutritional outcomes.

6.4.3 Maternal age

Mother's age has been found to be a predictor in birth outcomes, with children of adolescent mothers having a higher risk of undernutrition than nonadolescent mothers (Abdullah et al., 2007). Such mothers are also likely to be uneducated, increasing the risk of continuing malnutrition as the children grow older. Adolescence is regarded as a critical stage in physical development because it is the final time at which interventions might influence the effects of nutritional deficits (Chowdhury et al., 2006). In Bangladesh, adolescence is also a typical time for girls to become pregnant; hence a child's nutritional state during this period can foreshadow malnutrition. According to the Bangladesh Demographic and Health Survey (BDHS) 2022, 24% of women between the ages of 15 and 19 have started having children. Malnutrition is common among teenage girls and pregnant women in Bangladesh, with one-third of them having a low BMI and anemia (Ahmed et al., 2012). According to a recent household survey, stunting and thinness were common and persistent among teenage girls between the ages of 13 and 19 (Alam et al., 2010). It has been demonstrated that children of healthy mothers are less likely to be underweight than children of malnourished mothers, maybe as a result of thin mothers' insufficient breast milk production (Rayhan & Khan, 2006). Nutritional deficiencies were detected among teenage females working in garment industries. The underlying causes of malnutrition were connected to insufficient eating habits and a lack of essential micronutrients (Khan & Ahmed, 2005).

6.4.4 Child care giving

As children are vulnerable and rely on others for quality and quantity of care, mothers/caregivers have an important role in influencing their nutritional condition and overall health outcomes. Mothers and caregivers are central to determining the nutritional status and health outcomes of children, as they provide essential care, feeding, and emotional support during critical developmental stages. Their knowledge, attitudes, and practices around nutrition significantly affect children's dietary intake and overall health. Studies highlight that maternal education and empowerment are strongly associated with improved child nutrition and reduced rates of malnutrition and stunting (Smith & Haddad, 2015). Moreover, caregivers' ability to access healthcare, maintain hygiene, and manage illnesses directly impacts children's health and survival outcomes (UNICEF, 2019). Although depending on the child's age, maternal work outside the home may result in the neglect of exclusive breastfeeding, which can lead to undernutrition, children of working mothers had better nutritional outcomes than those of full-time housewives (Jesmin et al., 2011). Feeding practices can be classified as active, social, or responsive, and depending on the caregiver–child interaction during feeding practices and children response during feeding times may have different nutrition outcomes. Negative feeding behaviors, such as force feeding, were demonstrated to be ineffective (Moore et al., 2006). Therefore interventions targeting caregiver education and support, combined with community resources, are essential for fostering positive health outcomes in children.

6.5 Healthcare and sanitation

6.5.1 Access to healthcare

Access to healthcare is a critical determinant of nutritional status in Bangladesh, where limited healthcare services, particularly in rural areas, exacerbate malnutrition among vulnerable populations. Lack of preventive and curative healthcare contributes to infections, poor maternal health, and untreated illnesses, all of which can lead to malnutrition. Furthermore, lack of maternal and child health services leads to poor prenatal care, LBW, and inadequate child nutrition. Recurrent infections, such as diarrhea, pneumonia, and measles, weaken children's immune systems and hinder their ability to absorb nutrients (Morales et al., 2023). Untreated intestinal parasitic infections further deplete nutrients from the body. Poor maternal nutrition and healthcare during pregnancy increase the risk of malnourished infants. In addition, lack of awareness and access to supplements such as iron, folic acid, and calcium perpetuate cycles of malnutrition. Furthermore, low immunization rates leave children vulnerable to infections, whereas limited access to growth monitoring and early interventions for malnutrition delays treatment (Tette et al., 2015). Diarrhea, respiratory infections, and parasitic infestations exacerbate malnutrition by impairing nutrient absorption. Approximately 66% of Bangladeshis reside in rural regions, facing challenges such as inadequate healthcare infrastructure and interrupted access to essential health services (Akter & Kabir, 2023). This lack of access impedes the timely management of malnutrition and related health issues. Children from poorer households are at a higher risk of malnutrition, partly because of their limited capacity to access essential healthcare services, lack of potable water, and inadequate sanitation (Islam et al., 2019). Although child nutrition has steadily improved, with stunting rates dropping from 41% in 2011 to 24% in 2022, only 35% of children consume the minimum acceptable diet, and 44% of women of reproductive age are malnourished (USAID, 2023). Addressing these disparities requires strengthening healthcare infrastructure, enhancing service delivery in underserved areas, and implementing targeted interventions to improve both access to healthcare and nutritional outcomes across the country.

6.5.2 Healthcare infrastructure

Bangladesh's healthcare infrastructure is separated into three levels: medical universities, medical college hospitals, and specialized hospitals on the tertiary level. Secondary-level institutions include district hospitals, maternity, and child welfare clinics. Primary healthcare (PHC) providers include upazila health complexes, union health and family welfare centers, and community clinics (the lowest level of healthcare facilities). Poor healthcare and transportation infrastructure in rural areas hinder access to nutrition services and thus, various nongovernmental organizations (NGOs) and private institutions contribute to this healthcare network. Healthcare systems play a crucial role in addressing malnutrition in Bangladesh by providing essential services, education, and support to vulnerable populations. Integrated healthcare initiatives, such as community nutrition programs and maternal and child health services, are vital for early identification and treatment of malnutrition. For instance, programs like the National Nutrition Services (NNS) focus on promoting breastfeeding, improving complementary feeding, and providing micronutrient supplementation to children and mothers (Ahmed et al., 2021). In addition, healthcare facilities are instrumental in managing severe acute malnutrition (SAM) through therapeutic feeding programs and inpatient care (Islam et al., 2019). According to this study, 44.4% of pregnant women received four essential nutrition services, 22.6% of children had proper growth monitoring, 38.7% of caregivers received counseling on EBF, only 17.6% of health facilities had a dedicated space for counseling, and only 30% of healthcare providers received basic nutrition training. Adult weighing scales (96.2%), stadiometers (96.2%), and registers (90.5%) were present in the majority of facilities. Maternal nutrition-related social and behavior change communication (SBCC) resources were scarcer (69.8%). Overall, 64% of health facilities had vitamin A (postpartum) supplements, fewer than one-third had iron and folic acid (IFA) pills, and about half had calcium supplements. About one-third of facilities had IFA and calcium delivery requirements, whereas less than half had basic nutrition training guidelines. Strengthening healthcare infrastructure, increasing accessibility, and improving caregiver awareness can significantly enhance efforts to combat malnutrition and ensure better health outcomes for children in Bangladesh.

6.5.3 Sanitation and hygiene

Despite progress, 25% of the rural population lacks access to improved sanitation facilities (UNICEF, 2022). Although 97% of homes have a hand washing station, only 32% of rural households and 56% of urban households have both water and soap for hand washing, and only 38% of households have an upgraded latrine (NIPORT et al., 2019). On the other hand, contaminated water, open defecation, and poor hygiene practices increase exposure to diseases like diarrhea and intestinal worms, which impair nutrient absorption. Consumption of contaminated water leads to diseases such as cholera and diarrhea, which are significant contributors to malnutrition. Frequent illnesses deplete energy reserves and prevent the body from utilizing nutrients effectively (Lin et al., 2013). Although Bangladesh has made progress in reducing open defecation, but sanitation facilities are still inadequate in many rural and urban slums. Exposure to fecal contamination increases the risk of diseases that cause malnutrition. Persistent exposure to poor sanitation leads to a chronic condition where the intestinal lining is damaged, reducing the body's ability to absorb nutrients even in the presence of sufficient food. Frequent floods and cyclones disrupt access to clean water and sanitation.

6.6 Socioeconomic factors

6.6.1 *Poverty*

Poverty is a fundamental driver of undernutrition in Bangladesh, creating a cycle where limited financial resources restrict access to adequate food, healthcare, and education, thereby perpetuating malnutrition. Nearly 18.7% of the population lives below the poverty line (World Bank, 2022), limiting access to diverse and nutritious foods. According to studies conducted in Bangladesh, children from low-socioeconomic-status households regularly have a high proportion of undernutrition. Data indicates that children from the poorest households exhibit significantly higher rates of stunting, wasting, and underweight compared to those from wealthier families (Islam et al., 2019). Household income level can have unique temporal consequences on the risk of undernutrition since the risk of undernutrition in children changes as the EBF period ends and the child starts eating what the rest of the household is eating (Deolalikar, 2005). Rice and other high-calorie staples are frequently preferred by families over more costly, nutrient-dense foods like fruits, vegetables, and meats. Improvements in overall rates of child nutrition have been linked to higher living standards (Ahmed et al., 2012). Research of the causal dependence chains of undernutrition in Bangladesh found that one of the most significant factors contributing to child undernutrition is the household's economic situation (Foraita et al., 2008). According to Pryer et al. (2002) the low-income, most susceptible cluster—represented by female-headed, impoverished households—had the greatest rates of child undernutrition. Fair access to opportunities and resources is hampered by discrimination on the basis of caste, gender, ethnicity, or other social characteristics.

6.6.2 *Education*

Education plays a pivotal role in addressing undernutrition in Bangladesh, with both maternal and paternal education levels significantly influencing children's nutritional status. Studies have demonstrated that higher parental education correlates with reduced prevalence of childhood stunting and underweight. Specifically, children of educated parents are less likely to suffer from undernutrition, as educated mothers and fathers are more likely to ensure proper nutrition and medical care for their children (Nahar & Zahangir, 2024). Furthermore, maternal education has been associated with a reduction in child mortality rates, underscoring its importance in child health outcomes (Wu, 2022). These findings highlight the critical need for policies that promote education for both genders, as enhancing educational attainment among future parents can lead to substantial improvements in child nutrition and overall public health in Bangladesh. There is a lack of integration of nutrition education into school curricula. Insufficient community outreach programs to disseminate knowledge on balanced diets, maternal health, and infant feeding practices. Limited education, especially for women and girls, affects knowledge about nutrition, hygiene, and childcare practices. Communities may lack understanding of the importance of diverse, nutrient-rich diets or proper feeding practices.

6.6.3 Employment

Limited employment opportunities reduce purchasing power, affecting food security and dietary quality. Within low-income groups, different types of livelihoods can have differential impacts on a child's nutritional status. In addition, employment status, particularly maternal employment, significantly influences child nutrition in Bangladesh. Research indicates that children of employed mothers face a higher likelihood of malnutrition. For instance a study found that maternal employment is associated with an increased risk of child stunting in urban slum areas (Win et al., 2022). Similarly, another study reported that children of employed mothers have higher probabilities of being stunted, wasted, and underweight, with these impacts more pronounced among formal-working mothers (Hosen, 2023). These findings suggest that although employment can enhance household income, it may also limit the time mothers can dedicate to childcare and feeding practices, potentially leading to undernutrition. Therefore policies that support working mothers, such as providing access to quality childcare services and flexible working hours, are essential to mitigate the adverse effects of maternal employment on child nutrition in Bangladesh.

6.6.4 Gender disparities/cultural factors

Gender disparities and cultural factors significantly contribute to undernutrition in Bangladesh, particularly among children. Societal norms often prioritize male children, leading to unequal food distribution within households. This bias results in female children receiving less diverse and nutrient-rich diets, increasing their risk of undernutrition. A study analyzing the Bangladesh Multiple Indicator Cluster Survey found that approximately 61% of female children aged 6–23 months failed to meet MDD, compared to 57.8% of male children, indicating a significant gender disparity (Hossain et al., 2023a, 2023b). In addition, cultural practices that limit women's access to education and economic opportunities further exacerbate undernutrition. Women often have less decision-making power and access to resources, limiting their ability to care for themselves and their children. The ethnographic study found that women's decision-making, mobility, and reliance limits prevented them from participating in food provisioning. These limitations were more pronounced in rural areas, where women frequently had no say in how household food funds were allocated (Levay et al., 2013). Furthermore, women with limited education may lack essential knowledge about proper nutrition and childcare practices, adversely affecting their children's health. Addressing these challenges requires targeted interventions that promote gender equality, enhance women's access to education and resources, and challenge cultural norms that perpetuate discrimination, thereby improving nutritional outcomes for all children in Bangladesh.

6.6.5 *Environmental and natural factors*

Extreme weather events, rising temperatures, and shifting agricultural patterns impact food production and access. Deforestation, soil degradation, and water scarcity reduce agricultural productivity and food availability. Biodiversity loss reduces the access to diverse food sources, essential for balanced diets. Frequent floods and cyclones disrupt food production and availability. Climate change also related to nutrition security. Any climatic change has the potential to have detrimental effects on the security of food and nutrition. Our present eating patterns are causing greenhouse gas emissions (GHGE), which is causing the climate to change constantly. The nutrient makeup of some crops is predicted to vary as a result of climate change, which further complicates nutrition security. A metaanalysis of the data revealed that when C3 crops (such as wheat and rice) and legumes (such as field peas and soyabeans) were grown at increased CO_2 (levels anticipated for 2050), their concentrations of zinc, iron, and protein were significantly lower than when they were grown at ambient CO_2 levels (Myers et al, 2014). They found that the contents of zinc, iron, and protein were reduced by an average of 9.3%, 5.1%, and 6.3% in the edible part of wheat that was cultivated in warmer and higher CO_2 circumstances. In addition, the phytate concentration decreased, which might increase the bioavailability and partially offset the losses in iron and zinc. The phytate concentration did not significantly alter, although the reduction for rice was 3.3%, 5.2%, and 7.8%, respectively. In the meantime the amount, variety, and quality of food available to children and families have drastically decreased because of the climate crisis (such as extreme heat, droughts, and floods), biodiversity loss, and damage to water, air, and soil. This has increased food insecurity and nutrition poverty among vulnerable children, households, and populations. In addition, climate change has a negative impact on child care and feeding practices by, for example, taking women's labor away from child care. In addition, children are being exposed to potentially fatal childhood illnesses that affect nutrition, such as lung infections and diarrhea, as a result of rising global temperatures that are interfering with access to safe and clean water.

6.7 Interventions to improve child nutrition

Improving child nutrition in Bangladesh requires a multifaceted approach that addresses dietary intake, healthcare access, and socioeconomic factors. Key interventions include promoting EBF and appropriate complementary feeding practices, which are essential for optimal growth and development. In addition, integrating nutrition-specific interventions into existing maternal, neonatal, and child health programs has been effective in reducing food insecurity among pregnant and recently delivered women, thereby enhancing child nutrition outcomes (Frongillo et al., 2019). Furthermore, comprehensive intervention packages that provide nutrient-rich snacks, such as eggs and milk, have demonstrated improvements in linear growth and dietary diversity among infants (Ara et al., 2022). Micronutrient supplementation, such as vitamin A and iron, and food fortification programs can help combat deficiencies. Strengthening maternal nutrition during pregnancy and lactation ensures better birth outcomes and early childhood health. Enhancing access to safe water, sanitation, and hygiene (WASH) reduces the risk of infections like diarrhea, which deplete essential nutrients. Integrating behavior change communication (BCC) and community engagement ensures that families understand and adopt optimal nutrition practices, ultimately breaking the cycle of malnutrition. Implementing these strategies, alongside efforts to improve maternal education and economic opportunities, is crucial for combating undernutrition and promoting the well-being of children in Bangladesh.

6.7.1 Government initiatives

6.7.1.1 National Nutrition Program (NNP)

National Nutrition Program (NNP) focuses on reducing stunting and micronutrient deficiencies by established NNS in 2010 under the Ministry of Health and Family planning. NNS is bolstering the social mobilization strategy by supporting material development and production. This includes capacity development of individuals through on-the-job training to effectively implement the interventions. Control of vitamin A deficiency disorder, vitamin A supplementation and control and prevention of anemia, iron, and folate supplementation; control of iodine deficiency disorder (IDD) through the Salt Iodization Program; monitoring, evaluation, operations research, survey; School Nutritional Education Program; protection, promotion, and support of breastfeeding/IYCF; and community- and facility-based management of SAM (SAM and CMAM). In addition, NNS works to identify and choose core institutions and support the development of institutional capacity, such as updating or reviewing the curriculum to include nutrition for Medical College, MATS, Nursing Colleges/Training Institutes, and Institute of Health Technology; strengthening ties between outreach services and tertiary facilities; bolstering IPHN and pertinent institutions; working with other ministries; and supporting IPH for food safety and quality (including laboratory) activities. NNS training, such as SAM and IYCF, is already being implemented by tertiary institutions (ICMH and Medical Colleges). Through NNS, a short-term certificate program in nutrition would be implemented at IPHN.

6.7.1.2 School feeding programs

Children and adults of all ages should get nutrition education on how to improve their diets and lifestyles. Provide nutrition instruction, training, and technical assistance;

establish nutrition clubs, including school gardens for schoolchildren, adolescents, and their caregivers; promote school and community support for healthy eating and physical activity. It involves developing nutrition messages, supporting content, and guidelines for good eating in children. Obesity is becoming increasingly prevalent in Bangladesh, with many overweight youngsters attending metropolitan schools. Provide fortified lunches to boost nutrition and school attendance. Diets and materials, including exercise recommendations, must be designed to help people control their weight and live a healthy, active lifestyle.

6.7.1.3 Maternal and child health services

These promote breastfeeding, growth monitoring, and nutrition education. Maternal and child health services in Bangladesh have made significant strides over the past few decades, driven by a combination of government initiatives, NGO interventions, and international support. Key services include ANC, skilled birth attendance, postnatal care (PNC), immunization programs, and nutrition support. Community-based healthcare workers play a vital role in delivering these services to rural and underserved populations. The country has implemented programs such as the Expanded Programme on Immunization (EPI) and initiatives to promote institutional deliveries, which have reduced child mortality and maternal mortality rates. Efforts by organizations, such as Bangladesh Rural Advancement Committee (BRAC), UNICEF, and WHO, have enhanced maternal nutrition, EBF practices, and the management of childhood illnesses. Despite these achievements, challenges such as disparities in service access, inadequate healthcare infrastructure, and limited awareness about reproductive health persist. Continued investments in healthcare systems, education, and community engagement are essential to further improve maternal and child health outcomes in Bangladesh.

6.7.2 NGO and international efforts

Organizations, such as BRAC, UNICEF, Global Alliance for Improved Nutrition (GAIN), and World Food Programme (WFP), implement community-based nutrition programs, emphasizing:

6.7.2.1 Micronutrient supplementation

NGOs and international agencies play a pivotal role in micronutrient supplementation to combat malnutrition and prevent deficiencies, particularly in low- and middle-income countries. Programs, such as UNICEF's micronutrient initiative and WHO's efforts to promote universal fortification of staples, have significantly reduced deficiencies in vulnerable populations. Vitamin A supplementation campaigns, often led by NGOs in collaboration with governments, target children under 5 to reduce preventable blindness and mortality. Iron and folic acid supplementation programs for women of reproductive age address anemia and improve maternal and child health. Initiatives, such as the GAIN and Micronutrient Initiative (now Nutrition International), focus on fortifying foods such as salt with iodine, wheat flour with iron and folic acid, and cooking oil with vitamin D. These efforts are bolstered by partnerships with local communities, healthcare systems, and funding organizations like the Gates Foundation to ensure sustainable delivery and widespread impact. Through advocacy, innovation, and collaboration, these efforts contribute significantly to global progress in addressing micronutrient deficiencies: distribution of vitamin A, zinc, and iron supplements.

6.7.2.2 *Food fortification*

NGOs and international organizations have played a vital role in advancing food fortification efforts in Bangladesh to combat widespread micronutrient deficiencies. Key initiatives include the promotion of universal salt iodization, led by organizations such as UNICEF and the GAIN, which has significantly reduced IDD s. Nutrition International has collaborated with the government and local industries to fortify wheat flour and edible oils with essential nutrients such as iron, zinc, and vitamin A. The WFP has integrated fortified rice into school feeding programs and social safety nets, targeting vulnerable populations. Helen Keller International (HKI) has supported rice fortification and raised awareness about its benefits. These efforts are backed by international funding bodies, such as the Bill & Melinda Gates Foundation, and technical support from agencies like WHO. Despite challenges such as regulatory enforcement and public awareness, these partnerships have greatly contributed to improving nutrition and reducing hidden hunger across the country: fortified rice and oil initiatives to combat micronutrient deficiencies.

6.7.2.3 *WASH (water, sanitation, and hygiene)*

Programs to reduce disease transmission and improve sanitation: WASH initiatives are critical in Bangladesh, where waterborne diseases, poor sanitation, and inadequate hygiene practices significantly impact public health. Efforts by the government, NGOs, and international organizations have focused on improving access to safe drinking water, building sanitary latrines, and promoting hygiene education, particularly in rural and densely populated urban areas. Programs like the Department of Public Health Engineering (DPHE) and collaborations with organizations such as UNICEF, WaterAid, and BRAC have increased the use of tube wells and piped water systems while promoting handwashing practices and menstrual hygiene management. Despite progress, challenges such as arsenic contamination of groundwater, urban slum conditions, and climate change–related issues such as flooding and salinity intrusion continue to hinder WASH improvements. Strengthening infrastructure, ensuring sustainable water management, and fostering community involvement remain crucial to achieving universal WASH coverage and improving health outcomes in Bangladesh.

6.7.3 Behavior change communication (BCC)

BCC should develop campaign material and production to strengthen social mobilization on breastfeeding, complementary feeding, and dietary diversity. It can promote excellent health and nutrition practices through mass media campaigns, social mobilization, behavioral change, and communication initiatives at the health facility and community levels. Consistent transmission of vital messages to raise social consciousness via mass media, print media, and other channels. Specific behaviors to be targeted include counseling pregnant women on proper diet and care, promoting EBF for 6 months and continued breastfeeding for up to 2 years, introducing complementary foods of adequate nutritional quality and quantity after the age of 6 months, improving hygiene practices such as hand washing, and encouraging healthy habits among adolescents. Traditional techniques, such as street theater, drama, jari-shari, and courtyard drama, should all be investigated. BCC may involve religious leaders in nutrition advocacy and organization by hosting a nationwide nutrition day/week every year on significant nutrition themes at various levels, such as a nutrition fair, festival, folksongs, film presentation, discussion, essay competition, and so on. Adolescents, pregnant women, and nursing mothers receive nutrition education and counseling in addition to BCC messages on IYCF. These include topics such as the importance of deworming for health and nutrition, the use of micronutrient supplements (vitamin A, iron, folate, etc.), and personal hygiene and cleanliness, particularly during the preparation and feeding of food to infants and young children.

6.7.4 Mainstreaming gender into nutrition programming

Gender and nutrition are closely related in Bangladesh, where a woman's status has a big influence on her own health and her children's nutritional results. Therefore all people of the community and families who make decisions and have the power to influence the eating patterns of mothers, infants, and young children, as well as other nutrition behaviors, will be included in the health facility and community-based nutrition interventions. With an emphasis on the nutritional status of adolescent girls in the nation, this strategy will guarantee that men's and women's worries about the food and nutrition security of the home are seen as shared responsibilities for the nutritional well-being of all household members, men and women, and the community at large.

6.8 Scope of improvement

Reducing malnutrition in Bangladesh requires continued efforts and innovations across multiple domains. Despite progress in recent decades, significant gaps remain in addressing malnutrition comprehensively. Enhancing maternal and child nutrition programs through community-based interventions have shown promise in improving dietary diversity and reducing food insecurity (Seenithamby et al., 2021). Integrating nutrition education into health systems can empower communities to adopt better feeding practices, thereby promoting health and preventing malnutrition among children (Westerbotn et al., 2023). Strengthening social safety nets and integrating nutrition education into health systems can further empower communities to adopt better feeding practices. Addressing underlying socioeconomic challenges, such as poverty, gender disparities, and limited access to clean water and sanitation, is essential for sustained improvement. Investments in research, monitoring, and evaluation are also vital to identify barriers and tailor interventions to local needs. The synergy between governmental policies, nongovernmental initiatives, and community engagement offers a promising pathway to accelerate progress in reducing malnutrition in Bangladesh. By focusing on these areas, Bangladesh can make significant strides in reducing malnutrition and improving public health outcomes.

6.8.1 Microbiota-directed supplementary foods

Children with moderate acute malnutrition (MAM) and SAM exhibit altered gut microbial community development, as evidenced by changes in the representation of growth-associated bacterial taxa and microbial genes involved in several metabolic pathways. These disturbances result in microbial communities that mimic those of chronologically younger children. Standard nutritional therapies in children do not completely restore these disrupted community conditions. Recent research findings indicate that microbiota-directed meals, which aim to boost the representation and/or expressed metabolic functions of important gut bacteria, promote not only just weight gain but also linear growth and plasma indicators of a variety of developmental processes (Ishita et al., 2024). The study administered microbiota-directed complementary food (MDCF) to 124 Bangladeshi children with MAM for 2 years, which dramatically improved wasting and lowered stunting during follow-up. These findings show that microbiota-directed supplementary foods can be utilized to treat malnutrition (Ishita et al., 2024).

6.8.2 Enhancing community-based approaches

Community-based nutrition (CBN) services in selected areas and hard-to-reach areas: Each community clinic should be progressively equipped to provide comprehensive nutrition services alongside health and family planning services. Establishing partnerships with national and international NGOs is essential for delivering nutrition services in hard-to-reach areas such as remote regions, chars, and hill tracts. In these areas, partners support the implementation of Direct Nutrition Interventions under the NNS within health and family planning facilities. Program designs should remain flexible and diverse to adapt to the unique challenges of these regions.

The CBN services should include

- Regular growth monitoring for children under 2 years of age
- Nutrition education for mothers, adolescent girls, and newly married women
- Individual counseling for parents on child growth and development, childcare, immunization, etc.
- Counseling for pregnant women on self-care, well-being, nutrition, and healthy practices
- Micronutrient supplementation (vitamin A, iron–folate)
- Deworming for children and adolescent girls
- Referrals for children with SAM and other illnesses, as well as ANC and PNC for pregnant women

Mobilize community health workers to deliver nutrition education and monitor growth at the household level. Encourage local production and consumption of nutrient-rich foods.

6.8.2.1 Leveraging technology

Mobile health (mHealth) platforms offer an innovative and cost-effective way to disseminate nutrition information, particularly in regions with widespread mobile phone use but limited access to traditional healthcare services. By leveraging text messages, mobile applications, and interactive voice response systems, these platforms can deliver tailored nutrition advice, reminders for ANC and PNC, and guidance on breastfeeding and complementary feeding practices. In countries like Bangladesh, mHealth initiatives such as SMS-based counseling and app-driven awareness campaigns have proven effective in reaching rural and underserved populations. They can also provide real-time support during emergencies, such as managing acute malnutrition or addressing food security crises. Partnerships between governments, NGOs, and tech companies can enhance the reach and impact of these platforms, whereas integrating local languages and cultural contexts ensures relevance. Scaling up mHealth solutions can empower individuals with actionable knowledge, promote healthier practices, and improve overall nutritional outcomes, particularly for women and children. Use mobile health platforms to disseminate nutrition information and track service delivery. Implement digital monitoring systems for program evaluation.

6.8.2.2 Multisectoral collaboration

Malnutrition is inherently a multisectoral issue, and achieving lasting nutrition security requires coordinated, cross-sectoral efforts. This involves the continuous alignment of policies and strategies across various sectors and ministries.

In addition, critical nutrition messages will be distributed across all available information channels in partnership with the Ministry of Information. Linkages will be made with development programs, sanitation programs, and suitable technologies for enhancing food sources and forms, among other things, to avoid illness and diseases and maintain environmental sustainability. Create a connection with agricultural initiatives that can help small farming households meet their food needs. In contrast a cooperation with the agriculture sector will offer health education and orientation to agricultural workers to promote the production of safe, nutrient-dense food with the least amount of pesticide use. Along with the appropriate program under the ministry of fisheries and livestock, beneficiaries will be encouraged to engage in fish culture, poultry rearing, and dairy production to boost the availability and accessibility of foods high in protein. As malnutrition is thought to be caused by ignorance about food requirements at different stages of life, the nutritional worth of different foods, etc., it is imperative that nutrition be incorporated into both formal and informal education curricula in cooperation with the ministry of education. In the city and municipality areas, Local Government Engineering Department (LGED) is in charge of carrying out urban health projects. The health ministry can guarantee and offer technical assistance to carry out nutrition initiatives in urban areas by maintaining communication with the Ministry of LGED. Furthermore, to guarantee social protection, collaborations between the public and corporate sectors, academia, and NGOs are required.

6.8.2.3 Strengthening policies and programs

Strengthening policies and programs is essential to further reduce malnutrition in Bangladesh. The Second National Plan of Action for Nutrition (NPAN2) 2016–25 outlines comprehensive strategies to address various forms of malnutrition, including targets to increase the initiation of breastfeeding and improve dietary diversity among children. In addition, integrating nutrition-specific and nutrition-sensitive interventions into existing maternal, neonatal, and child health programs has proven effective in reducing food insecurity among pregnant and recently delivered women (USAID, 2021). Collaborative efforts involving government agencies, NGOs, and international partners have also contributed to significant reductions in child stunting through targeted nutrition programs (International Food Policy Research Institute (IFPRI), 2016). Integrate climate-resilient agricultural practices into nutrition programs. Continued investment in these policies and programs, along with robust monitoring and evaluation mechanisms, is crucial to sustain progress and achieve national nutrition goals in Bangladesh. Expand the scope and coverage of the NNP to include urban poor populations.

6.9 Conclusion

In conclusion the nutrition study of young children in Bangladesh highlights persistent challenges in achieving optimal nutritional outcomes, despite notable progress in recent years. Malnutrition remains a significant concern, with stunting, wasting, and micronutrient deficiencies prevalent among young children. The findings underscore the critical importance of addressing underlying factors such as poverty, education, and healthcare access. In addition, promoting EBF, improving complementary feeding practices, and enhancing dietary diversity are essential for sustainable improvements in child nutrition. The coordinated approach, integrating government policies, community-based programs, and international support, is necessary to combat malnutrition effectively. Strengthening monitoring and evaluation systems is also crucial to ensure the success of targeted interventions and to build a healthier future for the nation's children.

References

Abdullah, K., Malek, M.A., Faruque, A.S., Salam, M. A. and Ahmed, T. (2007). Health and nutritional status of children of adolescent mothers: experience from a diarrhoeal disease hospital in Bangladesh. Acta Paediatrica; 96.3, 396-400.

Alam, N., Roy, S.K., Ahmed, T. and Shamsir Ahmed, A.M. (2010). Nutritional status, dietary intake, and relevant knowledge of adolescent girls in rural Bangladesh. Journal of Health, Population and Nutrition; 28.1, 86-94.

Ahmed, M., Abedin, J., Alam, K. F, Al Mamun, A., Paul, R. C, Rahman, M., Iuliano, A. D, Sturm-Ramirez, K., Parashar, U., Luby, S. P, & Gurley, E. S. (2018). Incidence of acute diarrhea-associated death among children < 5 years of age in Bangladesh, 2010-12. *American Journal of Tropical Medicine and Hygiene, 98*(1), 281–286. doi:10.4269/ajtmh.17-0384.

Ahmed, T., et al. (2020). Understanding malnutrition trends in Bangladesh: Progress and challenges. *Journal of Public Health Nutrition, 23*(4), 556–567.

Ahmed, T., et al. (2021). Strategies to improve nutrition in Bangladesh: Achievements and future directions. *Food and Nutrition Bulletin, 42*(1), 1–13.

Akter, M., & Kabir, H. (2023). Health inequalities in rural and urban Bangladesh: The implications of digital health. *Mayo Clinic Proceedings: Digital Health, 1*(2), 201–202. doi:10.1016/j.mcpdig.2023.04.003.

Ara, G., Sanin, K. I., Khanam, M., Sarker, M. S. A., Tofail, F., Nahar, B., Chowdhury, I. A., Boitchi, A. B., Gibson, S., Afsana, K., Askari, S., & Ahmed, T. (2022). A comprehensive intervention package improves the linear growth of children under 2-years-old in rural Bangladesh: A community-based cluster randomized controlled trial. *Scientific Reports, 12*, 21962. doi:10.1038/s41598-022-26269-w.

Bangladesh Bureau of Statistics (BBS). (2019). Bangladesh multiple indicator cluster survey. 564. Bangladesh Bureau of Statistics.

Bhutta, Z. A., Das, J. K., Rizvi, A., Gaffey, M. F., Walker, N., Horton, S., Webb, P., Lartey, A., & Black, R. E.The Maternal and Child Nutrition Study Group. (2013). Evidence-based interventions for improvement of maternal and child nutrition: What can be done and at what cost ? *The Lancet, 382*(9890)), 452–477.

Black, R. E., et al. (2013). Maternal and child undernutrition and overweight in low-income and middle-income countries. *The Lancet, 382*(9890), 427–451.

Chowdhury, F., Khan, A.I., Hossain, M.I., Malek, M.A., Faruque, A.S.G., Ahmed, T. and Salam, M.A. (2006). Young children non-immunized against measles: Characteristics and programmatic implications. Acta Paediatrica, International Journal of Paediatrics; 95.1, 44-49.

Das, S. and Hossain, M.Z. (2008). Levels and determinants of child undernutrition in Bangladesh', Pakistan Journal of Statistics; 24.4, 301-323.

Deolalikar, A. (2005). Poverty and malnutrition in Bangladesh', Journal of Developing Societies; 21, 55.

Foraita, R., Klasen, S., & Pigeot, I. (2008). Using graphical chain models to analyze differences in structural correlates of undernutrition in Benin and Bangladesh. *Economics and Human Biology, 6*(3), 398–419.

Frongillo, E. A., Nguyen, P. H., Sanghvi, T., Mahmud, Z., Aktar, B., Alayon, S., & Menon, P. (2019). Nutrition interventions integrated into an existing maternal, neonatal, and child health program reduce food insecurity among recently delivered and pregnant women in Bangladesh. *The Journal of Nutrition, 149*(1), 159–166.

Haider, R., Rasheed, S., Sanghvi, T.G., Hassan, N., Pachon, H., Islam, S. and Jalal, C.S. (2010). Breastfeeding in infancy: identifying the program-relevant issues in Bangladesh. International Breastfeeding Journal; 5, 21.

Hosen, M. Z. (2023). Impact of maternal employment on children malnutrition status in Bangladesh: An empirical analysis. *Journal of Social and Economic Development, 25*(2), 500–530. doi:10.1007/s40847-023-00232-5.

Hossain, M. I., Islam, M. R., Saleheen, A. A. S., Rahman, A., Zinia, F. A., & Urmy, U. A. (2023a). Determining the risk factors of under-five morbidity in Bangladesh: A Bayesian logistic regression approach. *Discover Social Science and Health, 3*, 21. doi:10.1007/s44155-023-00052-2.

Hossain, M. I., Kabir, S., & Zinia, F. A. (2023b). Gender disparity in minimum dietary diversity failure among currently breastfed children aged 6–23 months in Bangladesh: Evidence from Bangladesh Multiple Indicator Cluster Survey, 2019. *Journal of Nutritional Science, 12*, e107. doi:10.1017/jns.2023.89.

International Food Policy Research Institute (IFPRI). (2016). *Strengthening food and nutrition policies and programs in Bangladesh by Janna de la Paz on October 21, 2016*. IFPRI Retrieved January 2025, from https://www.ifpri.org/blog/ifpri-strengthening-food-and-nutrition-policies-and-programs-bangladesh/ .

Ishita, M., Hibberd, M. C., Hartman, S. J., Hasan Hafizur Rahman, M., Mahfuz, M., Tafsir Hasan, S. M., Ashorn, P., Barratt, M. J., Ahmed, T., & Gordon, J. I. (2024). A microbiota-directed complementary food intervention in 12–18-month-old Bangladeshi children improves linear growth. *eBioMedicine, 104*, 105166. doi:10.1016/j.ebiom.2024.105166.

Islam, K. N, Sultana, S., Rahman, F., & Rahman, A. (2024). Exploring the impact of child underweight status on common childhood illnesses among children under five years in Bangladesh along with spatial analysis. *PLoS One, 19*(9), e0311183. doi:10.1371/journal.pone.0311183.

Islam, M. R, Rahman, M. S, Rahman, M. M, Nomura, S., de Silva, A., Lanerolle, P., & Rahman, M. M. (2019). Reducing childhood malnutrition in Bangladesh: The importance of addressing socio-economic inequalities. *Public Health Nutrition, 23*(1), 72–82. doi:10.1017/S136898001900140X.

Islam, M. A., Hasan, M. N., Ahammed, T., Anjum, A., Majumder, A., Noor-E-Alam Siddiqui, M., Mukharjee, S. K., Sultana, K. F., Sultana, S., Jakariya, M., Bhattacharya, P., Sarkodie, S. A., Dhama, K., Mumin, J., & Ahmed, F. (2022). Association of household fuel with acute respiratory infection (ARI) under-five years children in Bangladesh. *Frontiers in Public Health, 10*, 985445. doi:10.3389/fpubh.2022.985445.

Islam MR, Rahman MS, Rahman MM, Nomura S, de Silva A, Lanerolle, P, Jung J, Rahman MM. (2019). Reducing childhood malnutrition in Bangladesh: the importance of addressing socio-economic inequalities. Public Health Nutr. 23(1), 72-82. doi:10.1017/S136898001900140X.

Jesmin, A., Yamamoto, S.S., Malik, A.A. and Haque, M.A. (2011). Prevalence and determinants of chronic malnutrition among preschool children: a cross-sectional study in Dhaka City, Bangladesh. Journal of Health, Population and Nutrition 29.5, 494-499.

Khan, R.E.A. and Raza, M.A. (2013). Child malnutrition in developing economies: a case study of Bangladesh. Quality and Quantity; March 19, 1-20.

Khan, M.R. and Ahmed, F. (2005). Physical status, nutrient intake and dietary pattern of adolescent female factory workers in urban Bangladesh. Asia Pacific Journal of Clinical Nutrition; 14.1, 19-26.

Levay, A. V., Mumtaz, Z., Rashid, S. F., & Willows, N. (2013). Influence of gender roles and rising food prices on poor, pregnant women's eating and food provisioning practices in Dhaka, Bangladesh. *Reproductive Health, 10*(1), 53.

Lin, A., Bik, E. M., Costello, E. K., Dethlesfsen, L., Haque, R., Relman, D. A., & Singh, U. (2013). Distinct distal gut microbiome diversity and composition in healthy children from Bangladesh and the United States. *PLoS One, 8*(1), 1–19.

Magnani, R., Oot, L., Sethuraman, K., Kabir, G. and Rahman, S. (2015). USAID Office of Food forPeace Food Security Country Framework for Bangladesh (FY 2015-2019); Washington, DC: FHI 360/FANTA.

Moore, S., Prentice, A., Wagatsuma, Y., Fulford, A., Collinson, A., Raqib, R., Vahter, M., Persson, L., & Arifeen, S. (2006). Responsive complementary feeding in rural Bangladesh. *Social Science and Medicine, 62*(8), 1917–1919.

Morales, F., Montserrat-de la Paz, S., Leon, M. J, & Rivero-Pino, F. (2023). Effects of malnutrition on the immune system and infection and the role of nutritional strategies regarding improvements in children's health status: A literature review. *Nutrients, 16*(1), 1. doi:10.3390/nu16010001.

Myers, S. S., Zanobetti, A., Kloog, I., Huybers, P., Leakey, A. D. B., Bloom, A. J., Carlisle, E., Dietterich, L. H., Fitzgerald, G., Hasegawa, T., Holbrook, N. M., Nelson, R. L., Ottman, M. J., Raboy, V., Sakai, H., Sartor, K. A., Schwartz, J., Seneweera, S., Tausz, M., & Usui, Y. (2014). Increasing CO_2 threatens human nutrition. *Nature, 510*, 139–142.

Nahar, M. Z, & Zahangir, M. S (2024). The role of parental education and occupation on undernutrition among children under five in Bangladesh: A rural-urban comparison. *PLoS One, 19*(8), e0307257. doi:10.1371/journal.pone.0307257.

Nasreen, H.E., Kabir, Z.N., Forsell, Y. and Edhborg, M. (2010). Low birth weight in offspring of women with depressive and anxiety symptoms during pregnancy: results from a population based study in Bangladesh. BMC Public Health; 10, 51.

Nasreen, H.E., Kabir, Z.N., Forsell, Y. and Edhborg, M. (2013). Impact of maternal depressive symptoms and infant temperament on early infant growth and motor development: Results from a population based study in Bangladesh. Journal of Affective Disorders; 146.2, 254-61.

National Nutrition Service (NNS), Institute of Public Health Nutrition (IPHN), Directorate General of Health Services, Ministry of Health & Family Welfare, Government of Bangladesh. (2017). *National Low Birth Weight Survey Bangladesh, 2015*. Social Sector Management Foundation (SSMF).

NIPORT. (1997). *Bangladesh Demographic and Health Survey 1996–97*. NIPORT.

NIPORT. (2022). *Bangladesh Demographic and Health Survey (BDHS) 2022*. National Institute of Population Research and Training (NIPORT).

NIPORT 2019: National Institute of Population Research and Training (NIPORT), International Centre for Diarrhoeal Disease Research, Bangladesh (icddr,b), and Data for Impact. (2019). Bangladesh Adolescent Health and Wellbeing Survey 2019-20: Final Report. Dhaka, Bangladesh, and Chapel Hill, NC, USA: NIPORT, icddr,b, and Data for Impact.https://www.data4impactproject.org/publications/bangladesh-adolescent-health-and-wellbeing-survey-2019-20-final-report/.

NIPORT 2021: National Institute of Population Research and Training (NIPORT), Urban Health Survey 2021.Dhaka: National Institute of Population Research and Training (NIPORT). https://buhn.org/uploads/files/resources/reports/national/4_Bangladesh_Urban_Health_Survey_2021.pdf.

NIPORT. (2023). *Bangladesh Demographic and Health Survey 2022: Key indicators report*. NIPORT.

Rahman, A. E., Hossain, A. T., Siddique, A. B., Jabeen, S., Chisti, M. J., Dockrell, D. H., Nair, H., Jamil, K., Campbell, H., & El Arifeen, S. (2021). Child mortality in Bangladesh—Why, when, where and how? A national survey-based analysis. *Journal of Global Health, 11*, 04052. doi:10.7189/jogh.11.04052.

Pryer, J.A., Rogers, S., Normand, S. and Rahman, A. (2002). Livelihoods, nutrition and health in Dhaka slums' Study Urban Livelihoods Project. Public Health Nutrition; 5.5, 613-618.

Rayhan, M.I. and Khan, M.S.H. (2006). Factors causing malnutrition among under Five children in Bangladesh' Pakistan Journal of Nutrition; 5.6, 558-62.

Saha, K. K., Frongillo, E. A., Alam, D. S., Arifeen, S. E., Persson, L. A., & Rasmussen, K. M. (2008). Appropriate infant feeding practices result in better growth of infants and young children in rural Bangladesh. *The American Journal of Clinical Nutrition, 87*(6), 1852–1859. doi:10.1093/ajcn/87.6.1852.

Seenithamby, M., Saint-Geours, S. Y. J., Raza, W. A., & Chaudhery, D. (2021). *Multisectoral approach to reducing undernutrition in Bangladesh shows promise*. World Bank Blogs Retrieved January 2025, from https://blogs.worldbank.org/en/endpovertyinsouthasia/multisectoral-approach-reducing-undernutrition-bangladesh-shows-promise .

Smith, L. C., & Haddad, L. (2015). Reducing child undernutrition: Past drivers and priorities for the post-MDG era. *World Development, 68*, 180–204.

Tette, E. M, Sifah, E. K, & Nartey, E. T. (2015). Factors affecting malnutrition in children and the uptake of interventions to prevent the condition. *BMC Pediatrics, 15*, 189. doi:10.1186/s12887-015-0496-3.

UNICEF. (2019). *The state of the world's children 2019: Children, food, and nutrition*. UNICEF.

UNICEF. (2022). *State of the world's children: A statistical review*. UNICEF Publications.

UNICEF. (2024). *Child food poverty: Nutrition deprivation in early childhood*. UNICEF https://www.unicef.org/reports/child-food-poverty.

USAID. (2021). *Bangladesh: Nutrition profile*. USAID Retrieved January 2025, from https://www.usaid.gov/sites/default/files/2022-05/Copy_of_tagged_Bangladesh-Nutrition-Profile.pdf.

USAID. (2023). *USAID Bangladesh Health Strategy 2022-2027*. USAID https://www.usaid.gov/bangladesh/global-health/health-strategy-2022-2027.

Walker, S. P., Wachs, T. D., Grantham-McGregor, S., Black, M. M., Nelson, C. A., Huffman, S. L., Baker-Henningham, H., Chang, S. M., Hamadani, J. D., Lozoff, B., Meeks Gardner, J. M., Powell, C. A., Rahman, A., & Richter, L. (2011). Inequality in early childhood: Risk and protective factors for early child development. *The Lancet, 378*(9799), 1325–1338.

Westerbotn, M., Monfors, F., Reusser, J., & Tyrrell, M. (2023). Promoting health and preventing malnutrition among children in rural Bangladesh: A qualitative study. *Nursing Open, 10*(8), 5693–5700. doi:10.1002/nop2.1815.

Win, H., Shafique, S., Mizan, S., Wallenborn, J., Probst-Hensch, N., & Fink, G. (2022). Association between mother's work status and child stunting in urban slums: A cross-sectional assessment of 346 child-mother dyads in Dhaka, Bangladesh (2020). *Archives of Public Health, 80*, 192. doi:10.1186/s13690-022-00948-6.

World Bank. (2022). *Poverty and shared prosperity in South Asia*. World Bank Group.

World Health Organization (WHO). (2020). *Improving maternal mental health*. WHO.

World Health Organization (WHO). (2023). *Global nutrition report 2023: Progress and challenges*. WHO Press.

World Health Organization (WHO). (2024a). *Prevalence of overweight in children under 5 Country Bangladesh*. WHO Retrieved January 2025, from https://data.who.int/indicators/i/3AA5F44/64E2430 .

World Health Organization (WHO). (2024b). *Fact sheets—Malnutrition*. WHO https://www.who.int/news-room/fact-sheets/detail/malnutrition.

Wu, H. (2022). The effect of maternal education on child mortality in Bangladesh. *Population and Development Review, 48*(2), 475–503.

Nutrition and aging at tissue and cellular level: An update on the involvement of TRP ion channels

7

Abhishek Singh[a,b], *Rashmita Das*[b], *Luna Goswami*[a] *and Chandan Goswami*[b]

[a]School of Biotechnology, Kalinga Institute of Industrial Technology (KIIT) (Deemed to be University), Bhubaneswar, Odisha, India, [b]School of Biological Sciences, National Institute of Science Education and Research, HBNI, Jatni, Odisha, India

7.1 General introduction on TRP ion channels

The discovery of the mutant *trp* gene from *Drosophila* led to the identification of the first TRP (transient receptor potential) subfamily member (Cosens & Manning, 1969). TRP represents a type of polymodal cation channels that are extensively prevalent in many tissues and cells. TRP channels play important role in sensory perception and cell-to-cell communication. Later a large group of TRP ion channels has been identified in human as well as in other mammals. TRP ion channels are mainly present in animal kingdom, ranging from lower eukaryotes to human. TRP channels are also present in several fungi but are absent in higher plants. Further, TRP channels have been categorized into several subfamilies depending on their genomic sequences. These include TRPM (melastatin), TRPV (vanilloid), TRPC (canonical), TRPA (ankyrin), TRPN (NO-mechano-potential, NOMP) in group 1 subfamilies, and TRPML (mucolipin) and TRPP (polycystin) in group 2 subfamilies (Fig. 7.1), with each having their triggering mechanism and metabolic processes (Gardela et al., 2020). TRPY, another subfamily, comprises mainly yeast TRPs that have been distantly associated with both TRP groups.

TRP channels can be stimulated by different physical stimuli (such as temperature, mechanical force, and UV) as well as by a range of chemical compounds that are either natural or synthetic in origin. TRP channels are also known to be modulated by a series of endogenous factors and such molecules typically represents different lipids, steroids, neurotransmitters, gases, etc. (Caterina et al., 2016; Méndez-Reséndiz et al., 2020; Yang et al., 2017). Because of the ability of TRP channels to get modulated synergistically by physical and chemical factors, TRP channels form important signaling hubs that processes essential information for homeostatic and ecological–environmental response (Zhu et al., 2011).

Furthermore, TRPs are abundantly distributed throughout the different human tissues (Fig. 7.2). Despite years of research, the importance of TRP channels is still an underexplored area. However, investigation on TRP channels has garnered a lot of interest over the past three decades. Particularly the advancement of molecular biology

Nutritional Strategies, Predictive Models, and Sustainable Policies. DOI: https://doi.org/10.1016/B978-0-443-23671-6.00007-4

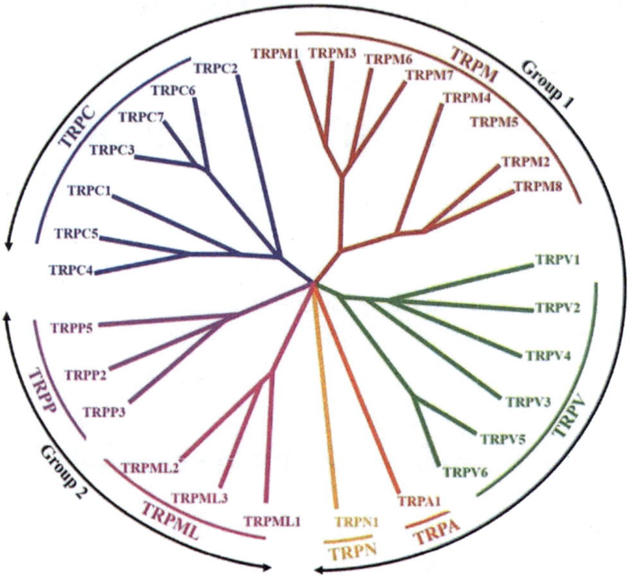

Figure 7.1 TRP ion channels subfamilies. Classifications of TRP channels based on the genomic sequences. Each color represents various TRP ion channel subfamilies.

and microscopy tools has enriched the scientific knowledge of TRPs. Furthermore, TRP channel alterations are being identified in a wide range of health conditions and in pathological situations, which, mainly, indicates the involvement of TRP channels in different diseases (Kaneko & Szallasi, 2014). Most significantly the modulation of the TRP channels could be useful for both prevention as well as treatment of medical conditions. The importance of TRP channels in overall health and disease is acknowledged by awarding the Nobel Prize in Physiology or Medicine 2021 to Prof. David Julius.

TRP channels are involved in a wide spectrum of biological events, including development, metabolism, physiology, and sensory functions (Zhang et al., 2023). TRP channels are critically important for different sensations such as for light, temperature, pressure, and pH and thus critical for detection and perception of different forms of pain. These channels also regulate important physiological functions such as regulation of cardiac functions, circulation and also fertilization (Earley & Brayden, 2015). Many health conditions that indicate chronic or transient health problem are associated with TRP channels. Pathophysiological conditions that are typically associated with altered immunity, such as infection, cancer, inflammatory bowel disease (IBD), different forms of autoimmunity are associated with TRP channels (Froghi et al., 2021; Yang et al., 2024a). Moreover, there are other health problems, such as gastrointestinal disorders, neurological disorders, skin disorders that have been linked to the dysfunction of TRP channels (Hong et al., 2020). Several pathological conditions that act as typical signature of aging, such as low bone density, low immunity, low hormonal levels,

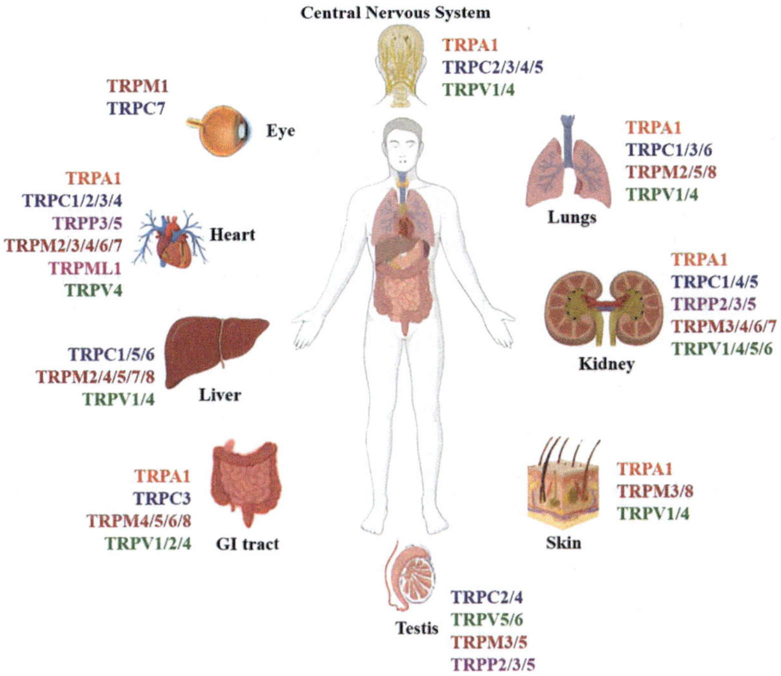

Figure 7.2 TRP channels are distributed throughout an individual's body. TRP channels are found throughout the human body's systems, including the lungs, liver, skin, neurons, and intestines. The multiple colors associated with the phrases stand for the various TRP groups.

reduced skin functions, abnormal cardiac functions, and reduced muscle strength and each of these are intimately related to TRP channel functions. Understandably, in age-related medical conditions, impaired cell functions can arise as a result of reduction in TRP channel expression and also altered functions in older persons (Lee et al., 2021).

7.2 TRP channels are involved in the process of habitat and food selection

TRP ion channels not only act as mare indicators for detecting external stimulus on the cell membrane, but these channels also induce feedback mechanisms that governs overall behavior and physiology. As a subset of TRP channels have the ability to get activated by changes in temperature, these channels have the unique property that is "thermo-gating." These thermo-gated TRP channels are involved in detection of environmental temperature. In a similar manner, several TRP channels have the ability to get activated in response to certain noxious products (such as toxins, venoms, odors, and volatile compounds) present in the nature (Vriens et al., 2008). TRP channels also response to certain metabolic intermediates (for example, steroids) that may accumulate from biochemical pathways and thus TRP channels are intimately linked to different metabolism also (Kumar et al., 2015). Therefore TRP channels are important to sense changes in the temperatures, pH-level and overall metabolism (Huang et al., 2023; Nilius, 2007). Because of all these reasons, TRP channels are frequently referred to as "molecular sensors" because these channels react to a broad range of external stimuli that can be either physical or chemical in nature. In addition, TRP channels are important for food choices, ecological responses and overall diverse health-related issues. The role of these ion channels in the selection of habitat, specifically regarding nutrition has direct impact on the aging at the organism, tissue and cellular levels, and such relationship is becoming more widely acknowledged. All these factors become critical to impact behavioral aspects that ensure preferred habitat and food selection and reject environments that are unpleasant and/or are likely to damage tissues/cells because of the presence of noxious physical conditions and potentially hazardous compounds.

7.3 Relationship of TRP channels with food and immunity

TRP channels are intimately related to food-uptake and modulation of immunity, especially innate immunity. For instance, TRPA1 and TRPV1 channels are linked to the control of sensations of fullness and hunger, indicating that these channels could affect food selection along with habitat selections depending on the accessibility of micronutrients (Jaffal & Abbas, 2021; Khalil et al., 2018). Several TRP channels are also expressed in specific regions of brain that regulates food uptake, an important regulation that is critical in pregnancy and lactation stage (Christie et al., 2018; Liu et al., 2022). These channels get activated in response to specific food products; bioactive components present in the foods. Such issues develop physiology-experienced and memory-based release of neurotransmitters that influence dietary routine, food preference, rejection of foods, directing people to prefer more conducive surroundings.

Moreover, TRP ion channels' importance in recognizing and responding to dietary contents has been demonstrated by their existence throughout a variety of physiological organs, particularly the gastrointestinal system. According to Morita et al. (2020), lipopolysaccharides (LPS) that exist in the cell walls of bacteria can stimulate the TRPA1 and TRPV4 channels (Morita et al., 2020). In fact, recent works indicate that LPS can act as pathogen-associated molecular patterns (PAMP) and TRPs can act as PAMP-responsive factors (Gauthier et al., 2022; Sahu & Goswami, 2023; Wu et al., 2023). This suggests that TRP channels have evolved with a function in sensing the existence of microorganisms (in food, environments, etc.) and these impacts on the selection of habitat by determining the secure nature of dietary sites. This sensory capability enables species to effectively gauge their environment, choose proper ecological niche that provides an adequate food supply whilst avoiding possibly toxic substances.

Beyond their canonical sensor roles, TRP ion channels are involved in the regulation of immune responses and especially contribute to pathogenicity-associated responses during infections as well as inflammatory processes. TRP ion channels are present in the populations of immune cells, especially in macrophages, T cells, natural killer (NK) cells, and other monocytes, making them easily responsive to all kinds of endogenous stimuli, for example, infectious agents as well as inflammatory mediators (Wu et al., 2023). As immune activation process is also coupled with slight increment in body temperature and enhanced Ca^{2+} influx in activated immune cells, most of the thermosensitive TRP channels are better suited for immune activation process (Majhi et al., 2015; Sahoo et al., 2019). Indeed, several reports confirmed that TRP channels play important roles in immune regulation and dietary supplement of specific bioactive compounds can greatly modulate the immune status. An example is the TRP ion channels which play an essential role in the tunneling of immunological responses, as well as in wound healing via regulation of proinflammatory cytokines and chemokines release (Bonsignore et al., 2024; Zheng et al., 2023). The interaction of TRP ion channels with the immunological signaling processes indicates how imperative TRP ion channels are in maintaining homeostatic balance and adjusting to the environmental stimuli.

TRP channels are essential for the operation of the systemic immunity, as demonstrated by the interaction between TLRs (Toll-like receptors) and TRP channels. TLRs and TRP channel expression in analogous cell types enable orchestrated defenses against infections (Morita et al., 2020). The approach that organisms react against pathogens within their surroundings might be influenced by such interplay, which could have a direct effect on niche selections. As a prime example, TRP channel stimulation in response to endotoxins released by bacteria might strengthen the body's immune system and possibly direct individuals into a healthier habitat.

The importance of TRP channels in choosing habitats is further emphasized by how they contribute through metabolic disorders and during the development of cancer. TRP channel activation has already been reported to alter across many malignancies, indicating that such channels could be potentially used as cancer therapy targets along with biological markers in the development of tumors (Chen et al., 2023; Yang & Kim, 2020). For example, TRPM8 as well as TRPV6 are both associated with prostate cancer, with the degree of expression correlated to the prognosis of the cancer (Gkika & Prevarskaya, 2011). Interaction among TRP channels and tumors emphasizes how external factors may influence the way cells behave and select their habitat, especially when it comes to dietary intake resources together with being exposed to carcinogenic compounds.

Moreover, TRP channels are essential for metabolic functions because they affect adipocyte activity and the distribution of nutrients (Bishnoi et al., 2018; Gao et al., 2019). Their function among Ca^{2+} mediated signaling pathways plays an important role in controlling metabolic processes such as storing fat and thermogenesis. Thus through regulating nutritional needs along with the consumption of energy, TRP channels might influence the selection of a habitat and eventually the ability of a species to flourish in its surroundings. TRPM8, which is triggered by menthol and cooler conditions, is involved in thermal regulation and might impact food selections depending on the perceived temperature (Cheng, 2018). The interaction of the TRP channels with food elements emphasizes how essential it is to comprehend the significance these channels represent in habitation and dietary routines, especially as people age.

Dietary routines may also modulate TRP channel activity, especially from nutritional intake in terms of macro- or micronutrients. Macronutrients, such as polyunsaturated omega-3 fatty acids (PUFA), undergo interactions with TRP channel for regulating pain and inflammatory responses; DHA (docosahexaenoic acid) leads to activation of TRPV1, whereas EPA (eicosapentaenoic acid) is responsible for inhibition (Matta et al., 2007). In addition, these are also responsible for the NLRP3 inflammasome suppression, which lowers IL-1β expression (Yan et al., 2013). On the other hand, elevated hyperglycemia (higher glucose level) stimulates TRPM2, which results in inflammation as well as oxidative stress (Yamamoto et al., 2011). Similarly, micronutrients also affect the activities of TRP channels. For example, the modulation of TRPM7 by zinc improves the activities of neutrophils as well as cytokines production (Prasad, 2008), whereas TRPM6/TRPM7 influenced by Mg^{2+} affects its cellular transportation and immunological homeostasis (Schmitz et al., 2003). Moreover, vitamin D facilitates TRPV6-mediated Ca^{2+}-transfer and augments antimicrobial activities (Gombart et al., 2020).

TRP channel activity gets less effective with aging in living things, which could have a direct effect on people's ability to react to external cues while making habitat selections. Both, adipose tissue and the autoimmune system have demonstrated age-related alteration in the function and expression of TRP channels (Zhu et al., 2011; Zsombok & Derbenev, 2016). Such a reduction could lead to greater vulnerability to medical conditions, such as tumors as well as metabolic syndrome, that are impacted by dietary changes and habitat selections.

There are a variety of studies currently in progress to analyze the potential medical benefits of affecting TRP channels in aging-related human or animal diseases. Several options to affect TRP ion channels to boost immunological activity, better metabolism, and assure proper aging. For example, pharmaceutical agonists and antagonists could be developed to stimulate or inhibit specific TRP ion channels, thereby reshaping healthy immune response system while ensuring a high quality of life during aging in humans (Zhang et al., 2023).

7.4 Expression and specific function of TRP channels in important tissues related to aging

The large number of TRP channels are well justified by their tissue- and/or developmental phase-specific expression and functions. This also accords well with the polymodal characteristics of these channels. Here we discuss few important tissues that are directly related to aging and related TRP channels that are expressed there.

7.4.1 Neuron and neurodegeneration

Aging is the most substantial contributory factor for neuron and neurodegeneration induce abnormal neurological conditions, which shows late onset and are mostly progressive in nature (Hong et al., 2020). Although the damage of nerve cells is unlikely in healthier neurological systems, it might be brought through external as well as internal stimulus in the majority of degenerative neurological conditions, wherein neural networks often lose its myelin layer and/or lose its capacity for retaining homeostatic balance primarily as a consequence of impairments in its neural phenology and activity (Chi et al., 2018). With their own pathology, neurodegenerative diseases, including epilepsy, amyotrophic lateral sclerosis, Parkinson's disease, Alzheimer's disease, and Huntington's disease, have demarcated the involvement of TRP ion channels in their pathophysiologies. As of now, Alzheimer's disease appears to be linked to TRPA1, TRPC1, TRPC3, TRPC6, TRPM2, TRPM7, TRPML1, TRPV1, and TRPV4. Parkinson's disease has been scientifically linked to TRPC1, TRPC3, TRPM2, TRPM7, and TRPV1. It has been demonstrated that Huntington's disease is influenced by TRPC1, TRPC5, and TRPV1. The involvement of TRPC4, TRPM2, TRPM3, TRPM7, and TRPML1 in amyotrophic lateral sclerosis has been thoroughly demonstrated. Similarly the involvement of TRPC1, TRPC3-7, TRPM2, TRPM7, TRPV1, TRPV4, and TRPA1 has been lined with epilepsy (Lee et al., 2021). These channels' dysfunction can contribute to neurons susceptibility and neurodegeneration, leading to the progression of neurological conditions. For example, antinociceptive effects are produced when TRPV1 expression is downregulated (Huang et al., 2020). Similarly, TRPV4, which mainly triggers neuropathic and inflammatory pain, showed considerable improvement in nociception in mice with TRPV4 knockouts (Brierley et al., 2008). The presence of TRPV4 in the mitochondria and its involvement in the regulation of mitochondrial function has been linked with the development neurodegeneration (Acharya et al., 2022). Despite significant progress has been gained toward comprehending the importance of TRP ion channels for neurological conditions, researchers nevertheless are still investigating for establishing a comprehensive knowledge of how such channels contribute to the onset and progression of such disorders.

Several studies highlight the importance of dietary intake influence (that is, vitamins, minerals, and antioxidants) on TRP channels regulation in relation to neurological disorders. Vitamin D deficiency has been associated with the Alzheimer's disease progression, because it controls TRPV channels and Ca^{2+} equilibrium through their receptors vitamin D receptor (VDR) (Gezen-Ak et al., 2013). Glutathione (GSH), an essential redox buffer, likewise minimizes oxidative injury within Alzheimer's disease via lowering TRPM2 stimulation (Belrose et al., 2012). A low level of Mg^{2+} leads to the pathophysiology of Parkinson's disease, which additionally affects TRPM7-mediated survival of neurons (Schmitz et al., 2003). TRPM7 regulating the Zn^{2+}-equilibrium plays an important role in epilepsy, and imbalance results in neurodegeneration (Tong et al., 2024). TRPA1 activated by turmeric's curcumin demonstrates antioxidant properties advantageous for premature aging and nerve inflammation (Nalli et al., 2017). Ca^{2+} operating as the major secondary messenger is critical in neurological activities. Ca^{2+} homeostasis in neurons is strictly controlled, and irregularities can have adverse effects. Neurodegeneration may arise from increased Ca^{2+} influx, which is frequently caused by overactivated TRP or NMDA receptors. This may cause mitochondria overexertion, oxidative damage, and apoptosis processes, which include the stimulation of proteases and caspases. On the contrary, low Ca^{2+} concentration suppresses signaling between synapses and neural excitability, resulting in decreased neuroplasticity and cognitive impairments (Gleichmann & Mattson, 2011). Therefore preserving ideal intracellular Ca^{2+} concentrations is essential to avoiding neurotoxicity as well as synaptic failures. According to these results, dietary modifications that modulate TRP channels may provide both medicinal as well as preventative approaches for various neurological disorders.

7.4.2 Eye cells and vision

Ophthalmic health or ocular vision is greatly impacted by aging, which can result in diseases, including age-related macular degeneration or incurable blindness (Ambati & Fowler, 2012). TRPs ion channels, such as TRPC1-4, TRPM1/3/7, TRPML1, TRPP2, TRPV2, and TRPV4, have been discovered within the retina of mice in addition to those that mediate retinal phototransduction for the eyes of *Drosophila* (Reinach et al., 2015). Although TRPV4 is responsible for apoptosis and Ca^{2+} flux modulation within the retinal ganglion cells (RGC) in mice, TRPV1 induces the elevated Ca^{2+} levels within cells and apoptosis of RGCs in rats (Ryskamp et al., 2011; Sappington et al., 2009). The retina of chickens also expresses TRPC1 and TRPC4 (Crousillac et al., 2003). Moreover, the TRPM1 was shown to be expressed on the dendrites of ON-bipolar cells in the human retina. TRPA1, TRPM8, and TRPV1 are expressed within the retinoblastoma. Healthier uvea exhibits an elevated expression of TRPA1, whereas uveal malignancies exhibit reduced TRPM8 expressions (Reinach et al., 2015). Mice, rats, and HCEC (human corneal epithelial cells) all expresses TRPV1-4. In addition, cornea sensory neurons exhibit temperature-sensitive TRPA1 and TRPM8 (Mergler et al., 2011; Parra et al., 2010). Conjunctival epithelial cells in humans have thermosensitive TRPV1, TRPV2, and TRPV4. So far, TRPA1 and TRPV1 (both having a crucial role in allergic conjunctivitis) have been discovered as facilitating conjunctivitis (Kwon et al., 2018). Therefore both adaptive and reactive behaviors to a broad spectrum of external triggers that jeopardize tissue equilibrium are dependent on the effective expression of ocular TRPs. When taken as a whole, these ion channels have enormous unexplored potential for making significant therapeutic advancements in eye illness.

7.4.3 Immune cells and inflammation

The human immune system is comprised up of bone marrow-derived innate leukocytes (such as macrophages, neutrophils, and NK cells) with adaptive lymphocytes (such as T and B cells). These immunological responses are affected by the widespread expression of TRP ion channels. A significant proportion of these immune cells move toward the site of the lesion whenever inflammatory processes begin (Yan et al., 2024). *Trpa1* & *Trpv1* mutant mice demonstrated a substantial reduction in IL-31-mediated pruritus, indicating a role for TRPA1 and TRPV1 in an immune system reaction (Cevikbas et al., 2014). Atherosclerosis macrophage in mice lacking lipoprotein E revealed higher levels for TRPA1 expression (Zhao et al., 2016). In addition, U937 (human macrophage) released more IL-8 and TNF-α when TRPA1 was activated. Through activating TRPM8, mice macrophages from the peritoneum demonstrated antiinflammatory properties (Khalil et al., 2016) and in addition blocked human's lymphocytes as well as monocytes from expressing cytokines that trigger inflammation, in vitro (Zhang et al., 2023). When RAW264.7 cell lines were experiencing inflammation, activating TRPV1 suppressed the NO, COX-2, PGE2, and iNOS discharge (Kim et al., 2003). Once TRPV4 was activated within in vitro conditions, T cells proliferated and produced the (IL-2, TNF-α, and IFN-γ) proinflammatory cytokines (Majhi et al., 2015). Among microglia, TRPM4 promotes inflammation, whereas, in T lymphocytes, mast cells, and macrophages, it has the opposite effect. With all these immune cells expressing TRPM7 extensively; within macrophages, they exhibit antiinflammatory properties, whereas, in T cells and mast cells, this has proinflammatory effects (Yan et al., 2024). Such results demonstrate that TRP channels play a crucial role among coordinating in immunological responses within immune system cells and contribute to immunomodulatory effects.

7.4.4 Bone cells and osteoporosis

Aging is a crucial parameter for maintaining bone homeostasis. Ion channel dysfunctions, when combined with age-related abnormalities involving bone development (osteoblast) and bone decomposition (osteoclast) can result in osteogenic diseases such as osteoporosis (Singh et al., 2024a). It has been widely accepted that intra- as well as extracellular Ca^{2+} signals are vital for regulating bone homeostasis (Singh et al., 2024b); therefore, ion channels perform a crucial role in this process (Jiao et al., 2019). As bones are essential for preserving systemic Ca^{2+} homeostasis, adequate blood Ca^{2+} levels are necessary for bone to perform its functions normally. Bone stores nearly 99% of the human body's Ca^{2+} that supports its mechanical and structural abilities. Thus adequate Ca^{2+} is required to bones to remain intact. Furthermore a crucial secondary signal of bones is intracellular Ca^{2+}. Numerous processes, such as differentiation, signal transmission and biomechanical transportation, permeability, and feeling for painful sensations, are believed to be regulated by intracellular Ca^{2+} signaling by neuronal endings, chondrocytes, osteoclasts, and osteoblasts. Ca^{2+} channels are playing an essential part in regulating intra- and extracellular Ca^{2+} equilibrium, which is crucial for bone development (Blair et al., 2007; Lieben & Carmeliet, 2012).

TRPV2 is anticipated to be the Ca^{2+} transportation in osteoclast which contributes to Ca^{2+} oscillations in vitro (Hwang & Putney, 2012). However, as osteoclasts differentiate, Ca^{2+} oscillations occurrences are substituted by continuous Ca^{2+}-influx through TRPV4 (Masuyama et al., 2012) and potentially TRPV5 (Chamoux et al., 2010). Osteoblasts' mechanotransduction signals are regulated by TRPM7 and TRPV4. These channels induce Ca^{2+}-influx in response to mechanical stresses and osmotic variations, which is essential for osteoblast survivability and functioning. The density of bones and microstructure are maintained via TRPV4's regulation of osteoblast development and activity of mitochondria (Acharya et al., 2023; Guilak et al., 2010; Rohde et al., 2019). In addition, TRP channel function has been linked with bone-formation capability because TRPM7 is necessary for the viability of mesenchymal stem cells produced from bone marrow that might transform into osteoblasts (Cheng et al., 2010). Particularly in cases of nutritional Ca^{2+} deficits, TRPV6 is essential in the absorption of Ca^{2+} in the intestine to maintain the mineralization of bones (Lieben et al., 2010). Despite having low degrees of expression in both osteoclasts and osteoblasts, TRPV6 is not explicitly involved in acquiring osteogenic Ca^{2+} or mineral deposition (Little et al., 2011;

Van der Eerden et al., 2012). It plays an indirect contribution to the metabolism of bones, mostly by making it easier for Ca^{2+} to move out of the colon. Conversely, TRPV5 improves Ca^{2+} reabsorption in the kidney, which is crucial for maintaining systemic Ca^{2+} homeostasis. Notably, osteoblasts were not expressing TRPV5. In addition, TRPV5 is found around the wrinkle's edge of osteoclasts that could help in resorption of bones (Jiao et al., 2019). Interestingly, TRPV5 and TRPV6 are two well-known Ca^{2+}-ion channels with great selectivity (Van Der Eerden et al., 2005). Expression of TRPV1 stimulates the differentiation process of both the cells, that is, osteoclast as well as osteoblasts. Furthermore, their development is inhibited by pharmacologic suppression of TRPV1 in vitro. In addition, through lowering the acceleration of the breakdown of bones as well as its development, in vivo inhibition of TRPV1 activities safeguards mice toward ovariectomy-induced decay of bones. TRPV1 could consequently have an immediate effect on the development of osteogenic cells (Lieben & Carmeliet, 2012). Therefore modulators of TRPV1 are currently employed in clinical management as a component of analgesics treatment.

Notably, optimum Ca^{2+} levels in serum as well as in intracellular environment are essential for proper Ca^{2+} signaling. Accordingly, Ca^{2+} deficiency leads to amplification of the deleterious effects of other ions, mainly due to the fact that optimum amount of Ca^{2+} ion imposes a biochemical competition with other divalent ions, which is linked with the physiological functions. Thus daily dietary calcium intake (mainly in the form of carbonates, citrates, and phosphates from highly Ca^{2+}-rich foods, which include dairy products, green leafy vegetables, and fortified cereals, as well as from seeds and nuts) is important. Through many biological processes, Ca^{2+} serves as a secondary transmitter. For example, Ca^{2+} is essential in healthy bones as well as function of other tissues (Singh et al., 2022). Ca^{2+} resorption, within renal cells and intestinal absorption depend mainly on TRPV channels, especially TRPV5 and TRPV6 (Lieben et al., 2012). By increasing TRPV6 expression, vitamin D promotes Ca^{2+} absorption as well as deposition of bone minerals. Furthermore, TRP channel-related function is modulated by nutraceuticals such as genistein (found from soy products) alongside resveratrol (present within grapes), which also promote osteoblast development and prevent osteoporosis. By activating estrogen-related mechanisms and signaling chains, including MAPK and PI3K, genistein promotes osteoblastogenesis (Cepeda et al., 2020). Resveratrol works by altering NF-κB pathway interactions to prevent osteoclastogenesis (Shakibaei et al., 2011). In addition, Mg^{2+}, through indirect means, communicates through TRP channels to promote bone tissue generation and lower the possibility of osteoporosis (Hao et al., 2024). Such nutrient-TRP channel associations point toward a potential nutrient-rich method to improve bone condition and Ca^{2+} equilibrium, indicating a comprehensive dietary change strategy that might prevent or address osteoporosis.

7.4.5 Adipocytes and adipogenesis

Adipose tissue, a crucial modulator of metabolic processes for energy, is greatly impacted by aging. Adipocyte physiology depends on a number of TRP ion channels, which affect insulin susceptibility, thermogenesis, and lipids accumulation. TRP ion channels also have a role in controlling inflammatory processes of adipose tissue that worsen throughout aging and contribute to metabolic diseases, including insulin intolerance and obesity (Bishnoi et al., 2018; Gao et al., 2019). TRPC1 inhibition within adipocytes could hinder Ca^{2+} entrance and differentiation. By triggering Ca^{2+} influx, TRPC3 could trigger the NF-KB signal transduction. Inhibition of TRPC4/TRPC5 via ML204 exacerbates liver steatosis, obesity-related fat deposits, dyslipidaemias, and elevated blood sugar levels. TRPC7-facilitated Ca^{2+} signaling capitalizes on MAPK and AKT pathways to prevent migrations and cell cycle development. When TRPV1 is overexpressed within developed 3T3-L1 preadipocytes, it increases the level of expression of several thermogenic genes. Expression of TRPV2 in brown adipocytes promotes differentiation as well as the process of thermogenesis (Wu et al., 2024). Expression of TRPV2 is more prevalent than TRPV1, TRPV3, TRPV4, and TRPM8 in mouse brown adipocytes. TRPV3 is already shown to be expressed in both brown and white adipose tissues. The obese mice (visceral adipose tissue), particularly those raised on a high-fat diet, showed an apparent downregulation of TRPV3 expressions. TRPV4 inhibits oxidation of mitochondria; TRPV4 deletion increased the level of expression for uncoupling protein 1 in adipocytes as well as showed reduced obesity when administered high-fat diets (Jiang et al., 2017). Moreover, when TRPM8 is activated in adipocytes, protein kinase A along with Ca^{2+} influx is triggered, which causes expression of uncoupling protein 1, β-oxidation, elongation as well as localization of mitochondria into droplets of lipids, and lipolysis (Sanders et al., 2021). Adipose tissue also expresses TRPP2 and its expression level is higher in mature adipocytes when compared to the preadipocytes. In addition, stimulation of TRPA1 causes rats to secrete adrenaline and prevents fat storage and obesity. TRPA1 governs brown adipose tissue's ability to produce heat via the central nervous system. Thus stimulation of TRPA1 using its ligands seems like a potential strategy for both the avoidance and cure of obesity among humans (Sun et al., 2021).

7.4.6 Gut tissue and nutrition uptake, IBD

Aging influencing the function and expression of the TRP ion channel can compromise the gut's potential to regulate inflammatory processes, and nutrient uptake as well as imbalance in gut homeostasis, thereby increasing the possibility of gut-related diseases that include IBD. TRPV4 is actively expressed in samples from human intestinal and colon cells such as Caco-2 and T84 as well as in mouse colons that are inflamed. TRPV4 activation within the gastrointestinal tract can raise the intracellular Ca^{2+} level thereby eventually, leading to chemokine secretion and colitis (D'Aldebert et al., 2011). Activating TRPV4 in the gastrointestinal tract can have a proinflammatory response while inhibiting TRPV4 selectively suppresses colitis and even reduces the discomfort caused by gastrointestinal inflammation in an IBD animal model (Fichna et al., 2012). Both the neuronal ends and immunologic cells were impacted by the increased expression of TRPV1 for people suffering from IBD, indicating the significance of TRPV1 for the pathophysiology of IBD as well as in colorectal immunological control of inflammations (Kun et al., 2014). TRPV1 expressing itself within the rectum is substantially raised in more than 20% of IBD patients, which makes it essential since it mediates pain associated with inflammation (Molodecky et al., 2012).

In addition, elevated TRPV1 expression has been observed in acute colitis animal models as well as individuals experiencing extreme occurrences of IBD (Engel et al., 2012). Sensory neuron in colons expresses TRPM8, which is linked with TRPA1 and TRPV1, which prevents their subsequent mechano- and chemo-sensory responses (Harrington et al., 2011). Within postinflammatory colorectal allergies rat models, enhanced TRPM8 expression considerably decreased the signs of colon allergies and diminished responsiveness toward mechanical stimulation (Adam et al., 2006). An important factor in the emergence of IBD is TRPA1. The colon afferent dorsal root ganglia (DRG) neuronal cells exhibit a higher level of expression of TRPA1. When TRPA1 is activated, the mucosal integrity within the colon epithelium prevents the generation of IL-10, IFN-γ, and nitric oxide, and markedly decreased nitrite concentrations (Zhang et al., 2023). Recent literature suggests that the cross-talk of the gut–brain for a number of enteroneuronal disorders is mediated by TRP ion channels that are sensitive to bacterial endotoxin, including TRPA1, TRPV1, TRPV4, TRPM3, and TRPM8. Furthermore, in vivo, it is demonstrated that knocking out either TRPA1 or TRPV1 or both has altered gut microbiota along with associated metabolic pathways (Yue & Xu, 2021).

TRP channels, including TRPV1, TRPV4, TRPM8, and TRPA1, modulate gastrointestinal movement, visceral discomfort, and inflammatory conditions, as well as the gut is essential for immunological control and nutrition intake (Dvornikova et al., 2024). Usually indigestible fibers, prebiotics, help to increase the number and productivity of healthy bacteria in the gut. TRP channel functionality is indirectly influenced by prebiotics via disturbances in the gut microbiota. Certain prebiotics, for example, have the ability to elevate the activation of TRPV1 and TRPA1 channels that may change gut movement and help create a better harmonious gastrointestinal microenvironment (Nagpal et al., 2020). Probiotic supplements (living microorganisms) are helpful for diseases like IBD because they can enhance the activity of the intestinal lining and reduce gut inflammation. These probiotics, when given in sufficient quantities, affect the development of TRP channels. For example, TRPV4 expression in mice was reduced indirectly under the influence of probiotic variant *Lactobacillus paracasei* F34-3 (F343) (Liu et al., 2024). Similarly, postbiotics (metabolic by-products obtained from probiotics) may also influence TRP channels expression. TRP channels are susceptible to short-chain fatty acids (SCFAs) like butyrate, a prevalent postbiotic created when the microbes in the gut ferment the fibers, to improve the integrity of barriers and lower inflammation within the gut (Shin et al., 2023). Prebiotics, probiotics, and postbiotics all regulate TRP channels, which promote gut health and help control IBD; however, it is still unknown how the gut microbiome and TRP interact directly. New findings could make personalized treatments for digestive diseases possible.

7.4.7 Liver and pancreas

Alteration in TRP ion channel expression and function within the liver and pancreas that are mainly responsible for maintaining a healthy metabolism and regulating cellular oxidation and inflammation may arise from age-related problems (Liu et al., 2023a). Interestingly, many TRP ion channels that are expressed within the liver get modulated and affect the disease onset and progressions with age-related health problems or aging. Numerous TRP ion channels, including TRPV1, TRPM2, along TRPC1, have been found expressing within liver cells and play an integral part in controlling inflammatory processes, oxidative damage control, and metabolic processes of lipids. In this context, capsaicin-induced stimulation of TRPV1 has been demonstrated to enhance insulin responsiveness, decrease triglyceride and lipid buildups, and alleviate nonalcoholic fatty liver disease (NAFLD) by modifying the pathways associated with lipid oxidations (Li et al., 2012; Liu et al., 2023b). Likewise, TRPM2, an ion channel that reacts with reactive oxygen species (ROS) and controls Ca^{2+} influx, is significantly expressed within hepatic cells while playing a role in damages caused by oxidation and apoptosis of hepatocytes in prolonged liver damage and old age (Liu et al., 2023b). Similarly, changes in the expression of TRPC6 have been linked with hepatocellular carcinoma and hepatic fibrosis (Rychkov & Barritt, 2011). Numerous studies have shown the TRP ion channel expression in pancreatic beta-cells performs a crucial part in their activities. TRPM5 and TRPM2 have a crucial role in releasing insulin within the pancreas, especially in the beta-cells of the human islets of Langerhans (Matos et al., 2022). TRPM5, a Ca^{2+}-activated channel, depolarizes the plasma membrane and promotes Ca^{2+} inflow to help glucose-driven insulin release (Brixel et al., 2010). TRPV2 has been associated with both insulin release as well as cell growth, and its activity is modulated via insulin's autocrine responses. Through regulating the amount of neuropeptide secretion, TRPV1 expression in neuronal sensory cells contributes to inflammatory processes and distress among pancreatic beta-cells (Uchida & Tominaga, 2011). Therefore gaining insight into these TRP ion channel functions may open new treatment options in aging-related metabolic diseases.

7.5 Molecular factors contributing to "aging" and the importance of TRP channels

Aging at individual level is a multifactorial phenomenon, and several factors such as nutritional deficits, infection, genotypes, other medical conditions, exposure to toxic and noxious chemicals, and reduced levels of steroids and hormones, all contribute to the aging. Accordingly, there are several molecular factors that contribute to the cellular aging. Here we discuss some of these key factors (not all) that are regulated by TRP channels and are linked with the aging.

7.5.1 ROS signaling

There are several reasons by which specific foods containing bioactive agents can contribute on ageing or act as antiageing. ROS generated within the cytosol as a well as within the specific subcellular organelles are considered a key reason related to ageing. Excess ROS production is linked to quicker aging, imposing the importance of antioxidants to present ageing. As the lifetime of ROS are short, excess ROS cause unwanted and uncontrolled "oxidation" of biomolecules, such as for DNA, lipids and proteins. ROS production causes DNA damage, a potential cause that such oxidations are covalent in nature and cause mostly irreversible or at least long-term changes in the molecules, leading to altered cellular functions (Cheignon et al., 2018). Often lipid peroxidation is also observed in cases where excess peroxide is produced. For example, lipid peroxidation in sperm membrane is observed and is linked with aging and/or lack of antioxidants.

7.5.2 Protein aggregation

Protein aggregation is often detrimental to cellular functions and specific cases of protein aggregation are linked to aging and pathophysiology. Few classic examples are aggregation of Tau protein, which is the molecular cause of neurodegeneration, which leads to the development of Alzheimer's disease. A less common example is Huntington's disease, which is also dependent on the presence of mutant gene (mHtt) (Yang et al., 2024b). Notably, TRP channels are involved in the Alzheimer's disease and other neurodegeneration processes. TRP channels are involved in the hyper activation of glial cells, demyelination process. TRP channels are also involved in neuroprotection and neuritogenesis, neuron-to-neuron contact formation. Thus TRP channels play a dual function in terms of neurodegeneration and neuroprotection.

7.5.3 pH homeostasis

Other factors that are related to aging are pH homeostasis of entire tissue and cells and even in the intracellular organelles. For example, maintenance of the low pH in the lysosome is crucial for healthy status of macrophages and thus a crucial determinant of the infection level of the entire body and overall immune function. In this context, TRP channels as well as other ion channels are important regulators of lysosomal functions.

7.5.4 Heavy metals

Exposure of tissues and cells to heavy metals is known to induce cellular toxicity and cause aging. At microscopic level, cells do not have specific ion channels and/or transports and pumps that can regulate the influx and efflux of majority of the heavy metals. Nevertheless, heavy metals can enter to the cells by using handful number of TRP ion channels because of two reasons. First, these channels have bigger pores (and such pores can also dilate depending on the ionic radius of the heavy metal), and these channels are nonspecific in nature (thus allowing the influx of different monovalent and divalent cations). Therefore TRP channels act as the "molecular routes" for heavy metal influx to the cells.

7.6 "Aging" at the subcellular levels and involvement of TRP channels

Aging at the subcellular level can be analyzed as degree of dysfunction of certain key subcellular organelle. In this section, we analyze few of these changes that occur in the subcellular organelles and are typically subject to regulation by TRP ion channels.

7.6.1 Mitochondria

Mitochondria not only act as the power house (because of the production of ATP-Adenosine Triphosphate) for cell but also act as major hub for several metabolisms. Such mitochondria-mediated metabolisms are required for production of key signaling molecules, such as NO, different ROS, steroids, and small peptides neurotransmitters (Murphy, 2008; Papadopoulos & Miller, 2012). In addition, mitochondria produce heat for the cell that is required for overall cellular thermal homeostasis. Therefore lack of mitochondrial numbers and/or functions, both results in lack of these essential factors, which leads to aging. Indeed, at present a series of diseases are known that are because of abnormal mitochondrial functions. Collectively such diseases are known as mitopathy. So far a large number of reports suggest present of TRP ion channels directly in mitochondria (such as TRPV4) and these channels regulate several mitochondrial functions (Acharya et al., 2025; Kumar et al., 2024a, 2024b).

7.6.2 Lysosome

Lysosomes are important organelles that are involved in the degradation and recycling of unwanted molecules, such as aggregated proteins, endocytosed receptors, and phagocytosed particles (such as bacteria) targeted for degradation. Lysosome-mediated degradation needs low pH (at the range of 3.5–5.5) at the lysosomal lumen, and such low acidic pH needs involvement of several lysosomal ion channels and ATP-dependent molecular pumps, a complex process that is still poorly understood. Nevertheless, malfunction of lysosomes can lead to serious compromization of the overall cellular functions. This can impose cellular stress and aging (Venkatachalam, 2022). Indeed, lysosomal disorders are hallmark of several diseases, commonly known as lysopathy. In this regard, TRP channels, such as TRPML and TRPV3, are present in the lysosomes and regulate lysosomal functions (Yadav & Goswami, 2017).

7.6.3 Endoplasmic reticulum (ER)

Endoplasmic reticulum (ER) is the subcellular organelles that is involved in the synthesis of transmembrane proteins, posttranslational modifications (such as glycosylation) and vesicle budding. ER content is also well distributed and ER function is also related to overall vesicular dynamics, maintenance of plasma membrane content and regulation of autophagy (Sukumaran et al., 2016). In that context, compromization of ER functions is directly related to several cellularmalfunctions that affects secretion of important products (such as enzymes, neurotransmitters, and hormones) by vesicles. Notably, ER functions are highly energy-dependent and thus close proximity to mitochondria or proper ER–mitochondrial contact formation is also important in the context of several diseases.

7.6.4 Epigenetic changes in the nucleus and DNA

Aging is directly related to the epigenetic changes in the DNA and thus gene expression. In this context, steroids and steroid-like molecules are also important. Total regulation of cellular metabolism, lipid profiles, and cytokine profiles is important. Notably, most of the TRP channels are involved in these cellular processes and thus can act as factors for cellular differentiation and aging.

7.7 Presence of ligands of TRP ion channels in the spices/foods/super foods

Spices, foods, and superfoods contain several phytochemicals and/or bioactive compounds that serve as either specific or nonspecific ligand for different TRP channels, making these channels biologically significant in various physiological conditions and therapeutic processes. This also makes TRP as molecular center for several nutraceuticals and food industry. As the number and types of all these plant/food-based components are very large, only selected few components that act as ligands of important TRP channels are discussed here in details (Fig. 7.3).

7.7.1 Capsinoids, capsaicinoids, and capsaicin

Capsinoids are a group of natural molecules that represent nonpungent analogues of capsaicin. Capsinoids have comparable biological actions, making them important constituents in superfoods, cuisines, and in spices. Capsaicinoids, including capsaicin, are abundant in varieties of peppers such as in *Capsicum annuum.* The contents of capsinoids and capsaicinoids in pepper plants are influenced by both environmental factors and genetic variations (Tarinta et al., 2023). The development of pepper hybrids with high capsaicinoid content is becoming increasingly important in food science, in agriculture and also for food preservation. In addition to their flavoring properties, capsinoids have gained attention for their health benefits. Investigation to study the impact of capsinoids on lipid profiles reveal that these compounds significantly reduced total cholesterol levels, making them beneficial for cardiovascular health (Amini et al., 2022). This effect was especially pronounced in fermented red pepper paste, a popular condiment in Asian cuisines. Capsaicin also serves as a natural food preservative as capsaicin in high concentration can act as an antimicrobial agent (mainly because of its high-hydrophobicity that causes membrane damage). Capsaicin is the bioactive component that gives chili peppers their spiciness and it has been extensively researched for its effect on the TRPV1 channel. In fact, the use of capsaicin as a neuro-stimulating agent helps to discover TRPV1, a mile stone work that was awarded with Noble prize (Caterina et al., 1997). Capsaicin has been demonstrated to activate TRPV1 specifically and thus initiates signaling for various biological processes such as pain perception, inflammatory regulation, immune activation, and in cancer progression. Capsaicin's potential to enhance exercise performance has also been explored. A randomized trial summarized positive effects of oral capsaicinoids and capsinoids supplementation on endurance, strength, and fatigue in high-intensity interval training (HIIT) (Sukan-Karaçağıl et al., 2023). Capsaicin's role in activating TRPV1 channels during exercise further underscores its ergogenic properties. These

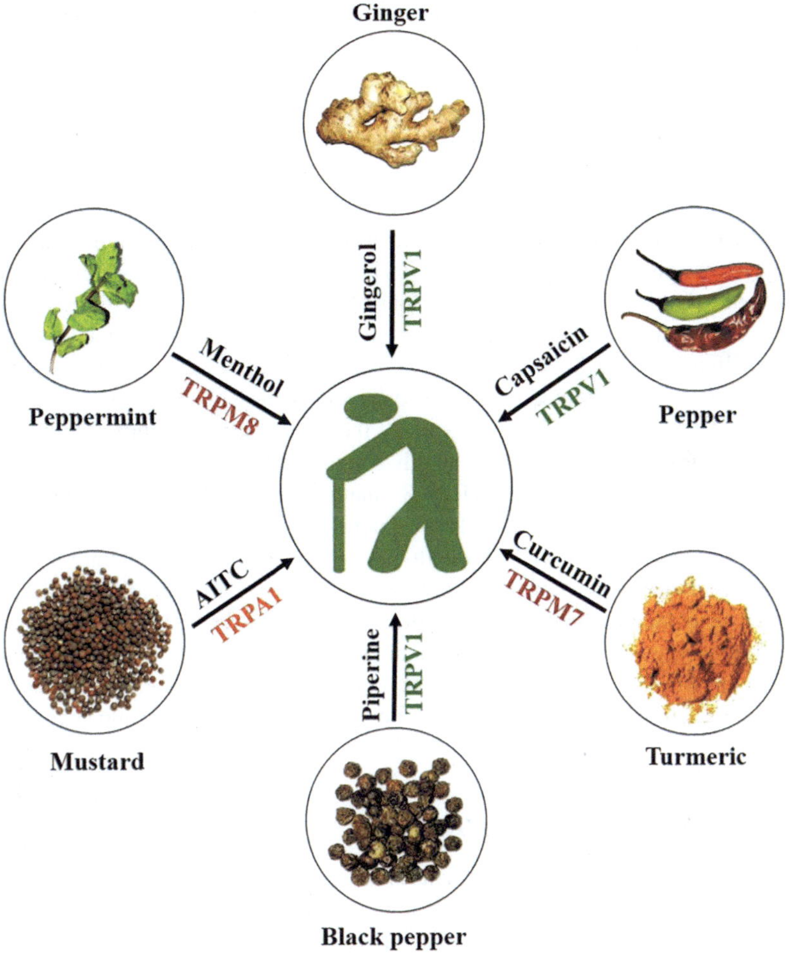

Figure 7.3 Natural dietary foods containing several phytochemicals and/or bioactive compounds serving as a specific or non-specific ligand for different TRP channels modulation affecting health and ageing processes. Only a few selected items are presented in this figure.

findings illustrate the diverse biological roles of capsaicin and capsinoids in superfoods, foods, and spices. From metabolic regulation to neuroprotection, these compounds offer promising health benefits when incorporated into the diet. Capsazepin is another bioactive component that is present in nonpungent chilli verities and act as an inhibitor of TRPV1 (Bevan et al., 1992).

7.7.2 Menthol

Menthol, a cooling compound found in many plants, is particularly associated with the mint family and acts as an activator of TRPM8 channel, thus inducing a cold sensation. Beyond its presence in mint and peppermint, recent studies have focused on its occurrence in a wider array of foods and superfoods in cosmetics and also in skin balm. *Mentha piperita* (peppermint) is a rich source in menthol, and its essential oils have been widely used not only in food flavoring but also in medicinal contexts.

Menthol also serves as an antifungal agent in food preservation. Antifungal activity of menthol combined with eugenol against *Aspergillus ochraceus* and *Aspergillus niger*, two fungi commonly found in stored cereals have been demonstrated (Ben Miri et al., 2023). Their findings revealed that menthol effectively reduced fungal growth and spore germination, providing evidence of its potential as a natural preservative. Further research into the flavor-modifying properties of menthol has revealed its sensory influence beyond mint. Menthol can also mask the bitter off-flavors of artificial sweeteners like acesulfame-K (Büchner et al., 2022). This highlights its role in enhancing the palatability of health-oriented beverages, particularly those using sugar alternatives.

A series of research works also explores the interaction of menthol with TRPM8 leading to sensory perception and health benefits. Menthol's cooling properties is extending to its interaction with TRPM8 channel, responsible for thermosensation. Menthol modulates thermal perception in neurons, showing that it attenuates cold-sensitive thermoreceptors, adding depth to our understanding of menthol's role in sensory experiences when consumed in foods and spices (Leijon et al., 2019). A recent report suggests menthol cools mitochondrial temperature that can have implication in preventing aging, especially against inflammation (Kumar et al., 2023). These studies underline menthol's significant role across food preservation, flavor enhancement, and sensory modulation, making it a valuable compound in both culinary and health-related applications.

7.7.3 Allyl isothiocyanate (AITC)

It is a sulfur-containing compound naturally present in cruciferous vegetables such as mustard, horseradish, and wasabi. Known for its distinctive pungency, AITC has attracted significant interest for its health-promoting properties, including anticancer, antimicrobial, and sensory effects. Application of AITC causes activation of TRPA1 ion channels in neurone as well as in different primary cells (such as in in T cell) leading to Ca^{2+} influx and multiple signaling events (Sahoo et al., 2019). However, excess of AITC and/or constitute TRPA1 activation can leads to proinflammatory condition or provide nociceptive signaling. Nevertheless, in addition to its role in cancer prevention, AITC exhibits potent antimicrobial activity. AITC in combination with eugenol effectively inhibits the growth of common fungal pathogens like *A. niger* in stored cereals, confirms that AITC antifungal effects (Ben Miri et al., 2023). This suggests that AITC can serve as a natural preservative in food systems, helping to extend shelf life while maintaining safety. AITC's impact on human sensory perception, particularly its interaction with taste and smell, is another area of research. It has been demonstrated that AITC can enhance the perception of saltiness in foods, potentially offering a strategy for reducing salt content without compromising flavor (Amyoony et al., 2024). This property has important implications for the development of healthier, low-sodium foods.

7.7.4 Gingerol

Gingerol is a major bioactive component present in ginger (*Zingiber officinale*). It is one of the key compounds responsible for the characteristic pungent taste of ginger and is present in several superfoods, foods, and spices. The growing interest in natural and functional foods has elevated the importance of bioactive compounds like gingerol in superfoods and spices. Ginger is widely used in traditional medicine and culinary practices, and its incorporation into foods such as ginger tea, smoothies, and ginger-flavored dishes reflects its importance as a functional food ingredient. Gingerol is known for its wide range of health benefits, including anti-inflammatory, antioxidant, and anticancer properties. Recent studies have explored its potential applications in various health contexts, emphasizing its importance in traditional and modern medicine. Gingerol exhibits strong antioxidant and anti-inflammatory properties. Gingerol also acts as a ligand for TRPV1. 6-Gingerol, a major variant, can alleviate hepatic steatosis and reduce oxidative stress, especially in the context of high-fat diets (Liu et al., 2023a). This highlights its role in liver protection and metabolic health. Moreover, 6-gingerol reduces brain infarct volume and inflammation in an ischemic stroke model, emphasizing its neuroprotective capabilities (Kongsui & Jittiwat., 2023). These findings underscore its potential in treating neurodegenerative diseases and preventing brain damage. Gingerol has also been studied for its anticancer properties. Gingerol has strong potential as nutraceutical. Gingerol has been found to inhibit cancer cell proliferation and induce apoptosis, positioning it as a promising candidate for integrative cancer therapies (Garza-Cadena et al., 2023).

Gingerol's benefits are also extend to gastrointestinal health, particularly in alleviating nausea and improving digestion. Gingerol ameliorates diabetic cardiomyopathy by reducing inflammation and oxidative stress through the Nrf2/HO-1 pathway, thereby promoting cardiovascular health (Wu et al., 2022). In conclusion, gingerol plays a significant role in promoting human health, offering a wide spectrum of biological activities from anti-inflammatory and antioxidant effects to potential anticancer properties. Its integration into superfoods and spices continues to drive its popularity as a natural therapeutic agent.

7.7.5 Piperine

Piperine is the primary bioactive compound found in superfoods, foods, and spices and it act on TRPV1. It is mainly found in black pepper (*Piper nigrum*), and is responsible for its pungent flavor and health-promoting properties and may have anticancer properties. Piperine is notable for its bioavailability-enhancing effects, as it improves the absorption of several nutrients and bioactive compounds, including curcumin, in the human body. Piperine interacts with DNA, specifically in human breast cancer cells (Rezaei et al., 2023). The study demonstrated that piperine induces cytotoxicity in cancer cells, increases lipid peroxidation, and activates caspase-3, a protein involved in apoptosis. Piperine has demonstrated efficacy in wound healing and inflammation management. Piperine-containing bioactive hydrogel has positive effects in a rat wound model (Alsareii et al., 2023). The results showed accelerated healing and reduced inflammation in wounds treated with piperine. Piperine has also neuroprotective effects. Synthetic piperine analogues have positive effects as it inhibits acetylcholinesterase (AChE) and butyrylcholinesterase (BChE), enzymes involved in Alzheimer's disease (Jaipea et al., 2023). Thus piperine analogues have potential applications for cognitive health and neurodegenerative disease management.

7.7.6 Curcumin

Curcumin, the principal bioactive compound in turmeric (*Curcuma longa*), is known for its diverse medicinal properties, including anti-inflammatory, antioxidant, and anticancer activities. Turmeric is commonly used in Asian cuisine and also as a traditional remedy for many health problems. Turmeric paste is also used in cosmetics for skin improvement and as an analgesic formulation. Curcumin is widely incorporated into superfoods and spices because of its health benefits. It has become an integral part of the functional food market, used in products such as turmeric lattes, smoothies, and health bars. Turmeric's ability to improve food appeal while offering health benefits has driven its popularity in both culinary and nutraceutical sectors. Curcumin can prevent and improves chronic diseases (Kunnumakkara et al., 2023). Curcumin affects several TRP channels such as TRPM7 and TRPV1 (Nalli et al., 2017). Curcumin has been found to inhibit the proliferation of cancer cells, reduce oxidative stress, and modulate immune responses, making it a powerful compound for health benefits. Curcumin–piperine supplementation improves glycaemic control, lipid profiles, and antioxidant status in patients with diabetes, obesity, and metabolic syndrome (Heidari et al., 2023). Curcumin reduces inflammation, acts as an anticancer compound, protect against neurodegenerative diseases, and support cardiovascular health. It is also effective as an analgesic in the case of chemotherapy-induced cytotoxicity. Application of curcumin as pharmaceutical, medicinal, and in food is effective in treating chronic diseases such as cancer and diabetes through its antioxidant and anti-inflammatory mechanisms (El-Saadony et al., 2023).

However, curcumin suffers from poor oral bioavailability. One of the main challenges associated with curcumin is its poor bioavailability because of rapid metabolism and low solubility in water. Coadministration of curcumin with piperine has been shown to significantly improve its bioabsorption. Various strategies have been developed to overcome these limitations. Use of nanotechnology to form specific nanoparticles and use of other agents such as cyclodextrins and novel polymorphic varieties can increase the bioavailability of curcumin.

7.8 Conclusion

It is important to note that TRP channels represent nonessential genes (as knockout animals survive without much difficulty, at least in controlled laboratory condition) that are present in all animals and often become subject to gene diversification and multiplication. However, the presence of TRP channels significantly improves the ability of animals to perform different tasks under certain conditions. This is also reflected in the "quality of cells" against several stressed and/or pathological conditions. Notably, TRP channels can be modulated by bioactive compounds present in the food ingredients even at very low concentrations.

There are immediate as well as long-term effects of consumption of certain bioactive agents that are present in the food and these actions are because of the modulation of TRP channels. Such effects are more prominent in case of routine consumption of specific food items. For example, consumption of capsaicin present in spicy food results in immediate activation of TRPV1 present in gut and also in the peripheral nerves associated with the digestive system. This results in an increase in body temperature, increase heartbeat, expansion of blood vessels. In an opposite manner, menthol, a food ingredient present in mint is known to induce an immediate cooling as well as analgesic effect. These immediate responses are mostly because of activation or inhibition of TRP channels present in peripheral neurons, especially in the gut.

However, regular and long-term consumption of food allows these bioactive compounds to reach to different organs and ideally affect TRP channels present in most part of the body. This can have profound physiological effects and such effects can be utilized for health benefits. For example, regular yet limited consumption of capsaicin through food may results in better fat-burn, increased immunity, lesser microbial load, better bone-density, and other health benefits. However, excess capsaicin can enhance inflammation and burning sensation. Long term consumption of gingerol (present in ginger and activates TRPV1) may have impact on bone density. Better cognitive functions can also be expected in case of regular consumption of certain spicy foods that target TRP channels. Specific food with bioactive compounds can also be utilized for treating depression and anxiety.

A proper understanding of bioactive compounds that are present in food, their bioavailability, effects on TRP channels and subsequent health benefits is critical for better health, prevention of age-related disorders and also for cure of certain pathological conditions. Notably the "calendar age of individual" and the "biological age of different organs or cells" are not same and often the second one aged faster than the first one in pathological conditions. Therefore recognizing the significance of TRP channels in the process of tissue and cell aging and how these channels communicate with dietary supplements is also important for establishing new treatment techniques for encouraging a healthy process of aging and/or tackling medical problems that are common in aged population.

Acknowledgments

Intramural funding from NISER is acknowledged. All authors acknowledge the supports from all the present lab members and their critical comments on the manuscript.

References

Acharya, T. K., Pal, S., Ghosh, A., Kumar, S., Kumar, S., Chattopadhyay, N., & Goswami, C. (2023). TRPV4 regulates osteoblast differentiation and mitochondrial function that are relevant for channelopathy. *Frontiers in Cell and Developmental Biology*, 11. https://doi.org/10.3389/FCELL.2023.1066788.

Acharya, T. K., Kumar, A., Kumar Majhi, R., Kumar, S., Chakraborty, R., Tiwari, A., Smalla, K. H., Liu, X., Chang, Y. T., Gundelfinger, E. D., & Goswami, C. (2022). TRPV4 acts as a mitochondrial Ca^{2+}-importer and regulates mitochondrial temperature and metabolism. *Mitochondrion, 67*, 38–58. https://doi.org/10.1016/J.MITO.2022.10.001.

Acharya, T. K., Mahapatra, P., Kumar, S., Dubey, N. K., Rajalaxmi, S., Ghosh, A., Kumar, A., & Goswami, C. (2025). Conserved and unique mitochondrial target sequence of TRPV4 can independently regulate mitochondrial functions. *Proteins, 93*(4), 908–919. https://doi.org/10.1002/prot.26772.

Adam, B., Liebregts, T., Best, J., Bechmann, L., Lackner, C., Neumann, J., Koehler, S., & Holtmann, G. (2006). A combination of peppermint oil and caraway oil attenuates the post-inflammatory visceral hyperalgesia in a rat model. *Scandinavian Journal of Gastroenterology, 41*(2), 155–160. https://doi.org/10.1080/00365520500206442.

Alsareii, S. A., Ahmad, J., Umar, A., Ahmad, M. Z., & Shaikh, I. A. (2023). Enhanced in vivo wound healing efficacy of a novel piperine-containing bioactive hydrogel in excision wound rat model. *Molecules, 28*(2), 545. https://doi.org/10.3390/molecules28020545.

Ambati, J., & Fowler, B. J. (2012). Mechanisms of age-related macular degeneration. *Neuron, 75*(1), 26–39. https://doi.org/10.1016/J.NEURON.2012.06.018.

Amini, M. R., Payandeh, N., Sheikhhossein, F., Alvani, M., Talebyan, A., Mohtashaminia, F., & Hekmatdoost, A. (2022). The effects of capsinoids and fermented red pepper paste supplementation on lipid profile: A systematic review and meta-analysis of randomized controlled trials. *Clinical Nutrition Research, 11*(4), 302. https://doi.org/10.7762/cnr.2022.11.4.302.

Amyoony, J., Gorman, M., Dabas, T., Moss, R., & McSweeney, M. B. (2024). The effect of allyl isothiocyanate addition on consumers' saltiness perception. *International Journal of Food Science & Technology, 59*(2), 950–958. https://doi.org/10.1111/IJFS.16855.

Belrose, J. C., Xie, Y. F., Gierszewski, L. J., MacDonald, J. F., & Jackson, M. F. (2012). Loss of glutathione homeostasis associated with neuronal senescence facilitates TRPM2 channel activation in cultured hippocampal pyramidal neurons. *Molecular Brain, 5*, 1–11. https://doi.org/10.1186/1756-6606-5-11.

Ben Miri, Y., Nouasri, A., Herrera, M., Djenane, D., & Ariño, A. (2023). Antifungal activity of menthol, eugenol and their combination against *Aspergillus ochraceus* and *Aspergillus niger* in vitro and in stored cereals. *Foods, 12*(11), 2108. https://doi.org/10.3390/FOODS12112108/S1.

Bevan, S., Hothi, S., Hughes, G., James, I. F., Rang, H. P., Shah, K., Walpole, C. S. J., & Yeats, J. C. (1992). Capsazepine: A competitive antagonist of the sensory neurone excitant capsaicin. *British Journal of Pharmacology, 107*(2), 544–552. https://doi.org/10.1111/J.1476-5381.1992.TB12781.X.

Bishnoi, M., Khare, P., Brown, L., & Panchal, S. K. (2018). Transient receptor potential (TRP) channels: A metabolic TR(i)P to obesity prevention and therapy. *Obesity Reviews, 19*(9), 1269–1292. https://doi.org/10.1111/OBR.12703.

Blair, H. C., Schlesinger, P. H., Huang, C. L. H., & Zaidi, M. (2007). Calcium signalling and calcium transport in bone disease. In E. Carafoli, & M. Brini (Eds.), *Calcium signalling and disease. Subcellular biochemistry* (p. 45). https://doi.org/10.1007/978-1-4020-6191-2_21.

Bonsignore, G., Martinotti, S., & Ranzato, E. (2024). Wound repair and Ca^{2+} signalling interplay: The role of Ca^{2+} channels in skin. *Cells, 13*(6), 491. https://doi.org/10.3390/CELLS13060491.

Brierley, S. M., Page, A. J., Hughes, P. A., Adam, B., Liebregts, T., Cooper, N. J., Holtmann, G., Liedtke, W., & Blackshaw, L. A. (2008). Selective role for TRPV4 ion channels in visceral sensory pathways. *Gastroenterology, 134*(7), 2059–2069. https://doi.org/10.1053/J.GASTRO.2008.01.074.

Brixel, L. R., Monteilh-Zoller, M. K., Ingenbrandt, C. S., Fleig, A., Penner, R., Enklaar, T., Zabel, B. U., & Prawitt, D. (2010). TRPM5 regulates glucose-stimulated insulin secretion. *Pflugers Archiv: European Journal of Physiology, 460*(1), 69–76. https://doi.org/10.1007/S00424-010-0835-Z.

Büchner, K., Haagen, J., Sastrosubroto, A., Kerpes, R., Freiherr, J., & Becker, T. (2022). Trigeminal stimulus menthol masks bitter off-flavor of artificial sweetener acesulfame-K. *Foods, 11*(18). https://doi.org/10.3390/FOODS11182734.

Caterina, M. J., Pang, Z., Szallasi, A., & Huang, S. M. (2016). TRP channels in skin biology and pathophysiology. *Pharmaceuticals, 9*(4), 77. https://doi.org/10.3390/PH9040077.

Caterina, M. J., Schumacher, M. A., Tominaga, M., Rosen, T. A., Levine, J. D., & Julius, D. (1997). The capsaicin receptor: A heat-activated ion channel in the pain pathway. *Nature, 389*(6653), 816–824. https://doi.org/10.1038/39807.

Cepeda, S. B., Sandoval, M. J., Crescitelli, M. C., Rauschemberger, M. B., & Massheimer, V. L. (2020). The isoflavone genistein enhances osteoblastogenesis: Signaling pathways involved. *Journal of Physiology and Biochemistry, 76*, 99–110. https://doi.org/10.1007/s13105-019-00722-3.

Cevikbas, F., Wang, X., Akiyama, T., Kempkes, C., Savinko, T., Antal, A., Kukova, G., Buhl, T., Ikoma, A., Buddenkotte, J., Soumelis, V., Feld, M., Alenius, H., Dillon, S. R., Carstens, E., Homey, B., Basbaum, A., & Steinhoff, M. (2014). A sensory neuron-expressed IL-31 receptor mediates T helper cell-dependent itch: Involvement of TRPV1 and TRPA1. *The Journal of Allergy and Clinical Immunology, 133*(2). https://doi.org/10.1016/J.JACI.2013.10.048.

Chamoux, E., Bisson, M., Payet, M. D., & Roux, S. (2010). TRPV-5 mediates a receptor activator of NF-κB (RANK) ligand-induced increase in cytosolic Ca2+ in human osteoclasts and down-regulates bone resorption. *The Journal of Biological Chemistry, 285*(33), 25354. https://doi.org/10.1074/JBC.M109.075234.

Cheignon, C., Tomas, M., Bonnefont-Rousselot, D., Faller, P., Hureau, C., & Collin, F. (2018). Oxidative stress and the amyloid beta peptide in Alzheimer's disease. *Redox Biology, 14*, 450–464. https://doi.org/10.1016/J.REDOX.2017.10.014.

Chen, Z., Zhao, Y., Tian, Y., Cao, R., & Shang, D. (2023). Pan-cancer analysis of the TRP family, especially TRPV4 and TRPC4, and its expression correlated with prognosis, tumor microenvironment, and treatment sensitivity. *Biomolecules, 13*(2). https://doi.org/10.3390/BIOM13020282.

Cheng, H., Feng, J. M., Figueiredo, M. L., Zhang, H., Nelson, P. L., Marigo, V., & Beck, A. (2010). Transient receptor potential melastatin type 7 channel is critical for the survival of bone marrow derived mesenchymal stem cells. *Stem Cells and Development, 19*(9), 1393–1403. https://doi.org/10.1089/SCD.2009.0262.

Cheng, W. (2018). TRP ion channels: From distribution to assembly. *Ion channels in health and sickness* https://doi.org/10.5772/INTECHOPEN.76479.

Chi, H., Chang, H. Y., & Sang, T. K. (2018). Neuronal cell death mechanisms in major neurodegenerative diseases. *International Journal of Molecular Sciences, 19*(10). https://doi.org/10.3390/IJMS19103082.

Christie, S., Wittert, G. A., Li, H., & Page, A. J. (2018). Involvement of TRPV1 channels in energy homeostasis. *Frontiers in Endocrinology, 9*, 420. https://doi.org/10.3389/FENDO.2018.00420.

Cosens, D. J., & Manning, A. (1969). Abnormal electroretinogram from a *Drosophila* mutant. *Nature, 224*(5216), 285–287. https://doi.org/10.1038/224285a0.

Crousillac, S., Lerouge, M., Rankin, M., & Gleason, E. (2003). Immunolocalization of TRPC channel subunits 1 and 4 in the chicken retina. *Visual Neuroscience, 20*(4), 453–463. https://doi.org/10.1017/S0952523803204107.

D'Aldebert, E., Cenac, N., Rousset, P., Martin, L., Rolland, C., Chapman, K., Selves, J., Alric, L., Vinel, J., & Vergnolle, N. (2011). Transient receptor potential vanilloid 4 activated inflammatory signals by intestinal epithelial cells and colitis in mice. *Gastroenterology, 140*(1), 275–285. https://doi.org/10.1053/J.GASTRO.2010.09.045.

Dvornikova, K. A., Platonova, O. N., & Bystrova, E. Y. (2024). The role of TRP channels in sepsis and colitis. *International Journal of Molecular Sciences, 25*(9), 4784. https://doi.org/10.3390/ijms25094784.

Earley, S., & Brayden, J. E. (2015). Transient receptor potential channels in the vasculature. *Physiological Reviews, 95*(2), 645–690. https://doi.org/10.1152/PHYSREV.00026.2014.

El-Saadony, M. T., Yang, T., Korma, S. A., Sitohy, M., Abd El-Mageed, T. A., Selim, S., Al Jaouni, S. K., Salem, H. M., Mahmmod, Y., Soliman, S. M., Mo'men, S. A. A., Mosa, W. F. A., El-Wafai, N. A., Abou-Aly, H. E., Sitohy, B., Abd El-Hack, M. E., El-Tarabily, K. A., & Saad, A. M. (2023). Impacts of turmeric and its principal bioactive curcumin on human health: Pharmaceutical, medicinal, and food applications: A comprehensive review. *Frontiers in Nutrition, 9*, 1040259. https://doi.org/10.3389/fnut.2022.1040259.

Engel, M. A., Khalil, M., Mueller-Tribbensee, S. M., Becker, C., Neuhuber, W. L., Neurath, M. F., & Reeh, P. W. (2012). The proximodistal aggravation of colitis depends on substance P released from TRPV1-expressing sensory neurons. *Journal of Gastroenterology, 47*(3), 256–265. https://doi.org/10.1007/S00535-011-0495-6.

Fichna, J., Mokrowiecka, A., Cygankiewicz, A. I., Zakrzewski, P. K., Malecka-Panas, E., Janecka, A., Krajewska, W. M., & Storr, M. A. (2012). Transient receptor potential vanilloid 4 blockade protects against experimental colitis in mice: A new strategy for inflammatory bowel diseases treatment? *Neurogastroenterology & Motility, 24*(11), e557–e560. https://doi.org/10.1111/J.1365-2982.2012.01999.X.

Froghi, S., Grant, C. R., Tandon, R., Quaglia, A., Davidson, B., & Fuller, B. (2021). New insights on the role of TRP channels in calcium signalling and immunomodulation: Review of pathways and implications for clinical practice. *Clinical Reviews in Allergy & Immunology, 60*(2), 271–292. https://doi.org/10.1007/S12016-020-08824-3.

Gao, P., Yan, Z., & Zhu, Z. (2019). The role of adipose TRP channels in the pathogenesis of obesity. *Journal of Cellular Physiology, 234*(8), 12483–12497. https://doi.org/10.1002/JCP.28106.

Gardela, J., Ruiz-Conca, M., Martinez, C. A., Wright, D., López-Béjar, M., Rodriguez-Martinez, H., & Alvarez-Rodriguez, M. (2020). The expression of cold-inducible RNA-binding protein mRNA in sow genital tract is modulated by natural mating, but not by seminal plasma. *International Journal of Molecular Sciences, 21*(15), 1–23. https://doi.org/10.3390/IJMS21155333.

Garza-Cadena, C., Ortega-Rivera, D. M., Machorro-García, G., Gonzalez-Zermeño, E. M., Homma-Dueñas, D., Plata-Gryl, M., & Castro-Muñoz, R. (2023). A comprehensive review on ginger (*Zingiber officinale*) as a potential source of nutraceuticals for food formulations: Towards the polishing of gingerol and other present biomolecules. *Food Chemistry, 413*, 135629. https://doi.org/10.1016/j.foodchem.2023.135629.

Gauthier, A. E., Rotjan, R. D., & Kagan, J. C. (2022). Lipopolysaccharide detection by the innate immune system may be an uncommon defence strategy used in nature. *Open Biology, 12*(10). https://doi.org/10.1098/RSOB.220146.

Gezen-Ak, D., Dursun, E., & Yilmazer, S. (2014). The effect of vitamin D treatment on nerve growth factor (NGF) release from hippocampal neurons. *Nöro Psikiyatri Arşivi, 51*(2), 157. https://doi.org/10.4274/npa.y7076.

Gkika, D., & Prevarskaya, N. (2011). TRP channels in prostate cancer: The good, the bad and the ugly? *Asian Journal of Andrology, 13*(5), 673. https://doi.org/10.1038/AJA.2011.18.

Gleichmann, M., & Mattson, M. P. (2011). Neuronal calcium homeostasis and dysregulation. *Antioxidants & Redox Signaling, 14*(7), 1261–1273. https://doi.org/10.1089/ars.2010.3386.

Gombart, A. F., Pierre, A., & Maggini, S. (2020). A review of micronutrients and the immune system–working in harmony to reduce the risk of infection. *Nutrients, 12*(1), 236. https://doi.org/10.3390/nu12010236.

Guilak, F., Leddy, H. A., & Liedtke, W. (2010). Transient receptor potential vanilloid 4: The sixth sense of the musculoskeletal system? *Annals of the New York Academy of Sciences, 1192*, 404. https://doi.org/10.1111/J.1749-6632.2010.05389.X.

Hao, Y., Yang, N., Sun, M., Yang, S., & Chen, X. (2024). The role of calcium channels in osteoporosis and their therapeutic potential. *Frontiers in Endocrinology, 15*, 1450328. https://doi.org/10.3389/fendo.2024.1450328.

Harrington, A. M., Hughes, P. A., Martin, C. M., Yang, J., Castro, J., Isaacs, N. J., Ashley Blackshaw, L., & Brierley, S. M. (2011). A novel role for TRPM8 in visceral afferent function. *Pain, 152*(7), 1459–1468. https://doi.org/10.1016/J.PAIN.2011.01.027.

Heidari, H., Bagherniya, M., Majeed, M., Sathyapalan, T., Jamialahmadi, T., & Sahebkar, A. (2023). Curcumin-piperine co-supplementation and human health: A comprehensive review of preclinical and clinical studies. *Phytotherapy Research, 37*(4), 1462–1487. https://doi.org/10.1002/ptr.7737.

Hong, C., Jeong, B., Park, H. J., Chung, J. Y., Lee, J. E., Kim, J., Shin, Y. C., & So, I. (2020). TRP channels as emerging therapeutic targets for neurodegenerative diseases. *Frontiers in Physiology, 11*, 521830. https://doi.org/10.3389/FPHYS.2020.00238/XML/NLM.

Huang, J., Korsunsky, A., Yazdani, M., & Chen, J. (2023). Targeting TRP channels: Recent advances in structure, ligand binding, and molecular mechanisms. *Frontiers in Molecular Neuroscience, 16*, 1334370. https://doi.org/10.3389/FNMOL.2023.1334370/XML/NLM.

Huang, Y. K., Lu, Y. G., Zhao, X., Zhang, J. B., Zhang, F. M., Chen, Y., Bi, L. B., Gu, J. H., Jiang, Z. J., Wu, X. M., Li, Q. Y., Liu, Y., Shen, J. X., & Liu, X. J. (2020). Cytokine activin C ameliorates chronic neuropathic pain in peripheral nerve injury rodents by modulating the TRPV1 channel. *British Journal of Pharmacology, 177*(24), 5642–5657. https://doi.org/10.1111/BPH.15284.

Hwang, S., & Putney, J. W. (2012). Orai1-mediated calcium entry plays a critical role in osteoclast differentiation and function by regulating activation of the transcription factor NFATc1. *The FASEB Journal, 26*(4), 1484–1492. https://doi.org/10.1096/FJ.11-194399.

Jaipea, S., Saehlim, N., Sutcharitruk, W., Athipornchai, A., Ingkaninan, K., & Saeeng, R. (2023). Synthesis of piperine analogues as AChE and BChE inhibitors for the treatment of Alzheimer's disease. *Phytochemistry Letters, 53*, 216–221. https://doi.org/10.1016/j.phytol.2023.01.004.

Jaffal, S. M., & Abbas, M. A. (2021). TRP channels in COVID-19 disease: Potential targets for prevention and treatment. *Chemico-Biological Interactions*, 345. https://doi.org/10.1016/J.CBI.2021.109567.

Jiang, C., Zhai, M., Yan, D., Li, D., Li, C., Zhang, Y., Xiao, L., Xiong, D., Deng, Q., & Sun, W. (2017). Dietary menthol-induced TRPM8 activation enhances WAT "browning" and ameliorates diet-induced obesity. *Oncotarget, 8*(43), 75114. https://doi.org/10.18632/ONCOTARGET.20540.

Jiao, D., Guo, S., Chen, Y., Zhan, Y., & An, H. (2019). Ion channels and bone homeostasis imbalance. *Biomedical Journal of Scientific & Technical Research, 16*(3), 1–6. https://doi.org/10.26717/BJSTR.2019.16.002862.

Kaneko, Y., & Szallasi, A. (2014). Transient receptor potential (TRP) channels: A clinical perspective. *British Journal of Pharmacology, 171*(10), 2474–2507. https://doi.org/10.1111/BPH.12414.

Khalil, M., Alliger, K., Weidinger, C., Yerinde, C., Wirtz, S., Becker, C., & Engel, M. A. (2018). Functional role of transient receptor potential channels in immune cells and epithelia. *Frontiers in Immunology, 9*, 174. https://doi.org/10.3389/fimmu.2018.00174.

Khalil, M., Babes, A., Lakra, R., Försch, S., Reeh, P. W., Wirtz, S., Becker, C., Neurath, M. F., & Engel, M. A. (2016). Transient receptor potential melastatin 8 ion channel in macrophages modulates colitis through a balance-shift in TNF-alpha and interleukin-10 production. *Mucosal Immunology, 9*(6), 1500–1513. https://doi.org/10.1038/MI.2016.16.

Kim, C. S., Kawada, T., Kim, B. S., Han, I. S., Choe, S. Y., Kurata, T., & Yu, R. (2003). Capsaicin exhibits anti-inflammatory property by inhibiting IkB-a degradation in LPS-stimulated peritoneal macrophages. *Cellular Signalling, 15*(3), 299–306. https://doi.org/10.1016/S0898-6568(02)00086-4.

Kongsui, R., & Jittiwat, J. (2023). Ameliorative effects of 6 gingerol in cerebral ischemia are mediated via the activation of antioxidant and anti-inflammatory pathways. *Biomedical Reports, 18*(4), 26. https://doi.org/10.3892/br.2023.1608.

Kumar, A., Kumari, S., Majhi, R. K., Swain, N., Yadav, M., & Goswami, C. (2015). Regulation of TRP channels by steroids: Implications in physiology and diseases. *General and Comparative Endocrinology, 220*, 23–32. https://doi.org/10.1016/J.YGCEN.2014.10.004.

Kumar, S., Acharya, T. K., Halder, R. R., Mahapatra, P., Chang, Y. T., & Goswami, C. (2023). Menthol causes mitochondrial Ca^{2+}-influx, affects structure-function relationship and cools mitochondria. *Life Sciences*, 331. https://doi.org/10.1016/J.LFS.2023.122032.

Kumar, S., Acharya, T. K., Kumar, S., Mahapatra, P., Chang, Y. T., & Goswami, C. (2024a). TRPV4 modulation affects mitochondrial parameters in adipocytes and its inhibition upregulates lipid accumulation. *Life Sciences, 358*, 123130. https://doi.org/10.1016/j.lfs.2024.123130.

Kumar, S., Acharya, T. K., Kumar, S., Rokade, T. P., Das, N. K., Chawla, S., Goswami, L., & Goswami, C. (2024b). TRPV4 activator-containing CMT-Hy hydrogel enhances bone tissue regeneration *in vivo* by enhancing mitochondrial health. *ACS Biomaterials Science & Engineering, 10*(4), 2367–2384. https://doi.org/10.1021/acsbiomaterials.3c01304.

Kun, J., Szitter, I., Kemény, Á., Perkecz, A., Kereskai, L., Pohóczky, K., Vincze, Á., Gódi, S., Szabó, I., Szolcsányi, J., Pintér, E., & Helyes, Z. (2014). Upregulation of the transient receptor potential ankyrin 1 ion channel in the inflamed human and mouse colon and its protective roles. *PLoS One, 9*(9). https://doi.org/10.1371/JOURNAL.PONE.0108164.

Kunnumakkara, A. B., Hegde, M., Parama, D., Girisa, S., Kumar, A., Daimary, U. D., Garodia, P., Yenisetti, S. C., Oommen, O. V., & Aggarwal, B. B. (2023). Role of turmeric and curcumin in prevention and treatment of chronic diseases: Lessons learned from clinical trials. *ACS Pharmacology & Translational Science, 6*(4), 447–518. https://doi.org/10.1021/acsptsci.2c00012.

Kwon, J. Y., Lee, H. S., & Joo, C. K. (2018). TRPV1 antagonist suppresses allergic conjunctivitis in a murine model. *Ocular Immunology and Inflammation, 26*(3), 440–448. https://doi.org/10.1080/09273948.2016.1231330.

Lee, K., Jo, Y. Y., Chung, G., Jung, J. H., Kim, Y. H., & Park, C. K. (2021). Functional importance of transient receptor potential (TRP) channels in neurological disorders. *Frontiers in Cell and Developmental Biology, 9*, 611773. https://doi.org/10.3389/FCELL.2021.611773.

Leijon, S., Neves, A. F., Breza, J. M., Simon, S. A., Chaudhari, N., & Roper, S. D. (2019). Oral thermosensing by murine trigeminal neurons: Modulation by capsaicin, menthol and mustard oil. *The Journal of Physiology, 597*(7), 2045–2061. https://doi.org/10.1113/jp277385.

Li, L., Chen, J., Ni, Y., Feng, X., Zhao, Z., Wang, P., Sun, J., Yu, H., Yan, Z., Liu, D., Nilius, B., & Zhu, Z. (2012). TRPV1 activation prevents nonalcoholic fatty liver through UCP2 upregulation in mice. *Pflugers Archiv: European Journal of Physiology, 463*(5), 727–732. https://doi.org/10.1007/S00424-012-1078-Y/METRICS.

Lieben, L., Benn, B. S., Ajibade, D., Stockmans, I., Moermans, K., Hediger, M. A., Peng, J. B., Christakos, S., Bouillon, R., & Carmeliet, G. (2010). Trpv6 mediates intestinal calcium absorption during calcium restriction and contributes to bone homeostasis. *Bone, 47*(2), 301–308. https://doi.org/10.1016/J.BONE.2010.04.595.

Lieben, L., & Carmeliet, G. (2012). The involvement of TRP channels in bone homeostasis. *Frontiers in Endocrinology, 3*, 29590. https://doi.org/10.3389/FENDO.2012.00099.

Little, R., Muimo, R., Robson, L., Harris, K., & Grabowski, P. S. (2011). The transient receptor potential ion channel TRPV6 is expressed at low levels in osteoblasts and has little role in osteoblast calcium uptake. *PLoS One, 6*(11). https://doi.org/10.1371/JOURNAL.PONE.0028166.

Liu, D., Mao, M., Liu, W., Xie, L., Zhong, X., Cao, W., & Chen, L. (2024). The role of the TRPV4 channel in intestinal physiology and pathology. *Journal of Inflammation Research*, 9307–9317. https://doi.org/10.2147/JIR.S483350.

Liu, Y., Lyu, Y., & Wang, H. (2022). TRP channels as molecular targets to relieve endocrine-related diseases. *Frontiers in Molecular Biosciences, 9*, 895814. https://doi.org/10.3389/FMOLB.2022.895814/FULL.

Liu, Y., Lyu, Y., Zhu, L., & Wang, H. (2023a). Role of TRP channels in liver-related diseases. *International Journal of Molecular Sciences, 24*(15), 12509. https://doi.org/10.3390/IJMS241512509.

Liu, Y., Li, D., Wang, S., Peng, Z., Tan, Q., He, Q., & Wang, J. (2023b). 6-Gingerol ameliorates hepatic steatosis, inflammation and oxidative stress in high-fat diet-fed mice through activating LKB1/AMPK signaling. *International Journal of Molecular Sciences, 24*(7), 6285. https://doi.org/10.3390/ijms24076285.

Majhi, R. K., Sahoo, S. S., Yadav, M., Pratheek, B. M., Chattopadhyay, S., & Goswami, C. (2015). Functional expression of TRPV channels in T cells and their implications in immune regulation. *The FEBS Journal, 282*(14), 2661–2681. https://doi.org/10.1111/FEBS.13306.

Masuyama, R., Mizuno, A., Komori, H., Kajiya, H., Uekawa, A., Kitaura, H., Okabe, K., Ohyama, K., & Komori, T. (2012). Calcium/calmodulin-signaling supports TRPV4 activation in osteoclasts and regulates bone mass. *Journal of Bone and Mineral Research, 27*(8), 1708–1721. https://doi.org/10.1002/JBMR.1629.

Matos, G. M., Andersson, B., & Islam, M. S. (2022). Expression of transient receptor potential channel genes and their isoforms in alpha-cells and beta-cells of human islets of Langerhans. *Journal of Diabetes Research, 2022*. https://doi.org/10.1155/2022/3975147.

Matta, J. A., Miyares, R. L., & Ahern, G. P. (2007). TRPV1 is a novel target for omega-3 polyunsaturated fatty acids. *The Journal of Physiology, 578*(2), 397–411. https://doi.org/10.1113/jphysiol.2006.121988.

Méndez-Reséndiz, K. A., Enciso-Pablo, Ó., González-Ramírez, R., Juárez-Contreras, R., Rosenbaum, T., & Morales-Lázaro, S. L. (2020). Steroids and TRP channels: A close relationship. *International Journal of Molecular Sciences, 21*(11), 3819. https://doi.org/10.3390/IJMS21113819.

Mergler, S., Garreis, F., Sahlmüller, M., Reinach, P. S., Paulsen, F., & Pleyer, U. (2011). Thermosensitive transient receptor potential channels in human corneal epithelial cells. *Journal of Cellular Physiology, 226*(7), 1828–1842. https://doi.org/10.1002/JCP.22514.

Molodecky, N. A., Soon, I. S., Rabi, D. M., Ghali, W. A., Ferris, M., Chernoff, G., Benchimol, E. I., Panaccione, R., Ghosh, S., Barkema, H. W., & Kaplan, G. G. (2012). Increasing incidence and prevalence of the inflammatory bowel diseases with time, based on systematic review. *Gastroenterology, 142*(1). https://doi.org/10.1053/J.GASTRO.2011.10.001.

Morita, T., Mitsuyama, K., Yamasaki, H., Mori, A., Yoshimura, T., Araki, T., Morita, M., Tsuruta, K., Yamasaki, S., Kuwaki, K., Yoshioka, S., Takedatsu, H., & Torimura, T. (2020). Gene expression of transient receptor potential channels in peripheral blood mononuclear cells of inflammatory bowel disease patients. *Journal of Clinical Medicine, 9*(8), 1–12. https://doi.org/10.3390/JCM9082643.

Murphy, M. P. (2008). How mitochondria produce reactive oxygen species. *Biochemical Journal, 417*(Pt 1), 1. https://doi.org/10.1042/BJ20081386.

Nagpal, R., Mishra, S. K., Deep, G., & Yadav, H. (2020). Role of TRP channels in shaping the gut microbiome. *Pathogens, 9*, 753. https://doi.org/10.3390/pathogens9090753.

Nalli, M., Ortar, G., Schiano Moriello, A., Di Marzo, V., & De Petrocellis, L. (2017). Effects of curcumin and curcumin analogues on TRP channels. *Fitoterapia, 122*, 126–131. https://doi.org/10.1016/j.fitote.2017.09.007.

Nilius, B. (2007). TRP channels in disease. *Biochimica et Biophysica Acta (BBA)—Molecular Basis of Disease, 1772*(8), 805–812. https://doi.org/10.1016/J.BBADIS.2007.02.002.

Papadopoulos, V., & Miller, W. L. (2012). Role of mitochondria in steroidogenesis. *Best Practice & Research Clinical Endocrinology & Metabolism, 26*(6), 771–790. https://doi.org/10.1016/J.BEEM.2012.05.002.

Parra, A., Madrid, R., Echevarria, D., Del Olmo, S., Morenilla-Palao, C., Acosta, M. C., Gallar, J., Dhaka, A., Viana, F., & Belmonte, C. (2010). Ocular surface wetness is regulated by TRPM8-dependent cold thermoreceptors of the cornea. *Nature Medicine, 16*(12), 1396–1399. https://doi.org/10.1038/NM.2264.

Prasad, A. S. (2008). Zinc in human health: Effect of zinc on immune cells. *Molecular Medicine, 14*, 353–357. https://doi.org/10.2119/2008-00033.Prasad.

Reinach, P. S., Mergler, S., Okada, Y., & Saika, S. (2015). Ocular transient receptor potential channel function in health and disease. *BMC Ophthalmology, 15*(Suppl 1). https://doi.org/10.1186/S12886-015-0135-7.

Rezaei, S., Meftah, H. S., Ebtehajpour, Y., Rahimi, H. R., & Chamani, J. (2024). Investigation on the effect of fluorescence quenching of calf thymus DNA by piperine: Caspase activation in the human breast cancer cell line studies. *DNA and Cell Biology, 43*(1), 26–38. https://doi.org/10.1089/dna.2023.0269.

Rohde, M., Ziebart, J., Kirschstein, T., Sellmann, T., Porath, K., Kühl, F., Delenda, B., Bahls, C., van Rienen, U., Bader, R., & Köhling, R. (2019). Human osteoblast migration in DC electrical fields depends on store operated Ca^{2+}-release and is correlated to upregulation of stretch-activated TRPM7 channels. *Frontiers in Bioengineering and Biotechnology, 7*, 422. https://doi.org/10.3389/FBIOE.2019.00422/FULL.

Rychkov, G. Y., & Barritt, G. J. (2011). Expression and function of TRP channels in liver cells. *Advances in Experimental Medicine and Biology, 704*, 667–686. https://doi.org/10.1007/978-94-007-0265-3_35.

Ryskamp, D. A., Witkovsky, P., Barabas, P., Huang, W., Koehler, C., Akimov, N. P., Lee, S. H., Chauhan, S., Xing, W., Rentería, R. C., Liedtke, W., & Križaj, D. (2011). The polymodal ion channel transient receptor potential vanilloid 4 modulates calcium flux, spiking rate, and apoptosis of mouse retinal ganglion cells. *The Journal of Neuroscience, 31*(19), 7089–7101. https://doi.org/10.1523/JNEUROSCI.0359-11.2011.

Sahoo, S. S., Majhi, R. K., Tiwari, A., Acharya, T., Kumar, P. S., Saha, S., Kumar, A., Goswami, C., & Chattopadhyay, S. (2019). Transient receptor potential ankyrin1 channel is endogenously expressed in T cells and is involved in immune functions. *Bioscience Reports, 39*(9), BSR20191437. https://doi.org/10.1042/BSR20191437.

Sahu, R. P., & Goswami, C. (2023). Presence of TRPV3 in macrophage lysosomes helps in skin wound healing against bacterial infection. *Experimental Dermatology, 32*(1), 60–74. https://doi.org/10.1111/EXD.14683.

Sanders, O. D., Rajagopal, J. A., & Rajagopal, L. (2021). Menthol to induce non-shivering thermogenesis via TRPM8/PKA signaling for treatment of obesity. *Journal of Obesity & Metabolic Syndrome, 30*(1), 4–11. https://doi.org/10.7570/JOMES20038.

Sappington, R. M., Sidorova, T., Long, D. J., & Calkins, D. J. (2009). TRPV1: Contribution to retinal ganglion cell apoptosis and increased intracellular Ca^{2+} with exposure to hydrostatic pressure. *Investigative Ophthalmology & Visual Science, 50*(2), 717–728. https://doi.org/10.1167/IOVS.08-2321.

Schmitz, C., Perraud, A. L., Johnson, C. O., Inabe, K., Smith, M. K., Penner, R., & Scharenberg, A. M. (2003). Regulation of vertebrate cellular Mg^{2+} homeostasis by TRPM7. *Cell, 114*(2), 191–200. https://doi.org/10.1016/S0092-8674(03)00556-7.

Shakibaei, M., Buhrmann, C., & Mobasheri, A. (2011). Resveratrol-mediated SIRT-1 interactions with p300 modulate receptor activator of NF-κB ligand (RANKL) activation of NF-κB signaling and inhibit osteoclastogenesis in bone-derived cells. *Journal of Biological Chemistry, 286*(13), 11492–11505. https://doi.org/10.1074/jbc.m110.198713.

Shin, Y., Han, S., Kwon, J., Ju, S., Choi, T. G., Kang, I., & Kim, S. S. (2023). Roles of short-chain fatty acids in inflammatory bowel disease. *Nutrients, 15*(20), 4466. https://doi.org/10.3390/nu15204466.

Singh, A., Kumar, S., Goswami, C., & Goswami, L. (2024a). Montmorillonite-reinforced xanthan gum-based biomaterial enhances biomineralization suitable for bone tissue engineering. *Materials Today Chemistry, 38*, 102067. https://doi.org/10.1016/j.mtchem.2024.102067.

Singh, A., Kumar, S., Acharya, T. K., Kumar, S., Chawla, S., Goswami, C., & Goswami, L. (2024b). Modulation of calcium-influx by carboxymethyl tamarind-gold nanoparticles promotes biomineralization for tissue regeneration. *International Journal of Biological Macromolecules, 264*, 130605. https://doi.org/10.1016/j.ijbiomac.2024.130605.

Singh, A., Kumar, S., Acharya, T. K., Goswami, C., & Goswami, L. (2022). Application of nanohydroxyapatite-polysaccharide based biomaterial for bone cell mineralization in tissue engineering. *Materials Today Communications, 31*, 103783. https://doi.org/10.1016/j.mtcomm.2022.103783.

Sukan-Karaçağıl, B., Akbulut, G., Açar, Y., & Demirkoparan, M. (2023). A little pepper-upper? Systematic review of randomized controlled studies on capsaicinoids, capsinoids, and exercise performance. *International Journal of Sport Nutrition and Exercise Metabolism, 33*(5), 291–301. https://doi.org/10.1123/ijsnem.2023-0016.

Sukumaran, P., Schaar, A., Sun, Y., & Singh, B. B. (2016). Functional role of TRP channels in modulating ER stress and autophagy. *Cell Calcium, 60*(2), 123–132. https://doi.org/10.1016/j.ceca.2016.02.012.

Sun, W., Luo, Y., Zhang, F., Tang, S., & Zhu, T. (2021). Involvement of TRP channels in adipocyte thermogenesis: An update. *Frontiers in Cell and Developmental Biology, 9*, 686173. https://doi.org/10.3389/FCELL.2021.686173/XML/NLM.

Tarinta, T., Chanthai, S., Nawata, E., & Techawongstien, S. (2023). Combining ability on yields, capsinoids and capsaicinoids in pepper varieties (*Capsicum annuum* L.). *Horticulturae, 9*(9), 1043. https://doi.org/10.3390/horticulturae9091043.

Tong, X., Tong, Y., Zheng, J., Shi, R., Liang, H., Li, M., & Guo, F. (2024). TRPM7 contributes to pyroptosis and its involvement in status epilepticus. *Journal of Neuroinflammation, 21*(1), 315. https://doi.org/10.1186/s12974-024-03292-4.

Uchida, K., & Tominaga, M. (2011). The role of thermosensitive TRP (transient receptor potential) channels in insulin secretion. *Endocrine Journal, 58*(12), 1021–1028. https://doi.org/10.1507/ENDOCRJ.EJ11-0130.

Van Der Eerden, B. C. J., Hoenderop, J. G. J., De Vries, T. J., Schoenmaker, T., Buurman, C. J., Uitterlinden, A. G., Pols, H. A. P., Bindels, R. J. M., & Van Leeuwen, J. P. T. M. (2005). The epithelial Ca^{2+} channel TRPV5 is essential for proper osteoclastic bone resorption. *Proceedings of the National Academy of Sciences of the United States of America, 102*(48), 17507–17512. https://doi.org/10.1073/PNAS.0505789102.

Van der Eerden, B. C. J., Weissgerber, P., Fratzl-Zelman, N., Olausson, J., Hoenderop, J. G. J., Schreuders-Koedam, M., Eijken, M., Roschger, P., De Vries, T. J., Chiba, H., Klaushofer, K., Flockerzi, V., Bindels, R. J. M., Freichel, M., & Van Leeuwen, J. P. T. M. (2012). The transient receptor potential channel TRPV6 is dynamically expressed in bone cells but is not crucial for bone mineralization in mice. *Journal of Cellular Physiology, 227*(5), 1951–1959. https://doi.org/10.1002/JCP.22923.

Venkatachalam, K. (2022). Regulation of aging and longevity by ion channels and transporters. *Cells, 11*(7), 1180. https://doi.org/10.3390/cells11071180.

Vriens, J., Nilius, B., & Vennekens, R. (2008). Herbal compounds and toxins modulating TRP channels. *Current Neuropharmacology, 6*(1), 79. https://doi.org/10.2174/157015908783769644.

Wu, F., Bu, S., & Wang, H. (2024). Role of TRP channels in metabolism-related diseases. *International Journal of Molecular Sciences, 25*(2). https://doi.org/10.3390/IJMS25020692.

Wu, J., Li, Z., Deng, Y., Lu, X., Luo, C., Mu, X., Zhang, T., Liu, Q., Tang, S., Li, J., An, Q., Fan, D., Xiang, Y., Wu, X., Hu, Y., Du, Q., Xu, J., & Xie, R. (2023). Function of TRP channels in monocytes/macrophages. *Frontiers in Immunology, 14*, 1187890. https://doi.org/10.3389/FIMMU.2023.1187890/XML/NLM.

Wu, S., Zhu, J., Wu, G., Hu, Z., Ying, P., Bao, Z., & Tan, X. (2022). 6-Gingerol alleviates ferroptosis and inflammation of diabetic cardiomyopathy via the Nrf2/HO-1 pathway. *Oxidative Medicine and Cellular Longevity, 2022*(1), 3027514. https://doi.org/10.1155/2022/3027514.

Yadav, M., & Goswami, C. (2017). TRPV3 mutants causing Olmsted syndrome induce impaired cell adhesion and nonfunctional lysosomes. *Channels (Austin), 11*(3), 196–208. https://doi.org/10.1080/19336950.2016.1249076.

Yamamoto, S., Shimizu, S., Kiyonaka, S., Takahashi, N., Wajima, T., Hara, Y., & Mori, Y. (2008). TRPM2-mediated Ca^{2+} influx induces chemokine production in monocytes that aggravates inflammatory neutrophil infiltration. *Nature Medicine, 14*(7), 738–747. https://doi.org/10.1038/nm1758.

Yan, Q., Gao, C., Li, M., Lan, R., Wei, S., Fan, R., & Cheng, W. (2024). TRP ion channels in immune cells and their implications for inflammation. *International Journal of Molecular Sciences, 25*(5). https://doi.org/10.3390/IJMS25052719.

Yan, Y., Jiang, W., Spinetti, T., Tardivel, A., Castillo, R., Bourquin, C., & Zhou, R. (2013). Omega-3 fatty acids prevent inflammation and metabolic disorder through inhibition of NLRP3 inflammasome activation. *Immunity, 38*(6), 1154–1163. https://doi.org/10.1016/j.immuni.2013.05.015.

Yang, B., Ma, D., Zhu, X., Wu, Z., An, Q., Zhao, J., Gao, X., & Zhang, L. (2024a). Roles of TRP and PIEZO receptors in autoimmune diseases. *Expert Reviews in Molecular Medicine, 26*, e10. https://doi.org/10.1017/ERM.2023.23.

Yang, D., & Kim, J. (2020). Emerging role of transient receptor potential (TRP) channels in cancer progression. *BMB Reports, 53*(3), 125–132. https://doi.org/10.5483/BMBREP.2020.53.3.016.

Yang, J., Zhi, W., & Wang, L. (2024b). Role of Tau protein in neurodegenerative diseases and development of its targeted drugs: A literature review. *Molecules, 29*, 2812. https://doi.org/10.3390/MOLECULES29122812.

Yang, P., Feng, J., Luo, J., Madison, M., & Hu, H. (2017). A critical role for TRP channels in the skin. In *Neurobiology of TRP channels* (pp. 95–111). https://doi.org/10.4324/9781315152837-6.

Yue, L., & Xu, H. (2021). TRP channels in health and disease at a glance. *Journal of Cell Science, 134*(13), jcs258372. https://doi.org/10.1242/JCS.258372.

Zhang, M., Ma, Y., Ye, X., Zhang, N., Pan, L., & Wang, B. (2023). TRP (transient receptor potential) ion channel family: Structures, biological functions and therapeutic interventions for diseases. *Signal Transduction and Targeted Therapy, 8*(1), 1–38. https://doi.org/10.1038/s41392-023-01464-x.

Zhao, J. F., Shyue, S. K., Kou, Y. R., Lu, T. M., & Lee, T. S. (2016). Transient receptor potential ankyrin 1 channel involved in atherosclerosis and macrophage-foam cell formation. *International Journal of Biological Sciences, 12*(7), 812–823. https://doi.org/10.7150/IJBS.15229.

Zheng, Y., Huang, Q., Zhang, Y., Geng, L., Wang, W., Zhang, H., He, X., & Li, Q. (2023). Multimodal roles of transient receptor potential channel activation in inducing pathological tissue scarification. *Frontiers in Immunology, 14*, 1237992. https://doi.org/10.3389/FIMMU.2023.1237992.

Zhu, Z., Luo, Z., Ma, S., & Liu, D. (2011). TRP channels and their implications in metabolic diseases. *Pflugers Archiv: European Journal of Physiology, 461*(2), 211–223. https://doi.org/10.1007/S00424-010-0902-5/METRICS.

Zsombok, A., & Derbenev, A. V. (2016). TRP channels as therapeutic targets in diabetes and obesity. *Pharmaceuticals (Basel), 9*(3). https://doi.org/10.3390/PH9030050.

Children's nutrition in COVID-19 pandemic in LMICs

8

Ipsa Mohapatra[a] *and Adrija Roy*[b,c]
[a] Department of Community Medicine, Kalinga Institute of Medical Sciences, Bhubaneswar, Odisha, India, [b] Department of Community Medicine, RVM Institute of Medical Sciences and Research Centre, Hyderabad, Telangana, India, [c] Achutha Menon Centre for Health Science Studies, Sree Chitra Tirunal Institute of Medical Sciences and Technology, Trivandrum, Kerala, India

8.1 Introduction

Development in any country is monitored by various direct and indirect indicators. The nutritional status of the population is directly linked to health and hence is an important measure of development and progress. The primary nutritional status indicators of malnutrition are underweight, short stature, overweight, and obesity. There has been a change in these indicators globally, including the low- and middle-income countries (LMICs) (Angkat et al., 2022; Headey & Ruel, 2020a; Ouma et al., 2021; Zhu et al., 2022). The Sustainable Development Goals (SDGs) have targets to be achieved by 2030. SDG 2 aims to create a world free of hunger, achieving food security, improved nutrition, and promoting sustainable agriculture; and SDG 3 aims to end hunger, food insecurity, and malnutrition in all its forms, by ensuring healthy lives and promoting wellbeing for all (Zhu et al., 2022).

The COVID-19 pandemic posed an unprecedented challenge with more than 122 million people facing hunger in the world since 2019; although the global hunger numbers have stalled between 2021 and 2022, there are still many places in the world facing food crises postpandemic, some other major drivers of food insecurity and malnutrition, being conflict, climate variability and extremes, and economic slowdowns, including the war in Ukraine (Headey & Ruel, 2020a; Zhu et al., 2022).

There still exists a wide variation in the global distribution of undernutrition between different income countries. In the year 2020 the highest prevalence (50%–55%) of childhood stunting was seen in low-income countries such as Timor, Burundi, and Eritrea, whereas it was as low as (1.5%–2.0%) in high-income countries, including Belgium, Australia, Greece, Germany, and Chile. Undernourishment continues to be a public health problem, contributing to increased mortality in children under 5 in low-income countries. In the year 2022, around 148.1 million children under 5 years of age were stunted, 45.0 million had wasting, and 37.0 million were overweight. Undernutrition is likely to be exacerbated by the socioeconomic disparities within these communities, making it more important to examine the determinants of these indicators

Nutritional Strategies, Predictive Models, and Sustainable Policies. DOI: https://doi.org/10.1016/B978-0-443-23671-6.00004-9

in these countries, using the most recently available data and if possible, compare how these have changed over time. It was predicted that the COVID-19 crisis would exacerbate maternal and child undernutrition and child mortality in LMICs (Headey & Ruel, 2020a; Zhu et al., 2022).

8.2 Effects of COVID-19 pandemic on nutritional status of infants and children in LMICs

The COVID-19 pandemic has had far-reaching impacts on child health, particularly in LMICs, where preexisting vulnerabilities were exacerbated. This section explores how the pandemic worsened stunting, wasting, micronutrient deficiencies, and disrupted essential nutrition programs, leading to a multifaceted nutrition crisis among infants and children.

8.2.1 Increase in stunting and wasting

Prevalence and severity: Stunting (low height-for-age) and wasting (low weight-for-height) are critical indicators of child malnutrition. Osendarp et al. (2021) estimated that the pandemic led to an additional 9.3 million children with wasting and 2.6 million with stunting globally, with the highest burden in LMICs. These conditions often coexisted with acute food insecurity, healthcare disruptions, and economic shocks.

Regional variations in LMICs:

- In Indonesia, Angkat et al. (2022) reported that reduced iron intake among children aged 24–35 months was strongly associated with stunting during the pandemic. Economic challenges limited access to iron-rich foods and supplements, particularly for low-income families (Angkat et al., 2022).
- In Central India, Wakode et al. (2024) observed a notable rise in stunting and wasting among children under 2 years of age. Healthcare service disruptions, reduced household incomes, and restricted food supply chains were the primary contributors (Wakode et al., 2024).

Contributing factors:

- Loss of livelihoods: Income losses limited household purchasing power, leading to reliance on low-cost, nutrient-poor diets.
- Healthcare service interruptions: Nutrition centers and growth monitoring programs were suspended in many regions.
- Food supply chain disruptions: Lockdowns impeded access to fresh produce, animal-source foods, and fortified products.

8.2.2 Micronutrient deficiencies

Micronutrient deficiencies, particularly of iron, vitamin A, and zinc, worsened during the pandemic because of disruptions in supplementation programs, fortified food supplies, and dietary diversity.

Iron deficiency and anemia:

- In Indonesia, Angkat et al. (2022) highlighted that reduced iron intake during the pandemic significantly contributed to stunting. Iron deficiency anemia, already a major public health concern, was exacerbated by limited access to iron-fortified foods and supplements.
- Similarly, studies in Kenya Ouma et al. (2021) reported increased anemia prevalence in pregnant women and children, linked to food insecurity.

Vitamin A and zinc deficiencies:

- In sub-Saharan Africa, coverage of vitamin A supplementation programs declined by 35%, increasing the risk of infections and visual impairment (Osendarp et al., 2021).
- Disruptions to the supply of fortified foods, including cereals and oils, deprive children of essential micronutrients critical for immune function and growth.

Impact of supplementation program disruptions: Programs like the Integrated Child Development Scheme (ICDS) in India and similar initiatives in Ethiopia were scaled back or halted, further reducing coverage of vitamin A, zinc, and iron supplementation (Khandelwal et al., 2022; McCann et al., 2023).

8.3 Impact on acute and chronic malnutrition

Severe acute malnutrition (SAM): SAM, characterized by extreme wasting, requires immediate treatment to prevent mortality. Ouedraogo et al. (2023) reported a sharp decline in admissions at outpatient malnutrition centers in Burkina Faso during the initial phases of the pandemic. Partial recovery was seen later in rural areas, but many children remained untreated.

Chronic malnutrition: Chronic malnutrition, reflected by stunting, has long-term impacts on growth, cognitive development, and productivity. The pandemic exacerbated chronic malnutrition because of

- Reduced access to healthcare for routine growth monitoring.
- Poor complementary feeding practices because of economic and food system challenges (Yanti & Fauziah, 2021; Zhu et al., 2022).

For instance, in Ethiopia, disruptions to food systems and rising food prices led to significant increases in chronic malnutrition (McCann et al., 2023).

8.4 Disruptions to growth monitoring and nutrition interventions

The pandemic severely disrupted essential child health services, including growth monitoring, screening for malnutrition, and the delivery of nutritional supplements.

Challenges in healthcare delivery:

- In India, Singh et al. (2021) found that institutional deliveries, antenatal care visits, and immunizations declined by approximately 20%, limiting opportunities to identify and treat malnutrition early.

- In Burkina Faso, outpatient malnutrition centers reported fewer follow-ups, leading to delays in care for malnourished children (Ouedraogo et al., 2023).

Impact of reduced access to nutrition centers: Many community-based nutrition programs, such as community-based management of acute malnutrition (CMAM), were modified. Wrabel et al. (2022) highlighted adaptations like the use of Family MUAC (mid-upper arm circumference) measurements to allow at-home screening during the pandemic.

8.5 Socioeconomic disparities and malnutrition

The pandemic magnified socioeconomic disparities, with the poorest households experiencing the worst nutritional outcomes.

Income losses and food insecurity:

- Ouma et al. (2021) reported that food insecurity in Kenya worsened because of income shocks, disproportionately affecting infants and pregnant women.
- In Indonesia, Yanti and Fauziah (2021) linked reduced family incomes to an increased prevalence of stunting among preschool children.

Inequitable impact on rural versus urban populations: Rural populations faced greater challenges accessing food and healthcare because of transportation restrictions and economic barriers. Urban slums, already prone to overcrowding and poor living conditions, experienced worsening food insecurity (Lubowa & Qali, 2024; Pradeilles et al., 2022).

Gender disparities: Girls were often deprived of food during shortages because of gender norms, leading to worse malnutrition outcomes in some regions (Ouma et al., 2021).

8.6 Increased mortality risks because of malnutrition

The combination of malnutrition and disruptions to healthcare services increased child mortality risks during the pandemic.

Indirect causes of child mortality:

- Roberton et al. (2020) projected significant increases in child mortality because of interruptions in healthcare services, particularly in LMICs.
- Malnutrition heightened susceptibility to infections such as diarrhea, pneumonia, and malaria, creating a vicious cycle of illness and undernutrition.

Synergistic impact of COVID-19 infections and malnutrition: Malnourished children, with weakened immune systems, were more vulnerable to severe COVID-19 infections. Studies in South Africa (Thsehla et al., 2023) emphasized that healthcare disruptions exacerbated this risk. A summary of key studies on the impact of COVID-19 on child nutrition and health in LMICs have been discussed in (Table 8.1).

Table 8.1 Summary of key studies on the impact of COVID-19 on child nutrition and health in LMICs.

Focus area	Key findings	Country	Author and references
Stunting and iron intake	Pandemic-related socioeconomic challenges reduced nutrient intake, particularly iron, contributing to stunting in children aged 24–35 months	Indonesia	Angkat et al. (2022)
Food security	Food insecurity worsened for vulnerable groups (infants and pregnant women) because of economic shocks. Household income loss significantly correlated with reduced dietary quality	Kenya	Ouma et al. (2021)
Global nutrition crisis	COVID-19 led to income losses, disruptions to food systems, and reduced healthcare access, increasing malnutrition and mortality risks. Declines in dietary quality and school feeding program suspensions strongly impacted LMICs	LMICs	Headey and Ruel (2020a)
Review of nutritional status, feeding practices	The narrative review highlights reduced breastfeeding support, diminished dietary diversity, and worsened food security in LMICs	LMICs	Zhu et al. (2022)

(continued on next page)

Table 8.1 Summary of key studies on the impact of COVID-19 on child nutrition and health in LMICs—cont'd

Focus area	Key findings	Country	Author and references
Modeling global undernutrition	Projections estimate 9.3 million additional wasted children, 2.6 million stunted, and 168,000 child deaths because of pandemic disruptions in LMICs	LMICs	Osendarp et al. (2021)
Malnutrition and supply chain disruptions	COVID-19 worsened malnutrition with 2.6 million stunted children, 9.3 million wasted, and $29.7 billion in productivity losses. Supply chain disruptions impacted food availability, delivery of RUTFs, and healthcare access	LMICs	Padhani and Bhutta (2022)
Maternal and child nutrition in LMICs	Lockdowns disrupted food systems, incomes, healthcare services, and social protection programs, worsening maternal and child health and pushing SDG targets out of reach	LMICs	Akseer et al. (2020)
Outpatient malnutrition centers	Malnutrition centers saw sharp declines in patient enrollment and follow-up during the pandemic, *with partial* recovery *in rural* areas after initial disruptions	Burkina Faso	Ouedraogo et al. (2023)

(*continued on next page*)

Maternal and child nutrition practices	Breastfeeding declined early in the pandemic because of misinformation and caregiver fears, but movement restrictions later increased exclusive breastfeeding. Job losses linked to food insecurity and dietary changes	Kenya	Ahoya et al. (2022)
Food insecurity and maternal nutrition	Government assistance and food aid programs during the pandemic prevented declines in breastfeeding and dietary quality, but nearly 47% of households reported moderate or severe food insecurity	Peru	Pradeilles et al. (2022)
Food security and maternal health	Food insecurity led to fewer meals, lower dietary diversity, and higher levels of maternal malnutrition	Uganda	Lubowa and Qali (2024)
Modeling indirect effects on maternal-child mortality	Predicted significant increases in child and maternal mortality because of healthcare service disruptions in LMICs	LMICs	Roberton et al. (2020)

(continued on next page)

Table 8.1 Summary of key studies on the impact of COVID-19 on child nutrition and health in LMICs—cont'd

Focus area	Key findings	Country	Author and references
Child health services	Pandemic reduced institutional deliveries, antenatal care visits, and immunizations by approximately 20%, worsening maternal and child health outcomes	India	Singh et al. (2021)
Global projections for undernutrition	COVID-19-related disruptions projected a significant rise in stunting, wasting, and maternal anemia across 118 LMICs, with long-term productivity losses	LMICs	Headey et al. (2020)
Food system disruptions	Pandemic amplified food security and supply chain disruptions in Ethiopia through reduced incomes, higher food prices, and limited agricultural outputs	Ethiopia	McCann et al. (2023)
Stunting and wasting	Increased rates of stunting and wasting linked to healthcare disruptions and reduced household incomes during the pandemic	India	Wakode et al. (2024)
Childhood malnutrition and mortality	Pandemic led to dietary quality decline and disruptions in food markets, healthcare systems, and school feeding programs, threatening SDG 2 and 3 progress	LMICs	

(continued on next page)

Stunting and feeding practices	Parental feeding challenges because of economic hardships greatly impacted children's nutritional status during the pandemic	Indonesia	Rahmatika et al. (2023)
CMAM program adaptations	Modified malnutrition protocols (for example, Family MUAC and reduced follow-up) allowed continued screening and treatment of malnutrition despite pandemic challenges, though disruptions persisted	LMICs	Wrabel et al. (2022)
Child nutrition and immunization	Approximately 14% stunted, 17% wasted, and 11% underweight children observed; malnutrition exacerbated by healthcare and food system disruptions	Nepal	Kayastha et al. (2022)
Child health disruptions in South Africa	Declines in immunizations and healthcare services during the pandemic most severely impacted children in poorer regions, increasing risks of severe malnutrition and associated diseases	South Africa	Thsehla et al. (2023)
Supply chain disruptions	Border closures disrupted supply chains for nutrition and health commodities, causing shortages of essential RMNCH services	Rwanda	Mutangana et al. (2022)

(*continued on next page*)

Table 8.1 Summary of key studies on the impact of COVID-19 on child nutrition and health in LMICs—cont'd

Focus area	Key findings	Country	Author and references
Maternal and child health	Healthcare disruptions related to COVID-19 impacted maternal and child health service provision globally, negatively affecting progress on SDG targets	Global	Dmello et al. (2020)
Service utilization trends	First 6 months of the pandemic showed dramatic declines in facility-based health services for children and mothers because of transportation restrictions and disease fears	Ethiopia	Bekele et al. (2022)
Family income and stunting	Reduced family incomes during COVID-19 were strongly linked to stunting prevalence among children under 5 because of limited access to nutritious foods	Indonesia	Yanti and Fauziah (2021)
Resilience in health and nutrition systems	Some maternal and child nutrition programs recovered after early declines because of coordinated interventions by NGOs and government	Ethiopia	Workicho et al. (2021)
Lessons from Ethiopian health systems	COVID-19 disrupted maternal and child health services, but efforts such as media campaigns, task forces, and community-led initiatives enabled partial recovery of health service utilization	Ethiopia	Tilahun et al. (2022)

(*continued on next page*)

Public nutrition services	Pandemic disrupted India's Integrated Child Development Scheme and public distribution systems for nutrition. Socioeconomic inequities compounded issues in accessing maternal and child nutrition services during the first 1000 days of life	India	Khandelwal et al. (2022)
Nutritional status of urban slum children	A repeated cross-sectional study found that HAZ (height-for-age) and WHZ (weight-for-height) significantly worsened post-COVID wave in Dhaka and Gazipur slums	Bangladesh	Wimo et al., 2022
Nutrition and food security trends during COVID	This review summarizes disruptions to food systems and nutrition services during COVID-19, noting reversals in gains on child undernutrition and food security	Bangladesh	Fahim et al. (2021)
Breastfeeding practices during COVID-19	Exclusive breastfeeding practices declined; maternal education, employment, and prior breastfeeding experience influenced outcomes	Pakistan	Fahim et al. (2021)

(continued on next page)

Table 8.1 Summary of key studies on the impact of COVID-19 on child nutrition and health in LMICs—cont'd

Focus area	Key findings	Country	Author and references
Nutrition and resilience during crisis	Nutrition-related behaviors adapted during crises like COVID-19 in Siargao, Philippines; emphasized need for "nutrition resilience plans"	Philippines	Bham et al. (2023)
Socioeconomic impact on nutrition	COVID-19 worsened food insecurity in Cambodia, affecting household dietary diversity and nutrition status, especially among vulnerable groups	Cambodia	Lasco et al. (2023)
Food insecurity and malnutrition in Haiti	COVID-19 and climate vulnerability worsened food insecurity and disrupted child nutrition services, threatening children's health and education outcomes	Haiti	UNESCO Haiti Proposal (World Food Programme (WFP), UNICEF, Asian Development Bank, 2022)

CMAM, community-based management of acute malnutrition; *LMICs*, low- and middle-income countries; *MUAC*, mid-upper arm circumference.

8.7 Case studies and regional examples

Jakarta, Indonesia: Angkat et al. (2022) demonstrated that stunting increased because of reduced iron intake during the pandemic.

Central India: Wakode et al. (2024) observed increased stunting and wasting because of limited healthcare access and reduced household incomes.

Kenya: Ouma et al. (2021) reported significant food insecurity, particularly among vulnerable groups, driven by economic hardships.

Peru: Pradeilles et al. (2022) found that government food assistance prevented complete dietary collapse but that nearly 47% of households still reported food insecurity.

Urban slums of Bangladesh: Wimo et al. (2022) reported that the nutritional status of children worsened after the first COVID-19 wave, with significant declines in height-for-age (HAZ) and weight-for-height (WHZ) scores in Dhaka and Gazipur urban slums.

Bangladesh (national): Fahim et al. (2021) documented broad disruptions to food systems and child nutrition services during COVID-19, noting reversals in prior gains against undernutrition and food insecurity.

Philippines (Siargao Island): Lasco et al. (2023) described adaptive community strategies to maintain child nutrition during crises like COVID-19, highlighting the need for "nutrition resilience plans."

8.8 Effects of COVID-19 pandemic on feeding practices of infants and children in LMICs

The COVID-19 pandemic has had profound impacts on Infant and Young Child Feeding (IYCF) practices, with lasting effects on the health and nutrition of children in LMICs. The pandemic disrupted breastfeeding, complementary feeding, and access to adequate nutrition, particularly for infants and young children. These disruptions have increased the prevalence of malnutrition, stunting, and wasting, and undermined progress toward achieving SDG 2 (Zero Hunger) and SDG 3 (Good Health and Well-being). This section explores how the COVID-19 pandemic affected IYCF practices in LMICs, focusing on breastfeeding, complementary feeding, and the broader nutrition landscape.

8.8.1 Impact on breastfeeding practices

Breastfeeding is one of the most important and cost-effective ways to ensure that infants receive adequate nutrition, particularly in the first 6 months of life. The WHO and UNICEF recommend exclusive breastfeeding for the first 6 months, followed by continued breastfeeding with complementary foods for up to 2 years or longer. However, the COVID-19 pandemic significantly disrupted breastfeeding practices across many LMICs.

8.8.1.1 Decline in exclusive breastfeeding rates

In the early stages of the pandemic, breastfeeding rates fell dramatically in some regions because of misinformation, fear of COVID-19 transmission, and healthcare system disruptions.

- **Misinformation and fear:** Many mothers were falsely advised that breastfeeding could transmit the virus, leading to an increase in the use of infant formula or other breast milk substitutes. For example, a study conducted by **Alive & Thrive** in **Bangladesh** found that nearly **22% of mothers** reduced or stopped breastfeeding because of COVID-19 fears (Ahoya et al., 2022).
- **Healthcare disruptions:** Routine antenatal and postnatal care services, which provide essential breastfeeding counseling, were disrupted as healthcare systems prioritized COVID-19 care. This disruption left many mothers without access to critical support for breastfeeding, particularly in rural and low-income areas.

8.8.1.2 Reduced breastfeeding support in healthcare settings

Healthcare workers, who typically provide crucial breastfeeding support and education, were overwhelmed or unavailable during the pandemic. This was particularly evident in LMICs, where health systems were already underresourced.

- In **Kenya**, early in the pandemic, many hospitals limited maternity services, and breastfeeding support was either unavailable or minimal. This led to an increase in the use of breast milk substitutes, particularly in urban areas with higher access to such products (Ahoya et al., 2022).
- In contrast, **Nepal** saw a **14% decline in breastfeeding** rates during the early stages of the pandemic but later experienced a slight improvement because of the implementation of community-based programs promoting breastfeeding and restrictions on the sale of breast milk substitutes (Kayastha et al., 2022).

8.8.1.3 Recovery in breastfeeding practices

Despite these early setbacks, some regions saw a recovery in breastfeeding rates as governments and organizations implemented policies to support breastfeeding.

- In **South Asia**, for example, public health campaigns and social media initiatives were launched to counteract misinformation and encourage continued breastfeeding.
- **India's ICDS** adapted to the pandemic by promoting breastfeeding through mobile messaging services and local community workers. These efforts helped raise awareness and encourage exclusive breastfeeding during the lockdown period (Khandelwal et al., 2022).

8.8.2 Challenges to complementary feeding practices

Complementary feeding (the introduction of solid and semisolid foods after 6 months of age) is essential to ensure that infants and young children receive the nutrients they need to grow and develop. The pandemic severely disrupted complementary feeding practices, leading to a decline in dietary diversity and an increase in malnutrition.

8.8.2.1 *Economic hardships and dietary diversity*

The COVID-19 pandemic induced severe economic challenges in many LMICs, leading to increased poverty and food insecurity. This directly impacted complementary feeding practices, as many families could no longer afford diverse, nutritious foods for their children.

- In **Kenya**, a study by Ouma et al. (2021) revealed that **household income losses** were significantly associated with reduced dietary quality for young children. Families faced limited access to animal-source foods, fruits, and vegetables, resulting in poor nutrition for infants and young children.
- Similarly, in **Peru, nearly 47% of households** reported moderate to severe food insecurity during the pandemic. This directly impacted children's diets, with families unable to access the diverse foods needed to meet the nutritional requirements of growing children (Pradeilles et al., 2022).

8.8.2.2 *Food supply chain disruptions*

The disruption of food supply chains further compounded challenges to complementary feeding.

- In **Ethiopia** the pandemic severely impacted food availability because of disruptions in agriculture and food markets. Supply chain breakdowns led to shortages of key foods such as fruits, vegetables, and animal products, which are vital for young children's nutrition (McCann et al., 2023).
- In **Nigeria** a study found that the consumption of **animal-source foods**—which are rich in protein and micronutrients—declined by **20%** during the pandemic, as families prioritized cheaper staple foods such as rice and maize (Ahoya et al., 2022).

8.8.2.3 *Reduction in access to food programs*

Many food assistance programs that provide complementary foods for vulnerable populations were disrupted or discontinued during the pandemic.

- The **Mid-Day Meal Scheme** in **India** faced significant disruptions, particularly during school closures. This was a major source of nutrition for millions of children in rural and urban areas, and its cessation led to a rise in food insecurity among school-aged children (Khandelwal et al., 2022).
- In **Bangladesh** the government attempted to mitigate the impact by distributing take-home rations to children enrolled in school feeding programs, but logistical challenges and delayed distribution meant that not all children received adequate nutrition (Roberton et al., 2020).

8.8.3 *Socioeconomic inequities and impact on feeding practices*

The COVID-19 pandemic disproportionately impacted already marginalized populations, further exacerbating existing inequities in child nutrition.

- **Gender disparities:** In many LMICs, girls often received less food than boys during times of food scarcity, leading to worsened nutrition outcomes for girls (Ouma et al., 2021).

- **Rural versus urban disparities:** Rural populations faced more severe disruptions to food access, healthcare, and nutrition programs compared to urban populations. The **World Food Programme (WFP)** reported that urban poor populations in LMICs had relatively better access to food assistance and nutrition support services compared to their rural counterparts (Headey et al., 2020).

8.8.4 Impact on child health and immunization because of feeding disruptions

Malnutrition because of disrupted feeding practices directly impacts child health and immunity.

- **Increased vulnerability to infections:** Children who do not receive proper nutrition are more susceptible to infections such as pneumonia, diarrhea, and malaria. These conditions can lead to a vicious cycle of illness and undernutrition, which significantly increases the risk of mortality.
- **Immunization gaps:** The pandemic disrupted routine immunization services, leaving children unprotected against vaccine-preventable diseases. A **WHO** report found that **68 countries** had significant disruptions in immunization services during the pandemic, which led to increased risks of malnutrition-related diseases in children (Wakode et al., 2024).

8.8.5 Strategies for supporting IYCF during crises

As the pandemic highlighted the vulnerabilities of existing IYCF practices, several strategies were identified to support and strengthen these practices during crises:

8.8.5.1 Community-based approaches

- Local community health workers, especially in rural areas, have been instrumental in disseminating accurate information about breastfeeding and complementary feeding. Programs such as **baby-friendly community initiatives (BFCIs) and local breastfeeding support groups** have shown promise in increasing breastfeeding rates and improving complementary feeding practices.

8.8.5.2 Digital platforms for information dissemination

- Mobile technology has played a key role in maintaining communication and providing nutritional information. In **India** the use of digital platforms for nutrition counseling helped mitigate the impact of restricted movement during lockdowns (Khandelwal et al., 2022).

8.8.5.3 Resilience-building measures for nutrition systems

- Governments and international organizations need to invest in building resilient nutrition systems that can withstand future shocks. This includes ensuring the continuity of essential nutrition programs, improving access to diversified foods, and integrating nutrition services into broader health systems.

8.9 Effects of COVID-19 pandemic on access to food for infants and children in LMICs

Food access is a fundamental determinant of child nutrition and well-being. The COVID-19 pandemic exacerbated food insecurity in **LMICs** by triggering a cascade of economic shocks, disrupting food supply chains, and driving food prices higher. These factors combined to create significant barriers to adequate nutrition for infants, children, and vulnerable populations. The repercussions were especially severe for children, whose access to nutritious food is directly linked to their growth, development, and long-term health outcomes.

8.9.1 Food insecurity and economic hardships

8.9.1.1 Loss of livelihoods and economic shocks

The COVID-19 pandemic triggered widespread **economic hardship**, particularly through the **loss of livelihoods** and the **disruption of informal sector jobs**, which are prevalent in many LMICs. Lockdowns, travel restrictions, and social distancing measures led to business closures, job losses, and economic slowdowns, pushing many families into poverty.

- In **Kenya,**Ouma et al. (2021) reported a significant correlation between **income loss and reduced dietary quality**, particularly for vulnerable groups such as **infants and pregnant women.** The loss of income meant that families had less purchasing power to buy diverse, nutritious foods. Instead, they were forced to rely on cheaper, less nutritious staples, exacerbating malnutrition (Ouma et al., 2021). The inability to purchase fresh fruits, vegetables, and animal-source foods—critical components of a balanced diet—led to increased **micronutrient deficiencies**, particularly among young children.
- Similarly, in **Uganda**, the pandemic's economic impact led to **worsened food insecurity**, as many families struggled to access food even when it was available. A study by Lubowa and Qali (2024) revealed that **food insecurity** was associated with **reduced meal frequency** and **lower dietary diversity** among mothers and children, contributing to an increase in both **stunting** and **wasting**. This decrease in food access disproportionately affected children in rural areas, where household incomes are generally lower, and the availability of diverse, nutrient-rich foods is limited.

8.9.1.2 Decline in household food access

With many families losing their primary sources of income during the pandemic the lack of financial resources meant fewer options for purchasing food, particularly those with high nutritional value. Families were often forced to prioritize **cheap, high-calorie** foods over **nutrient-dense** alternatives such as fruits, vegetables, and meats.

- In **Bangladesh**, research conducted by **Alive & Thrive** showed that **children's diets** became less diverse because of economic stress, and many families replaced nutrient-rich meals with rice and other low-cost foods. This contributed to **micronutrient deficiencies** such as **iron**

deficiency anemia and **vitamin A deficiency**, which are both linked to poor child growth and development (Roberton et al., 2020).

- In **Nigeria** a study found that **low-income families** were particularly impacted by rising food prices during the pandemic. **Animal-source foods**, which are essential for healthy child development, became unaffordable, leading to a **significant decline** in their consumption (Ahoya et al., 2022). The **lack of dietary diversity** during this period worsened **child malnutrition** and stunting, especially in infants aged 6–24 months, whose nutritional needs for growth and development are highest.

8.9.2 School feeding program disruptions

School feeding programs have long been an important tool in combating child malnutrition in LMICs, providing children with **regular meals** that meet their **daily nutritional requirements.** The **closure of schools** because of the pandemic created a large void in nutrition provision for millions of children who depend on these programs. These disruptions, combined with **logistical challenges**, led to **widespread malnutrition** and **food insecurity.**

8.9.2.1 The role of school feeding programs in LMICs

School feeding programs, particularly **mid-day meals,** provide a vital source of nutrition for children, especially in **low-income households.** These programs not only help children meet their immediate nutritional needs but also play a crucial role in promoting **school attendance** and supporting **cognitive development.**

- According to the **WFP**, over **368 million children globally** missed out on their **school meals** during the pandemic because of school closures (Headey & Ruel, 2020a). The loss of these meals increased the risk of **malnutrition**, particularly among school-aged children in **rural** and **disadvantaged urban areas** where families face **severe food insecurity.**

8.9.2.2 Disruptions in India's Integrated Child Development Scheme (ICDS)

In **India** the **ICDS**, a flagship nutrition program that provides **mid-day meals, nutritional supplements**, and **immunization** services to children, was severely disrupted during the pandemic. As schools closed, millions of children who relied on these meals were left without regular access to **balanced, nutritious food.**

- The government attempted to implement **take-home rations** as an alternative. However, **logistical challenges** and **inefficiencies** in distribution meant that **many vulnerable children** in remote or underserved areas did not receive adequate food supplies. The delays and **incomplete rations** led to **increased food insecurity**, further exacerbating the malnutrition crisis in children (Khandelwal et al., 2022).
- Moreover, in rural areas, **migrant workers** and their families, who often depend on the school feeding programs for their children's daily meals, experienced heightened vulnerability. With mobility restrictions in place, these families were unable to access the **rations** or any alternate food assistance programs. This situation resulted in significant **disruptions** to children's **access to nutrition** and **well-being** (Khandelwal et al., 2022).

8.9.2.3 Global efforts to address disruptions: Food rations and take-home programs

In response to the disruption of school feeding programs, several LMICs implemented **emergency food assistance** measures, such as food rations and **take-home meal packages.** Although these efforts were well-intentioned, they faced **logistical challenges** that hindered their ability to reach the most vulnerable children.

- For instance, **Brazil** expanded its **emergency food assistance programs** to provide **food baskets** to children in areas affected by school closures. However, transportation restrictions and **supply chain bottlenecks** limited the timely distribution of food, and many families were unable to access the assistance on time (Headey & Ruel, 2020a).
- In **South Africa** the government launched an initiative to distribute **food parcels** to **children in vulnerable households**. However, the demand far exceeded the supply, and logistical difficulties meant that only a portion of children received the full benefit of these programs (Osendarp et al., 2021).

Despite these efforts the **lack of consistency** in food delivery and **regional disparities** in distribution meant that many children missed out on essential nutrition, leading to a **worsening of malnutrition.**

8.9.3 Long-term consequences of disruptions to food access

The disruptions to food access and nutrition services during the COVID-19 pandemic will have long-term consequences for children in LMICs. The **temporary loss of school meals** and reductions in **dietary diversity** will likely result in lasting developmental consequences, including

8.9.3.1 Increased rates of malnutrition

The **long-term effects of food insecurity** and the disruptions in feeding programs are expected to increase the prevalence of **chronic malnutrition** (stunting) and **acute malnutrition** (wasting). Malnutrition in early childhood has lifelong effects, including **impaired cognitive development, reduced educational outcomes**, and **increased susceptibility to infections.**

- According to McCann et al. (2023)**, food insecurity** has been linked to **higher rates of stunting,** which in turn affects **cognitive development** and the overall **quality of life** for children in LMICs.

8.9.3.2 Vulnerable populations at greater risk

Children from **marginalized communities**, including **refugees, migrant workers**, and those in **rural or conflict-affected areas**, were the most vulnerable during the pandemic. These children are more likely to experience **food insecurity** and **malnutrition,** which have long-lasting effects on their growth, learning, and development.

8.10 Factors affecting the nutrition supply chain

8.10.1 Agricultural and supply chain disruptions

The COVID-19 pandemic led to significant disruptions in **agricultural production** and the **global food supply chain**, adversely affecting food availability and access in LMICs. These disruptions worsened malnutrition by limiting access to diverse and nutritious foods, particularly in regions where agriculture is the primary livelihood and food source.

8.10.1.1 Lockdowns and labor shortages affecting agricultural production

- **In Ethiopia**, lockdowns and labor shortages disrupted agricultural activities, leading to a decline in food availability. As farmers were unable to work because of movement restrictions and health concerns, the production of **fruits, vegetables, and animal-source foods** decreased significantly. These types of foods are critical for providing essential nutrients, and their reduction has direct consequences on the **health and nutrition** of children. The lack of access to fresh produce resulted in a shift toward **staple grains** (for example, rice and maize), which are low in protein and essential micronutrients, leading to **increased malnutrition rates** (McCann et al., 2023).
- **In India** the nationwide lockdown disrupted food production and distribution, particularly affecting **smallholder farmers** who were unable to access markets, leading to reduced food availability and higher prices for fresh produce. This resulted in **increased food insecurity** and worsened **child malnutrition**, especially in rural areas where access to diverse foods was already limited (Khandelwal et al., 2022).

8.10.1.2 Impact on food distribution and supply chains

The pandemic also led to disruptions in the distribution of food, exacerbated by transport restrictions and reduced market access. These factors affected the **flow of food from producers to consumers**, making it difficult for LMIC populations to access essential foods.

- In **Burkina Faso** the movement restrictions and fears of infection led to sharp declines in **patient enrollment at malnutrition treatment centers**. These centers, which provide therapeutic food and healthcare services to malnourished children, experienced a reduction in capacity because of transportation challenges and the need for physical distancing to prevent the spread of COVID-19 (Ouedraogo et al., 2023).
- In **Ethiopia** the disruption of essential health services for maternal and child nutrition was significant. Outpatient nutrition centers were affected, and there was a decline in the availability of nutrition support services because of a lack of healthcare personnel and logistical support. However, these disruptions were mitigated by coordinated efforts from the government and international NGOs, which helped restore some level of healthcare service and nutrition support (Bekele et al., 2022; Workicho et al., 2021).

8.10.2 Healthcare and nutrition program interruptions

The pandemic also disrupted healthcare and nutrition programs, particularly those focused on **maternal and child health**. These interruptions had far-reaching impacts on child nutrition, worsening malnutrition, and increasing the risk of illness.

8.10.2.1 Declines in healthcare and nutrition services

- In **Burkina Faso**, outpatient malnutrition centers experienced significant declines in patient enrollment. These facilities, which play a vital role in screening, diagnosing, and treating severe malnutrition, saw a reduction in access to care because of **transportation challenges** and **fears of infection** among healthcare workers and families (Ouedraogo et al., 2023). As a result, many children did not receive timely treatment for malnutrition, leading to increased cases of severe malnutrition and mortality in some areas.
- In **Ethiopia**, essential health services for maternal and child nutrition declined during the pandemic. The interruptions were partly mitigated by efforts from government bodies and NGOs, such as providing modified malnutrition treatment and integrating community health workers to maintain care access (Bekele et al., 2022; Workicho et al., 2021). Despite these efforts the pandemic highlighted critical gaps in healthcare provision, especially in remote and rural areas where access to nutrition support is already limited.

8.10.2.2 Indirect effects of malnutrition on child health

The **disruption of healthcare services** because of the pandemic had **indirect impacts on child health**, especially for children under 5 years of age. The lack of routine immunizations and growth monitoring exacerbated malnutrition and increased the risk of infections among children, contributing to higher rates of **morbidity** and **mortality**.

- In **South Africa**, healthcare disruptions and delays in immunization campaigns led to a decline in vaccine coverage, which heightened the risk of severe malnutrition and associated diseases such as pneumonia and diarrhea (Thsehla et al., 2023). These conditions, often preventable through proper nutrition and healthcare, became more common among malnourished children, further perpetuating a cycle of poor health outcomes.
- Modeling studies conducted during the pandemic predicted that **an additional 168,000 child deaths globally** could be attributed to healthcare service disruptions, highlighting the profound indirect impacts of the pandemic on child health and nutrition (Roberton et al., 2020).

8.10.3 Modified malnutrition screening and treatment protocols

The pandemic led to the adaptation of existing nutrition and health programs to maintain essential services despite the challenges of lockdowns, social distancing, and healthcare worker shortages.

8.10.3.1 The use of family MUAC (middle upper arm circumference) and community-based screening

To address disruptions in malnutrition screening and treatment, healthcare providers implemented modified protocols, such as **Family MUAC** for at-home screening of malnutrition. This approach enabled the continued detection and treatment of malnutrition without the need for face-to-face consultations.

- In **Burkina Faso** the shift to using Family MUAC significantly increased access to screening for acute malnutrition, particularly in areas where traditional health facilities were inaccessible or operating at reduced capacity because of COVID-19. The approach helped maintain continuity of care, despite the challenges of the pandemic, and ensured that some children received necessary nutritional support despite the crisis (Wrabel et al., 2022).
- Similarly, in **Ethiopia,** efforts by the government and international NGOs helped restore some healthcare services and provided training and support to community health workers. These initiatives allowed for the continued distribution of essential nutrition supplies and immunizations, helping to mitigate the impacts of the pandemic on maternal and child health (Bekele et al., 2022; Workicho et al., 2021).

8.11 Indirect impact on children's health because of COVID-19 pandemic

The indirect health impacts of disrupted nutrition supply chains have been far-reaching, contributing to **higher rates of malnutrition-related diseases** and increased **child mortality** in LMICs.

8.11.1 Increased child mortality because of malnutrition

The combined effects of **food insecurity, economic shocks,** and the **disruption of nutrition services** have contributed to an increase in **child mortality** from preventable causes such as **diarrhea, respiratory infections,** and **pneumonia.**

- Studies predict that the **indirect effects of COVID-19,** such as **disrupted nutrition services,** could lead to **an additional 168,000 child deaths** annually in LMICs, exacerbating the **malnutrition burden** (Osendarp et al., 2021; Roberton et al., 2020).

8.11.2 Heightened vulnerability of marginalized groups

Children from **marginalized groups,** such as those living in **refugee camps, conflict zones**, or **slum areas**, have been the hardest hit by the pandemic's disruptions to the nutrition supply chain. These children, who often rely on **external aid** or **community programs** for nutrition, have been disproportionately affected by the breakdown in food and health services (Mutangana et al., 2022).

8.12 Conclusion

The COVID-19 pandemic has exposed the deep vulnerabilities of low-LMICs, particularly in the realm of child nutrition. The crisis has exacerbated existing challenges related to malnutrition, food insecurity, and inadequate healthcare access, leading to a significant rise in stunting, wasting, and micronutrient deficiencies among children. The disruptions to food supply chains, economic stability, and essential nutrition programs have compounded these issues, creating a cascade of negative effects on children's health. The pandemic has disrupted key feeding practices, such as breastfeeding and complementary feeding, which are crucial for infant and child survival, and has hampered access to diverse, nutritious foods. Healthcare service interruptions further exacerbated the situation, leading to higher mortality rates from preventable diseases such as diarrhea, pneumonia, and malnutrition-related complications. Vulnerable groups, including those living in poverty, refugees, and conflict zones, have been disproportionately affected by these disruptions, amplifying existing socioeconomic inequalities. The long-term effects of the pandemic on maternal and child health are still unfolding, with the full scope of damage likely to be felt for years to come. The pandemic has highlighted the urgent need for stronger, more resilient food systems, improved healthcare infrastructure, and more robust social protection mechanisms to protect children's nutrition during future crises. The path forward must focus on building resilience in both food and health systems to safeguard the well-being of the most vulnerable populations.

References

Ahoya, B., Kavle, J. A., Kiige, L., Gathi, C., Samburu, B., Maina, L., ... Codjia, P. (2022). How COVID-19 affected food systems, health service delivery and maternal and infant nutrition practices: Implications for moving forward in Kenya. *Maternal & Child Nutrition, 19*(2), e13466. https://doi.org/10.1111/mcn.13466.

Akseer, N., Kandru, G., Keats, E. C., & Bhutta, Z. A. (2020). COVID-19 pandemic and mitigation strategies: Implications for maternal and child health and nutrition. *American Journal of Clinical Nutrition, 112*(2), 251–256. https://doi.org/10.1093/ajcn/nqaa171.

Angkat, A.H., Chandra, D.N., & Hardiany, N. S. (2022). Relationship between iron intake and iron status to stunted in children aged 24-35 months during the COVID-19 pandemic in Jakarta. World Nutrition Journal, 5(S3), 35. https://doi.org/10.25220/WNJ.V05.S3.0023

Bekele, C., Bekele, D., Hunegnaw, B. M., Van Wickle, K., Ashenafi, F., Korte, M., ... Chan, G. J. (2022). *Impact of COVID-19 pandemic on utilization of facility-based essential maternal and child health services in North Shewa Zone, Ethiopia. medRxiv* https://doi.org/10.1101/2022.01.10.22268794.

Bham, S. Q., Khan, K. M. A., Munaver, S. A., & Sharif, U. H. A. (2023). Breastfeeding practices in nursing mothers during COVID-19 pandemic: Dual center study in Karachi, Pakistan. *Pakistan Journal of Medical Sciences, 39*(2), 467–473. https://doi.org/10.12669/pjms.39.2.6707.

Dmello, B. S., Housseine, N., van den Akker, T., van Roosmalen, J., & Maaløe, N. (2020). Impact of COVID-19 on maternal and child health. *The Lancet Global Health, 8*(10), e1259. https://doi.org/10.1016/S2214-109X(20)30328-4.

Fahim, S.M., Hossain, M.S., Sen, S., Das, S., Hosssain, M., Ahmed, T., Rahman, S.M.M., Rahman, M.K., & Alam, S. (2021). Nutrition and food security in Bangladesh: Achievements, challenges, and impact of the COVID-19 pandemic. The Journal of Infectious Diseases, 224(Suppl. 7), S901–S909. https://doi.org/10.1093/infdis/jiab473

Headey, D., Heidkamp, R., Osendarp, S., Ruel, M., Scott, N., Black, R., … Walker, N. (2020). Impacts of COVID-19 on childhood malnutrition and nutrition-related mortality. *The Lancet, 396*(10250), 519–521. https://doi.org/10.1016/S0140-6736(20)31647-0.

Headey, D., & Ruel, M. (2020a). The COVID-19 nutrition crisis: What to expect and how to protect. In J. Swinnen, & J. McDermott (Eds.), *COVID-19 and global food security* (pp. 38–41). International Food Policy Research Institute (IFPRI) https://doi.org/10.2499/p15738coll2.133762_08.

Kayastha, P., Chikanbanjar, V. K., Panday, R. K., & Manandhar, S. R. (2022). Nutritional and immunisation status of children visiting hospital during COVID-19 pandemic in Kathmandu, Nepal. *Journal of Kathmandu Medical College, 11*(1), 4–7. https://doi.org/10.3126/jkmc.v11i1.45486.

Khandelwal, S., Mehra, M., & Singh, A. (2022). Impact on public health nutrition services due to COVID-19 pandemic in India: A scoping review of primary studies on health and social security determinants affecting the first 1000 days of life. *International Journal of Environmental Research and Public Health, 19*(21), 13973. https://doi.org/10.3390/ijerph192113973.

Lasco, G., Yu, V. G., Compra, J. M., Leuangvilay, P., Suphanchaimat, R., Zhang, Y., & Javier, C. (2023). Nutrition in times of crisis: A qualitative study in Siargao Island, Philippines, during the COVID-19 pandemic. *Acta Medica Philippina, 57*(5). https://doi.org/10.47895/amp.vi0.4963.

Lubowa, M., & Qali, I. A. (2024). Effect of COVID-19 pandemic on food security and maternal nutrition status of selected peri-urban and urban communities in Mbale, Uganda. *Journal of Food Innovation, Nutrition & Environmental Sciences, 1*(1), 1–10. https://doi.org/10.70851/v83hw171.

McCann, J., Sinno, L., Ramadhan, E., Assefa, N., Berhane, H. Y., Madzorera, I., & Fawzi, W. (2023). COVID-19 disruptions of food systems and nutrition services in Ethiopia: Evidence of the impacts and policy responses. *Annals of Global Health, 89*(1), 30. https://doi.org/10.5334/aogh.3980.

Mutangana, A., Ntakirutimana, O., Mwali, A. K., & Radeny, S. (2022). Supporting Rwanda's COVID-19 response and mitigating its impact on maternal, newborn, and child health and malaria service delivery. *IntraHealth International* https://www.intrahealth.org/sites/default/files/attachment-files/tb1supportingrwandacovid19rev-5-22hr-d.pdf.

Osendarp, S., Akuoku, J. K., Black, R. E., Headey, D., Ruel, M., Scott, N., … Heidkamp, R. (2021). The COVID-19 crisis will exacerbate maternal and child undernutrition and child mortality in low- and middle-income countries. *Nature Food, 2*(7), 476–484. https://doi.org/10.1038/s43016-021-00319-4.

Ouedraogo, P., Pietra, V., & Schumacher, R. (2023). Impact of COVID-19 on outpatient malnutrition centers in urban and rural Burkina Faso. *American Journal of Tropical Medicine and Hygiene, 109*(2), 460–465. https://doi.org/10.4269/ajtmh.22-0714.

Ouma, P. O., Robinson, O., Mugalavai, V. K., & Onkware, A. O. (2021). Food security status during the COVID-19 pandemic among vulnerable groups in Keiyo South, Elgeyo Marakwet County, Kenya. *International Journal of Scientific and Research Publications.*

Padhani, Z., & Bhutta, Z. (2022). Tackling protein-calorie malnutrition during world crises. Annals of Nutrition & Metabolism, 78(Suppl 2), 19–26. https://doi.org/10.1159/000522242.

Pradeilles, R., Pareja, R., Creed-Kanashiro, H. M., Griffiths, P. L., Holdsworth, M., Verdezoto, N., … Rousham, E. K. (2022). Diet and food insecurity among mothers, infants, and young children in Peru before and during COVID-19: A panel survey. *Maternal & Child Nutrition, 18*(3), e13343. https://doi.org/10.1111/mcn.13343.

Rahmatika, Q. T., Mulyono, S., & Rahmadiyah, D. C. (2023). Feeding practices and child stunting during the COVID-19 pandemic: A qualitative study. *Journal of Public Health in Africa, 14*(5), e2580. https://doi.org/10.4081/jphia.2023.2580.

Roberton, T., Carter, E. D., Chou, V. B., Stegmuller, A. R., Jackson, B. D., Tam, Y., … Walker, N. (2020). Early estimates of the indirect effects of the COVID-19 pandemic on maternal and child mortality in low-income and middle-income countries: A modelling study. *The Lancet Global Health, 8*(7), e901–e908. https://doi.org/10.1016/S2214-109X(20)30229-1.

Singh, A. K., Jain, P. K., Singh, N. P., Kumar, S., Bajpai, P. K., Singh, S., & Jha, M. (2021). Impact of COVID-19 pandemic on maternal and child health services in Uttar Pradesh, India. *Journal of Family Medicine and Primary Care, 10*(1), 509–513. https://doi.org/10.4103/jfmpc.jfmpc_1550_20.

Thsehla, E., Balusik, A., Boachie, M. K., Tombe-Mdewa, W., Kabudula, C., Du Toit, J., … Hofman, K. (2023). Indirect effects of COVID-19 on maternal and child health in South Africa. *Global Health Action, 16*(1), 2153442. https://doi.org/10.1080/16549716.2022.2153442.

Tilahun, B., Nigusie, A., Zelalem, M., & Mekonnen, Z. A. (2022). Effect of COVID-19 pandemic on maternal and child health services and strategies for effective service implementation in Ethiopia. *Journal of Multidisciplinary Healthcare, 15*, 2781–2795. https://doi.org/10.2147/JMDH.S390750.

Wakode, N., Bajpai, K., Trushna, T., Wakode, S., Garg, K., & Wakode, A. (2024). Influence of sociodemographic factors on stunting, wasting, and underweight among children under two years of age born during the COVID-19 pandemic in central India: A cross-sectional study. *Cureus, 16*(3), e56381. https://doi.org/10.7759/cureus.56381.

Wimo, H., Shafique, S., Probst-Hensch, N., & Gneiting, F. (2022). Change in nutritional status of urban slum children before and after the first COVID-19 wave in Bangladesh: A repeated cross-sectional assessment. *PLOS Global Public Health, 2*(7), e0000456.

Workicho, A., Kershaw, M. J., Berhanu, L., Kebede, M., & Kennedy, E. (2021). Essential health and nutrition service provision during the COVID-19 pandemic: Lessons from select Ethiopian Woredas. *Current Developments in Nutrition, 5*(4), nzab024. https://doi.org/10.1093/cdn/nzab024.

World Food Programme (WFP), UNICEF, Asian Development Bank. (2022). *COVID-19 socio-economic impact assessment in Cambodia—Phase 1 report.* WFP Cambodia Retrieved April 20, 2025, from https://www.wfp.org/publications/2022-covid-19-socio-economic-impact-assessment-cambodia-phase-1-report .

Wrabel, M., Stokes-Walters, R., King, S., Funnell, G., & Stobaugh, H. (2022). Programmatic adaptations to acute malnutrition screening and treatment during the COVID-19 pandemic. *Maternal & Child Nutrition, 18*(4), e13406. https://doi.org/10.1111/mcn.13406.

Yanti, T., & Fauziah, D. A. (2021). The effect of family income on stunting incident in preschool children at Bogor City during COVID-19 pandemic. *Indian Journal of Public Health Research & Development, 12*(2), 407–412. https://doi.org/10.37506/ijphrd.v12i2.14167.

Zhu, P. H., Mhango, S. N., Vinnakota, A., Mansour, M., & Coss-Bu, J. A. (2022). Effects of COVID-19 pandemic on nutritional status, feeding practices, and access to food among infants and children in lower and middle-income countries: A narrative review. *Current Tropical Medicine Reports, 9*(4), 197–206. https://doi.org/10.1007/s40475-022-00271-8.

Section II

Strategies for special populations

Nutritional status of women and children in Northeast India

9

Saranyadevi S[a], *Lekshmi Gangadhar*[b], *Selva Kumar T*[c,d] *and Raju Sasikumar*[d]
[a]Computational Biology and Therapeutics Lab, Saveetha College of Physiotherapy, Saveetha Institute of Medical and Technical Sciences (SIMATS), Saveetha University, Thandalam, Chennai, Tamil Nadu, India, [b]NanoDot Research Private Limited, Nagercoil, Tamil Nadu, India, [c]Vel Tech Rangarajan Dr. Sagunthala R&D Institute of Science and Technology, Chennai, Tamil Nadu, India, [d]Department of Agribusiness Management and Food Technology, North-Eastern Hill University, Tura, Meghalaya, India

9.1 Introduction

The significance of nutritional health cannot be overstated, particularly for women and children, because it is an integral part of human development. This is particularly the case in Northeast India, which is famous for its numerous cultures, high diversity, and natural landscapes, which are characterized by its stark developmental issues (Meshram et al., 2017). To this end, women's and children's nutritional condition plays a dominant role in affecting individual health, family well-being, and overall societal advancement. It is a matter that has to be carefully studied and addressed by targeted intervention because of its prime importance in interrupting the cycle of poverty and hunger across generations (Wells et al., 2021). The region of Northeast India is constituted by eight states: Arunachal Pradesh, Assam, Manipur, Meghalaya, Mizoram, Nagaland, Sikkim, and Tripura, which are distinguished by their immense cultural diversity, difficult terrain, and socioeconomic vulnerabilities. Especially for children and women, who are the most vulnerable groups in society, the nutritional indicators of the region tend to lag behind the national average (Chatterjee & Rai, 2024). This chapter examines the nutritional status among women and children of Northeastern India, the primary causes, issues, and measures to decrease nutritional inequalities.

The "dual burden of malnutrition," or the simultaneous presence of undernutrition and overnutrition, is one aspect that distinguishes Northeast India's nutritional landscape. Undernutrition manifests as wasting, stunted growth, and micronutrient deficiency among many women and children (Seferidi et al., 2022). However, in some urban and semiurban areas of the region, the prevalence of noncommunicable diseases (NCDs), including diabetes and obesity, that are associated with overnutrition is rising. Policymakers and medical professionals face a great deal of difficulty in addressing the requirements of people at both extremes of the dietary spectrum because of this dual burden. Women significantly influence the family's nutritional results. However,

Nutritional Strategies, Predictive Models, and Sustainable Policies. DOI: https://doi.org/10.1016/B978-0-443-23671-6.00008-6

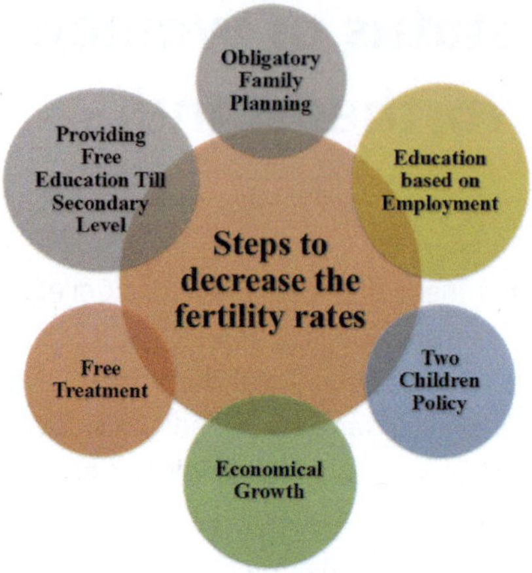

Figure 9.1 Stages to lessening fertility rates in poor women. Northeast India's nutritional status and dietary patterns are closely linked to its environmental and sociocultural setting. The traditional diets, which focus on foods that are easily accessible within the region, such as fermented foods, bamboo shoots, and wild greens, contain many nutritional advantages but typically lack sufficient calories and protein for adolescents and pregnant women. The geographical difficulties of the region and recurring natural calamities, which act as major hurdles in accessing healthcare and food security, significantly increase the vulnerability to malnutrition (Manik et al., 2024). Over time, various government and nongovernmental efforts have been initiated to tackle Northeast India's nutritional issues. Through schemes such as Poshan Abhiyaan, the Mid-Day Meal Scheme, and the Integrated Child Development Services (ICDS), some progress led to enhancing nutritional outcomes.

some issues, such as early marriage, high reproduction rates, gender-based inequities, and restricted access to healthcare and education, frequently result in their nutritional condition being impaired in Northeast India (Bhuiyan et al., 2024). Iron deficiency anemia hurts their health, productivity, and ability to child rear. Furthermore, food taboos and practices among certain communities might further limit women's access to an adequate diet (Kumar et al., 2022).

9.1.1 Decreasing fertility rates of women in Northeast India

Declining fertility among poor women occurs through several phases. The first 1000 days of life, between conception and the child's second birthday, is a developmentally critical phase. Fig. 9.1 exemplifies the various stages of lessening fertility rates in poor women. In Northeast India, poor nutrition during this phase is prevalent and has long-term implications such as cognitive impairment, reduced learning ability, and susceptibility to diseases. Underweight, stunting, and wasting continue to be extremely prevalent among children below 5 years in many states of the region, as highlighted by the National Family Health Survey-5 (NFHS-5), pointing toward the imperative need for successful interventions (Likhar & Patil, 2022).

However, the region's specific needs and challenges require locally tailored approaches addressing the root socioeconomic causes of malnutrition, taking advantage of community participation, and involving local expertise. The nutritional health of women and children in Northeast India is an indicator of broader developmental disparities that must be met immediately (Narayan et al., 2019). To address these problems, there is a need for a multisectoral intervention involving social welfare, education, health, and agriculture. It also demands enhanced investment in research, infrastructure construction, and capacity development to come up with fair and sustainable solutions. The groundwork for a thorough examination of the determinants of nutritional status in Northeast India, the effects of malnutrition on the health of individuals and society, and the measures to attain long-term changes is established in this chapter. We can set the stage for a healthier, more sustainable future for the women and children in the region by developing an overall awareness of the special potential and challenges of the region.

9.2 Nutritional status of NER

Data on the dietary status of the NFHS is trustworthy. Comparing NFHS 1, 2, 3, 4, and 5 indicates that underweight prevalence among children aged under 5 has decreased by 21.3% in India. Assam recorded the highest percentage of underweight children aged under 5 (50.40) in 1992–93 (NFHS-1). Moreover, underweight children aged under 5 in 2019–20 have a higher rate than the national standard. Among the states with a high percentage of underweight children, Arunachal Pradesh and Tripura have significantly reduced their percentage of underweight children from 1992–93 to 2019–20, even surpassing the national average (Jha et al., 2024). Nagaland has only managed to decline by 1.8%; therefore, there is not a noticeable decrease. According to the NFHS-5, acute malnutrition or wasting in children under 5 is 19.30% in India, whereas Northeastern States (NESs) like Assam have higher rates than the national average (21.70%). The aforementioned signs are all the result of inadequately planned and executed nutrition programs (Chakraborty et al., 2021). Since 1992–93, there has been a 1.8% increase in acute malnutrition. Except for Mizoram, Meghalaya, and Nagaland, NESs have been able to lower the rates by about 6%–7%. In addition, Assam saw a dramatic 10% rise in acute malnutrition between 1992–93 and 2019–20. All NESs and India have been successful in reducing stunting in children under 5, except Nagaland, where stunting has slightly increased by 0.30%. Children's stunting has decreased by 25.90% in Arunachal Pradesh, compared to 16.50% throughout India, which is better than the national average. Although some states perform well, other states have insufficient or no access to food (Narayanan et al., 2024). Overall, 45% of child fatalities worldwide are because of undernutrition, which results from inadequate nutrient consumption. Stronger immunity in children is largely dependent on proper feeding habits and enough nutrition. India placed 94th out of 107 countries in the global hunger index, much behind Bangladesh, Pakistan, and Nepal (Ngaihte & Kaur, 2020). Fig. 9.1 displays the theoretical framework linking agricultural practices, time usage, and nutrition consequences.

Research from both developed and developing nations demonstrates that children with two parents have better developmental outcomes when compared to children with a single parent and that parental presence promotes a child's healthy development (Amato, 2001). Moreover, the child's nutritional status is slightly impacted by parental out-migration (Lei et al., 2020). The census data indicates that the number of female migrants has increased over time. Moving from one location to another causes changes in the dietary features of migrants. The existing body of research on women and nutrition has typically depended on measures of empowerment such as income control and women's education (Anastasiadou et al., 2023).

Studies explicitly examining women's nutrition are scarce in India. At the national level, women's exposure to land reforms and agricultural employment has been used to account for nutritional components. The majority have used equality and household spending as stand-ins for health and nutrition. Using secondary data from NFHS, we examine the nutritional and health status of women in NESs in this section. Food instability and a lack of proper health services exacerbate the issue of undernutrition and malnutrition. The NFHS-5 estimates that 15–49-year-old Indian women have an 18.70% body mass index (BMI) (Jha et al., 2024). Table 9.1 clearly shows the women's nutritional status in Northeast India.

Despite being one of the NESs with the smallest population, Arunachal Pradesh is found to have the highest percentage of women with a high-risk waist-to-hip ratio. Except for Mizoram, all NESs reported higher percentages of women with a high-risk waist-to-hip ratio than the national norm. Premature birth and infant death are concerns associated with anemia during pregnancy (Anastasiadou et al., 2023). Although not particularly the proportion of pregnant women who are anemic has decreased for NESs during 1998–99. The number of anemic pregnant women in India is steadily rising. Compared to the other Northeast Indian states, Nagaland had a notably lower number of pregnant women who were anemic. In addition, estimates of anemic pregnant women are higher in Tripura and Assam than the national average.

9.2.1 Challenges faced by women and children of Northeast India

9.2.1.1 Socioeconomic barriers

Maternal nutrition significantly influences the mother's and her children's health and well-being. Women in Northeast India had varied degrees of dietary inadequacies, per the NFHS-5 (2019–21). To provide for their children and other family members, women in low-income households frequently forgo their nutritional needs. This prioritizing leads to undernutrition, especially during critical life stages such as pregnancy and lactation (Nguyen et al., 2021). Low household income limits access to a range of nutrient-dense meals, which can result in deficiencies in essential nutrients, including iron, calcium, and vitamins. Women often have less control over home finances, making it difficult for them to meet their personal dietary needs. Women's negotiating position for better nutrition is weakened because their informal labor and caregiving contributions to home income are usually undervalued (Vilar-Compte et al., 2021).

Table 9.1 Women's Nutritional Status in Northeast India.

S. no.	Places (age 15–49 years)	Year	Below normal BMI of women	Overweight women	Higher risk of waist-to-hip ratio	Anemic pregnant women	References
1	Arunachal Pradesh	2019–20	5.7	23.9	68.9	27.9	Agrawal & Mishra, 2004
		2015–16	8.5	18.8	NA	37.8	
2	Assam	2019–20	17.6	15.2	67.2	54.2	Das et al. (2024)
		2015–16	25.7	13.2	NA	44.8	
3	Manipur	2019–20	7.2	34.1	65.7	32.4	Thanglen and Maheo (2022)
		2015–16	8.8	26	NA	26	
4	Meghalaya	2019–20	10.8	11.5	60.6	45	Let et al. (2023)
		2015–16	12.1	12.2	NA	53.3	
5	Mizoram	2019–20	5.3	24.2	47.6	34	Girotra et al. (2023)
		2015–16	8.4	21	NA	27	
6	Nagaland	2019–20	11.1	14.4	62	22.2	Tantri et al. (2022)
		2015–16	12.3	16.2	NA	32.7	
7	Sikkim	2019–20	5.8	34.7	75.6	40.7	Gahlawat (2024)
		2015–16	6.4	26.7	NA	23.6	
		2015–16	22.9	20.6	NA	50.40	

BMI, body mass index.

Poor-income children sometimes struggle to consume a balanced diet, resulting in meals that are calorie-dense but nutrient-poor. Seasonal fluctuations in food availability cause unequal access to proper nutrition, particularly in farming families. The common tendency of low-income families to consume cheaper staple foods such as rice or wheat, vegetables, and foods rich in protein results in a lack of vital minerals such as iron and zinc and vitamins (Lee et al., 2023).

9.2.1.2 Cultural and gender norms

Cultural norms often dictate that women should eat last and in smaller portions, leading to inadequate nutrient intake. Women typically eat fewer nutrient-dense foods because of gender biases in food distribution, especially in patriarchal environments. Social pressure to maintain a specific body type might lead to women adopting unhealthy eating habits or restricted diets. Myths and cultural taboos about eating during pregnancy and nursing can have a detrimental effect on the nutrition of both the mother and the fetus (Harris-Fry et al., 2022).

9.2.1.3 Body mass index

Identifies those who are at risk for health problems associated with being overweight or underweight. It aids in directing clinician judgments about medication, exercise, and food. Frequently acts as a preliminary metric before more thorough evaluations such as waist-to-hip ratio or body fat percentage. Although trends show regional variances, a sizable minority of women in the region is underweight (BMI < 18.5). States such as Assam and Meghalaya, for example, have greater prevalence rates than Sikkim and Mizoram (Bradley et al., 2023).

9.2.1.4 Limitations of body mass index

Despite its widespread use, BMI has several drawbacks. Bone, muscle, and fat mass are all included in BMI. Athletes with a lot of muscle mass, for instance, could have a high BMI yet little body fat. BMI does not take into consideration the fact that central obesity, or fat around the abdomen, is more harmful than fat dispersed elsewhere. In elderly persons with reduced muscular mass, BMI may exaggerate fatness. At the same BMI, different ethnic groups have varying amounts of body fat (e.g., Asians may have larger percentages of fat at lower BMIs than Caucasians). Other health indicators, such as blood pressure, cholesterol, and blood sugar levels, are not into account (Callahan et al., 2023).

9.2.1.5 Anemia

A medical disease known as anemia occurs when the body lacks enough healthy red blood cells to supply tissues and organs with enough oxygen. Weakness, exhaustion, and other symptoms may result from this. A prevalent ailment can range in severity from mild to severe. In most jurisdictions, anemia affects more than 50% of women who are of reproductive age, which is still a major concern. Poor hygiene habits, low access to healthcare, and iron-deficient diets are some of the factors that contribute to anemia (Chaparro et al., 2019).

9.2.1.6 Prevention of anemia

9.2.1.6.1 Healthy diet

Include foods rich in iron, including spinach, beans, lentils, chicken, shellfish, and red meat. Intake of vitamin C-rich foods, such as citrus fruits, to improve the absorption of iron. Consume foods high in B12, such as dairy products, eggs, and fortified cereals. Incorporate foods high in folate, such as leafy greens, almonds, and seeds. For those with long-term conditions or those who are at risk (such as expectant mothers), routine examinations are especially crucial. Treat ailments such as stomach problems, heavy periods, or ulcers (Ford et al., 2019).

9.2.1.6.2 Micronutrient deficiencies

Deficiencies in essential nutrients, which include vitamin A, vitamin D, and iodine, are frequent because of an inadequate number of varied diets and a poor consumption of fruits, vegetables, and fortified foods. Many women of reproductive age suffer from a high frequency of vitamin A insufficiency, which hurts maternal health and pregnancy outcomes. Physical and cognitive developments are hampered by inadequate consumption of vital nutrients such as iron, iodine, and zinc. Iron, zinc, vitamin A, and iodine shortages in children can result in impaired immunity, delayed growth, and heightened vulnerability to infections.

9.2.1.6.3 Underweight and overweight

Growing rates of overweight and obesity indicate a dual burden of malnutrition, even if undernutrition is still a concern. Low birth weight (LBW) babies, who are more prone to suffer from stunting, wasting, and undernutrition, are more likely to be born to malnourished mothers. Pregnancy-related malnutrition has an impact on fetal development, which can cause long-term health and developmental issues for the unborn child. In Northeast India, stunting, wasting, and underweight are some of the symptoms of childhood malnutrition. In places such as Meghalaya (47.2%) and Arunachal Pradesh (34.3%), stunting rates (low height-for-age) continue to be dangerously high. This is caused in part by suboptimal baby feeding habits, chronic malnutrition, and poor maternal health.

9.2.1.6.4 Limited access to healthcare and nutrition education

Many women of Northeast states of India have limited access to healthcare facilities that provide essential nutrition guidance, supplementation, and monitoring during pregnancy and lactation. In rural communities, women can struggle to receive basic treatments because medical centers are underfunded or far from the communities. As they lack knowledge about balanced diets, portion sizes, and nutrition needs, most women cannot make healthy dietary choices (Srivastava et al., 2015).

9.2.1.6.5 Impact of workload and time poverty

In many cases, women are in charge of both taking care of the home and making a living. This hectic work leaves little time for self-care activities such as cooking and maintaining a nutritious diet. Although they exert a great deal of physical energy, women who work in the informal economy and agriculture usually do not consume enough calories and nutrients to meet their energy needs (Mussida & Patimo, 2021). Especially in rural areas, women's time for meal preparation and nutritional planning is limited because they spend a lot of time fetching water, gathering firewood, and performing other labor-intensive tasks.

9.2.1.6.6 Poor sanitation and health conditions

The danger of waterborne infections, which hinder the absorption of nutrients and result in illness, is increased by inadequate sanitation and a lack of access to safe drinking water. Diseases such as urinary tract infections and reproductive tract infections, to which women are particularly vulnerable, further impair their nutritional status. Intestinal worms and other parasite diseases, sometimes linked to poor sanitation, induce nutritional loss, especially iron, which leads to anemia (Hutton & Chase, 2017).

9.2.1.6.7 Impact of climate change and food security

Subsistence farming is a major source of income for many women. Droughts, floods, and erratic weather patterns brought on by climate change impede food production and availability. Women farmers frequently lack access to resources such as loans, high-quality seeds, and modern agricultural techniques, which hinders their ability to grow nutrient-dense crops (Kumar et al., 2021). Seasonal food shortages, particularly during lean agricultural years, cause cyclic undernutrition among women in many rural areas.

9.2.1.6.8 Limited government and policy support

Most government programs that are designed to improve women's nutrition do not reach the most vulnerable because of poor implementation, illiteracy, or corruption. The programs tend to concentrate on calorie consumption without addressing the requirement for micronutrient-dense food. As policies tend to neglect the interlinked challenges of gender, poverty, and nutrition, most women do not have specialist solutions (Kumar, 2017).

9.2.1.6.9 Adolescent malnutrition

Teenage girls who are malnourished will end up as undernourished mothers, fueling the cycle of hunger from generation to generation. Teen pregnancies and early marriages in certain regions, where adolescent girls are deprived of the nutrition necessary for work, make it more pronounced.

9.2.1.6.10 Psychological stress and mental health

Chronic stress resulting from poverty, domestic violence, and gender discrimination impacts hunger, digestion, and absorption of nutrients. As they are less likely to pay attention to their nutritional requirements, undernourishment is more likely among women with mental illnesses. A comprehensive response is needed to tackle women's issues in reaching satisfactory nutritional status. Social protection, gender empowerment, healthcare, and education must be incorporated into policies and programs to provide women with equal access to opportunities and resources (Siddiqui et al., 2020). To enhance women's nutritional status and well-being, addressing unhealthy cultural norms, raising awareness of women's specific nutritional requirements, and enhancing the delivery of healthcare are all required.

9.2.1.6.11 Infant and young child feeding practices

Many children are either not nursed or are exposed to complementary foods too early or too late, despite international recommendations that they should only be breastfed for the first 6 months of life. Societal conventions, maternity leave restrictions, and insufficient breastfeeding support networks frequently discourage the best nursing techniques. Nutrient shortages might result from the introduction of complementary foods after 6 months, which are frequently hazardous or nutritionally insufficient. Suboptimal feeding habits may result from caregivers' ignorance of the value of nutritional diversification (Torles & Raju, 2018). Optimal growth is impeded by inadequate nursing and supplemental feeding methods. The nutrition of children is greatly impacted by inadequate breastfeeding and supplemental feeding techniques. According to NFHS-5 statistics, states such as Nagaland and Arunachal Pradesh have lower-than-ideal rates of early breastfeeding initiation (within an hour of delivery). In addition, different states have different exclusive breastfeeding rates for the first 6 months, with some falling short of the national goal (Lakhanpaul et al., 2022).

9.3 Factors contributing to poor nutritional status

Some issues that affect people of all ages and socioeconomic backgrounds cause poor nutritional status in India. These elements fall under the following general categories: social, economic, cultural, environmental, and healthcare-related. A variety of interconnected factors, such as structural impediments, dietary practices, health status, and socioeconomic circumstances, all have an impact on poor nutritional status (Agurs-Collins et al., 2024). A thorough examination of these elements is provided below.

9.3.1 Poverty and food insecurity

Access to wholesome food, potable water, and medical treatment is restricted by poverty. Cheap, high-calorie, low-nutrient foods are commonly consumed by low-income households, which can lead to deficiencies in vital nutrients, including protein, vitamins, and minerals. Seasonal food shortages, increasing food prices, and low agricultural productivity, particularly in rural and poor areas, worsen food insecurity. Food-insecure households can miss meals or eat insufficient quantities of food, which could impact their overall nutritional status (Siddiqui et al., 2020).

9.3.2 Poor dietary practices

Inadequate nursing practices such as premature cessation or nonexclusive breastfeeding in the first 6 months deprive infants of vital nutrients. Inadequate complementary feeding practices like the presentation of meals that are nutritionally poor or late introduction to solid foods can also cause undernutrition in early childhood. Micronutrients such as iron, zinc, and vitamins are essential but not in diets made up primarily of staple foods such as wheat, rice, or maize (Paintal et al., 2016). This is prevalent in poor households where fruits, vegetables, and animal-based foods are out of reach. Micronutrient deficiencies and increased obesity are brought about by increased intake of processed, high-calorie, low-nutrient foods in urban settings.

9.3.3 Lack of nutrition education and awareness

Especially in rural and underserved populations, individuals are unaware of the significance of nutritional variety and well-balanced meals. This usually results in a dependence on conventional, yet nutritionally poor, eating habits. Cultural myths and beliefs regarding certain foods, for example, the avoidance of fish or eggs during pregnancy or adolescence, could lead to avoidable vitamin deficiencies. Misconceptions regarding food needs and serving sizes usually result in inappropriate food selection, which can cause overnutrition or undernutrition (Weerasekara et al., 2020).

9.3.4 Gender inequality

In most patriarchal settings, females and girls consume last and least, resulting in an inadequate nutrient supply. This intrahousehold food inequality disproportionately disadvantages pregnant and breastfeeding women, leading to increased maternal and child undernutrition (Seferidi et al., 2022). Sex-preferential desire for male children could lead to the neglect of females' nutritional requirements, entrenching hunger cycles for generations.

9.3.5 Health and disease burden

Prevalent diseases that cause loss of nutrition and reduced absorption, such as measles, respiratory infections, diarrhea, and malaria, worsen undernutrition. For instance, diarrhea causes extensive loss of fluids and electrolytes, and intestinal parasites lower the absorption of iron and protein. Diabetes, hypertension, and cancer are some of the conditions that impair the body's capacity to utilize nourishment. Malnutrition can result as a side effect of medications such as appetite suppressants or chemotherapy (Ibrahim et al., 2017). These issues lead to increased metabolic needs, reduced appetite, and compromised nutrient absorption, and it becomes challenging to sustain proper nutritional status.

9.3.6 Poor sanitation and hygiene

The ability of the body to absorb and utilize nutrients is impaired by diarrhea and parasite infections, which are more probable where there is poor sanitation and contaminated water sources. For instance, children who have repeated diarrhea are more susceptible to developing stunted growth. Prolonged exposure to unhygienic conditions

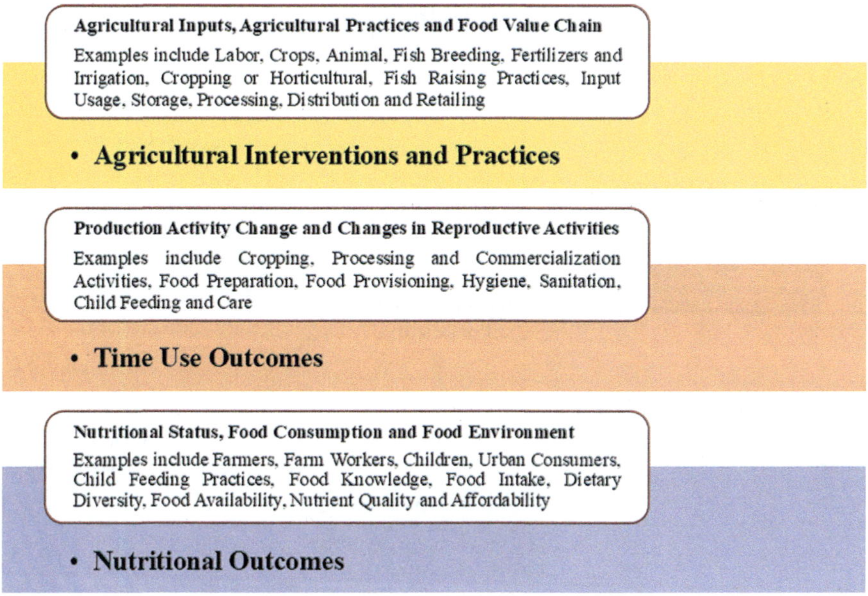

Figure 9.2 Theoretical framework connecting agricultural practices, time usage, and nutrition consequences.

results in environmental enteropathy, an illness that has intestinal inflammation, which impairs the absorption of food.

9.3.7 Maternal malnutrition

Malnourished mothers are likely to deliver LBW children, who are likely to experience stunting, wasting, and developmental impairments. Maternal malnutrition during pregnancy and breastfeeding impacts infant nutrition by lowering the quality of breast milk. The cycle of starvation continues when malnourished girls grow up to become malnourished mothers who give birth to malnourished children (Budge et al., 2019). Fig. 9.2 shows the global hunger index and malnutrition in India.

9.3.8 Weak implementation of nutrition programs

Government initiatives to combat hunger, such as school meal schemes and supplementary feeding programs, are at times inaccessible to the most needy because of logistical constraints, corruption, or lack of information. Program gaps caused by a lack of effective methods for measuring the impact of nutrition interventions weaken the overall effectiveness of the programs. Poor funding and personnel in public health systems also hamper the provision of nutrition-specific and nutrition-sensitive interventions (Fig. 9.3).

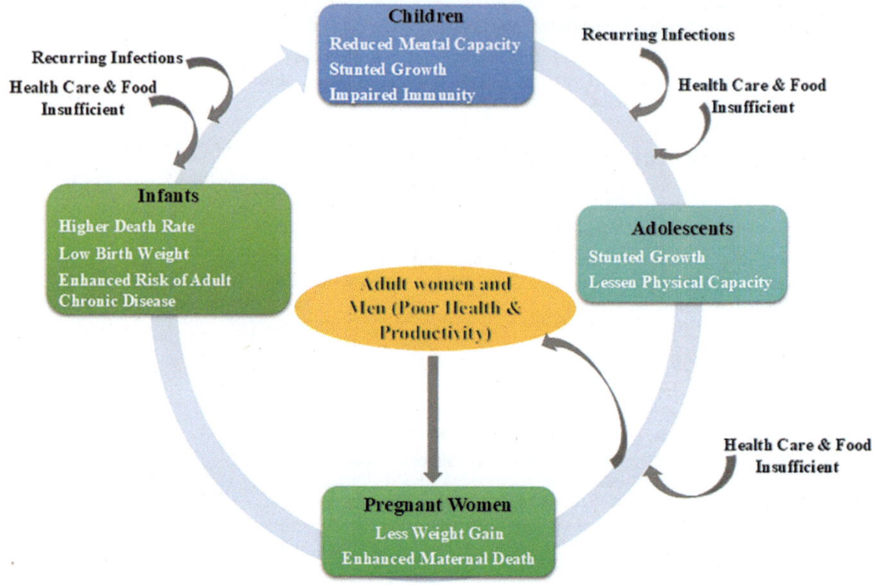

Figure 9.3 Global hunger index and malnutrition in Northeast India.

9.3.9 Micronutrient deficiencies

Even with adequate caloric consumption, "hidden hunger" occurs because of diets with inadequate essential micronutrients such as iron, iodine, zinc, and vitamin A. The deficiencies have serious implications that are often overlooked, such as compromised immunity, mental development, and general growth. This is common among women and children and decreases energy levels, cognitive ability, and productivity (Sinha et al., 2018). It compromises the immune system and enhances vulnerability to infection, and it is a primary cause of preventable blindness.

9.3.10 Climate change and environmental factors

Lower farm production caused by unpredictable weather conditions, floods, droughts, and soil erosion results in food scarcity and price inflation. This has a particular impact on poor families because it limits their access to nutritious food (Godde et al., 2021). Apart from displacing individuals and disrupting food supply chains, disasters tend to heighten dependency on emergency food aid, which tends to be of poor quality and variety.

9.3.11 Urbanization and lifestyle changes

Urbanization and increased consumption of processed and convenience foods rich in unhealthy fats, sugar, and salt have led to an increase in NCDs such as diabetes and obesity. As urban lifestyles cause a reduction in physical activity, undernutrition tends to be present alongside overweight and obesity in most civilizations (Casari et al., 2022).

9.3.12 Political and economic instability

Armed conflicts and political instability compel individuals to move, destroy food production, and restrict access to food and healthcare. Malnutrition is a significant threat for refugees and internally displaced persons. Because of disparities in wealth and resource distribution, poor communities are subject to structural obstacles to proper nutrition.

9.3.13 Psychological and emotional stress

Food instability and erratic eating behaviors are common among children raised in stressful or neglectful situations, which further compromises their nutritional condition. Stress, depression, and other mental health issues can influence eating behaviors, resulting in either overnutrition or malnutrition. To address the issues that contribute to nutritional deficiency, there should be a multisectoral approach that involves poverty reduction, education, healthcare, sanitation, and sustainable agriculture (Myers, 2020). To break the vicious cycle of malnutrition and produce a healthier and more productive populace, addressing gender disparities, increasing access to healthcare, strengthening communities through nutrition education, and promoting public health interventions must be prioritized.

9.4 Government policies and interventions

The Indian government has implemented several comprehensive policies and programs to correct the age-old problem of poor nutritional status throughout the nation. The policies seek to lower food insecurity, malnutrition, and micronutrient deficiency by targeting vulnerable groups such as women, children, and poor communities. One of the flagship schemes, the Integrated Child Development Services (ICDS), was launched in 1975 and offers health tests, supplementary nutrition, preschool education, immunizations, and services to children under 6 years, pregnant women, and lactating mothers (Nichols, 2020). Along a similar line, children in government and government-aided schools are provided free ready meals under the Mid-Day Meal Scheme, initiated in 1995 to ensure their nutritional well-being and school enrollment. The Poshan Abhiyaan (National Nutrition Mission) was initiated by the government in 2018 to tackle stunting, anemia, and undernutrition. An IT-enabled scheme focuses on intersectoral convergence, real-time monitoring, and community participation to approach nutritional issues with a more integrated strategy.

In addition, the National Food Security Act (NFSA) of 2013 significantly curtails hunger by distributing subsidized food grains to nearly two-thirds of India's population under the public distribution system (PDS). To improve nutrition and minimize wage loss during pregnancy the Pradhan Mantri Matru Vandana Yojana (PMMVY) scheme provides funds to pregnant and lactating mothers. Anemia Mukt Bharat (AMB) was initiated in 2018 to lower anemia by addressing specific health problems through deworming interventions, fortified meals, and iron and folic acid supplements (Puri, 2022). The Food Safety and Standards Authority of India (FSSAI) supports food fortification programs aimed at enhancing staple foods such as rice, wheat, milk, and salt with necessary micronutrients to combat "hidden hunger" because of deficiencies of vitamins and minerals.

The government also tackles nutrition-related issues to lifestyle through programs such as the Eat Right India Movement, which encourages safe, nutrient-rich, and sustainable diets and against the consumption of transfats, added sweets, and high-sodium foods. Focusing on nutritional awareness and early interventions the National Program for Prevention and Control of Cancer, Diabetes, Cardiovascular Diseases, and Stroke (NPCDCS) addresses NCDs related to malnutrition, including diabetes and hypertension. Programs such as Mission Poshan 2.0 aim to enhance children's nutritional status, particularly among disadvantaged and rural populations, by incorporating clean water and sanitation programs with supplemental nutrition programs.

Despite such stringent criteria the efficacy of the program is limited by issues such as inadequate coverage, ignorance among beneficiaries, budgetary limitations, and errors in implementation and monitoring. For example, extensive rural and remote regions are often plagued by restricted access to healthcare facilities and logistical challenges in providing benefits. To bridge these gaps the government is emphasizing intersectoral coordination among the sanitation, education, and health sectors and leveraging technology to obtain data in real-time, including local communities, for the purpose of improved outreach (Maxim et al., 2021). These measures must be reinforced, funding be expanded, and public–private partnerships be promoted to ensure that India's nutrition-related policies provide the intended outcomes and assist the broader goal of sustainable development.

Bottom of form: Although ICDS provides extra nutrition and early education, their implementation is challenging in remote areas. The National Nutrition Mission (Poshan Abhiyaan) intends to enhance the nutrition of mothers and children, but Northeast India calls for regional approaches. PDS ensures food security, but it requires more effective targeting.

9.5 Strategies for improvement

Existing initiatives such as the Mid-Day Meal Scheme, Poshan Abhiyaan, and the ICDS must be improved with regional modifications. Along with food fortification programs, it is important to provide regular iron, folic acid, and vitamin A supplements. Dietary gaps can be addressed with the support of awareness initiatives that promote the intake of nutrient-dense, locally accessible foods (Thakur et al., 2023).

Enhancing service delivery can be achieved by teaching community health workers how to monitor growth and offer dietary counseling. Family nutrition can be indirectly improved by programs that support women's education, skill development, and economic independence. To overcome cultural barriers and encourage the best feeding practices, customized communication tactics are essential. Geographical obstacles can be solved by utilizing technology for telemedicine, early warning systems, and nutrition monitoring. Digital platforms and mobile applications can help spread information and provide services. Adapt nutrition regulations to the particular requirements of the area (Dewida et al., 2023). To guarantee the efficacy of initiatives, reinforce monitoring and assessment systems and develop disaster-resilient food systems to reduce their impacts.

Enhancing the nutritional status of women involves a multipronged strategy addressing their specific dietary, health, and socioeconomic needs at various stages of life. One such strategy is creating awareness about balanced nutrition through education campaigns highlighting the significance of vitamins, minerals, and macronutrients critical to women's health, including iron, calcium, folic acid, and protein. Health programs need to target adolescents, pregnant and lactating women, and menopausal women, providing specific dietary advice to address their nutritional requirements. Fortification of staple foods with critical micronutrients can also minimize deficiencies in populations with low dietary diversity. Facilitating access to low-cost, nutritious food through community-based agricultural schemes and social welfare programs is also crucial, especially for poor households. Overcoming cultural and gender-based constraints is also vital, ensuring women are free to make food choices and are given priority within household food allocation. Incorporating nutritional advice into healthcare services and maternal care can further improve outcomes by detecting and correcting deficiencies early. Working with policymakers to develop supportive environments that promote healthy eating habits, combined with efforts to enhance water, sanitation, and hygiene (WASH) practices, can comprehensively improve the nutritional status of women and contribute to their overall health.

9.5.1 Awareness and education about balanced nutrition

One of the most important strategies to enhance nutrition is increasing awareness regarding the need for a balanced diet. Educational campaigns should be directed at women, mothers, caregivers, and adolescents to encourage knowledge regarding key nutrients such as iron, calcium, folic acid, vitamins, and proteins. Educational interventions should highlight the importance of nutrient-rich foods, portion control, and the risks of malnutrition and obesity. Schools can play an important role in nutrition literacy among children by including dietary education in the curriculum. Women, especially pregnant and lactating women, require education on their higher nutritional needs to ensure healthy pregnancy and breastfeeding.

9.5.2 Maternal and child healthcare services

Access to good healthcare services is crucial in enhancing nutrition for women and children. Prenatal and postnatal checkups should comprise nutritional evaluation, counseling, and supplementation when necessary. Supplementation with iron and folic acid during pregnancy has the potential to decrease anemia, a prevalent nutritional deficiency in women. Health workers should also track the development and growth of children to detect and treat nutritional deficiencies early. Immunization and deworming interventions are also essential because they prevent diseases that may impair nutrient uptake and general well-being.

9.5.3 Breastfeeding and infant and young child feeding practices

The best infant and young child feeding practices are necessary to decrease malnutrition and ensure healthy development. Exclusive breastfeeding up to the age of 6 months gives the child all the required nutrients and a strong immune system. Continued breastfeeding and the introduction of complementary foods in appropriate amounts until 2 years or more are important for healthy growth and development. Breastfeeding promotion can be enhanced by developing workplaces that are friendly to mothers, offering lactation rooms, and enforcing national policies that support and promote breastfeeding.

9.5.4 Food fortification and supplementation programs

Food fortification is an affordable means of preventing micronutrient deficiencies in high-risk populations. Fortification of staple foods such as wheat flour, rice, and cooking oil with key vitamins and minerals can be used to combat iron, iodine, vitamin A, and folic acid deficiencies. Governments must also fund the distribution of micronutrient powders and supplements to at-risk groups, particularly pregnant and lactating women and children under 5 years. Effective fortification programs depend on robust regulatory systems, quality control measures, and public education campaigns.

9.5.5 Food security and nutritious food access

Food security is important to enhance the nutritional well-being of women and children. People must have constant access to cheap, safe, and nutritious food. Governments and nongovernmental organizations can ensure food security by providing support to local agricultural activities, enhancing food distribution systems, and offering subsidies on nutritious food. Urban farming and community farming schemes enable women to produce vegetables for themselves, which ensures nutrition and food security for the household. Food wastage should also be curbed and storage methods enhanced so that fresh produce is available throughout the year.

9.5.6 Social protection programs

Social protection interventions such as cash transfers, food support, and school feeding schemes are important in enhancing the nutrition of women and children in poor communities. These interventions contribute to lowering economic constraints to the consumption of nutritious food and healthcare services. School meal schemes are especially useful in enhancing the nutritional intake and school enrollment of children. Integrating social protection programs with nutrition education can further increase their effectiveness by promoting healthier diets.

9.5.7 Water, sanitation, and hygiene interventions

Clean water access, better sanitation, and hygiene habits are necessary for the prevention of infections that lead to malnutrition. Water contamination and lack of proper hygiene enhance the risk of diarrheal diseases, which hamper the utilization of nutrients. WASH community-based interventions have the potential to minimize disease burden and nutritional status improvements. Women and girls, who are usually responsible for water collection from household sources and managing hygiene, must be empowered through WASH education campaigns and infrastructure development.

9.5.8 Women empowerment and gender equality

Enfranchising women is perhaps the single most powerful approach to enhancing both women's and children's nutrition. Women in control of resources within their homes are more apt to spend their money on education, health, and quality foods for their families. Promoting policies favorable to women's education, income, and voice is key to achieving gender equity and enhanced nutrition. Facilitating women's access to land, credit, and fertilizers can boost household food security as well.

9.5.9 Community-based nutrition programs

Programs at the community level offer a vehicle for delivering nutrition services to women and children directly. Community health workers may be involved in community-based programs to conduct nutritional counseling, growth monitoring, and supplementation. Community kitchens and nutrition clubs can also facilitate the exchange of knowledge and better food choices. Local leaders and stakeholders are involved in such programs to ensure that they are acceptable culturally and have adequate support.

9.5.10 Policy and governance for nutrition

There is a need for strong political will and well-coordinated policies to enhance nutrition outcomes. National nutrition strategies should be implemented by governments that bring together the efforts of different sectors, such as health, education, agriculture, and social welfare. Monitoring and evaluation systems are needed to monitor progress and hold people accountable. Technical assistance and innovative solutions can be offered by international organizations and research institutions through collaboration.

9.5.11 Evaluation and monitoring of nutrition programs

Ongoing monitoring and evaluation of nutrition programs are necessary to determine their effects and areas for improvement. Data collection and analysis enable policymakers to make informed decisions and allocate resources based on evidence. Involvement of the community in monitoring activities can guarantee that programs are responsive to local needs. To enhance the nutritional status of women and children, comprehensive strategies that address the root causes of malnutrition and promote long-term solutions are required. Social protection, food security, healthcare, education, and women's empowerment are all crucial components of these programs. Using a collaborative and multisectoral approach, governments, organizations, and communities may work together to create an environment where women and children can thrive with healthy eating and overall well-being.

9.6 Conclusion

To counter the nutritional challenges faced by women and children in Northeast India a multisectoral approach that includes technology innovation, community engagement, and legislative action is needed. By identifying its specific context and adapting treatments accordingly, it is possible to enhance the health and well-being of the region's most vulnerable groups. Yet, factors such as poverty, poor healthcare facilities, food insecurity, and traditional diets substantially increase the risk of malnutrition among vulnerable groups, even though the region is rich in natural resources and cultural diversity. Especially among rural and tribal communities, early marriage, high reproductive rates, and poor access to healthcare and education increase the risks of undernutrition, anemia, and micronutrient deficiencies among women and children. Government programs such as the NFSA, Poshan Abhiyaan, and ICDS have brought about remarkable improvement in nutritional outcomes, yet issues remain because of weak implementation, low outreach, and sociocultural heterogeneity. To address these problems, there is a need for a holistic approach, one that improves the systems providing healthcare and nutrition, encourages community engagement, and raises public awareness and education. Encouraging the use of nutrient-dense foods that are locally produced and leveraging the agricultural potential of the region to produce local foods are additional strategies to enhance dietary diversity. Strategic investments, community-led interventions, and targeted policy actions can efficiently counter the nutritional challenges that women and children in Northeast India encounter, opening doors to communities becoming healthier and more resilient.

Acknowledgments

The authors thank NanoDot Research Private Limited, Nagercoil, for their support.

References

Agrawal, P., & Mishra, V. (2004). Covariates of overweight and obesity among women in north India (East-West). *Center Working Papers, Population and Health*: 116. Honolulu, HI: East-West Center.

Agurs-Collins, T., Alvidrez, J., Ferreira, S. E., Evans, M., Gibbs, K., Kowtha, B., Pratt, C., Reedy, J., Shams-White, M., & Brown, A. G. (2024). Perspective: Nutrition health disparities framework: A model to advance health equity. *Advances in Nutrition, 15*(4), 100194.

Amato, P. R. (2001). Children of divorce in the 1990s: An update of the Amato and Keith (1991) meta-analysis. *Journal of Family Psychology, 15*(3), 355.

Anastasiadou, A., Kim, J., Sanlitürk, A. E., de Valk, H., & Zagheni, E. (2023). *Sex-and gender-based differences in the migration process: A systematic literature review*. Max Planck Institute for Demographic Research.

Bhuiyan, M. A., Galdes, N., Cuschieri, S., & Hu, P. (2024). A comparative systematic review of risk factors, prevalence, and challenges contributing to non-communicable diseases in South Asia, Africa, and Caribbeans. *Journal of Health, Population, and Nutrition, 43*(1), 140.

Bradley, M., Melchor, J., Carr, R., & Karjoo, S. (2023). Obesity and malnutrition in children and adults: A clinical review. *Obesity Pillars, 8*, 100087.

Budge, S., Parker, A. H., Hutchings, P. T., & Garbutt, C. (2019). Environmental enteric dysfunction and child stunting. *Nutrition Reviews, 77*(4), 240–253.

Callahan, E. A. (2023). The science, strengths, and limitations of body mass index. In *Translating knowledge of foundational drivers of obesity into practice: Proceedings of a workshop series*. US: National Academies Press.

Casari, S., Di Paola, M., Banci, E., Diallo, S., Scarallo, L., Renzo, S., Gori, A., Renzi, S., Paci, M., de Mast, Q., & Pecht, T. (2022). Changing dietary habits: The impact of urbanization and rising socio-economic status in families from Burkina Faso in Sub-Saharan Africa. *Nutrients, 14*(9), 1782.

Chakraborty, R., Devikrishna, N. B., Chauhan, A., & Mishra, N. L. *Acute malnutrition worsened among children: NFHS-5. Down to Earth*. https://www.downtoearth.org.in/health/acute-malnutrition-worsened-among-children-nfhs-5-74987.

Chaparro, C. M., & Suchdev, P. S. (2019). Anemia epidemiology, pathophysiology, and etiology in low-and middle-income countries. *Annals of the New York Academy of Sciences, 1450*(1), 15–31.

Chatterjee, A., & Rai, S. K. (2024). The issue of identity in the context of North East India: A survey. Library of Progress-Library Science. *Information Technology & Computer, 44*(3), 6558–6565.

Das, M., Verma, M., Barman, P., & Behera, D. K. (2024). Prevalence of anaemia among married women with recent birth history and high-risk fertility behaviour: Secondary data analysis of the National Family Health Survey-India (2019–21). *BMJ Open, 14*(1), e073395.

Dewidar, O., John, J., Baqar, A., Madani, M. T., Saad, A., Riddle, A., Ota, E., Kung'u, J. K., Arabi, M., Raut, M. K., & Klobodu, S. S. (2023). Effectiveness of nutrition counseling for pregnant women in low-and middle-income countries to improve maternal and infant behavioral, nutritional, and health outcomes: A systematic review. *Campbell Systematic Reviews, 19*(4), e1361.

Ford, K. L., Jorgenson, D. J., Landry, E. J., & Whiting, S. J. (2019). Vitamin and mineral supplement use in medically complex, community-living, older adults. *Applied Physiology, Nutrition and Metabolism, 44*(4), 450–453.

Gahlawat, K. (2024). National Family Health Survey-5 (Phase-II) India: A review of selected maternal and child health indicators in India. In Proceedings of the 2nd ICSSR Conference on India Towards Viksit Bharat (2047) (pp. 13–14). Bharati Vidyapeeth's Institute of Computer Applications and Management (BVICAM), New Delhi, India.

Girotra, S., Malik, M., Roy, S., & Basu, S. (2023). Utilization and determinants of adequate quality antenatal care services in India: Evidence from the National Family Health Survey (NFHS-5) (2019-21). *BMC Pregnancy and Childbirth, 23*(1), 800.

Godde, C. M., Mason-D'Croz, D., Mayberry, D. E., Thornton, P. K., & Herrero, M. (2021). Impacts of climate change on the livestock food supply chain; a review of the evidence. *Global Food Security, 28*, 100488.

Harris-Fry, H., Lamson, L., Roett, K., & Katz, E. (2022). Reducing gender bias in household consumption data: Implications for food fortification policy. *Food Policy, 110*, 102279.

Hutton, G., & Chase, C. (2017). Water Supply, Sanitation, and Hygiene. In C. N. Mock, R. Nugent, O. Kobusingye, & K. R. Smith (Eds.), Injury Prevention and Environmental Health (3rd ed.). The International Bank for Reconstruction and Development.

Ibrahim, M. K., Zambruni, M., Melby, C. L., & Melby, P. C. (2017). Impact of childhood malnutrition on host defense and infection. *Clinical Microbiology Reviews, 30*(4), 919–971.

Jha, A., & Chandrakar, A. (2024). A Comparative Study of National Family Health Survey-4 and National Family Health Survey-5 of nutritional indicators in Chhattisgarh. *Cureus, 16*(3), e55524.

Kumar, A., Nagar, S., & Anand, S. (2021). Climate change and existential threats. In S. Singh, P. Singh, S. Rangabhashiyam, & K. K. Srivastava (Eds.), *Global Climate Change* (pp. 1–31). Elsevier.

Kumar, P. (2017). Food and nutrition security in India: The way forward. *Agricultural Economics Research Review, 30*(1), 1–21.

Kumar, S. B., Arnipalli, S. R., Mehta, P., Carrau, S., & Ziouzenkova, O. (2022). Iron deficiency anemia: Efficacy and limitations of nutritional and comprehensive mitigation strategies. *Nutrients, 14*(14), 2976.

Lakhanpaul, M., Roy, S., Benton, L., Lall, M., Khanna, R., Vijay, V. K., Sharma, S., Manikam, L., Santwani, N., Reddy, H., & Chaturvedi, H. (2022). Why India is struggling to feed their young children? A qualitative analysis for tribal communities. *BMJ Open, 12*(7), e051558.

Lee, H., Oldewage-Theron, W., Lyford, C., & Shine, S. (2023). Nutrition and health challenges among low-income families of young children in the post COVID-19 era: A qualitative study. *Nutrition Research and Practice, 17*(6), 1185.

Lei, L., Desai, S., & Chen, F. (2020). Fathers' migration and nutritional status of children in India: Do the effects vary by community context? *Demographic Research, 43*, 545.

Let, S., Tiwari, S., Singh, A., & Chakrabarty, M. (2023). Spatiotemporal change in wealth-based inequalities in overweight/obesity among women of reproductive age in India, 2015–2021. *Clinical Epidemiology and Global Health, 24*, 101458.

Likhar, A., & Patil, M. S. (2022). Importance of maternal nutrition in the first 1,000 days of life and its effects on child development: A narrative review. *Cureus, 14*(10), e30083.

Manik, S., Ramani, A., Majumder, R., Hossain, S., & Hazra, T. (2024). Traditional foods for festivity: Linking food diversity with socio-cultural aspects. In S. Roy, P. Nisha, & R. Chakraborty (Eds.), *Traditional foods: The reinvented superfoods* (pp. 69–88). Springer.

Maxim, L., Mazzocchi, M., Van den Broucke, S., Zollo, F., Robinson, T., Rogers, C., Vrbos, D., Zamariola, G., & Smith, A.European Food Safety Authority (EFSA). (2021). Technical assistance in the field of risk communication. *EFSA Journal, 19*(4), e06574.

Meshram, I. I., Kodavanti, M. R., Rachkulla, H. K., Nagalla, B., & Kakani, S. R.National Nutrition Monitoring Bureau Study Group. (2017). Trends in nutrient intakes, nutritional status, and correlates of undernutrition among rural children below 5 years of age: The National Nutrition Monitoring Bureau Survey 2012. *Journal of Postgraduate Medicine, 63*(2), 84–91.

Mussida, C., & Patimo, R. (2021). Women's family care responsibilities, employment and health: A tale of two countries. *JFEI, 42*(3), 489–507.

Myers, C. A. (2020). Food insecurity and psychological distress: A review of the recent literature. *Current Nutrition Reports, 9*(2), 107–118.

Ngaihte, D. P., & Kaur, R. (2020). Nutritional deficiencies in North-East India: A weak shield against the virus. *Outlook Poshan, 2*.

Narayanan, M., Karlsson, O., Kumar, A., Pullum, T. W., Kim, R., & Subramanian, S. V. (2024). Prevalence of severe and moderate anthropometric failure among children in India, 1993–2021. *Maternal & Child Nutrition, 21*(2), e13751.

Narayan, J., John, D., & Ramadas, N. (2019). Malnutrition in India: Status and government initiatives. *Journal of Public Health Policy, 40*, 126–141.

Nichols, C. (2020). Nutrition sensitive agriculture: An equity-based analysis from India. *World Development, 133*, 105004.

Nguyen, P. H., Kachwaha, S., Tran, L. M., Sanghvi, T., Ghosh, S., Kulkarni, B., Beesabathuni, K., Menon, P., & Sethi, V. (2021). Maternal diets in India: Gaps, barriers, and opportunities. *Nutrients, 13*(10), 3534.

Paintal, K., & Aguayo, V. M. (2016). Feeding practices for infants and young children during and after common illness. Evidence from South Asia. *Maternal & Child Nutrition, 12*, 39–71.

Puri, R. (2022). *India's National Food Security Act (NFSA): Early experiences. Food Governance in India* (pp. 1–18). Leveraging Agriculture for Nutrition in South Asia (LANSA).

Seferidi, P., Hone, T., Duran, A. C., Bernabe-Ortiz, A., & Millett, C. (2022). Global inequalities in the double burden of malnutrition and associations with globalisation: A multilevel analysis of Demographic and Health Surveys from 55 low-income and middle-income countries, 1992–2018. *The Lancet Global Health, 10*(4), e482–e490.

Siddiqui, F., Salam, R. A., Lassi, Z. S., & Das, J. K. (2020). The intertwined relationship between malnutrition and poverty. *Frontiers in Public Health, 8*, 453.

Sinha, B., Taneja, S., Chowdhury, R., Mazumder, S., Rongsen-Chandola, T., Upadhyay, R. P., Martines, J., Bhandari, N., & Bhan, M. K. (2018). Low-birthweight infants born to short-stature mothers are at additional risk of stunting and poor growth velocity: Evidence from secondary data analyses. *Maternal & Child Nutrition, 14*(1), e12504.

Srivastava, A., Avan, B. I., Rajbangshi, P., & Bhattacharyya, S. (2015). Determinants of women's satisfaction with maternal health care: A review of literature from developing countries. *BMC Pregnancy and Childbirth, 15*, 1–12.

Tantri, M. L., Kambara, C., & Bhat, H. (2022). *Nutritional Status of Women and Children in North Eastern States. Working Papers, 552*. Bangalore: Institute for Social and Economic Change.

Thakur, S., Singh, A., Insa, B., & Sharma, S. (2023). Food fortification in India as malnutrition concern: A global approach. *Sustainable Food Technology, 1*(5), 681–695.

Thanglen, H., & Maheo, L. M. (2022). Prevalence of obesity and hypertension and its associated risk factors among chiru females of Manipur. *Indian Journal of Public Health, 66*(1), 3–8.

Torlesse, H., & Raju, D. (2018). *Feeding of infants and young children in South Asia (World Bank Policy Research Working Paper 8655)*. World Bank.

Vilar-Compte, M., Burrola-Méndez, S., Lozano-Marrufo, A., Ferré-Eguiluz, I., Flores, D., Gaitán-Rossi, P., Teruel, G., & Pérez-Escamilla, R. (2021). Urban poverty and nutrition challenges associated with accessibility to a healthy diet: A global systematic literature review. *International Journal for Equity in Health, 20*, 1–19.

Weerasekara, P. C., Withanachchi, C. R., Ginigaddara, G. A. S., & Ploeger, A. (2020). Understanding dietary diversity, dietary practices and changes in food patterns in marginalised societies in Sri Lanka. *Foods, 9*(11), 1659.

Wells, J. C., Marphatia, A. A., Amable, G., Siervo, M., Friis, H., Miranda, J. J., Haisma, H. H., & Raubenheimer, D. (2021). The future of human malnutrition: Rebalancing agency for better nutritional health. *Global Health, 17*, 1–25.

Predictive modeling for cancer protective nutrition

10

Meghna Sarkar[a], *Sohini Mukherjee*[a], *Aoife Ward-Gahlawat*[b] *and Soumya R. Mohapatra*[a]
[a]School of Biotechnology, Kalinga Institute of Industrial Technology (KIIT) (Deemed to be University), Bhubaneswar , Odisha, India, [b]German Cancer Research Center (DKFZ) and National Center for Tumor Diseases (NCT), Heidelberg, Germany

10.1 Introduction

"Nutraceuticals," a term coined in 1989 by Dr. Stephen De Felice, refers to the combination of nutritional and pharmaceutical concepts. The term may vary from country to country, but they are generally considered biologically active compounds derived from various food sources. They add benefits to our diet beyond providing a basic level of nutrition and contribute to the prevention and treatment of diseases (Nasri et al., 2014; Puri et al., 2022). Nutraceuticals can be categorized as dietary supplements that consist of vitamins, minerals, and amino acids to provide health benefits. They are available in the form of powders, capsules, etc. (Nasri et al., 2014; Ruby et al., 2021), and second as functional foods, for example, probiotic yoghurts, fortified cereals, which are enhanced versions of foods with added bioactive components to benefit the health (Ruby et al., 2021). The next category is medicinal foods, which are specially designed to address dietary requirements in disease conditions and are provided under medical guidance (Aronson, 2017; Ruby et al., 2021), and lastly, recombinant nutraceuticals, which involve biotechnological modification in food to enhance its nutritional value (Ruby et al., 2021). For example, golden rice contains beta-carotene, the precursor of vitamin A, and it helps address the vitamin A deficiency in populations (Alali et al., 2021).

A balanced diet plays a major role in the reduction of cancer risk and proves how important it is to treat and manage cancer effectively. A diet rich in whole grains, vegetables, fruits, and healthy fats contributes to lower incidences of cancer. Furthermore a plant-based diet is associated with a reduced risk of cancer, such as colorectal or breast cancer (Bahrami, 2023; Parsons et al., 2023). In colorectal cancer, for example, food containing fiber from whole grains is associated with promoting the helpful microbiota of the gut and reducing inflammation. As a result, the incidence of cancer has been reduced (Slavin, 2004).

In addition to macronutrients, lower incidences of such cancers have also been attributed to the active metabolite of vitamin D, that is, 1,25(OH)2D, which acts by inhibiting angiogenesis, regulating cell growth and proliferation, and reducing metastatic potential (Wong et al., 2015). Moreover, it was found that certain phytochemicals in fruits and vegetables possess antioxidant properties, enabling

Nutritional Strategies, Predictive Models, and Sustainable Policies. DOI: https://doi.org/10.1016/B978-0-443-23671-6.00011-6

the reduction of oxidative stress associated with carcinogenesis by neutralizing free radicals (Kaur et al., 2018). On the other hand, cancer patients who suffer from issues of malnourishment are less responsive to the chemotherapy and immunotherapy provided and often require nutritional interventions during their treatment (Bossi et al., 2022; Narimatsu & Yaguchi, 2022). It has recently been demonstrated that a well-balanced diet can enhance recovery and significantly mitigate the side effects of chemotherapy (Donaldson, 2004). At the same time, maintaining an overall healthy weight through adequate nutrition consumption is a cancer preventive measure. Risks of breast, endometrial, and colorectal cancers are highly associated with obesity (Calle & Thun, 2004). Thus maintaining good health protects individuals from metabolic diseases and reduces the risk of obesity-associated cancers (Boeing, 2013).

In parallel, predictive modeling plays a crucial role in cancer prevention by analyzing complex dietary, clinical, and biological data to better understand cancer risks and develop effective prevention strategies. Applying machine learning, systems biology, and statistical models is needed to integrate epidemiological, omics, and clinical data to verify correlations between nutrition and cancer occurrence (Richter & Khoshgoftaar, 2018; Suzuki et al., 2009). Such models can study and consider a patient's clinical history to identify high-risk individuals for chronic diseases, allowing for potential interventions to be made earlier (Bahrami, 2023). Certain models can be used in multiple healthcare settings to predict disease progression rate and ensure proper treatment outcomes (Hinduja et al., 2023). In clinical settings, these models facilitate better chronic disease management and patient outcomes by enabling personalized treatment plans (Hinduja et al., 2023). Animal models also play an important part in preclinical studies (Suzuki et al., 2009), whereas clinical studies help bridge the gap between research and translating the results, thus giving rise to personalized nutrition plans tailored to each individual's needs (Malcomson & Mathers, 2023). Despite challenges in data integration and result translation, predictive modeling has revolutionized the field of personalized nutrition strategies, thereby improving cancer prevention and health outcomes.

In this chapter, we are going to explore more on details of predictive modeling tools and how they can be linked with nutraceuticals to prevent cancer.

10.2 Role of nutrition in cancer prevention

10.2.1 Properties of nutraceuticals in cancer prevention

The antioxidative properties of nutraceuticals are crucial in preventing cancer, as they are known to neutralize the effects of free radicals, which would otherwise damage DNA and cellular structures through oxidative stress. Dietary antioxidants, such as carotenoids and vitamin C, not only scavenge free radicals but also enhance the body's defense mechanisms against toxins, thereby reducing the risk of cancer. For example, certain carotenoids present in vegetables or fruits have been shown to exhibit defensive mechanisms against cancers of the stomach, lungs, and colon by mitigating oxidative stress and influencing cellular health (Divella et al., 2020; Donaldson, 2004). Next are the antiinflammatory effects, where a nutritious diet can reduce the risk of chronic inflammation, a risk factor in cancer development. As an example, omega-3 fatty acids have been shown to inhibit proinflammatory eicosanoids produced by the COX-2 pathway (Talib et al., 2023). Compounds, such as curcumin and resveratrol, have been found to exert antiinflammatory actions through modulation of inflammation-related pathways and reduction in the production of cytokinin, thus contributing toward anticancer effects (Di Napoli et al., 2023; Divella et al., 2020). Yet another property is epigenetic modulation. Epigenetics can be defined as an alteration in gene expression without modifying the DNA sequence. Nutrients, such as folate, polyphenols, and certain other bioactive compounds, can influence epigenetic changes, including DNA methylation and histone modifications (acetylation and methylation). Thus, owing to these modifications, certain tumor suppressor genes can be activated, and certain oncogenes can also be silenced. The Mediterranean diet is rich in these compounds and has been associated with causing favorable epigenetic modifications that may reduce the risk of cancer (Bahrami, 2023; Divella et al., 2020). Certain phytochemicals have been found to act as epigenetic modifiers, restoring the normal functioning of genes in cancer cells and thereby preventing tumor growth (Di Napoli et al., 2023).

10.2.2 Types of nutraceuticals in cancer prevention

10.2.2.1 Vitamins and minerals

Some vitamins, such as vitamins C and D, play major roles in cancer prevention as they possess antioxidative, antiinflammatory, and immunity-boosting properties (Talib et al., 2023; Thomas et al., 2015), thereby reducing cancer risk. Minerals such as selenium and zinc play a crucial role in DNA damage repair and immune function. Lastly, calcium is another mineral that plays a role in enhancing cellular health and reducing the risk of colorectal cancer (Talib et al., 2023).

10.2.2.2 Probiotics and prebiotics

According to the FAO/WHO, probiotics are defined as living microorganisms that stimulate health benefits to the consumer when administered in definite amounts. *Lactobacillus* sp. is a probiotic that functions to improve gut health and regulate immune responses. It serves as a promising intervention in cancer prevention. They are associated with improving gut microbiota balance, thereby reducing chemotherapy's harmful effects (Di Napoli et al., 2023). Prebiotics are nondigestible substances that selectively stimulate the growth function of various beneficial microorganisms in the gut, providing health benefits (Hutkins et al., 2016). They support the functioning of the immune system, decrease inflammation, and thus reduce the risk of cancer development (Bahrami, 2023; Di Napoli et al., 2023).

10.2.2.3 Animal-based compounds

Certain animal-based products have also portrayed cancer prevention mechanisms. Animal sources, including marine and terrestrial organisms, provide bioactive peptides that exhibit anticancer mechanisms, such as inducing apoptosis in cancer cells and enhancing immune responses. Furthermore animal-derived products also have the potential to inhibit tumor cell migration and growth, thereby enabling efficient therapeutic intervention (Noble et al., 2020; Qu et al., 2023; Wang et al., 2017). As an example a compound derived from the toad *Bufo gargarizans*, named bufalin, has been found to exhibit anticancer properties by hindering tumor proliferation, growth, and migration, and inducing apoptosis, particularly in head and neck cancer. It is also involved in modulating immune responses by targeting the beta-catenin signaling pathway (Mhaidly et al., 2024).

10.2.2.4 Plant-based compounds

Several plant-based compounds have been shown to have anticancer properties, for example, resveratrol and curcumin (from the spice turmeric). Curcumin is known to have antiinflammatory and antioxidative properties and is also involved in regulating many signaling pathways associated with cell proliferation and apoptosis. In tumor models, it has been shown to arrest the cell cycle and induce apoptosis, thereby inhibiting tumor growth (Di Napoli et al., 2023; Divella et al., 2020). Similarly, resveratrol exhibits epigenetic effects and regulates gene expression associated with cancer progression (Bahrami, 2023; Talib et al., 2023). When combined with other nutraceuticals, both of these compounds exhibit significant synergistic effects in cancer prevention strategies. For example, omega-3 fatty acids function as antiinflammatory agents and play a role in cancer prevention. They undergo this process by altering the composition of cell membranes and various signaling mechanisms that play a role in inflammation and apoptosis. It has been found that omega-3-containing foods can not only increase the effectiveness of chemotherapy but also reduce other potential side effects of cancer treatment on the patient (Di Napoli et al., 2023; Talib et al., 2023).

In a nutshell, nutrients hold immense value and contribute to cancer prevention through their antiinflammatory, antioxidative, and epigenetic effects. Prebiotics, probiotics, animal-based, and plant-based compounds have significant potential to exert protective effects against cancer.

10.2.3 Types of nutraceuticals in cancer treatment

Nutraceuticals, in addition to having cancer-preventive properties, are also instrumental in enhancing the outcomes of conventional cancer therapies. These natural, biologically active components show antioxidative, immuno-modulatory, and antiinflammatory properties. Compounds like curcumin, resveratrol, and other polyphenols have significantly improved chemotherapy outcomes, as they are involved in regulating signaling mechanisms that contribute to cancer progression (Di Napoli et al., 2023; Maiuolo et al., 2021). Several phytochemicals and vitamins have been reported for their effectiveness in the prevention of cancer (Table 10.1) as well as efficacy in the treatment of cancers, some of which are listed in Table 10.2.

Table 10.1 Vitamins, minerals, and phytochemicals reported in cancer prevention.

Nutrient type	Nutrient	Properties	Food sources	Role in cancer prevention
Vitamins	Vitamin C	Antioxidant, antiinflammatory	Citrus fruits, strawberries	Supports immune system and DNA repair mechanisms and reduces oxidative stress, thereby lowering cancer risk (Talib et al., 2023; Thomas et al., 2015)
	Vitamin E	Antioxidant, boosts immune system	Spinach, seeds, nuts, broccoli	Modulates inflammation, protects cells from damage caused by oxidative stress, thereby reducing cancer risk (Talib et al., 2023; Rudzińska et al., 2023)
Phytochemicals	Curcumin (turmeric)	Antiinflammatory, antioxidant	Turmeric root	Induces apoptosis and inhibits tumor growth and development, thereby providing anticancer properties (Rathee et al., 2024; Rudzińska et al., 2023)
	Lycopene	Antioxidant	Tomatoes, watermelon, pink grapefruit	Acts as an antioxidant and shows protective effects against cancer, particularly prostate and lung cancers (Rathee et al., 2024; Thomas et al., 2015)
	Flavonoids	Antioxidant, antiinflammatory	Berries, apples, onions, tea	Inhibits cancer growth and proliferation and reduces inflammation (Rathee et al., 2024; Rudzińska et al., 2023)

(*continued on next page*)

Table 10.1 Vitamins, minerals, and phytochemicals reported in cancer prevention—cont'd

Nutrient type	Nutrient	Properties	Food sources	Role in cancer prevention
	Anthocyanins	Antioxidant	Blueberries, blackberries, red cabbage	Associated with reduced cancer risk by acting as an antioxidant and an antiinflammatory agent (Rathee et al., 2024; Rudzińska et al., 2023)
Minerals	Selenium	Antioxidant	Brazil nuts, seafood, grains	Acts as an antioxidant, involved in DNA repair mechanisms, and thereby reduces cancer risk (Talib et al., 2023; Thomas et al., 2015)
	Zinc	Immune support	Meat, shellfish, legumes	Provides immune support, and deficiency can lead to increased cancer risk (Talib et al., 2023; Thomas et al., 2015)
	Calcium	Cellular function and bone health	Dairy products, leafy greens	Improves cellular function and is associated with reducing the risk of colorectal cancer (Rudzińska et al., 2023; Talib et al., 2023)

Table 10.2 Vitamins used to treat cancers.

Vitamin	Types of cancer treated	Citations
Vitamin A	Lung cancer, prostate cancer, breast cancer, bladder cancer	Talib et al. (2023), Tratnjek et al. (2021)
Vitamin C	Colorectal cancer, pancreatic cancer, breast cancer	Talib et al. (2023)
Vitamin D	Colorectal cancer, breast cancer, prostate cancer, skin cancer	Wong et al. (2015)
Vitamin E	Prostate cancer, colorectal cancer	Talib et al. (2023)

10.3 Predictive modeling in cancer-protective nutrition

The process of developing, assessing, and validating a model to most precisely predict the likelihood of an event is known as predictive modeling (Bae & Park, 2020). Several studies have used predictive modeling as an effective tool for cancer prediction. One such study by Kalia et al. (2024) enhanced breast cancer risk prediction (with 23,518 cases and 22,832 controls) in all non-Hispanic White women using prediction modeling. Another study by Tota et al. (2019) highlighted the use of predictive models to identify individuals at a higher risk of oropharynx cancer in the United States. Predictive models have also been extensively employed to study the survival outcomes in cancer patients (Chow et al., 2008; Goshayeshi et al., 2017). The process for predictive modelling involving an iterative cycle currently used in cancer research is depicted in Fig. 10.1.

Predictive modeling in cancer-protective nutrition utilizes advanced computational tools to analyze complex dietary and biological data on the effects of specific nutrients, dietary patterns, and nutraceuticals that can influence the risk of cancer development and progression (Shiao et al., 2018). Predictive modeling primarily depends on three major approaches: machine learning, statistical models, and systems biology (Toma & Wei, 2023). Machine learning utilizes data-driven algorithms to identify distinct patterns and construct models that can predict the outcome, specifically the effect of specific diets and nutrients on cancer prevention. Through numerous studies, it is evident that machine learning methods can enhance the accuracy of cancer detection, recurrence, and mortality by 15%–25% (Cruz & Wishart, 2006). The models use a wide range of datasets, including genomic, proteomic, and dietary data, to uncover correlations and improve predictions (Richter & Khoshgoftaar, 2018). Techniques such as supervised techniques (Afsari et al., 2021) help predict cancer risks, while unsupervised techniques (Panduranga Vital et al., 2019) uncover hidden patterns in the data, including dietary factors associated with a lower risk of cancer.

Statistical models establish mathematical correlations that help understand the relationship between dietary nutrients and the risk of developing cancer. The statistical model can be further divided into three types: (1) regression models that are used to understand the relation between specific nutrients and the risk of developing cancer (Shiao et al., 2018); (2) survival models that study the connections between how nutrition influences the progression and recurrence of cancer (Chen et al., 2012);

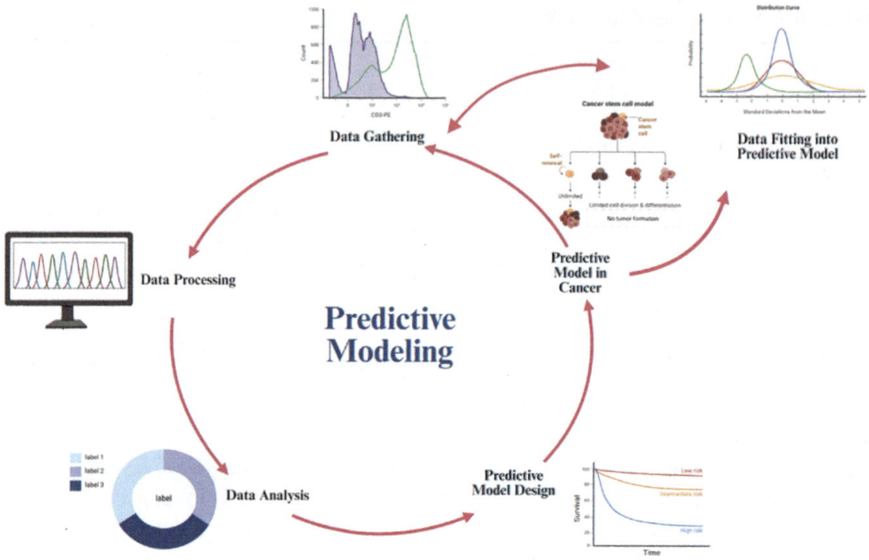

Figure 10.1 This figure illustrates the predictive modeling process in cancer research, which encompasses data gathering, processing, analysis, predictive model design, and its application. Predictive modeling contributes to data collection and refinement, enabling continuous improvement in cancer diagnosis and treatment methods.

and (3) Bayesian models that are very useful when working with sparse data since they consider uncertainties and include previous research (Edefonti et al., 2024). To model the intricate relationships between nutrients, metabolic pathways, and biological systems linked to cancer, systems biology techniques combine a variety of biological data (Badimon et al., 2017). Dynamic simulations examine how nutrients affect cellular functions, while network modeling finds links between dietary elements and biochemical processes (Khilwani & Singh, 2023). Personalized dietary recommendations based on each person's metabolic profile and cancer risk are made possible by multiomics integration, which integrates genomic, proteomic, and metabolomic data (Murphy, 2020; Lampe et al., 2013).

Predictive modeling derives information from various high-quality databases to find the relationship between nutrition and cancer development. A list of various databases suitable for data extraction in predictive modeling is listed in Table 10.3. The databases contain a wide range of information, integrating nutrition science, molecular biology, and clinical research to create an adequate model that provides proper insights (Zheng et al., 2024). The databases comprise epidemiological studies from the fields of molecular biology, clinical research, and integrative nutrient science. Epidemiological studies give large-scale data on lifestyle, dietary information, and cancer occurrence in a particular region (Doll, 2017). Omics data, including transcriptomics, proteomics, metabolomics, and genomics, are essential for understanding how dietary factors influence the molecular pathways associated with cancer. This data

Table 10.3 Types of databases.

Database type	Key contributions	Examples
Epidemiological studies	Large-scale data on lifestyle, dietary information, and cancer occurrence in a particular region	Epidemiological evidence shows that the consumption of tea helps in the reduction of certain types of cancer, such as those of upper gastrointestinal tract and breast cancer (Yuan et al., 2011) The relationship between intake of antioxidants and cancer risk was studied with the help of epidemiological studies in aerodigestive tract cancer, lung cancer, and uterine cervix cancer (Flagg et al., 1995)
Omics databases	Includes transcriptomics, proteomics, metabolomics, and genomics data Provides insights on metabolic profiles, gene–nutrient interactions, and cancer biomarkers	Various articles show the usage of omics data in different types of cancer research, such as breast cancer (Kalita-De Croft et al., 2016) and lung cancer (Balbin et al., 2013). Prostate cancer (Zhang et al., 2020) and many more
Clinical databases	Detailed patient profiles, clinical registers, and clinical trial results Offers a detailed insight into cancer progression and outcomes of nutritional interventions	Clinical databases are an indispensable factor for the advancement of various cancer research such as breast cancer (Hwang, 2021)
Dietary databases	Help evaluate the impact of specific nutrients or dietary patterns in cancer development	Several research have taken the help of dietary database to assess the link between dietary patterns and cancer occurrence such as in colorectal cancer (Thiébaut et al., 2007) and hepatocellular carcinoma (Yang et al., 2019)

provides an understanding of metabolic profiles, gene–nutrient interactions, and cancer biomarkers (Vlachavas et al., 2021). Clinical studies provide detailed information on patient profiles, clinical registers, and clinical trials, offering a comprehensive insight into cancer progression, trial results, and nutritional breakthroughs (Greenwald, 2004).

10.4 Animal studies in cancer protective nutrition

Various animal models have been utilized to investigate nutraceuticals as potential therapeutic approaches for cancer. The chosen animal model should possess certain qualities; first and foremost, the model must be able to replicate the disease process that occurs in humans to some extent. Second the animal model used should be readily available so that rigorous experiments can be conducted in multiple sets, and it should also be accessible to other researchers for replication of the experimental prototype. Third the models should meet the biological requirements for easy maintenance and use in experiments according to the guidelines for research animal welfare (Institute of Laboratory Animal Resources & Committee on Care and Use of Laboratory Animals, 1986). The most widely used animal models in cancer research are purpose-bred rodents, such as mice and rats. They provide the optimal environment to carry out experiments that unravel the connection between nutrition and cancer prevention. Some of the advantages of using them are that they are easy to handle, have a low maintenance cost, have a genome that is defined so it is easy to manipulate, have easily available reagents that are specific to the species, have availability of transplantable cell lines, and have the availability of immune-suppressive cell lines that allow the transplantation of cancer cells from human patients (de Jong & Maina, 2010).

Scientists have demonstrated the effect of dietary modifications on cancer occurrence in animal models. For example, obesity is linked to an increased occurrence of cancer (Basen-Engquist & Chang, 2011). A decrease in calorie intake and a diet focused on vegetables, fruits, whole grains, and certain nutrients have been shown to inhibit tumor growth and development. Moreover, data have shown that certain nutrients, such as sulforaphane, a phytochemical compound found in cruciferous vegetables such as broccoli, cauliflower, and cabbage, have been seen to possess antitumor effects in mice (Donaldson, 2004). Most cruciferous vegetables, especially cabbages, are known to activate the transcription factor aryl hydrocarbon receptor (AhR) because of the presence of indole-derived compounds and their metabolites. These bioactive compounds influence AhR signaling, which, in turn, plays a crucial role in immune regulation, xenobiotic metabolism, and eventually cancer protection (Wang et al., 2018).

Another AhR activator, anthocyanins, is a type of flavonoid found in several plant-based foods and has shown promising chemopreventive effects against breast and colorectal cancer in rodent models (Bars-Cortina et al., 2022). Similarly, green tree polyphenols, which are phenolic compounds as suggested by the name, especially epigallocatechin gallate (EGCG) found in green tea, certain kinds of fruits such as cranberries, strawberries, blueberries, cherries, kiwi, and even nuts, have shown a potential role in the treatment of various types of cancer in preclinical studies (Sharifi-Rad et al., 2020; Wei et al., 2018).

Though animal models have been an invaluable asset, they also possess certain inherent limitations. Animals and humans have major physiological differences in metabolism, immune system function, and overall anatomy. This can lead to inaccurate predictions on how a drug or treatment will work in humans. As tumors are highly heterogeneous, animal models often fail to represent the exact intricacy, genetic factors, environment, and immunological factors that lead to the development of cancer in humans (de Jong & Maina, 2010; Mak et al., 2014). Another limitation is that, despite extensive research, drugs or treatments that have shown excellent results in animal models may fail to successfully translate those results into human clinical trials (Hartung, 2008). Moreover, another reason links directly to ethical considerations: The use of animals in research is required to ensure animal welfare and avoid unnecessary suffering. To maintain a balance between scientific growth and ethical responsibility, ethical considerations also emphasize the importance of humane methods driven by principles such as the 3Rs concept, that is, replacement, reduction, and refinement (Shim & Kim, 2022). Despite all its limitations the animal model is irreplaceable for advancing research and understanding the role of nutrition in cancer prevention.

10.5 Clinical studies and human models

Clinical studies and human models play a crucial role in developing cancer-protective nutrition and effectively bridging the gap between research and application. Epidemiological studies have demonstrated the effect of nutrition on the risk of cancer occurrence. Various large-scale cohort studies, such as the Nurses' Health Studies (NHS), Multiethnic Cohort Studies, and the European Prospective Investigation into Cancer and Nutrition (EPIC), have provided data on the relationship between nutrition and cancer risk among various populations (Riboli, 1992, 1997). Several studies have suggested that the Mediterranean diet, which essentially includes fruits, whole grains, vegetables, nuts, beans, and legumes, reduces the risk of cancer. It has also been observed that minimizing the intake of refined sugar, processed foods, and refined meats decreases cancer incidences (Ubago-Guisado et al., 2021). These studies link nutrition to the factors that can directly affect the cause of cancer.

Although epidemiological studies provide valuable data, clinical studies give insight into whether a particular form of prevention is effective on humans. One such insight was the reporting of vitamin D deficiency, which has been linked to the development of cancer (Holick, 2006). Vitamin D's ability to regulate cell proliferation, differentiation, and immune response adds to its preventive effects. Although supplements can be a good alternative for people with a deficiency, they typically provide only about 400 IU of vitamin D, whereas the body requires approximately 3000–5000 IU of vitamin D to meet its daily needs (Barger-Lux et al., 1998). Nowadays, researchers have agreed that 1000 IU of vitamin D is required daily (Tangpricha et al., 2003). Another compound known as curcumin is obtained from the plant *Curcuma longa*, which is said to have potential anticancer properties. Curcumin suppresses the development, progression, and metastasis of various malignancies. It also prevents carcinogenesis by interfering with two key factors: tumor development and angiogenesis (Hamzehzadeh et al., 2018). The first use of curcumin against cancer dates back to 1982, as reported by Kuttan et al. Kuttan et al. conducted a clinical trial involving 62 patients with external cancerous lesions. It was observed that topical curcumin had the most effect. Evidence showed a reduction in smell, itching, lesion size, and pain (Kuttan et al., 1987). Curcumin was shown to be effective in treating colorectal cancer, pancreatic cancer, head and neck squamous cell carcinoma, oral carcinoma, and many more (Hamzehzadeh et al., 2018).

Although clinical trials provide valuable data, predictive modeling enables us to integrate these findings into personalized nutrient and cancer risk prevention. A personalized nutrient plan tailored to an individual's needs, which includes genetic makeup, metabolic requirements, lifestyle, and individual dietary preferences. A professional can utilize data from clinical trials and epidemiological studies to create personalized diet plans and recommend specific nutrient intakes, thereby reducing the overall risk factor for a particular population (Kaput, 2008; Malcomson & Mathers, 2023; Rahman et al., 2020). Thus, by considering the challenges of data integration, the translational gap, and ethical concerns, as well as the integration of clinical trial data with epidemiological studies, predictive modeling has the power to revolutionize the field of cancer-protective nutrition. This approach to dietary recommendations is evidence-based and tailored to an individual's needs, thus improving the rate of cancer prevention and overall health outcomes (Malcomson & Mathers, 2023).

10.6 Challenges in predictive modeling

Multiple challenges can hinder the functioning of predictive modeling in cancer-protective nutrition, primarily including the integration of data and data heterogeneity. It becomes challenging to develop a single model that can effectively inform the nutritional requirements of patients and their cancer risk profiles, given the diverse data on diet, demographics, and clinically variable patient parameters. This problem is further exacerbated by regulatory and ethical considerations that concern patients' data privacy, thereby hindering the sharing of data and collaboration among researchers (Frank, 2024; Zheng et al., 2024). In addition, a discontinuity exists between the predictive models and their implementation in clinical practice scenarios. No doubt that machine learning and various other algorithms have paved the way for analyzing nutritional risks and benefits, but their implementation in clinical practices becomes difficult because of the various levels of learning and training that the professionals possess and the requirements for comprehensibility of model outputs (Guida et al., 2023; Yu et al., 2024). Predictive models can also be less effective because of the limitation of providing high-end data in clinical settings, which is important for accurate predictions (Frank, 2024). Containment of these constraints requires a concerted effort toward improving the quality of data, ensuring adherence to ethics, and devising training programs that will empower healthcare professionals to use the various predictive tools in their management of cancer nutrition.

10.7 Future directions

Personalized cancer prevention strategies, informed by cancer-protective nutrition, are advancing with the advent of innovative approaches in predictive modeling. The integration of varied data types, including omics data (that is, genomics, proteomics, and metabolomics), is made possible by artificial intelligence (AI) and deep learning, which are the leading techniques at present. Researchers can analyze complex biological processes and simultaneously identify patterns with the help of these advanced modeling approaches, which are commonly overlooked by traditional methods. Deep learning frameworks, for example, can integrate multiomics data to create molecular networks that can clarify arbitrary pathways responsible for cancer progression, thus increasing accuracy as compared to single-omics-based analysis (Ozaki et al., 2024; Zhou et al., 2023).

Furthermore predictive models offer the opportunity to develop personalized treatment strategies by considering individual risk factors and specific biological markers to inform nutritional interventions. Healthcare providers, by harnessing the power of AI, can develop targeted nutritional plans owing to their unique genetic and metabolic patterns, thereby significantly reducing malnutrition related to cancer and upgrading treatment aftermath (Ozaki et al., 2024; Zheng et al., 2024). The role of the microbiome is also receiving attention in the context of predictive modeling. As highlighted by some recent studies, alterations in gut microbiota can have an impact on nutrient metabolism and immune responses, thus affecting the risks of cancer and its progression. Microbiome data could be integrated into predictive models, which can provide information on how dietary changes can impact the development of cancer, its progression, and, as a result, patient outcomes (Alsharif, 2024; Zheng et al., 2024).

To sum up, future research on predictive models for protective nutrition in cancer will be benchmarked by incorporating AI-mediated approaches that couple with multiomics data and consider individualized microbiome profiles. This comprehensive perspective will resolve the challenge, improve the effectiveness of cancer prevention practices, and promote the utilization of nutrition tailored to the patient in oncological care, with the ultimate goal of improving patient healthcare and prognosis.

10.8 Conclusion

Nutrition plays a crucial role in cancer prevention, and nutraceuticals offer several benefits in reducing cancer incidence and enhancing treatment outcomes. Several bioactive compounds, including vitamins, minerals, and polyphenols, contribute to enhanced cellular health, as demonstrated in various clinical and preclinical studies. Predictive modeling, on the other hand, is also an essential tool in understanding the relationship between diet, genetics, and the risk of cancer occurrence. Machine learning, statistical models, and systems biology integrate data from various fields, including epidemiological studies, omics data, and clinical data, to create personalized dietary recommendations for each patient. AI further assesses cancer risk and aids in early detection, as well as personalized nutritional interventions.

Despite all this progress, certain challenges, such as data heterogeneity, ethical considerations, and a major translational gap, remain. This calls for interdisciplinary cooperation to test models, standardize data, and integrate microbiome profiling for a more profound understanding. Future treatments should focus on improving predictive models, conducting more clinical trials, and utilizing AI to ensure more personalized treatments, ultimately aiming for more effective preventive strategies. This collaboration between nutraceuticals and predictive modeling presents a promising future in cancer prevention.

References

Afsari, B., Kuo, A., Zhang, Y., Li, L., Lahouel, K., Danilova, L., Favorov, A., Rosenquist, T., Grollman, A. P., Kinzler, K. W., Cope, L., Vogelstein, B., & Tomasetti, C. (2021). Supervised mutational signatures for obesity and other tissue-specific etiological factors in cancer. *eLife, 10*, 1–71. doi:10.7554/eLife.61082.

Alali, M., Alqubaisy, M., Aljaafari, M. N., Alali, A. O., Baqais, L., Molouki, A., Abushelaibi, A., Lai, K. S., & Lim, S. H. E. (2021). Nutraceuticals: Transformation of conventional foods into health promoters/disease preventers and safety considerations. *Molecules, 26*(9). doi:10.3390/molecules26092540.

Alsharif, F. (2024). Artificial intelligence in oncology: Applications, challenges and future frontiers. *International Journal of Pharmaceutical Investigation, 14*(3), 647–656. doi:10.5530/ijpi.14.3.76.

Aronson, J. K. (2017). Defining 'nutraceuticals': Neither nutritious nor pharmaceutical. *British Journal of Clinical Pharmacology, 83*(1), 8–19. doi:10.1111/bcp.12935.

Badimon, L., Vilahur, G., & Padro, T. (2017). Systems biology approaches to understand the effects of nutrition and promote health. *British Journal of Clinical Pharmacology, 83*(1), 38–45. doi:10.1111/bcp.12965.

Bae, Y. H., & Park, K. (2020). Advanced drug delivery 2020 and beyond: Perspectives on the future. *Advanced Drug Delivery Reviews, 158*, 4–16. doi:10.1016/j.addr.2020.06.018.

Bahrami, H. (2023). Nutrition for cancer prevention and control: A review of dietary risk factors and protective measures. *Cancer Screening and Prevention, 2*(4), 250–259. doi:10.14218/csp.2023.00008.

Balbin, O. A., Prensner, J. R., Sahu, A., Yocum, A., Shankar, S., Malik, R., Fermin, D., Dhanasekaran, S. M., Chandler, B., Thomas, D., Beer, D. G., Cao, X., Nesvizhskii, A. I., & Chinnaiyan, A. M. (2013). Reconstructing targetable pathways in lung cancer by integrating diverse omics data. *Nature Communications, 4*. doi:10.1038/ncomms3617.

Barger-Lux, M. J., Heaney, R. P., Dowell, T. C. C., & Holick, M. F. (1998). Vitamin D and its major metabolites: Serum levels after graded oral dosing in healthy men. *Osteoporosis International, 8*(3), 222–230. doi:10.1007/s001980050058.

Bars-Cortina, D., Sakhawat, A., Piñol-Felis, C., & Motilva, M. J. (2022). Chemopreventive effects of anthocyanins on colorectal and breast cancer: A review. *Seminars in Cancer Biology, 81*, 241–258. doi:10.1016/j.semcancer.2020.12.013.

Basen-Engquist, K., & Chang, M. (2011). Obesity and cancer risk: Recent review and evidence. *Current Oncology Reports, 13*(1), 71–76. doi:10.1007/s11912-010-0139-7.

Boeing, H. (2013). Obesity and cancer – The update 2013. *Best Practice & Research Clinical Endocrinology & Metabolism, 27*(2), 219–227. doi:10.1016/j.beem.2013.04.005.

Bossi, P., De Luca, R., Ciani, O., D'Angelo, E., & Caccialanza, R. (2022). Malnutrition management in oncology: An expert view on controversial issues and future perspectives. *Frontiers in Oncology, 12*. doi:10.3389/fonc.2022.910770.

Calle, E. E., & Thun, M. J. (2004). Obesity and cancer. *Oncogene, 23*(38), 6365–6378. doi:10.1038/sj.onc.1207751.

Committee on Care and Use of Laboratory Animals. (1986). *Guide for the care and use of laboratory animals (Issue 86)*. US Department of Health and Human Services, Public Health Service, National Institutes of Health.

Chen, H. C., Kodell, R. L., Cheng, K. F., & Chen, J. J. (2012). Assessment of performance of survival prediction models for cancer prognosis. *BMC Medical Research Methodology, 12*. doi:10.1186/1471-2288-12-102.

Chow, E., Abdolell, M., Panzarella, T., Harris, K., Bezjak, A., Warde, P., & Tannock, I. (2008). Predictive model for survival in patients with advanced cancer. *Journal of Clinical Oncology, 26*(36), 5863–5869. doi:10.1200/JCO.2008.17.1363.

Cruz, J. A., & Wishart, D. S. (2006). Applications of machine learning in cancer prediction and prognosis. *Cancer Informatics, 2*, 59–77. doi:10.1177/117693510600200030.

Di Napoli, R., Balzano, N., Mascolo, A., Cimmino, C., Vitiello, A., Zovi, A., Capuano, A., & Boccellino, M. (2023). What is the role of nutraceutical products in cancer patients? A systematic review of randomized clinical trials. *Nutrients, 15*(14). doi:10.3390/nu15143249.

Divella, R., Daniele, A., Savino, E., & Paradiso, A. (2020). Anticancer effects of nutraceuticals in the Mediterranean diet: An epigenetic diet model. *Cancer Genomics – Proteomics, 17*(4), 335–350. doi:10.21873/cgp.20193.

Doll, R. (2017). *The prevention of cancer: Pointers from epidemiology* (pp. 1–143). Taylor and Francis. doi:10.4324/9781315134178.

Donaldson, M. S. (2004). Nutrition and cancer: A review of the evidence for an anticancer diet. *Nutrition Journal, 3*, 19. doi:10.1186/1475-2891-3-19.

Edefonti, V., De Vito, R., Parpinel, M., & Ferraroni, M. (2024). Dietary patterns and cancer risk: An overview with focus on methods. *The New England Journal of Statistics in Data Science, 2*(1), 30–53.

Flagg, E. W., Coates, R. J., & Greenberg, R. S. (1995). Epidemiologic studies of antioxidants and cancer in humans. *Journal of the American College of Nutrition, 14*(5), 419–427. doi:10.1080/07315724.1995.10718532.

Frank, E. (2024). *The impact of predictive modeling in improving the prognosis of patients with colorectal cancer*. EasyChair.

Goshayeshi, L., Hoseini, B., Yousefli, Z., Khooie, A., Etminani, K., Esmaeilzadeh, A., & Golabpour, A. (2017). Predictive model for survival in patients with gastric cancer. *Electronic Physician, 9*(12), 6035–6042. doi:10.19082/6035.

Greenwald, P. (2004). Clinical trials in cancer prevention: Current results and perspectives for the future. *The Journal of Nutrition, 134*(12), 3507S. doi:10.1093/jn/134.12.3507s.

Guida, F., Andreozzi, L., Zama, D., Prete, A., Masetti, R., Fabi, M., & Lanari, M. (2023). Innovative strategies to predict and prevent the risk for malnutrition in child, adolescent, and young adult cancer survivors. *Frontiers in Nutrition, 10*. doi:10.3389/fnut.2023.1332881.

Hamzehzadeh, L., Atkin, S. L., Majeed, M., Butler, A. E., & Sahebkar, A. (2018). The versatile role of curcumin in cancer prevention and treatment: A focus on PI3K/AKT pathway. *Journal of Cellular Physiology, 233*(10), 6530–6537. doi:10.1002/jcp.26620.

Hartung, T. (2008). Thoughts on limitations of animal models. *Parkinsonism & Related Disorders, 14*(2), S81. doi:10.1016/j.parkreldis.2008.04.003.

Hinduja, D. B., Dhanu, A. S., Swamy, G. G., Murugesan, K., Elango, B., Murali, U., Rashid, M., Mathanmohun, M., & Basalingappa, K. M. (2023). Diet and nutrition strategies for cancer prevention: A comprehensive review. *Research in Biotechnology*, 12–18. doi:10.25081/rib.2023.v14.8618.

Holick, M. F. (2006). Vitamin D: Its role in cancer prevention and treatment. *Progress in Biophysics and Molecular Biology, 92*(1), 49–59. doi:10.1016/j.pbiomolbio.2006.02.014.

Hutkins, R. W., Krumbeck, J. A., Bindels, L. B., Cani, P. D., Fahey, G., Goh, Y. J., Hamaker, B., Martens, E. C., Mills, D. A., Rastal, R. A., Vaughan, E., & Sanders, M. E. (2016). Prebiotics: Why definitions matter. *Current Opinion in Biotechnology, 37*, 1–7. doi:10.1016/j.copbio.2015.09.001.

Hwang, K. T. (2021). Clinical databases for breast cancer research. *Advances in Experimental Medicine and Biology, 1187*, 493–509. doi:10.1007/978-981-32-9620-6_26.

de Jong, M., & Maina, T. (2010). Of mice and humans: Are they the same?—Implications in cancer translational research: Table 1. *Journal of Nuclear Medicine, 51*(4), 501–504. doi:10.2967/jnumed.109.065706.

Kalia, S. S., Boddicker, N. J., Yadav, S., Huang, H., Na, J., Hu, C., ... Kraft, P. (2024). Development of a breast cancer risk prediction model integrating monogenic, polygenic, and epidemiologic risk. *Cancer Epidemiology, Biomarkers & Prevention, 33*(11), 1490–1499. doi:10.1158/1055-9965.EPI-24-0594.

Kalita-De Croft, P., Al-Ejeh, F., Reed, A. E. M. C., Saunus, J. M., & Lakhani, S. R. (2016). Omics approaches in breast cancer research and clinical practice. *Advances in Anatomic Pathology, 23*(6), 356–367. doi:10.1097/PAP.0000000000000128.

Kaput, J. (2008). Nutrigenomics research for personalized nutrition and medicine. *Current Opinion in Biotechnology, 19*(2), 110–120. doi:10.1016/j.copbio.2008.02.005.

Kaur, V., Kumar, M., Kumar, A., Kaur, K., Dhillon, V. S., & Kaur, S. (2018). Pharmacotherapeutic potential of phytochemicals: Implications in cancer chemoprevention and future perspectives. *Biomedicine and Pharmacotherapy, 97*, 564–586. doi:10.1016/j.biopha.2017.10.124.

Khilwani, R., & Singh, S. (2023). Systems biology and cytokines potential role in lung cancer immunotherapy targeting autophagic axis. *Biomedicines, 11*(10), 2706. doi:10.3390/biomedicines11102706.

Kuttan, R., Sudheeran, P. C., & Josph, C. D. (1987). Turmeric and curcumin as topical agents in cancer therapy. *Tumori, 73*(1), 29–31. doi:10.1177/030089168707300105.

Lampe, J. W., Navarro, S. L., Hullar, M. A. J., & Shojaie, A. (2013). Inter-individual differences in response to dietary intervention: Integrating omics platforms towards personalised dietary recommendations. *Proceedings of the Nutrition Society, 72*(2), 207–218. doi:10.1017/S0029665113000025.

Maiuolo, J., Gliozzi, M., Carresi, C., Musolino, V., Oppedisano, F., Scarano, F., Nucera, S., Scicchitano, M., Bosco, F., Macri, R., Ruga, S., Cardamone, A., Coppoletta, A., Mollace, A., Cognetti, F., & Mollace, V. (2021). Nutraceuticals and cancer: Potential for natural polyphenols. *Nutrients, 13*(11), 3834. doi:10.3390/nu13113834.

Mak, I. W. Y., Evaniew, N., & Ghert, M. (2014). Lost in translation: Animal models and clinical trials in cancer treatment. *American Journal of Translational Research, 6*(2), 114–118. http://www.ajtr.org/files/ajtr1312010.pdf.

Malcomson, F. C., & Mathers, J. C. (2023). Translation of nutrigenomic research for personalised and precision nutrition for cancer prevention and for cancer survivors. *Redox Biology, 62*, 102710. doi:10.1016/j.redox.2023.102710.

Mhaidly, N., Barake, N., Trelcat, A., Journe, F., Saussez, S., & Descamps, G. é (2024). Bufalin suppresses head and neck cancer development by modulating immune responses and targeting the β-catenin signaling pathway. *Cancers, 16*(15), 2739. doi:10.3390/cancers16152739.

Murphy, R. (2020). An integrative approach to assessing diet–cancer relationships. *Metabolites, 10*(4), 123. doi:10.3390/metabo10040123.

Narimatsu, H., & Yaguchi, Y. T. (2022). The role of diet and nutrition in cancer: Prevention, treatment, and survival. *Nutrients, 14*(16). doi:10.3390/nu14163329.

Nasri, H., Baradaran, A., Shirzad, H., & Kopaei, M. R. (2014). New concepts in nutraceuticals as alternative for pharmaceuticals. *International Journal of Preventive Medicine, 5*(12), 1487–1499. http://ijpm.mui.ac.ir/index.php/ijpm/article/download/1450/1733.

Noble, K., Rohaj, A., Abegglen, L. M., & Schiffman, J. D. (2020). Cancer therapeutics inspired by defense mechanisms in the animal kingdom. *Evolutionary Applications, 13*(7), 1681–1700. doi:10.1111/eva.12963.

Ozaki, Y., Broughton, P., Abdollahi, H., Valafar, H., & Blenda, A. V. (2024). Integrating omics data and AI for cancer diagnosis and prognosis. *Cancers, 16*(13). doi:10.3390/cancers16132448.

Panduranga Vital, T., Dileep Kumar, K., Bhagya Sri, H. V., & Murali Krishna, M. (2019). Analysis of cancer data set with statistical and unsupervised machine learning methods. In *Smart Intelligent Computing and Applications* (pp. 267–276). Singapore: Springer. https://doi.org/10.1007/978-981-13-1921-1_27.

Parsons, H. M., Forte, M. L., Abdi, H. I., Brandt, S., Claussen, A. M., Wilt, T., Klein, M., Ester, E., Landsteiner, A., Shaukut, A., Sibley, S. S., Slavin, J., Sowerby, C., Ng, W., & Butler, M. (2023). Nutrition as prevention for improved cancer health outcomes: A systematic literature review. *JNCI Cancer Spectrum, 7*(3). doi:10.1093/jncics/pkad035.

Puri, V., Nagpal, M., Singh, I., Singh, M., Dhingra, G. A., Huanbutta, K., Dheer, D., Sharma, A., & Sangnim, T. (2022). A comprehensive review on nutraceuticals: Therapy support and formulation challenges. *Nutrients, 14*(21). doi:10.3390/nu14214637.

Qu, B., Yuan, J., Liu, X., Zhang, S., Ma, X., & Lu, L. (2023). Anticancer activities of natural antimicrobial peptides from animals. *Frontiers in Microbiology, 14*. doi:10.3389/fmicb.2023.1321386.

Rahman, A., Chakraborty, S., & Kabir, Y. (2020). Harnessing personalized nutrigenomics for cancer prevention and treatment through diet-gene interaction. In *Functional foods in cancer prevention and therapy* (pp. 387–403). Elsevier. doi:10.1016/B978-0-12-816151-7.00019-3.

Rathee, S., Patil, U. K., & Jain, S. K. (2024). Exploring the potential of dietary phytochemicals in cancer prevention: A comprehensive review. *Journal of Exploratory Research in Pharmacology, 9*(1), 51–64. doi:10.14218/jerp.2023.00050.

Riboli, E. (1997). The EPIC Project: Rationale and study design. European Prospective Investigation into Cancer and Nutrition. *International Journal of Epidemiology, 26*(90001), 6S. doi:10.1093/ije/26.suppl_1.S6.

Riboli, E. (1992). Nutrition and cancer: Background and rationale of the European Prospective Investigation into Cancer and Nutrition (EPIC). *Annals of Oncology, 3*(10), 783–791. doi:10.1093/oxfordjournals.annonc.a058097.

Richter, A. N., & Khoshgoftaar, T. M. (2018). A review of statistical and machine learning methods for modeling cancer risk using structured clinical data. *Artificial Intelligence in Medicine, 90*, 1–14. doi:10.1016/j.artmed.2018.06.002.

Ruby, S., Prakash, S., Kumar, V. P., Kumar, T. P., & Prathab, S. (2021). A comprehensive review on nutraceuticals. *International Journal of Pharmaceutical Sciences Review and Research., 68*(2). doi:10.47583/ijpsrr.2021.v68i02.021.

Rudzińska, A., Juchaniuk, P., Oberda, J., Wiśniewska, J., Wojdan, W., Szklener, K., & Mańdziuk, S. (2023). Phytochemicals in cancer treatment and cancer prevention—Review on epidemiological data and clinical trials. *Nutrients, 15*(8), 1896. doi:10.3390/nu15081896.

Sharifi-Rad, M., Pezzani, R., Redaelli, M., Zorzan, M., Imran, M., Khalil, A. A., Salehi, B., Sharopov, F., Cho, W. C., & Sharifi-Rad, J. (2020). Preclinical pharmacological activities of epigallocatechin-3-gallate in signaling pathways: An update on cancer. *Molecules, 25*(3). doi:10.3390/molecules25030467.

Shiao, S. P. K., Grayson, J., Lie, A., & Yu, C. H. (2018). Personalized nutrition—Genes, diet, and related interactive parameters as predictors of cancer in multiethnic colorectal cancer families. *Nutrients, 10*(6). doi:10.3390/nu10060795.

Shim, J., & Kim, J. (2022). Considerations for experimental animal ethics in the research planning and evaluation process. *Kosin Medical Journal, 37*(4), 271–277. doi:10.7180/kmj.22.139.

Slavin, J. (2004). Whole grains and human health. *Nutrition Research Reviews, 17*(1), 99–110. doi:10.1079/nrr200374.

Suzuki, Y., Yeung, A. C., & Ikeno, F. (2009). The pre-clinical animal model in the translational research of interventional cardiology. *JACC Cardiovascular Interventions, 2*(5), 373–383. doi:10.1016/j.jcin.2009.03.004.

Talib, W. H., Ahmed Jum'AH, D. A., Attallah, Z. S., Jallad, M. S., Al Kury, L. T., Hadi, R. W., & Mahmod, A. I. (2023). Role of vitamins A, C, D, E in cancer prevention and therapy: Therapeutic potentials and mechanisms of action. *Frontiers in Nutrition, 10.* doi:10.3389/fnut.2023.1281879.

Tangpricha, V., Koutkia, P., Rieke, S. M., Chen, T. C., Perez, A. A., & Holick, M. F. (2003). Fortification of orange juice with vitamin D: A novel approach for enhancing vitamin D nutritional health. *American Journal of Clinical Nutrition, 77*(6), 1478–1483. doi:10.1093/ajcn/77.6.1478.

Thiébaut, A. C. M., Kipnis, V., Chang, S. C., Subar, A. F., Thompson, F. E., Rosenberg, P. S., Hollenbeck, A. R., Leitzmann, M., & Schatzkin, A. (2007). Dietary fat and postmenopausal invasive breast cancer in the national institutes of health – AARP diet and health study cohort. *Journal of the National Cancer Institute, 99*(6), 451–462. doi:10.1093/jnci/djk094.

Thomas, R., Butler, E., Macchi, F., & Williams, M. (2015). Phytochemicals in cancer prevention and management? *British Journal of Medical Practitioners, 8*(2). http://bjmp.org/files/2015-8-2/bjmp-2015-8-2-a815.pdf.

Toma, M., & Wei, O. C. (2023). Predictive modeling in medicine. *Encyclopedia, 3*(2), 590–601. doi:10.3390/encyclopedia3020042.

Tota, J. E., Gillison, M. L., Katki, H. A., Kahle, L., Pickard, R. K., Xiao, W., … Chaturvedi, A. K. (2019). Development and validation of an individualized risk prediction model for oropharynx cancer in the US population. *Cancer, 125*(24), 4407–4416. doi:10.1002/cncr.32412.

Tratnjek, L., Jeruc, J., Romih, R., & Zupančič, D. aša (2021). Vitamin A and retinoids in bladder cancer chemoprevention and treatment: A narrative review of current evidence, challenges and future prospects. *International Journal of Molecular Sciences, 22*(7), 3510. doi:10.3390/ijms22073510.

Ubago-Guisado, E., Rodríguez-Barranco, M., Ching-López, A., Petrova, D., Molina-Montes, E., Amiano, P., Barricarte-Gurrea, A., Chirlaque, M. D., Agudo, A., & Sánchez, M. J. (2021). Evidence update on the relationship between diet and the most common cancers from the European Prospective Investigation into Cancer and Nutrition (EPIC) study: A systematic review. *Nutrients, 13*(10). doi:10.3390/nu13103582.

Vlachavas, E. I., Bohn, J., Ückert, F., & Nürnberg, S. (2021). A detailed catalogue of multi-omics methodologies for identification of putative biomarkers and causal molecular networks in translational cancer research. *International Journal of Molecular Sciences, 22*(6), 1–41. doi:10.3390/ijms22062822.

Wang, L., Dong, C., Li, X., Han, W., & Su, X. (2017). Anticancer potential of bioactive peptides from animal sources (review). *Oncology Reports, 38*(2), 637–651. doi:10.3892/or.2017.5778.

Wang, T. T. Y., Pham, Q., & Kim, Y. S. (2018). Elucidating the role of CD84 and AHR in modulation of LPS-induced cytokines production by cruciferous vegetable-derived compounds indole-3-carbinol and 3,3′-diindolylmethane. *International Journal of Molecular Sciences, 19*(2). doi:10.3390/ijms19020339.

Wei, R., Mao, L., Xu, P., Zheng, X., Hackman, R. M., MacKenzie, G. G., & Wang, Y. (2018). Suppressing glucose metabolism with epigallocatechin-3-gallate (EGCG) reduces breast cancer cell growth in preclinical models. *Food and Function, 9*(11), 5682–5696. doi:10.1039/c8fo01397g.

Wong, G., Lim, W. H., Lewis, J., Craig, J. C., Turner, R., Zhu, K., Lim, E. M., & Prince, R. (2015). Vitamin D and cancer mortality in elderly women. *BMC Cancer, 15*(1), 106. doi:10.1186/s12885-015-1112-5.

Yang, W., Ma, Y., Liu, Y., Smith-Warner, S. A., Simon, T. G., Chong, D. Q., Qi, Q., Meyerhardt, J. A., Giovannucci, E. L., Chan, A. T., & Zhang, X. (2019). Association of intake of whole grains and dietary fiber with risk of hepatocellular carcinoma in US adults. *JAMA Oncology, 5*(6), 879–886. doi:10.1001/jamaoncol.2018.7159.

Yu, J., Soh, K. L., He, L., Wang, P., & Cao, Y. (2024). Development of a short-term nutritional risk prediction model for hepatocellular carcinoma patients: A retrospective cohort study. *Scientific Reports, 14*(1). doi:10.1038/s41598-024-54456-4.

Yuan, J. M., Sun, C., & Butler, L. M. (2011). Tea and cancer prevention: Epidemiological studies. *Pharmacological Research, 64*(2), 123–135. doi:10.1016/j.phrs.2011.03.002.

Zhang, E., Zhang, M., Shi, C., Sun, L., Shan, L., Zhang, H., & Song, Y. (2020). An overview of advances in multi-omics analysis in prostate cancer. *Life Sciences, 260*, 118376. doi:10.1016/j.lfs.2020.118376.

Zheng, P., Wang, B. o, Luo, Y., Duan, R., & Feng, T. (2024). Research progress on predictive models for malnutrition in cancer patients. *Frontiers in Nutrition, 11*. doi:10.3389/fnut.2024.1438941.

Zhou, A., Zhang, C., & Eminaga, O. (2023). Advances in deep learning-based cancer outcome prediction using multi-omics data. *Annals of Proteomics and Bioinformatics, 7*(1), 010–013. doi:10.29328/journal.apb.1001020.

Predictive modeling and quantitative risk assessment toward assured microbiological food safety in tropical countries

11

Ursula Gonzales-Barron and Vasco Cadavez
CIMO, LA SusTEC, Instituto Politécnico de Bragança, Bragança, Portugal

11.1 Predictive microbial modeling foundations and outlook

Predictive microbiology is a field that uses mathematical models to predict how microorganisms will respond to various environmental conditions, particularly in food. It leverages the principle that microbial behavior is reproducible under specific circumstances, allowing for estimations of growth, survival, and inactivation. Predictive microbiology is widely used in the food industry to assess food safety and quality, estimate shelf life, and optimize processing and storage conditions (Ross et al., 1999). The three major model tiers in predictive microbiology include

1. **Primary models**, which describe microbial dynamics over time under constant conditions (e.g., logistic, Gompertz, Baranyi, and Roberts). These sigmoidal models account for the lag, exponential, and stationary phases of microbial growth. Among them the Baranyi–Roberts model is particularly valued for its mechanistic basis and accurate description of lag phase dynamics (Albert & Mafart, 2005; Huang, 2013; Lo Grasso et al., 2023).
2. **Secondary models**, which relate model parameters of primary models—such as maximum specific growth rate (μ_{max}) or lag time duration (λ)—to environmental variables such as temperature, pH, and water activity (Rosso et al., 1995). The Ratkowsky square-root model is a common secondary model used to describe the temperature dependence of μ_{max} (Ratkowsky et al., 1982): where T is the temperature and T_{min} is the theoretical minimum temperature for microbial growth.
3. **Tertiary models**, which integrate primary and secondary models into decision-support tools, are often embedded in interactive software tools such as ComBase, Sym'Previus, PMM-Lab, and IPMP (Huang, 2017; Tenenhaus-Aziza & Ellouze, 2015).

In addition, **dynamic models** have been developed to describe microbial growth or inactivation under fluctuating environmental conditions. These models often take the form of differential equations and require numerical methods for their solution. In the R software, packages, such as deSolve and bioinactivation, support this type of modeling. These models are not only predictive but can also be mechanistic, allowing the interpretation of microbial responses through biologically meaningful parameters such as specific growth rate, lag time duration, and decimal reduction time (D value) (Peñalver-Soto et al., 2019; Shama et al., 2005).

Nutritional Strategies, Predictive Models, and Sustainable Policies. DOI: https://doi.org/10.1016/B978-0-443-23671-6.00012-8

Despite their success, nonlinear regression used in fitting such models introduces statistical challenges. Issues such as parameter nonidentifiability, correlation, and model nonlinearity require careful numerical handling (Bolker et al., 2013; Ratkowsky, 1993). Software environments, such as R and AD Model Builder, are widely used for this purpose, offering reproducibility, transparency, and access to open-source modeling tools (Bolker et al., 2013).

11.1.1 Experimental design

An often-overlooked but critical component of predictive microbiology is the design of experiments. Poorly designed experiments lead to weak parameter estimates and unreliable models. The use of optimal experimental design (OED) frameworks, such as D-optimal and A-optimal designs, helps maximize information gain while minimizing experimental effort. These methods are increasingly applied in microbial inactivation studies, especially in complex systems with many interacting variables (Ratkowsky, 1993).

Moreover, recent work has emphasized the need for standardized protocols for model fitting, validation, and performance reporting. The use of model selection criteria (Akaike Information Criterion, Bayesian Information Criterion), residual diagnostics, and goodness-of-fit statistics is vital to ensure model robustness and transparency (Peñalver-Soto et al., 2019).

11.1.2 From determinism to stochasticity and machine learning

Traditionally, predictive models have been deterministic, describing average microbial responses. However, recent studies emphasize the need to account for variability and stochastic behavior—especially when dealing with low initial microbial counts or heterogeneous populations. Stochastic models, including individual-based approaches and Bayesian frameworks, offer improved capacity to quantify uncertainty and biological variability (Koseki et al., 2021; Liu et al., 2022).

Machine learning (ML) and artificial intelligence (AI) are now at the forefront of predictive microbiology. These data-driven methods can extract patterns from complex datasets, predict microbial growth or inactivation without explicit mechanistic assumptions, and integrate multiple sources of data (e.g., genomics and sensor data) (Liu et al., 2022; Taiwo et al., 2024). Techniques such as random forests, support vector machines (SVMs), and neural networks are being used to enhance prediction accuracy, especially when experimental data are limited or noisy.

11.1.3 Toward integrated, sustainable, and context-aware models

The future of predictive microbiology also lies in integration and localization. Geographic information systems (GIS), climate databases, and food chain mapping can be integrated with microbial models to forecast risks spatially and temporally, helping public health authorities anticipate outbreaks or contamination hotspots

(Taiwo et al., 2024). Sustainable food system modeling—combining microbial, environmental, and socioeconomic data—can also inform policy and innovation in low-resource settings.

In this context, predictive microbiology is not just a scientific tool but a critical enabler for food security, consumer protection, and sustainable food system development in tropical regions. Ongoing collaboration between microbiologists, data scientists, engineers, and local stakeholders will be key to tailoring these tools to the unique challenges and opportunities in the Global South.

11.1.4 Key applications of predictive modeling

Predictive modeling of microorganisms is widely applied in the field of food safety.

11.1.4.1 Microbial behavior prediction

Predictive models in microbiology aim to quantitatively describe the dynamics of microbial populations in food systems. Predictive models for microbial behavior constitute a powerful toolset for understanding and forecasting microbial responses in foods. As such, predictive modeling is fundamental for estimating shelf life, managing food spoilage, and designing food safety interventions. A variety of tools are available for modeling microbial behavior. For instance, ComBase Predictor (https://www.combase.cc) is a web-based tool for microbial growth predictions; PMM-Lab is an open-source platform for managing and analyzing predictive microbiology data. The R software also contains a number of packages useful in microbial dynamics predictions; namely, (1) nls.microbio: for fitting primary models in integrated and differential form; (2) bioinactivation: for modeling microbial inactivation, including the Weibull and Bigelow models; (3) growthrates and grofit: for nonlinear regression and spline-based growth curve fitting; and (4) bioOED: for OED in microbial inactivation studies.

When selecting the most appropriate predictive microbiology model, some considerations should be paid attention to. The choice of model should balance biological realism, parsimony, and statistical robustness. As emphasized earlier by Ratkowsky (1993), parameters should be interpretable, models should be close to linear to ensure reliable parameter estimation, and care must be taken to avoid overfitting, especially with limited data. Furthermore, attention should be paid to

1. Experimental design: Factorial and optimal design methods (e.g., Box–Behnken, central composite design) are used to ensure the collection of informative data points.
2. Data quality: Accurate enumeration methods (e.g., plate count, optical density) and sufficient replication are necessary for reliable model fitting.

11.1.4.2 Quantitative risk assessment

Risk assessment is a central pillar of food safety management. It provides a structured approach for evaluating the potential for microbial hazards to cause harm, particularly in the context of consumer exposure. Quantitative microbial risk assessment (QMRA) models allow food safety professionals to estimate public health risk from microbial contamination; evaluate the impact of interventions; and support data-driven food policy and regulatory decisions. Predictive microbiology plays a vital role in QMRA by supplying mathematical models that describe microbial dynamics throughout the food supply chain. Risk assessment consists of four steps:

1. **Hazard identification:** Recognition of microbial pathogens of concern (e.g., *Listeria monocytogenes, Salmonella* spp., and *Escherichia coli* O157:H7).
2. **Hazard characterization:** Quantification of the dose–response relationship, describing the probability of illness given a specific dose.
3. **Exposure assessment:** Estimation of the frequency and level of pathogen ingestion by consumers, accounting for production, storage, and preparation conditions.
4. **Risk characterization:** Integration of the above steps to estimate the likelihood and severity of adverse health effects.

Predictive models are essential for exposure assessment, as they describe microbial growth, survival, or inactivation across food processing and handling scenarios. These models enable simulation of pathogen levels from farm to fork, which are then linked to dose–response models to estimate risk. Predictive models for risk assessment often follow a chain-of-events structure. A simplified conceptual example for *L. monocytogenes* in ready-to-eat (RTE) foods covering retail and consumer handling is as follows: (1) growth during chilled storage; (2) temperature abuse during transport; (3) recontamination during slicing; (4) survival during home refrigeration; and (5) final ingestion dose estimation.

Several studies illustrate the use of predictive models in real-world QMRA applications. For instance: (1) RTE **salads**: Modeling *L. monocytogenes* growth during refrigerated storage helped define regulatory shelf life limits (Bernardo et al., 2020); (2) **thermal processing of infant formula**: Inactivation kinetics of *Cronobacter sakazakii* were modeled to validate process lethality (Zhang et al., 2020); (3) **street foods in tropical settings**: Exposure assessments modeled contamination and temperature abuse in informal market chains (Barro et al., 2012).

Each step is described using deterministic or stochastic models. Deterministic models use point estimates (e.g., constant storage temperature), whereas stochastic models incorporate uncertainty and variability using distributions and simulations (e.g., Monte Carlo methods). In the R software, packages, such as mc2d, fitdistrplus, and rriskDistributions, are commonly used for probabilistic risk modeling.

11.1.4.3 Application in HACCP

Predictive microbiology is instrumental in supporting hazard analysis and critical control point (HACCP) systems. It assists in (1) identifying critical control points (CCPs) where interventions are most effective; (2) defining critical limits, such as safe storage times and temperatures; and (3) validating processing steps, such as thermal treatments. For example, the lethality of heat treatments can be evaluated using the Bigelow model, which is a secondary model that describes the death of a microorganism as a function of temperature.

11.1.4.4 Optimization of food safety practices

Beyond understanding microbial behavior and assessing risk, predictive models serve as powerful tools for optimizing food safety strategies. Through simulation, sensitivity analysis, and scenario testing, these models guide decisions that reduce contamination risks, enhance shelf life, and improve the efficacy of interventions—often while minimizing economic and environmental costs. Predictive microbiology supports the design and optimization of food processing and preservation methods, including

1. Thermal processing: Determining the time–temperature combinations necessary for achieving desired log reductions of pathogens, while preserving product quality.
2. Refrigeration and cold chain management: Modeling microbial growth under fluctuating temperature profiles to identify acceptable time–temperature limits.
3. Formulation design: Exploring combinations of pH, water activity, salt content, and preservatives to achieve hurdle effects.
4. Cleaning and sanitation schedules: Modeling microbial biofilm regrowth to optimize cleaning frequency and sanitizer application.

11.1.5 Economic and environmental benefits of predictive microbiology modeling

Predictive modeling contributes to the **rationalization of food safety systems** because it reduces the need for excessive thermal or chemical treatments and helps minimize product recalls and waste because of better process control. Furthermore, predictive microbiology supports the development of eco-efficient processes (e.g., energy-efficient chilling or pasteurization schedules) and enhances the shelf-life prediction accuracy, which helps balance product turnover and food waste (Membre & Kubaczka, 2005).

Models can also enable industries to test new processing or packaging options before implementation. For instance the impact of switching from vacuum to modified-atmosphere packaging on *Clostridium botulinum* growth in seafood products can be assessed using secondary models that relate μ_{max} to oxygen concentration and temperature (Arritt et al., 2007).

11.1.6 Integration of predictive microbiology modeling with emerging technologies

Advanced modeling frameworks, including decision support systems (DSSs), integrate predictive models with real-time data to support operational decisions. These tools often include **simulation engines** based on microbial growth/inactivation equations; **optimization routines** using criteria such as microbial safety margin, cost, and environmental load; and **user interfaces** for nonexperts in production environments. The best example of a DSS-based tool is Sym'Previus, which has been developed in France for shelf life prediction, hurdle technology design, and contamination risk simulation.

The optimization of food safety practices is increasingly enhanced by coupling predictive models with emerging technologies, such as (1) **real-time sensors** (e.g., temperature, humidity, and microbial load) (Zhang & Li, 2023); (2) **geospatial and temporal datasets** (e.g., GIS for contamination mapping) (Beni et al., 2011); (3) **AI** and **ML** algorithms that learn from past production data to recommend optimal safety actions (Smith & Doe, 2025). For example, ML algorithms can identify hidden patterns in temperature abuse incidents or predict failure points in HACCP plans (Zhang & Li, 2023).

Although optimization through modeling offers great potential, several considerations must be addressed (1) **model validation**: Predicted outcomes should be tested under real-life conditions (Oscar, 2011); (2) **data quality**: Garbage in, garbage out—accurate, representative data is key (Membre & Kubaczka, 2005); (3) **regulatory acceptance**: Optimization-based decisions must align with food safety regulations (EFSA, 2023); and (4) **uncertainty**: Model predictions should account for biological variability and parameter uncertainty (Akkermans et al., 2018). In this context the use of stochastic models and sensitivity analyses is recommended to evaluate how input uncertainty propagates to outcomes.

11.2 Recent advances of predictive microbiology

The field of predictive microbiology has undergone a significant transformation in recent years, driven by innovations in computational tools, data science, and molecular technologies. Recent advances that have expanded the scope and power of predictive microbiology encompass: (1) molecular and geospatial tools, which improve model input quality; (2) AI and Bayesian statistics, which expand modeling flexibility and uncertainty quantification; (3) dynamic and multipathway models for increased representativeness of reality; and (4) accessible interfaces, which enhance uptake by diverse stakeholders. These advances are addressing previous limitations and enabling more accurate, flexible, and context-specific modeling of microbial behavior in food systems, including those in tropical regions.

11.2.1 Integration of omics technologies

Genomics, transcriptomics, proteomics, and metabolomics are revolutionizing our understanding of microbial physiology and stress responses. In predictive microbiology, these technologies: (1) enhance the characterization of microbial species and strains, including their heat resistance, acid tolerance, and growth kinetics (Membre & Kubaczka, 2005; Posthuma-Trumpie et al., 2017); (2) allow for the identification of sublethal injury mechanisms, important for modeling recovery and regrowth in mildly processed foods (Casey et al., 2014; Metris et al., 2011); and (3) support the development of strain-specific models, replacing broad assumptions with genome-informed predictions (Noor et al., 2019). For instance, integration of transcriptomic data into growth models may reveal how *L. monocytogenes* upregulates certain genes under cold stress, thereby refining secondary model parameter estimates at low temperatures (Dlusskaya et al., 2011; Oliver et al., 2015).

11.2.2 Spatial modeling with GIS and remote sensing

GIS and remote sensing data are increasingly integrated with predictive models to assess contamination risks in space and time. Applications include (1) mapping microbial risk zones based on environmental variables, e.g., temperature, moisture, animal density (Arora et al., 2023); (2) modeling contamination pathways in irrigation systems or aquaculture (Falconer et al., 2019); and (3) forecasting seasonal variation in pathogen loads on crops and raw materials (FDA, 2014). This spatial-temporal modeling enables targeted interventions and surveillance, particularly valuable in expansive or undermonitored regions (Ahmed et al., 2025).

11.2.3 Dynamic and mechanistic modeling

Traditional isothermal models are being supplemented or replaced by dynamic models capable of simulating nonisothermal or fluctuating environments, typical of real-world food chains. Advances include the use of differential equation solvers for nonisothermal growth/inactivation (e.g., the use of the package deSolve in R); omnibus models that combine multiple stages (growth, inactivation, and regrowth) in a single framework (Pennone et al., 2021); and multispecies models to account for microbial competition, using frameworks such as the Jameson effect or Lotka–Volterra equations (Cornu et al., 2011). These developments improve model realism and adaptability to diverse food matrices and processing histories.

11.2.4 Artificial intelligence (AI) and machine learning (ML)

AI and ML are transforming the modeling landscape by enabling nonparametric predictions without needing explicit kinetic equations. Through their solvers, it is possible to handle complex, high-dimensional datasets, such as consumer behavior, weather data, and microbial ecology, while discovering new relationships or predictors through unsupervised learning, e.g., clustering contamination patterns (Li et al., 2021). The most commonly used ML algorithms in predictive microbiology include (1) random forests for classification; (2) SVM for pattern recognition in microbial responses; and (3) neural networks for modeling nonlinear growth curves or shelf life estimates (Li et al., 2023). Such models are now being integrated into early-warning systems and smart processing lines (Shehzad et al., 2025).

11.2.5 Bayesian modeling and probabilistic inference

Bayesian approaches are gaining popularity because of their ability to incorporate prior knowledge, quantify uncertainty, and update predictions as new data become available. Instead of single point estimates, Bayesian modeling provides posterior distributions of model parameters, thereby quantifying the uncertainty of key parameters. Furthermore, Bayesian modeling enables the extraction of credible intervals for risk assessment outputs, whereas enhanced model comparisons can be carried out through Bayesian factors. These frameworks are particularly valuable when data are sparse or noisy—a common challenge in tropical and developing regions. For instance, Bayesian spatio-temporal models have been employed to estimate malaria incidence in regions with sparse health data, demonstrating their effectiveness in such contexts (Li et al., 2021). In addition, Bayesian methods have been applied to food safety risk assessments, offering a probabilistic framework that accommodates uncertainty and facilitates the integration of diverse data sources (Wang et al., 2022).

11.2.6 User friendly interfaces and mobile applications

To increase adoption, especially in small food businesses and government agencies, predictive modeling tools are being packaged into **shiny apps** with visual input sliders and downloadable reports; **mobile apps** that run offline and guide shelf-life decisions in field settings; and **plug-and-play DSSs** for processors and regulators. Examples include R-based **shiny interfaces** for growth model fitting (FSQA, 2022) and scenario simulation (WHO, 2023); and mobile DSS for food vendors in Latin America and Southeast Asia that help manage chilled foods without electricity (Anonymous, 2022).

11.3 The tropical challenge: Complexity and data gaps

Many tropical countries face unique food safety challenges because of their environmental, socioeconomic, and infrastructural characteristics. These challenges can hinder the effectiveness of predictive models unless contextual factors are considered in their development and application.

- **Climatic pressures**: High ambient temperatures and humidity favor rapid microbial growth, reducing the effectiveness of standard cold-chain approaches (Koseki et al., 2021).
- **Informal food sectors**: Much of the food is produced, processed, and sold through informal channels with limited regulatory oversight and hygienic practices.
- **Data scarcity**: The calibration and validation of models require localized microbial kinetic data, which are often unavailable or poorly documented in tropical contexts (Taiwo et al., 2024).

These challenges call for robust models capable of capturing variability and uncertainty under real-world, dynamic conditions. For instance, models developed in temperate regions may not accurately reflect microbial behavior in tropical conditions unless revalidated or reparameterized with region-specific data (Peñalver-Soto et al., 2019).

11.3.1 Environmental complexity

Tropical environments are characterized by consistently high temperatures, elevated humidity, and pronounced seasonal rainfall patterns. These conditions accelerate microbial growth and spoilage kinetics, often beyond the ranges used to calibrate conventional models. For instance, microbial growth curves derived from isothermal studies at 4°C–30°C may underestimate the actual growth of *Salmonella* or *L. monocytogenes* at 35°C–42°C, common in many tropical food markets and storage settings. High ambient temperatures (often above 30°C) will reduce the lag phase and dramatically increase growth rate, whereas high humidity promotes condensation and surface moisture, favoring microbial adhesion and proliferation. Furthermore, power instability, if present, will lead to cold-chain disruptions, contributing to unintentional temperature abuse.

11.3.2 Informal and unregulated markets

A substantial portion of food in tropical countries is sold in informal markets, often with minimal regulatory oversight in terms of hygiene. These settings pose modeling difficulties because of lack of temperature control during handling and transport, minimal data recording (e.g., no time–temperature logs), and variable consumer handling and storage practices. Such unpredictability adds both variability (natural fluctuation) and uncertainty (lack of knowledge) to model inputs, which must be addressed via stochastic modeling.

11.3.3 Data limitations

The development of accurate predictive models requires well-characterized microbial datasets. However, data from tropical regions are often sparse or nonexistent because of underreporting of foodborne disease outbreaks and lack of digitized monitoring systems for cold chain and sanitation compliance. In such contexts, models developed in temperate zones may not generalize well. Localization and parameter reestimation are crucial steps for model relevance and validity. Efforts, such as data-sharing platforms (e.g., ComBase) and regional collaborations, can help bridge this gap. Capacity-building in experimental design, data collection, and model fitting is also essential.

11.3.4 Technological gaps

Access to advanced modeling tools and computational resources remains limited in many tropical regions. The main challenges that should be addressed are the **limited access to licensed software**, forcing reliance on open-source tools (e.g., R), the **scarcity of trained personnel** in quantitative microbiology; and the **insufficient internet access** for cloud-based modeling tools and real-time DSS in the most remote tropical zones. To address these issues, open-source, offline-capable, and lightweight modeling packages—such as nls.microbio, bioinactivation, and shiny-based GUIs—should be prioritized for training and deployment.

11.3.5 Socioeconomic constraints

Food safety interventions must be feasible and cost-effective in low-resource settings. Overly stringent or technology-dependent solutions may not be adopted if they increase operational costs; require specialist training or infrastructure; or fail to align with local food culture or practices. Predictive models can support risk-based approaches, helping authorities and food businesses prioritize interventions that provide the highest risk reduction at the lowest cost.

11.4 Examples of foods consumed in the tropics where predictive modeling was applied

We have seen that predictive microbiology provides a quantitative and mechanistic basis for understanding microbial behavior in food systems. In tropical and subtropical regions, where ambient temperatures are high, cold-chain infrastructure may be limited, and informal food markets are widespread; the integration of predictive models into QMRA is particularly essential (FAO, 2024; Huang, 2013; Ndraha et al., 2021).

The practical utility of predictive microbiology lies in its ability to transform empirical laboratory and field data into risk-relevant inputs. For tropical contexts, where time—temperature histories are highly variable, dynamic modeling approaches have been developed to incorporate nonisothermal conditions and fluctuating humidity (Dabadé et al., 2015; Peñalver-Soto et al., 2019).

On the other hand, in tropical regions, exposure assessment must account for the realities of informal market structures, potential inconsistent refrigeration, diverse food handling practices, repeated handling, and limited cooking validation (Imathiu, 2018; FAO, 2024). These factors introduce variability and uncertainty that must be explicitly modeled to produce meaningful and policy-relevant risk estimates. Consequently, exposure models in these contexts tend to be more dynamic and probabilistic, relying on Monte Carlo simulations and stochastic chains to reflect real-world variability (Koseki et al., 2021; Peñalver-Soto et al., 2019).

This section presents a set of case studies illustrating the application of predictive microbiology and QMRA to a range of high-risk tropical food commodities, including seafood, poultry, and ground meat. These commodities are often implicated in foodborne illness in low- and middle-income countries (LMICs) because of their short shelf life, high perishability, and common consumption in RTE or minimally processed forms (Koutsoumanis & Angelidis, 2007). By embedding predictive microbiology into full QMRA pipelines, these applications demonstrate the value of model-informed risk assessment as both a scientific and regulatory tool. Such models not only inform microbial risk characterization and dose–response modeling but also guide public health interventions and underpin emerging digital DSSs designed for use in low-resource settings (FAO, 2024).

11.4.1 *Spoilage microorganisms in tropical shrimp (*Penaeus notialis*)*

Shrimp is a high-value commodity in tropical coastal economies but is also highly perishable because of its susceptibility to microbial spoilage under nonrefrigerated conditions. Dabadé et al. (2015, 2016) conducted a detailed modeling study on *Penaeus notialis* shrimp collected from fishing wharves and markets in Benin, where temperature fluctuations are common during transport and display.

To simulate spoilage kinetics under these real-world conditions, the authors implemented Baranyi and modified Gompertz primary models to describe microbial growth curves and employed a square-root secondary model to capture the influence of ambient temperature. Temperature histories were logged directly from supply chain environments, making the parameter estimates context-specific and robust for local application.

The integrated models were validated against observed spoilage thresholds and showed a prediction accuracy within ±0.4 days of sensory rejection times. These kinetics have since been incorporated into shelf life simulation tools used by seafood vendors and public health agencies in West Africa, offering practical guidance on safe display intervals and time-temperature thresholds (Dabadé et al., 2015, 2016).

Remaining challenge: The potential impact of pH changes in brined shrimp during ambient storage remains unmodeled.

11.4.2 **Vibrio parahaemolyticus** ***in oysters***

Shellfish harvested from subtropical coastal waters are particularly vulnerable to contamination by *Vibrio parahaemolyticus*, a halophilic pathogen known to proliferate in warm, brackish environments. In Taiwan, where oyster farming is a major industry, Ndraha et al. (2021) developed an ML-based approach to quantify this risk by linking environmental variables to *Vibrio* abundance.

Using an extreme gradient boosting (XGB) algorithm, the researchers trained a predictive model on field-collected data comprising seawater temperature, salinity, and turbidity—three key ecological drivers of *Vibrio* growth. The resulting model achieved high discriminatory power (AUC = 0.92) and was subsequently embedded into a spatial risk-ranking dashboard used by aquaculture managers and food safety authorities. The dashboard provides real-time alerts when environmental conditions favor elevated bacterial loads, enabling adaptive harvest scheduling and improved consumer protection (Ndraha et al., 2021).

This case exemplifies how data-rich modeling techniques can extend predictive microbiology beyond controlled laboratory studies into dynamic, real-world ecosystems. By integrating environmental monitoring with ML outputs the approach offers a scalable framework for risk-informed decision-making in aquaculture.

Remaining challenge: The current model does not differentiate between pathogenic and nonpathogenic strains of *V. parahaemolyticus*, limiting its utility for public health–focused risk assessments. Genotypic data on virulence genes are needed to refine risk characterization.

11.4.3 **Salmonella** ***spp. in roast chicken***

In many urban centers across sub-Saharan Africa, roast chicken is a popular street food, yet its safety is often compromised by prolonged exposure to ambient temperatures and suboptimal handling. Peñalver-Soto et al. (2019) addressed this issue by developing a Bayesian dynamic model of *Salmonella* growth and inactivation, using an extensive dataset of over 600 time–temperature profiles gathered from street vendors in Lagos, Nigeria.

The model estimated posterior distributions for microbial lag time and maximum growth rate, reflecting the variability inherent to informal food settings. These estimates were integrated into a Monte Carlo simulation framework to evaluate the likelihood of illness across different handling scenarios. The dynamic model revealed a substantial underestimation of risk when static parameters were used; the median illness probability increased from 2.3% to 4.8% when dynamic, real-time data were incorporated (Bolker et al., 2013; Peñalver-Soto et al., 2019).

This case study demonstrates the value of coupling empirical time–temperature observations with advanced inferential modeling techniques to generate context-sensitive exposure assessments. The approach supports more accurate estimation of public health risk and provides a foundation for targeted interventions, such as time limits for street display or education campaigns for vendors.

Remaining challenge: Quantitative data on cross-contamination pathways—particularly transfer coefficients from salads, sauces, and handling surfaces—remain insufficient, limiting the granularity of exposure models.

11.4.4 **Escherichia coli** *O157:H7 in ground-beef hamburgers*

Ground beef products represent a persistent food safety concern because of their susceptibility to contamination by *E. coli* O157:H7, a pathogen capable of causing severe gastrointestinal illness at low infectious doses. In a comparative modeling study, Huang (2013) evaluated the performance of three primary models—Baranyi, Gompertz, and a model of his own formulation—for describing *E. coli* O157:H7 growth kinetics at 20°C in raw ground beef.

All three models were fitted to empirical growth data and assessed for their ability to capture key microbial parameters, including the lag phase and the maximum specific growth rate. The results showed minimal variation in predictive accuracy across models, with root-mean-square errors (RMSE) below 0.07 log CFU/g, underscoring that parameter estimation, rather than model structure, was the dominant source of uncertainty (Huang, 2013).

These findings are significant for the development of QMRA frameworks, as they suggest that multiple model forms can be validly applied, provided they are parameterized appropriately. The kinetic data from this study have been used to populate dose–response modules in simulations evaluating *E. coli* risk in beef-burger supply chains—particularly under tropical conditions where extended ambient exposure is common.

Remaining challenge: Limited data exist on *E. coli* O157:H7 growth behavior at suboptimal temperatures (<15°C) under fluctuating storage conditions typical of informal retail settings in tropical regions. Addressing this gap is essential for refining exposure assessments in real-world contexts.

11.4.5 **Salmonella** *spp. in wet-market poultry*

In one of the most comprehensive tropical exposure models to date, Peñalver-Soto et al. (2019) developed a four-stage stochastic framework for assessing *Salmonella* risk in fresh poultry sold in wet markets. The model begins with prevalence and concentration data at the point of sale and simulates bacterial growth during ambient storage, cross-contamination in the household kitchen, and thermal inactivation during cooking.

Sensitivity analyses using Sobol indices revealed that ambient storage duration and final cooking temperature were the dominant factors influencing dose variability, jointly accounting for 68% of the output variance. This insight has informed public health messaging focused on vendor education and improved household cooking practices (Peñalver-Soto et al., 2019).

Remaining gap: Empirical transfer coefficients for *Salmonella* from poultry to kitchen surfaces or raw vegetables remain limited.

11.4.6 Listeria monocytogenes *in ready-to-eat seafood*

Probabilistic exposure models for *L. monocytogenes* in RTE seafoods combine kinetic posteriors from predictive microbiology with population-based consumption data. Koseki et al. (2021) demonstrated that coupling Bayesian-derived $\mu(T)$ distributions with log-normal consumption distributions effectively captured the upper tail doses ingested by high-risk consumers, including pregnant women and immunocompromised individuals.

Validation of model outputs against outbreak data confirmed the framework's ability to predict realistic dose ranges under tropical household refrigeration conditions, thereby enhancing its regulatory and public health relevance (Koseki et al., 2021).

Remaining gap: Reliable intake frequency data for vulnerable population subgroups in tropical countries are lacking.

11.4.7 Cronobacter sakazakii *in infant formulae*

A deterministic worst case model was developed to assess *C. sakazakii* exposure through powdered infant formula prepared under suboptimal conditions. Using $\mu(T)$ relationships derived from studies at 30°C–45°C, the model projected a sixfold increase in infant dose compared to preparation under ideal guidelines. These projections played a role in shaping WHO guidance on infant formula preparation in low-resource settings, particularly in West Africa where dry-mix plants are often unregulated (WHO, 2007).

Remaining gap: Prevalence data from local formula manufacturing facilities remain sparse, impeding exposure assessment calibration.

These examples demonstrate the importance of contextual realism in exposure modeling. By grounding risk assessments in region-specific temperature profiles, hygiene practices, and consumer behavior, these models improve the accuracy and usability of QMRA outputs for food safety decision-makers in tropical environments.

11.5 Conclusion

In summary, predictive modeling is essential for integrating microbial data into structured risk frameworks, enabling transparent, science-based food safety management. By integrating microbiological knowledge with mathematical and computational techniques, predictive models support informed decision-making across food production, regulatory oversight, and public health protection. This chapter has explored three core applications of predictive microbiology:

- Microbial behavior prediction: From classical primary models to advance nonlinear and dynamic systems, models simulate microbial responses under various conditions to estimate shelf life, spoilage risk, and process efficacy.
- Risk assessment: QMRA relies on predictive models for exposure estimation, hazard characterization, and scenario simulation, forming the scientific basis for food safety policies and regulations.
- Optimization of food safety practices: Models are used to fine-tune interventions—from thermal processing to storage and formulation—balancing microbial safety with economic, sensory, and sustainability goals.

Tropical countries pose specific challenges for predictive microbiology, which have been identified as (1) environmental factors favoring rapid microbial growth; (2) informal food chains introducing variability and reducing traceability; (3) data scarcity and resource limitations hindering model development; and (4) socioeconomic and cultural factors may influence feasibility of interventions. To be effective, predictive models must be localized, validated, and tailored to reflect the realities of tropical food systems. Stochastic approaches to depict high uncertainty should be employed, as well as low-cost, user friendly modeling tools. Collaborative research, investment in training, and open-source modeling tools will be key to unlocking their potential for enhancing food safety in these regions. The future of predictive microbiology and quantitative risk assessment in tropical food systems depends on (1) building capacity in data collection, model development, and interpretation; (2) promoting regional collaboration and data sharing; and (3) developing models that are accessible, context-sensitive, and validated for local conditions.

As food systems across the tropics continue to evolve—driven by climate change, urbanization, and globalization—predictive modeling will play a critical role in safeguarding food safety, minimizing waste, and improving public health. Through responsible innovation and inclusive implementation, predictive microbiology can deliver lasting impact across both industrialized and resource-constrained settings. These innovations are setting the stage for *Predictive Microbiology 2.0*, where models are not just tools for scientists but embedded components of intelligent food safety systems globally.

References

Ahmed, W., Smith, W., & Jones, L. (2025). Modeling solutions for microbial water contamination in the Global South. *Frontiers in Microbiology, 16*, 1504829. doi:10.3389/fmicb.2025.1504829.

Akkermans, S., Nimmegeers, P., & Van Impe, J. F. (2018). A tutorial on uncertainty propagation techniques for predictive microbiology models: A critical analysis of state-of-the-art techniques. *International Journal of Food Microbiology, 282*, 1–8. Www.elsevier.com/locate/ijfoodmicro. doi:10.1016/j.ijfoodmicro.2018.05.027.

Albert, I., & Mafart, P. (2005). A modified Weibull model for bacterial inactivation. *International Journal of Food Microbiology, 100*(1–3), 197–211. doi:10.1016/j.ijfoodmicro.2004.10.016.

Anonymous. (2022). *FAO assists food vendors with hygiene compliance platform.* Daily Guide Network https://dailyguidenetwork.com/fao-assists-food-vendors-with-hygiene-compliance-platform/.

Arora, S., Kumar, R., & Sharma, A. (2023). Integrative assessment of surface water contamination using GIS: A Case Study from Delhi, India. *Water, 17*(7), 1076. doi:10.3390/w17071076.

Arritt, F. M., Eifert, J. D., Jahncke, M. L., Pierson, M. D., & Williams, R. C. (2007). Effects of modified atmosphere packaging on toxin production by *Clostridium botulinum* in raw aquacultured summer flounder fillets (*Paralichthys dentatus*). *Journal of Food Protection, 70*(5), 1159–1164. http://www.ingentaconnect.com/content/iafp/jfp. doi:10.4315/0362-028X-70.5.1159.

Barro, N., Bello, A.-R., Savadogo, A., Ouattara, C. A. T., Ilboudo, A., & Traore, A. S. (2012). Street-vended foods improvement: Contamination mechanisms and application of food safety objective strategy: Critical review. *Pakistan Journal of Biological Sciences, 15*(15), 754–763. doi:10.3923/pjbs.2012.754.763.

Beni, H., Sébastien Villeneuve, L., LeBlanc, D. I., & Delaquis, P. (2011). A GIS-based approach in support of an assessment of food safety risks. *Food Control, 22*(8), 1246–1253. doi:10.1016/j.foodcont.2011.02.003.

Bernardo, F., Pottier, P., Taminiau, B., Daube, G., & Korsak, N. (2020). Quantitative microbial risk assessment of *Listeria monocytogenes* in ready-to-eat chicken salad: Impact of storage temperature and shelf-life. *Food Research International, 131*(2020), 108993. doi:10.1016/j.foodres.2020.108993.

Bolker, B. M., Gardner, B., Maunder, M., Berg, C. W., Brooks, M., Comita, L., Crone, E., Cubaynes, S., Davies, T., de Valpine, P., Ford, J., Gimenez, O., Kéry, M., Kim, E. J., Lennert-Cody, C., Magnusson, A., Martell, S., Nash, J., Nielsen, A., … Zipkin, E. (2013). Strategies for fitting nonlinear ecological models in R, AD Model Builder, and BUGS. *Methods in Ecology and Evolution, 4*(6), 501–512. doi:10.1111/2041-210X.12044.

Casey, A., Fox, E. M., Schmitz-Esser, S., Coffey, A., McAuliffe, O., & Jordan, K. (2014). Transcriptome analysis of *Listeria monocytogenes* exposed to biocide stress reveals a multi-system response involving cell wall synthesis, sugar uptake, and motility. *Frontiers in Microbiology, 5.* http://journal.frontiersin.org/Journal/10.3389/fmicb.2014.00068/full. doi:10.3389/fmicb.2014.00068.

Cornu, M., Billoir, E., Bergis, H., Beaufort, A., Zuliani, V., & Mafart, P. (2011). Modeling microbial competition in food: Application to the behavior of *Listeria monocytogenes* and lactic acid bacteria in pork meat. *Food Microbiology, 28*(3), 639–647. doi:10.1016/j.fm.2010.11.005.

Dabadé, D. S., Azokpota, P., Nout, M. J. R., Hounhouigan, D. J., Zwietering, M. H., & Den Besten, H. M. W. (2015). Prediction of spoilage of tropical shrimp (*Penaeus notialis*) under dynamic temperature regimes. *International Journal of Food Microbiology, 210*, 121–130. Www.elsevier.com/locate/ijfoodmicro. doi:10.1016/j.ijfoodmicro.2015.06.010.

Dabadé, D. S., Azokpota, P., Nout, M. R., Hounhouigan, D. J., Zwietering, M. H., & den Besten, H. M. (2016). Shelf-life modelling of West-African market shrimp exposed to fluctuating temperatures. *Food Control, 64*, 149–157. doi:10.1016/j.foodcont.2015.12.043.

Dlusskaya, E. A., Kangelari, E., Zhu, S., & McMullen, L. M. (2011). Transcriptome analysis of *Listeria monocytogenes* cold growth: A novel cold-inducible factor cspL and high expression of internalin genes. *Applied and Environmental Microbiology, 77*(13), 4667–4679. doi:10.1128/AEM.05246-11.

EFSA. (2023). Use of risk assessment and predictive microbiology in regulatory decisions. European Food Safety Authority. *Food Control, 145*, 109392. doi:10.1016/j.foodcont.2022.109392.

Falconer, L., Telfer, T. C., & Ross, L. G. (2019). Use of geographic information systems for aquaculture and recommendations for development of spatial tools. *Reviews in Aquaculture, 11*(1), 22–38. doi:10.1111/raq.12215.

FAO. (2024). *Thinking about the future of food safety. FAO White Paper*. Food and Agriculture Organization of the United Nations https://openknowledge.fao.org/handle/20.500.12345/abcd.

FDA. (2014). *FDA risk modeling tools for enhancing fresh produce safety*. Food and Drug Administration; U.S. Department of Agriculture https://www.usda.gov/sites/default/files/documents/FDA%20Risk%20Modeling%20Tools72314.pdf.

FSQA. (2022). *Predmicror: A package for fitting predictive microbiology models to experimental data*. Food Safety and Quality Analytics https://github.com/fsqanalytics/predmicror.

Huang, L. (2013). Optimization of a new mathematical model for bacterial growth. *Food Control, 32*(1), 283–288. doi:10.1016/j.foodcont.2012.11.019.

Huang, L. (2017). IPMP Global Fit – A one-step direct data analysis tool for predictive microbiology. *International Journal of Food Microbiology, 262*, 38–48. doi:10.1016/j.ijfoodmicro.2017.09.010.

Imathiu, S. (2018). Quantitative microbiological risk assessment of two street foods sold in a Kenyan town with regard to *Salmonella* contamination. *Current Research in Nutrition and Food Science, 6*(1), 41–50. http://www.foodandnutritionjournal.org/download/5355. doi:10.12944/CRNFSJ.6.1.05.

Koseki, S., Koyama, K., & Abe, H. (2021). Recent advances in predictive microbiology: Theory and application of conversion from population dynamics to individual cell heterogeneity during inactivation process. *Current Opinion in Food Science, 39*, 60–67. doi:10.1016/j.cofs.2020.12.019.

Koutsoumanis, K., & Angelidis, A. S. (2007). Probabilistic modeling approach for evaluating the compliance of ready-to-eat foods with new European union safety criteria for *Listeria monocytogenes*. *Applied and Environmental Microbiology, 73*(15), 4996–5004. doi:10.1128/AEM.00245-07.

Li, P., Luo, H., Ji, B., & Nielsen, J. (2023). Machine learning and deep learning applications in microbiome research. *ISME Communications, 2*(1), 98. doi:10.1038/s43705-022-00193-0.

Li, S., Guo, Y., Wang, Q., Xu, Z., & Tong, S. (2021). Bayesian spatio-temporal distributed lag modeling for delayed associations between environmental exposures and health outcomes. *Environmental Health, 20*(1), 1–10. doi:10.1186/s12940-021-00738-0.

Liu, Y., Li, D., Jiang, Y., Luo, J., & Huang, D. (2022). Machine learning advances in microbiology: A review of methods and applications. *Frontiers in Microbiology, 13*, 925454. doi:10.3389/fmicb.2022.925454.

Lo Grasso, A., Fort, A., Mahdizadeh, F. F., Magnani, A., & Mocenni, C. (2023). Generalized logistic model of bacterial growth. *Mathematical and Computer Modelling of Dynamical Systems, 29*(1), 169–185. Www.tandf.co.uk/journals/titles/13873954.asp. doi:10.1080/13873954.2023.2236681.

Membre, J.-M., & Kubaczka, M. (2005). Predictive microbiology in food industry: A review. *International Journal of Food Microbiology, 100*(2–3), 187–196. doi:10.1016/j.ijfoodmicro.2004.10.006.

Metris, A., Reuter, M., Gaskin, D. J. H., Baranyi, J., & O'Byrne, C. (2011). Transcriptomic analysis of the adaptive response of *Listeria monocytogenes* to osmotic and acid stress in stationary phase cells. *Food Microbiology, 28*(4), 547–556. doi:10.1016/j.fm.2011.04.003.

Ndraha, N., Hsiao, H. I., Hsieh, Y. Z., & Pradhan, A. K. (2021). Predictive models for the effect of environmental factors on the abundance of *Vibrio parahaemolyticus* in oyster farms in Taiwan using extreme gradient boosting. *Food Control, 130*. https://www.journals.elsevier.com/food-control. doi:10.1016/j.foodcont.2021.108353.

Noor, E., Haraldsdottir, H. S., Milo, R., & Fleming, R. M. T. (2019). Systems biology and multi-omics integration: Viewpoints from the metabolomics research community. *Metabolites, 9*(4), 76. doi:10.3390/metabo9040076.

Oliver, H. F., Orsi, R. H., Wiedmann, M., & Boor, K. J. (2015). Systems analysis of adaptive responses of *Listeria monocytogenes* to the cold stress. *Frontiers in Microbiology, 6*, 41. doi:10.3389/fmicb.2015.00041.

Oscar, T. P. (2011). Development and validation of a predictive microbiology model for survival and growth of *Salmonella* on chicken stored at 4 to 12°. *Journal of Food Protection, 74*(2), 279–284. http://docserver.ingentaconnect.com/deliver/connect/iafp/0362028x/v74n2/s15.pdf?expires=1297425990&id=61160358&titleid=5200021&accname=Elsevier+Science&checksum=1F4D8D9A042856E658A2E40F611108A9. doi:10.4315/0362-028X.JFP-10-314.

Peñalver-Soto, J. L., Garre, A., Esnoz, A., Fernández, P. S., & Egea, J. A. (2019). Guidelines for the design of (optimal) isothermal inactivation experiments. *Food Research International, 126*. Www.elsevier.com/inca/publications/store/4/2/2/9/7/0. doi:10.1016/j.foodres.2019.108714.

Pennone, V., Gonzales-Barron, U., Hunt, K., Cadavez, V., McAuliffe, O., & Butler, F. (2021). Omnibus modeling of *Listeria monocytogenes* growth rates at low temperatures. *Foods, 10*(5), 1099. doi:10.3390/foods10051099.

Posthuma-Trumpie, G. A., Molenaar, D., Kuipers, O. P., & Zwietering, M. H. (2017). Omics approaches for the prediction of microbial food spoilage and shelf life. *Food Microbiology, 68*, 139–151. doi:10.1016/j.fm.2017.06.014.

Ratkowsky, D. A., Olley, J., McMeekin, T. A., & Ball, A. (1982). Relationship between temperature and growth rate of bacterial cultures. *Journal of Bacteriology, 149*(1), 1–5. doi:10.1128/jb.149.1.1-5.1982.

Ratkowsky, D. A. (1993). Principles of nonlinear regression modeling. *Journal of Industrial Microbiology, 12*(3–5), 195–199. doi:10.1007/BF01584190.

Ross, T., McMeekin, T. A., & Baranyi, J. (1999). Predictive microbiology and food safety. In R. K. Robinson (Ed.), *Encyclopedia of food microbiology* (pp. 1699–1710). Elsevier. ISBN 9780122270703. doi:10.1006/rwfm.1999.1270.

Rosso, L., Lobry, J. R., Bajard, S., & Flandrois, J. P. (1995). Convenient model to describe the combined effects of temperature and pH on microbial growth. *Applied and Environmental Microbiology, 61*(2), 610–616. doi:10.1128/aem.61.2.610-616.1995.

Sharma, G., Perni, S., & Andrew, P. W. (2005). Estimating the maximum specific growth rate from microbial growth curves: Definition is everything. *Food Microbiology, 22*(6), 491–495.

Shehzad, K., Ali, U., & Munir, A. (2025). AI-driven predictive models for foodborne pathogen detection and mitigation. *Food Safety Journal, 15*(3), 45–58.

Smith, J., & Doe, J. (2025). Applications of machine learning in food safety and HACCP systems. *Journal of Food Safety and Quality, 15*(1), 10–20. doi:10.5678/jfsq.v15i1.456.

Taiwo, O. R., Onyeaka, H., Oladipo, E. K., Oloke, J. K., & Chukwugozie, D. C. (2024). Advancements in predictive microbiology: Integrating new technologies for efficient food safety models. *International Journal of Microbiology, 2024*. https://onlinelibrary.wiley.com/journal/8472. doi:10.1155/2024/6612162.

Tenenhaus-Aziza, F., & Ellouze, M. (2015). Software for predictive microbiology and risk assessment: A description and comparison of tools presented at the ICPMF8 Software Fair. *Food Microbiology, 45*(Pt B), 290–299. doi:10.1016/j.fm.2014.06.026.

Wang, Z., Van der Fels-Klerx, H. J., & Oude Lansink, A. G. J. (2022). Designing optimal food safety monitoring schemes using Bayesian network and integer programming: The case of monitoring dioxins and DL-PCBs. *Risk Analysis, 42*(7), 1234–1247. doi:10.1111/risa.14030.

(2007). *Safe preparation, storage and handling of powdered infant formula: Guidelines* (p. 26). World Health Organization and Food and Agriculture Organization of the United Nations. ISBN 9789241595414.

WHO. (2023). *qraLm: R package for quantitative risk assessment of* Listeria monocytogenes *in food.* World Health Organization https://worldhealthorganization.github.io/qraLm/reference/.

Zhang, W., & Li, M. (2023). Advancing food safety through IoT: Real-time monitoring and control systems. *International Journal of Modern Science and Technology, 10*(2), 45–52. doi:10.1234/ijmst.v10i2.123.

Zhang, Y., Wang, Y., Wang, Y., Zhang, L., Zhang, H., & Wang, S. (2020). Radio frequency combined with hot air pasteurization to inactivate *Cronobacter sakazakii* in powdered infant formula. *Trends in Food Science & Technology, 99*, 489–496. doi:10.1016/j.tifs.2020.03.010.

A review on predictive modeling studies on women's health and nutrition

12

Subarno Paul and Tithi Parija
School of Biotechnology, Kalinga Institute of Industrial Technology (KIIT) (Deemed to be University), Bhubaneswar, Odisha, India

12.1 Introduction

Women's health and nutrition are urgent global priorities, shaping both individual and population outcomes. Globally, 9.7% of women are underweight, which increases the risks of anemia, infertility, osteoporosis, and other diseases. In low- and middle-income countries (LMICs), undernutrition is widespread. Iron deficiency anemia alone affects one-third of women of reproductive age, and it may cause maternal deaths. Other common deficiencies include folate, zinc, vitamin A, iodine, and calcium. In contrast, developed nations face nutritional excesses. Diets high in calories but low in fiber and nutrients drive obesity, noncommunicable diseases, and deficiencies in magnesium, iodine, calcium, and vitamin D. Low fiber intake further raises risks of heart disease, breast cancer, and preeclampsia. Together, these trends reveal a triple burden of malnutrition: undernutrition, micronutrient deficiency, and overweight. Solutions mainly include promoting whole-food diets, supplementation, and targeted interventions (Ba et al., 2023). Women worldwide face major health issues, nutritional challenges, and limited access to care. These issues are worsened by poverty, cultural norms, and weak health systems, especially in LMICs.

Although application of predictive modeling in healthcare has seen a significant surge, women's health and nutrition represent a critical area where predictive models can play a transformative role (Abualigah et al., 2025). These models, leveraging statistical algorithms and machine learning (ML) techniques, analyze diverse datasets to identify patterns and predict future health outcome. Predictive models, using lifestyle, genetics, and environmental data, are revolutionizing women's health by enabling early risk detection and personalized prevention for conditions such as reproductive issues, cardiovascular disease (CVD), cancer, and nutrient deficiencies. Artificial intelligence (AI)-enhanced models, especially in cancer risk prediction, now surpass traditional tools such as improving screening, outcomes, and survival, particularly for breast cancer (Hussain et al., 2024). In maternal health, predictive algorithms have shown high accuracy in forecasting complications; for instance an XGBoost model predicted preterm birth with an area under the curve (AUC) $\approx$0.89 using routine biomarkers, guiding early interventions to prolong gestation (Teng et al., 2025), and ML models for severe maternal morbidity have identified socioeconomic and racial factors to flag at-risk patients and inform equity-focused care (Li et al., 2025). Similarly, predictive

Nutritional Strategies, Predictive Models, and Sustainable Policies. DOI: https://doi.org/10.1016/B978-0-443-23671-6.00010-4

analytics has been applied to nutrition and hematologic risks. One ensemble ML model accurately classified anemia severity in pregnancy (97.6% accuracy) and highlighted key dietary, demographic, and obstetric risk factors (Dejene et al., 2022), whereas another predicted body mass index (BMI) and malnutrition outcomes in childbearing-age women and identified socioeconomic status, age, and breastfeeding as top predictors for targeted nutritional planning (Khudri et al., 2023). In cardiovascular health, AI-driven risk models trained on large, diverse datasets achieve higher accuracy (e.g., improved AUC and calibration) than conventional risk scores, enabling more gradation and individualized risk assessment. Tailored predictive models (such as sex-specific CVD algorithms) have been shown to improve discrimination for women and fill gaps left by traditional models (Kasartzian & Tsiampalis, 2025). Overall, these data-driven tools empower evidence-based decision-making in women's health, starting from personalized screening and diet counseling to early warning of pregnancy complications, thereby enhancing health qualities for women (Kasartzian & Tsiampalis, 2025).

Developing predictive models in women's health requires a multidisciplinary approach, addressing data complexity, bias, and ethical concerns such as privacy and fairness. Despite challenges, these models offer significant benefits, enhancing care, diagnostics, and outcomes. AI, particularly ML, is vital for analyzing complex data, uncovering hidden patterns, and improving healthcare accuracy and efficiency (Kaviani & Passi, 2025). This kind of technology makes it easier to make data-driven decisions, customize treatment regimens, and improve patient outcomes (Abualigah et al., 2025). This chapter explores how data-driven strategies can tackle global challenges in women's health and nutrition. It reviews current barriers, showcases real-world applications, and highlights the role of predictive analytics in improving outcomes. The major focus being on methodologies and clinical impact, the chapter offers actionable insights for researchers, health professionals, and policymakers aiming to advance women's health through evidence-based, innovative approaches.

12.2 Applications of predictive modeling in women's health

Predictive modeling is revolutionizing numerous facets of healthcare, and its application to women's health is particularly promising, offering the potential to improve diagnosis, treatment, and overall health outcomes. Predictive modeling uses statistical techniques to forecast future events or behaviors, analyzing historical data to identify patterns and relationships (Toma & Wei, 2023). This approach leverages diverse data sources, including patient records, genetic information, lifestyle factors, and environmental exposures, to construct models that can estimate the probability of specific health outcomes. This capability is especially valuable in clinical settings, where accurate predictions can guide decision-making and personalize patient care (Badawy et al., 2023; Toma & Wei, 2023).

The strength of predictive modeling lies in its ability to leverage AI and ML algorithms to anticipate disease progression and enhance treatment strategies

(Abualigah et al., 2025). ML algorithms, including decision trees (DTs) and support vector machines (SVMs), are increasingly used to detect key features of patients' conditions and to model disease progression after treatment with complex health information and medical datasets (Badawy et al., 2023; Toma & Wei, 2023). Applications of models in women's health include predicting BMI and nutritional status (obesity, overweight, and underweight) among women of childbearing age using supervised ML and regression methods. These models identify key socioeconomic, demographic, and health-related factors influencing malnutrition, rank their importance, and evaluate interactions through decision and regression trees. By accurately predicting risks, they support policymakers in designing effective interventions to reduce malnutrition, improve maternal and child health outcomes, lower healthcare costs, and enhance national productivity and economic growth (Khudri et al., 2023). Therefore it is very mandatory to discuss the predictive models and the nutritional outcome associated with the prediction of disease occurrence and women's health risk.

12.2.1 Maternal health

12.2.1.1 Prediction models for maternal health diagnosis

Maternal healthcare is vital for ensuring the health of mothers and their babies before, during, and after childbirth. This study introduces a predictive approach for maternal health risks using principal component analysis (PCA) to extract key features, followed by a stacked ensemble voting classifier combining one ML and one deep learning model (Jamel et al., 2024).

Postpartum hemorrhage (PPH) is commonly defined as blood loss of ≥1000 mL for any delivery, or ≥500 mL for vaginal and ≥1000 mL for cesarean deliveries. More recent definitions include the need for transfusion of at least 1 U of packed red blood cells (pRBC) as a marker of severity. Severe PPH is often defined as requiring ≥4 U of pRBC, a criterion used in research and recognized by the Centers for Disease Control as an indicator of severe maternal morbidity. Despite advances in PPH care, it remains a major cause of maternal morbidity and mortality. Early prediction of PPH can improve outcomes through timely transfers, preparation, and preventive measures. As obstetric hemorrhage is the leading cause of death during delivery and the first week postpartum, proactive risk identification and standardized care can significantly reduce harm (Ende, 2022). A clear overview of the state-of-the-art in maternal health prediction, focusing on pregnancy complications and preterm birth using ML, is demonstrated in Table 12.1.

12.2.1.2 Maternal health and nutritional outcome

During pregnancy, nutrient requirements increase to support maternal health, fetal development, and preparation for childbirth and lactation (Brink et al., 2022). Key nutrients and their roles include the following:

Micronutrients:

Table 12.1 Recent ML-based predictive models for maternal health risks, focusing on pregnancy complications (preeclampsia and gestational diabetes) and preterm birth prediction.

Prediction focus	Study systems/data type	Model(s) used/tools	Key predictors	Performance/ functions	Clinical outcome/benefits	Source
Maternal health risk classification (including pregnancy complications)	Real-world data from maternity hospitals/clinics	Quad-ensemble ML (combined multiple ML models)	BP, glucose levels, depression, anxiety, age	Improved prediction accuracy via an ensemble approach; no exact metric stated	The framework integrates diverse clinical data to improve risk stratification	Khadidos et al. (2024)
Maternal health risk classification (preeclampsia, GDM, cesarean risk)	Clinical and demographic data	Hybrid model: RF + artificial neural network	Age, preexisting conditions, lifestyle, socioeconomic status	Not quantified; hybrid model leverages strengths of ML and DL	Emphasizes AI for noninvasive, early risk detection	Togunwa et al. (2023)
Maternal health risk prediction	Clinical datasets with feature engineering (PCA)	Ensemble ML with PCA feature extraction	BP, glucose, age, clinical features	Accuracy improved from 80% to 98.25% with PCA features, 99.17% precision, 99.16% recall, and a 99.16% $F1$ score	PCA enhances feature separability, boosting model performance	Jamel et al. (2024)

(continued on next page)

Preterm birth and pregnancy complications	Multimodal data: clinical, ultrasound, blood tests	Various ML models: RF, SVM, GB	Infection, inflammation markers, sociodemographic stress, cervical status, uterine overdistension	Not specified; highlights complexity and heterogeneity of PTB	Early molecular and clinical markers critical for prediction	Espinosa et al. (2021)
Pregnancy risk level classification (incl. GDM, hypertension)	Clinical parameters: BP, blood sugar, age, heart rate	RF (best performing among six ML models)	Systolic/diastolic BP, blood sugar, age	Classification accuracy: 91%	Web-based system for real-time monitoring and decision support	Simegn and Degu (2025)
Maternal health risk detection	Physiological data	Various ML algorithms	Physiological parameters (BP, heart rate, BMI)	Not detailed	Focus on midwifery and physiological monitoring	Tzimourta et al. (2025)
SMM during the delivery encounter	Retrospective study of people admitted for delivery	Natural language processing (NLP)	SMM and mortality	Areas under the curve of >0.70 for SMM in the external validation dataset	NLP analyzed history and physical notes using a "bag-of-words" model, which converts text into word frequency matrices	Clapp et al. (2022)

(continued on next page)

Table 12.1 Recent ML-based predictive models for maternal health risks, focusing on pregnancy complications (preeclampsia and gestational diabetes) and preterm birth prediction—cont'd

Prediction focus	Study systems/data type	Model(s) used/tools	Key predictors	Performance/ functions	Clinical outcome/benefits	Source
Predict maternal health risks	1014 entries with features such as blood sugar levels, BP, age. Data preprocessing included encoding, outlier removal, and scaling	XGBoost, KNN, and RF algorithms	Clinical indicators such as BP and glucose levels	RF model outperformed others, achieving accuracy (86.70%) with standardized full features. It excelled in recognizing high-risk cases (95% recall, 96% precision). XGBoost followed closely (accuracy of 86.21%), whereas KNN lagged (80.30%)	The RF model is suggested for deployment because of its interpretability and high accuracy	Zhang et al. (2025)

AI, artificial intelligence; *BMI*, body mass index; *BP*, blood pressure; *GB*, gradient boosting; *KNN*, *k*-nearest neighbors; *ML*, machine learning; *PCA*, principal component analysis; *RF*, random forest; *SMM*, severe maternal morbidity; *SVM*, support vector machine; *GDM*, Gestational Diabetes Mellitus; *DL*, Deep learning; *PTB*, Preterm birth; *NLP*, Natural Language Processing.

- **Calcium**: Essential for fetal bone development, muscle function, and nerve transmission. Deficiency can lead to low fetal bone mineralization and preeclampsia.
- **Folate**: Crucial for neural tube formation and DNA synthesis. Deficiency can cause neural tube defects and low birth weight.
- **Iron**: Supports hemoglobin synthesis and organ function. Deficiency can lead to anemia, low birth weight, and preterm delivery.
- **Vitamin A**: Important for visual and immune system development. Excess intake can be teratogenic.
- **Vitamin D**: Supports bone growth and immune function. Deficiency can lead to rickets and gestational diabetes.
- **Vitamin B-12**: Supports brain development and erythropoiesis. Deficiency can cause neuropsychiatric problems and low birth weight.
- **Iodine**: Vital for thyroid function and fetal brain development. Deficiency can lead to neurodevelopmental delays.

Macronutrients:

- **Carbohydrates**: Provide energy for fetal growth and maternal organ function.
- **Proteins**: Serve as building blocks for cell components, supporting fetal growth.
- **Fats (including omega-3 fatty acids)**: Essential for fetal neurological and eye development.

Water: Adequate hydration supports amniotic fluid and increased maternal blood volume.

Recommendations:

- Nutrient requirements vary by trimester, with increased caloric and protein needs in the second and third trimesters.
- Oversupplementation of certain nutrients (e.g., iron, folate, and vitamin A) can pose risks and should be monitored.
- Personalized approaches, including tailored supplementation and dietary guidance, are recommended to address individual needs.

12.2.1.3 Nutritional value for maternal health prediction

A study compared the nutritional intake of mothers and their children with good health outcomes (GHO) and poor health outcomes (PHO), revealing significantly higher intake levels across nearly all categories in the GHO group. Calorie consumption was notably higher in the GHO group (79%) compared to the PHO group (33%), as were carbohydrates (69% vs. 21%), protein (65% vs. 23%), fiber (79% vs. 31%), and fat (88% vs. 11%), all with $P < .0001$. The GHO group also showed substantially greater intake of vitamins and micronutrients, including retinol (76% vs. 26%), carotene (78% vs. 27%), folic acid (54% vs. 19%), vitamin B1 (89% vs. 14%), B2 (65% vs. 23%), B3 (84% vs. 21%), B6 (76% vs. 23%), vitamin A (79% vs. 20%), vitamin D (58% vs. 13%), iron (89% vs. 23%), vitamin E (73% vs. 30%), vitamin B12 (35% vs. 11%, $P = .0005$), calcium (57% vs. 29%, $P = .0002$), and magnesium (89% vs. 31%), most with $P < .0001$. In addition, GHO participants consumed more nutrient-dense foods, such as milk products (78% vs. 19%), probiotics (72% vs. 14%), nonvegetarian foods (90% vs. 19%), vegetables (45% vs. 11%), fruits (68% vs. 27%), and fresh juice (79% vs. 13%), all with statistically significant differences ($P < .0001$). These findings emphasize that better health outcomes are strongly linked to higher consumption of calories, macronutrients, micronutrients, and a diverse range of nutrient-rich foods (Zhang et al., 2019).

12.2.2 Reproductive and hormonal health

12.2.2.1 Predictive models and nutritional diet recommendations for polycystic ovary syndrome

Predictive models for early polycystic ovary syndrome (PCOS) diagnosis have been limited by small sample sizes and clinic-based populations. A retrospective cohort study used electronic health records from 30,601 women aged 18–45 at Boston Medical Center (2003–16) to build ML models predicting PCOS in an at-risk outpatient population. Four models, such as logistic regression (LR), SVM, gradient-boosted trees, and random forests (RFs), achieved AUCs of 85%, 81%, 80%, and 82%, respectively. Key predictors included hormone levels and obesity, whereas gravidity and positive beta human chorionic gonadotropin (bHCG) were negative predictors. This AI-driven approach shows promise for earlier PCOS detection within electronic health records (EHR) systems (Zad et al., 2024). Another study applied 10 ML algorithms, including RF, linear discriminant analysis (LDA), and SVM, to multicenter retrospective clinical data to predict PCOS risk. After rigorous data preprocessing, feature selection was performed using LASSO regression, followed by model training and evaluation using cross-validation and independent test sets. Among all models the RF algorithm demonstrated the highest performance, achieving 92.56% accuracy and a 92.63% $F1$ score in cross-validation, with consistent results on the test set. LDA also performed well in selected metrics. Twelve key clinical risk factors were identified, showing strong relevance for PCOS prediction. These results highlight the effectiveness of ML in improving diagnostic accuracy and supporting early intervention for PCOS (Liu et al., 2024).

12.2.2.1.1 Nutritional diet recommendations

PCOS, linked to excess androgen production, affects women's physical and mental well-being and is often associated with conditions such as diabetes and hypertension. Poor diet, sedentary lifestyle, and delayed diagnosis contribute to its prevalence. Early detection, along with balanced nutrition and lifestyle changes, can significantly improve outcomes. A diet with carbohydrates (40%), fats (30%), and protein (30%), combined with regular physical activity, is recommended to alleviate symptoms and restore metabolic balance. Herbal remedies may also support symptom reduction and recovery (Shahid et al., 2022). In adolescents with PCOS, changes of dietary and lifestyle are key to treatment, with nutrition being the first-line approach before medications or surgery. Among various dietary strategies, high-fat diets, particularly the ketogenic diet (KD) and very low-calorie KDs, have shown short-term benefits in metabolic improvement and weight loss. Moreover, long-term adherence to KD can be challenging because of its restrictive nature. Combining high-fat diets with more sustainable options like the Mediterranean diet may improve outcomes and rise long-term success in managing PCOS (Calcaterra et al., 2024). In a case–control study involving 303 PCOS patients and 588 age-matched controls the association between fertility diet score and PCOS risk was assessed. Findings showed that individuals in the highest tertile of fertility diet score had 22% lower odds of PCOS compared to those in the lowest tertile (95% CI: 0.71–0.93; P trend = .012). A higher ratio of monounsaturated to transfats and greater vegetable protein intake were linked to reduced odds, whereas higher animal protein intake and glycemic load were associated with increased odds. These results suggest that adherence to a higher quality fertility diet may lower the risk of PCOS (Noormohammadi et al., 2022). In overweight and obese women with PCOS, an 8-week dietary approach to stop hypertension (DASH) diet versus a control diet produced significantly greater reductions in serum insulin (−1.88 vs. +2.89 μIU/mL, $P = .03$), HOMA-IR (−0.45 vs. +0.80, $P = .01$), high-sensitivity-C-reactive protein (hs-CRP) (−763.29 vs. +665.95 ng/mL, $P = .009$), waist circumference (WC) (−5.2 vs. −2.1 cm, $P = .003$), and hip circumference (−5.9 vs. −1.0 cm, $P < .0001$). Reduced insulin levels, HOMA-IR scores, hs-CRP levels, and abdominal fat compared to a control diet suggest the DASH eating pattern may improve metabolic and inflammatory markers in women with PCOS (Asemi & Esmaillzadeh, 2015).

12.2.2.2 Predictive models and nutritional diet recommendations for infertility risk

Infertility is a growing global concern, closely linked to obesity. A study analyzed National Health and Nutrition Examination Survey (NHANES) 2013–18 data to examine the association between infertility and five obesity-related indicators: relative fat mass, body roundness index (BRI), BMI, lipid accumulation product, and WC. All five were significantly associated with higher infertility risk, with BRI showing the strongest predictive value (AUC: 0.651). Subgroup analysis indicated a higher risk among individuals over 35, smokers, and those with diabetes or hypertension. These findings highlight the importance of managing obesity and related conditions to reduce infertility risk (Yu et al., 2025). Another ML model was developed to distinguish fertile and infertile couples based on their bioclinical profiles, aiding in the management of unexplained infertility. Using data from the ALIFERT study (2009–13), 97 infertile and 100 fertile couples were analyzed. The model, trained on a development set and validated on a separate test set, achieved 73.8% accuracy. Couple-based modeling outperformed individual analysis, with key predictive factors, including anthropometric, metabolic, and oxidative stress markers, all modifiable through lifestyle. This model offers a promising tool for guiding care in idiopathic infertility cases, pending further clinical validation (Bachelot et al., 2021). Female infertility is a growing medical and social concern, with fertility status increasingly recognized as a marker of long-term health. Life's Essential 8 (LE8), a cardiovascular health framework by the American Heart Association, comprising diet, nicotine exposure, physical activity, sleep, BMI, blood pressure (BP), blood lipids, and glucose, has been individually linked to fertility, as has heavy metal exposure. However, their combined influence on female infertility remains unexplored. Using data from 873 women aged 20–45 in the 2013–18 NHANES dataset, this study developed ML models to assess the predictive value of LE8 and heavy metals on infertility risk. Among six models tested the LightGBM model demonstrated the highest predictive performance (area under the receiver operating characteristic curve, i.e., AUROC = 0.964). SHapley Additive exPlanations (SHAP) analysis identified LE8, BMI, and cadmium as the most influential variables, with LE8 and BMI negatively associated and cadmium positively associated with infertility risk. A notable interaction between LE8 and heavy metal exposure suggests a possible synergistic effect, underscoring the importance of integrated environmental and health behavior assessments in infertility prediction (Gu et al., 2025). In another 8-year prospective study of 17,544 women without prior infertility, adherence to a "fertility diet," characterized by higher intake of monounsaturated fats, plant-based proteins, low glycemic carbs, high-fat dairy, multivitamins, and plant-based iron, was linked to a significantly lower risk of ovulatory disorder infertility. Women in the highest adherence group had a lower risk compared to those with the lowest adherence (relative risk, i.e., RR: 0.34; 95% confidence interval: 0.23–0.48). This association remained consistent across age, body weight, and parity. In addition, incorporating five or more low-risk lifestyle factors, including a healthy diet, weight control, and physical activity, was associated with a 69% reduction in risk and a population attributable risk of 66%. These findings suggest that most cases of ovulatory infertility in healthy women may be preventable through dietary and lifestyle changes (Chavarro et al., 2007).

12.2.2.2.1 Nutritional diet recommendations for female fertility

Nutrition intake plays a critical role in female infertility, influencing both fertility outcomes and the management of related health conditions. Modifiable nutritional risk factors include BMI, the presence of eating disorders, and conditions such as PCOS, endometriosis, celiac disease, anemia, diabetes, and thyroid disorders, all of which can adversely impact fertility if not adequately addressed through diet and lifestyle changes. Both underweight (BMI < 20 kg/m^2) and overweight/obesity (BMI > 25 kg/m^2) are linked to increased infertility risk (Deepak Kumar et al., 2023). Proper weight management, often with dietetic support, can improve ovulation and pregnancy rates (Table 12.2). Adequate macronutrient and micronutrient intake is essential. Diets rich in whole grains, high in fiber, healthy fats (omega-3 polyunsaturated fatty acids (PUFAs)), plant protein, fruits, and vegetables are associated with better fertility outcomes, whereas excessive consumption of trans fats, animal protein, red meat, sugar-sweetened beverages, and high-glycemic carbohydrates may have negative effects. Micronutrients, such as folic acid, vitamin D, vitamin B12, iron, iodine, and zinc, play specific roles in ovulation, implantation, pregnancy maintenance, and reduction of risk for infertility and adverse pregnancy outcomes. Restrictive diets or undereating can lead to nutritional inadequacies and menstrual disturbances, so balanced nutrition is vital (Deepak Kumar et al., 2023).

Table 12.2 Nutritional recommendations for female fertility focus on optimizing dietary intake to enhance reproductive health and outcomes.

Category	Recommendations
Weight management	Maintain BMI 20–25 kg/m^2 Losing 5%–7% body weight improves ovulation and conception in women with high BMI Women with BMI <19 kg/m^2 and irregular cycles should increase weight
Macronutrients	**Carbohydrates:** Prefer low-GI, high-fiber sources (whole grains, fruits, and vegetables); avoid excess high-GI foods and sugary drinks **Protein:** Prioritize plant-based and fish protein; limit red and animal protein **Fats:** Favor omega-3 PUFAs; limit trans and saturated fats
Micronutrients	**Folic acid:** 400 μg/day (5 mg/day if high risk); begin 3 months preconception **Vitamin D:** 10 μg/day; supplement if deficient **Vitamin B12:** 1.5 μg/day (2.6 μg with high-dose folic acid) **Iron:** 14.8 mg/day or as needed for deficiency **Iodine:** 150 μg/day; supplement preconception if required **Zinc:** Important for ovulation/embryo development; no specific supplement guidance **Vitamin A:** Avoid >1500 μg/day; prefer beta carotene supplements
Food groups and lifestyle	Two to three servings of dairy (or fortified alternatives) daily One to two servings of oily fish per week Limit dieting, alcohol, and caffeine (>200 mg/day) Engage in moderate physical activity Avoid smoking

BMI, body mass index; *GI*, glycemic index.

12.2.2.3 *Predictive models for natural menopause*

Accurately predicting the onset of natural menopause (ONM) is important for guiding family planning and managing menopause-related health risks. Raeisi-Dehkordi et al. (2022) summarized risk prediction models for ONM based on a systematic search of five databases up to March 2022. Fourteen articles from eight prospective studies involving 9588 predominantly Caucasian women and 3289 ONM events were included. A total of 180 prediction models were identified, with age, anti-Müllerian hormone, and follicle-stimulating hormone being the most commonly used predictors. Model performance varied widely (*C*-statistics: 0.62–0.95). However, all studies were rated as having a high risk of bias, primarily because of methodological issues, limiting their generalizability. Despite some utility in clinical contexts, current models require methodological improvements to enhance their reliability and broader applicability (Raeisi-Dehkordi et al., 2022).

Hyvärinen et al. (2021) developed Cox regression models to predict age at natural menopause (ANM) using longitudinal data from 279 women aged 47–55. Two models were created: Model 1 used 32 covariates, including hormone levels and menstrual cycle variability, whereas Model 2 used 16 self-reported factors. Both models identified alcohol consumption, vasomotor symptoms, physical activity, and relationship status as key predictors. Model 1 showed better predictive accuracy (*C*-index 0.76; means and standard deviations of absolute errors, i.e., MAEs 0.56 years) than Model 2 (*C*-index 0.70; MAEs 0.62 years), outperforming prediction by sample mean. Findings suggest that, beyond hormonal markers, lifestyle and socioeconomic factors enhance ANM prediction, supporting improved clinical decisions on contraception and menopausal treatment in perimenopausal women (Hyvärinen et al., 2021).

12.2.2.3.1 Nutritional diet recommendations for natural menopause

During menopause, nutritional management should begin with an assessment of body composition to determine individual nutritional status. Maintaining a healthy weight is essential and can be supported by adequate nutrient intake and, when necessary, reducing daily energy intake by 500–700 kcal to manage overweight or obesity. Regular physical activity is also strongly recommended (Erdélyi et al., 2023).

Dietary recommendations include protein intake of 0.8–1.2 g/kg of body weight per day. Key nutrients, such as calcium, vitamin D, vitamin C, vitamin B n-3 LCPUFA, and omega-3 fatty acids, should be prioritized. Vegetable consumption should reach 300–400 g/day (3–4 portions), and fruit intake should be 100–200 g (1–2 portions). Legumes, such as beans, peas, lentils, chickpeas, and soy, should be consumed at least once a week. Low-fat dairy products, including around half a liter of milk per day, are recommended as calcium sources. Red meat intake should be limited to 350–500 g/week, prepared by boiling, steaming, or frying. Deep-sea fish should be consumed at least twice per week, with each serving around 100–120 g. A daily intake of 30 g of unsalted nuts or oily seeds is advised, along with 30–45 g of dietary fiber from whole grains and fiber-rich cereals (Erdélyi et al., 2023).

Certain foods and habits should be avoided during menopause. These include simple, fast-acting sugars, sugary and alcoholic beverages, smoking, excessive salt (limit to 5 g/day), sedentary behavior, and saturated fats, which should not exceed 10% of total daily energy intake (Erdélyi et al., 2023).

12.2.3 Osteoporosis in women's health and its nutritional impact

Osteoporosis is a major public health concern, leading to significant illness and death. Despite its importance the role of calcium and vitamin D in maintaining bone health is often underestimated by both patients and healthcare providers. Adequate intake is essential through diet or supplements and forms the foundation of osteoporosis care. Recent guidelines emphasize increased vitamin D intake, and adherence to calcium and vitamin D therapy is crucial for preventing fractures. The updated NOF guidelines include the use of a new algorithm on absolute fracture risk which is termed as FRAX. Tools like the FRAX algorithm help determine when to add medications, but continued use of calcium and vitamin D remains necessary for optimal treatment. The "bricks and mortar" analogy is a useful way to explain their supportive role in bone strength to patients (Sunyecz, 2008).

12.2.3.1 Application of predictive models of osteoporosis

Traditional approaches to fracture risk stratification, such as using a fixed bone mineral content (BMC) threshold, fail to account for the continuous nature of fracture risk and influencing factors like age. Normative data expressed as percentiles or z-scores describe bone status but do not directly quantify fracture probability. More advanced models now treat fracture risk as a continuum, incorporating BMC, age, treatment duration, and survival probability. These models, such as the remaining lifetime fracture probability, provide more accurate estimates of future fracture risk and help guide treatment duration and cost-effectiveness (Ross et al., 1990). An ML model was developed to predict osteoporosis risk using routinely collected clinical data, excluding dual-energy X-ray absorptiometry (DXA) measurements to improve accessibility. Using NHANES 2007–14 data from 7924 adults aged $\geq$50 years (20.6% with osteoporosis) a stacking ensemble of gradient boosting (GB), RF, XGBoost, and LightGBM with an LR metaclassifier achieved 93% accuracy and an AUC of 0.94. Key predictors included age, arm muscle circumference, body weight, gender, BMI, and calcium intake, alongside other biologically relevant factors. The model's strong performance and reliance on easily obtained data highlight its potential as a cost-effective screening tool, especially in DXA-limited settings (Carvalho & Gavaia, 2025). Another study showed that RF, SVM, and artificial neural network (ANN) models showed the highest predictive accuracy, indicating their potential for earlier osteoporosis detection in clinical settings. They briefly demonstrated that in women (n = 2929), ML models achieved AUROCs of 0.781 (ANN), 0.807 (SVM), 0.811 (RF), 0.767 [k-nearest neighbors (KNN)], and 0.772 (LR), all outperforming the traditional osteoporosis self-assessment tool for Asians model except KNN (Ou Yang et al., 2021). A cross-sectional study of 401 randomly selected women used a validated health belief model–based questionnaire to identify predictors of osteoporosis preventive behaviors. Walking behavior was significantly associated with perceived susceptibility and motivation, whereas nutrition behavior correlated positively with perceived susceptibility and self-efficacy and negatively with perceived barriers. The model explained 29.1% of variance in walking and 20.2% in nutrition behaviors, supporting its use for designing prevention-focused educational interventions (Jeihooni et al., 2017). In Hyejin's study on female students, health belief model constructs explained 6.7% of the variance in osteoporosis preventive behaviors, whereas a study in Yazd students reported 29%. These findings suggest that the model's structure can serve as a reference framework for developing educational interventions to promote osteoporosis prevention behaviors among women (Jeihooni et al., 2017).

12.2.3.2 Nutrition and osteoporosis

In postmenopausal women aged 55–65 a prediction model incorporating serotonin, vitamins K, A, and D3, and bone turnover markers achieved 79.8% training accuracy and 72.5% validation accuracy. Vitamin K and serotonin emerged as key predictors, underscoring the critical role of nutrition-related factors in osteoporosis risk assessment (Wang et al., 2025). A study found that adequate calcium intake is directly linked to higher bone mass density, whereas calcium deficiency, especially with high phosphorus, can damage bone tissue. Vitamin D levels below 20 ng/mL reduce bone density and increase fracture risk. Excess protein promotes calcium loss, and saturated fats show an inverse correlation with bone density. Deficiencies in vitamin K, magnesium, copper, and zinc impair bone mineralization. Overall, balanced intake of calcium (1200 mg/day), vitamin D (600 IU), protein, magnesium, and vitamin K is crucial for osteoporosis prevention and treatment (Hejazi et al., 2020).

12.2.4 Arthritis

Arthritis refers to inflammation of the joints and causes pain, swelling, and stiffness. Its two most common forms differ fundamentally: in osteoarthritis (OA), joint cartilage gradually breaks down from age or use, whereas rheumatoid arthritis (RA) is an autoimmune disease in which the body's immune system attacks the joint lining. Modern predictive models (e.g., statistical or AI-driven risk calculators) can analyze patient data and risk factors to estimate an individual's likelihood of developing arthritis or how rapidly it may progress, thereby helping clinicians with earlier diagnosis, prognosis, and personalized treatment planning (Kerkhof et al., 2014; Shadick, 2006).

12.2.4.1 Osteoarthritis

12.2.4.1.1 Traditional regression-based prediction models for knee osteoarthritis

A Bayesian LR model was developed using data from 1822 participants in North Nottinghamshire, United Kingdom, to predict incident knee pain, defined as self-reported pain on most days for at least 1 month. Calibration was acceptable (Hosmer and Lemeshow test, i.e., HLT, $P = .52$), and internal performance yielded an receiver operating characteristic curve (ROC) of 0.70 with high sensitivity (94%) but low specificity (32%). External validation in the OA initiative (OAI) dataset showed reduced performance (ROC = 0.54, sensitivity = 73%, specificity = 31%). The authors noted the outcome definition was prone to recall bias, and external validity was poor (Fernandes et al., 2017). Garriga et al. (2020) employed LR in the Chingford 1000 Women study (n = 649) to predict incident radiographic knee OA, defined as progression to KL grade > 2. Although calibration was reported as good, no statistics were provided. A radiographic model achieved an AUC of 0.797, and a clinical model reached 0.692. No external validation was performed. Limitations included the women-only cohort, lifestyle changes since the 1980s–1990s, and lack of validation (Garriga et al., 2020). Joseph et al. (2018) analyzed 641 OAI participants using LR to predict moderate-to-severe radiographic or symptomatic OA, defined as progression to KL grade 3–4, Western Ontario and McMaster Universities arthritis index (WOMAC) pain score > 5, or total knee replacement (TKR). AUC values for three models ranged from 0.67 to 0.72, without calibration assessment or external validation. Limitations included the inclusion of at-risk early OA subjects, sole reliance on T2 composite imaging, and ignoring potential interknee interactions (Joseph et al., 2018). Kerkhof et al. (2014) used the Rotterdam Study (n = 929) to model incident knee OA, defined as KL progression from <2 to ≥2. LR models showed calibration P-values between .19 and .90 and AUC values between 0.66 and 0.79. External validation in RS-II (AUC = 0.86) and the Chingford study (AUC = 0.76) showed good performance. Knee injury history and physical activity were not included (Kerkhof et al., 2014). Kinds et al. (2012) analyzed 1002 participants from the CHECK study in the Netherlands. Incident OA was defined either radiographically (KL grade 2) or clinically (painful knee in the highest three WOMAC quintiles). Models achieved AUCs of 0.64 (clinical), 0.74 (clinical + radiographic), and 0.70 (KL grades 0–1). No calibration statistics or external validation was reported. Inclusion of at-risk rather than established OA subjects and participant-level WOMAC measurement were noted limitations (Kinds et al., 2012). Kraus et al. (2017) used OAI data (n = 600) with LR to predict clinically relevant OA (radiographic and pain progression combined). The AUC was 0.586; no calibration or external validation was performed. Biomarker levels may have been influenced by other joints (Kraus et al., 2017). In 192 knee OA patients (53% female) followed 24 months, higher baseline IL-6 quartiles were significantly associated with greater total knee bone marrow lesions (BMLs) and with BML progression (trend $P < .01$ and $P = .05$, adjusted). Elevated IL-17F and IL-23 (highest quartiles) predicted increased BML scores in women only (IL-17F $P = .04$; IL-23 $P = .01$), whereas IL-17A showed no significant association in either sex (Zhu et al., 2017).

A study with 407 participants in the prevention of knee osteoarthritis in overweight females (PROOF) predicted frequent knee pain or symptomatic OA. Calibration was excellent (HLT = 0.92–0.93), and AUC ranged from 0.63 (basic) to 0.71 (backward selection). External validation in the Rotterdam Study yielded an AUC of 0.71. Loss to follow-up and missed cases between time points were key limitations (Landsmeer et al., 2019). Another model (553 OAI participants) predicted structural OA progression (medial joint space loss between 36 and 48 months). LR models with bone mineral density features improved AUC from 0.65 to 0.73. No external validation was performed; the cohort included at-risk individuals (LaValley et al., 2017). Van Oudenaarde et al. used the CHECK study (n = 148) to model KL ≥ 2 or Total Knee Arthroplasty (TKA) occurrence. Calibration was good (HLT = 0.645), with an AUC of 0.722 (optimism-corrected = 0.685). Sensitivity and specificity were both ~66%. No external validation; small sample size and inclusion of OA patients limited robustness (Van Oudenaarde et al., 2017). Takahashi et al. (2010) studied 2158 Japanese participants, predicting OA from clinical and radiographic findings (JSN and osteophytes) using LR. AUC ranged from 0.554 to 0.685, with no calibration or external validation. Only three genes were studied in a nonrepresentative sample (Takahashi et al., 2010). Halilaj et al. (2018) applied LASSO regression to 1243 OAI participants to predict radiographic (AUC = 0.86) and pain progression (AUC = 0.95). Calibration and external validation were absent. Model interpretability was limited, and baseline data quality was poor (Halilaj et al., 2018).

12.2.4.1.2 ML Prediction models for knee osteoarthritis

An RF model predicting early OA was trained using ranked guided iterative feature elimination and PCA (incident pain, lateral JSN ≥ 1 mm, medial JSN ≥ 1 mm, or KL ≥ 2) by analyzing 407 PROOF participants. The model achieved an AUC of 0.823. Limitations included restriction to obese women and absence of external validation (Lazzarini et al., 2017). Ashinsky et al. (2017) used a weighted neighborhood deep convolutional histogram regression model (WN(D-CHRM)) on 68 OAI participants to classify symptomatic OA (WOMAC-based definition). The model reached 75% accuracy, with 74% sensitivity and 76% specificity. The small sample size, long processing times, use of only a central MRI slice, and dependency of the registration method on the target image were key limitations, and no external validation was performed (Ashinsky et al., 2017). Du et al. (2018) studied 100 OAI participants, applying PCA for dimensionality reduction and testing ANN, SVM, RF, and naïve Bayes classifiers to predict OA progression (KL grade change and joint space narrowing). ROC values ranged from 0.651 (SVM) to 0.761 (ANN). No external validation was conducted, and the study was constrained by its small sample size (Du et al., 2018). Interestingly a model used 5749 Korean National Health and Nutrition Examination Survey (KNHANES) participants with PCA-based dimensionality reduction and feed-forward neural networks to identify early OA, defined as self-reported physician diagnosis. The model achieved an AUC of 0.768. Limitations included reliance on self-reported diagnosis, lack of longitudinal data, predominantly binary input features, exclusion of treated OA patients, and no external validation (Lim et al., 2019). Long et al. (2017) used KNN on 176 participants to classify OA severity based on knee injury and osteoarthritis outcome score (KOOS) scores, biomechanical parameters, and combined features. AUCs were 0.82 (self-reported outcomes), 0.92 (biomechanical), and 1.00 (combined). The study was cross-sectional, small in sample size, and lacked external validation (Long et al., 2017). Sheng et al. (2019) trained a Bayesian network on 157 residents of the Kongjiang community, China, using self-reported OA diagnoses. The model achieved an AUC of 0.78, with 76% accuracy, 73% sensitivity, and

78% specificity. The sample was small and nonrepresentative; the study was cross-sectional (Sheng et al., 2019). In addition, a research group used both convolutional neural networks with LR and GB machines (GBM) on 2711 OAI and 2129 multicenter osteoarthritis study participants to predict OA progression (KL grade increase). AUCs were 0.75 (LR) and 0.76 (GBM). Limitations included reliance on standardized radiographs with frame positioning, missing data imputation in the LR test evaluation, and use of total WOMAC scores (Tiulpin et al., 2019). Zhong et al. (2016) applied KNN to 182 OAI participants to predict symptomatic OA progression (WOMAC score change > 10 over 3 years). Accuracy was 84%, with 77% sensitivity and 90% specificity. The small sample size and absence of external validation were limitations (Zhong et al., 2016).

12.2.4.1.3 Nutritional supplement in osteoarthritis

Current evidence suggests that nutrition can play a supportive role in alleviating OA symptoms in women, although its ability to modify the underlying disease process remains unproven. Several nutraceuticals and dietary compounds have been investigated, with varying levels of evidence for their efficacy and safety.

Avocado soybean unsaponifiables (ASUs) have the strongest evidence base among the reviewed interventions. Randomized controlled trials in knee and hip OA indicate that ASUs can improve pain and function while reducing the need for nonsteroidal antiinflammatory drugs (NSAIDs). Although there is no convincing evidence that ASUs slow structural joint degeneration, they appear to be safe and well-tolerated, with minimal reported side effects. **Methylsulfonylmethane (MSM)** has moderate evidence supporting its use, particularly for knee OA. Doses of approximately 3 g twice a day have been associated with pain reduction and functional improvement. However, data on long-term safety and sustained efficacy are limited, highlighting the need for further investigation. **SKI306X**, a multiherbal extract preparation, also has moderate evidence for symptom relief in knee OA. Clinical studies suggest good tolerability, but as with MSM, more robust and long-term data are required to confirm its role in routine management. **Vitamin C** supplementation, especially in the form of calcium ascorbate at high doses, has been explored for OA symptom management. Limited evidence suggests a potential reduction in pain, but high-dose regimens are controversial because of conflicting animal data and possible safety concerns. Current recommendations favor meeting, but not exceeding, standard daily intake levels through diet or supplementation. Other nutraceuticals, including **green-lipped mussel extracts, bromelain, and ginger**, have shown inconsistent or low-quality evidence for mild symptom relief. Although some studies report modest benefits, the overall strength of the evidence is insufficient for strong recommendations, and certain products may carry a higher risk of adverse effects (Ameye & Chee, 2006).

General dietary advice for women with OA emphasizes weight management, a nutrient-dense diet rich in fruits and vegetables for antioxidant support, and the considered use of well-studied nutraceuticals for symptom relief. Importantly, there is a continued need for high-quality research on nutritional interventions specifically targeting women with OA to clarify optimal dietary strategies and supplement use.

12.2.4.2 *Rheumatoid arthritis*

RA affects about 1.3 million Americans, with women affected 2.5 times more often than men (Hu et al., 2017). Although its causes are not fully understood, both genetic and environmental factors, including diet, influence RA risk. Evidence suggests that alcohol, fish, olive oil, and cooked vegetables may be protective, whereas red meat and sugar-sweetened beverages may increase risk (Hu et al., 2017).

In a cohort of 692 methotrexate-naïve RA patients (192 men and 500 women) initiating methotrexate between 2014 and 2022, baseline prognostic nutritional index (PNI), clinical, and laboratory parameters were recorded and monitored every 3 months for 1 year. Associations between baseline PNI and disease activity score using C-reactive protein (DAS28-CRP) and its change (cDAS28) were assessed using linear and multivariate regression. ROC analysis was performed to identify a PNI cutoff for predicting remission at 1 year. Baseline PNI was significantly correlated with DAS28-CRP at initiation and at all follow-up points, as well as with health assessment questionnaire disability index, pain score, estimated glomerular filtration ratio (eGFR), hemoglobin, platelet count, matrix metalloproteinase-3, and inflammatory activity. cDAS28 at all intervals showed significant associations with baseline PNI and DAS28-CRP. ROC analysis identified a PNI > 44.21 as a predictor of 1-year remission (AUC=0.582). These findings suggest that baseline PNI is linked to both baseline and short-term changes in RA disease activity after methotrexate initiation (Yoshii, 2024).

12.2.4.2.1 Association between dietary quality and rheumatoid arthritis risk in the Nurses' Health Studies

A pooled analysis from the Nurses' Health Studies (NHS) (1984–2012) and NHS-II (1991–2013) examined the association between cumulative alternative healthy eating index-2010 (AHEI-2010) scores and incident RA. Across 3.68 million person-years, women in the highest quartile of dietary quality consistently demonstrated lower hazard ratios (HRs) for RA compared with those in the lowest quartile, although results were not statistically significant in the overall cohort. In the age-adjusted model the HR for RA in the highest versus lowest quartile was 0.86 (95% CI 0.72–1.03; *P*-trend = .11). This association was slightly strengthened in the multivariable-adjusted model accounting for lifestyle, reproductive, and hormonal factors (HR 0.85, 95% CI 0.70–1.02; *P*-trend = .08) and was minimally affected by further BMI adjustment (HR 0.87, 95% CI 0.73–1.05; *P*-trend = .16). When stratified by RA serostatus the inverse association appeared in both seropositive and seronegative RA, though neither reached statistical significance. For seropositive RA the multivariable-adjusted HR comparing the highest to the lowest diet quality quartile was 0.88 (95% CI 0.70–1.12; *P*-trend = .34), and for seronegative RA it was 0.78 (95% CI 0.58–1.06; *P*-trend = .10). Additional BMI adjustment slightly attenuated these estimates. Overall, higher long-term dietary quality was associated with a trend toward reduced RA risk, with more pronounced effects for seronegative RA, though limited by statistical power. It suggested potential benefits of a healthier diet in RA prevention, warranting further investigation in age- and serostatus-specific analyses (Hu et al., 2017).

12.2.4.2.2 Baseline characteristics across dietary quality quartiles in the Nurses' Health Studies

Analysis of the NHS, 1984 (n = 76,597) and NHS-II, 1991 (n = 93,392) revealed clear sociodemographic and lifestyle gradients across quartiles of the Alternative Healthy Eating Index-2010 (AHEI-2010). In both cohorts, higher diet quality scores were associated with older age, lower BMI, higher socioeconomic status, and greater physical activity. In the NHS, mean age increased from 49.3 years in the lowest quartile to 52.4 years in the highest, whereas BMI decreased from 25.4 to 24.4 kg/m^2. Similar patterns were seen in NHS-II, where age rose from 35.9 to 37.3 years and BMI fell from 25.3 to 23.9 kg/m^2. Median family income increased progressively across quartiles in both cohorts. Healthy eating patterns were also linked to favorable health behaviors. Physical activity increased markedly with AHEI-2010 quartile from 4.6 to 11.1 MET-hours/week in the NHS and from 8.3 to 19.4 in NHS-II, whereas smoking prevalence declined (NHS: 30.3% to 18.1%; NHS-II: 14.7% to 9.8%). Alcohol intake rose modestly with diet quality, as did multivitamin use. Reproductive and hormonal factors showed mixed associations. In the NHS, higher quartiles were slightly more likely to report early menarche, oral contraceptive use, and postmenopausal hormone therapy, whereas parity decreased with diet quality. In NHS-II, parity similarly declined, but breastfeeding rates peaked in mid-quartiles. Total energy intake declined across quartiles in both studies, from ~1900 kcal/day in the lowest quartile to ~1600–1700 kcal/day in the highest. Overall, these patterns suggest that higher long-term diet quality is correlated with a constellation of healthier lifestyle behaviors and socioeconomic advantages, alongside modest differences in reproductive characteristics (Hu et al., 2017).

12.2.4.2.3 Dietary components and rheumatoid arthritis risk in women

In pooled analyses from NHS and NHS-II, several individual components of the Alternative Healthy Eating Index-2010 showed distinct associations with RA risk in women aged ≤55 years. Lower intakes of red/processed meat and sodium were strongly associated with reduced RA risk. Women in the highest versus lowest quartile of red/processed meat consumption had a 36%–42% lower risk after full adjustment (HR ≈ 0.64; P-trend = .002). For sodium the highest quartile was associated with a 29% lower risk (HR ≈ 0.71; P-trend = .07). Moderate alcohol consumption (0.5–1.5 drinks/day) was also protective (HR ≈ 0.73; P-trend = .013). Other components—including sugar-sweetened beverages, transfat, nuts, vegetables, fruits, polyunsaturated fat, whole grains, and long-chain omega-3 fats—showed no statistically significant associations with RA in this age group. These findings suggest that limiting red/processed meat and sodium, and maintaining moderate alcohol intake, may contribute to lower RA risk in younger women (Hu et al., 2017).

A study assessed whether baseline CRP levels predict RA risk in 27,939 healthy women from the Women's Health Study. Over 9.9 years, 90 confirmed RA cases occurred, but no significant association was found between CRP tertiles and RA risk, even when stratified by time to diagnosis. A single CRP measurement did not predict incident RA (Shadick, 2006). In a study of 93 RA patients and matched controls, mid-arm muscular circumference and serum albumin were significantly lower in RA, especially in functional class IV, despite higher reported energy and nutrient intake. Nutritional parameters correlated inversely with disease activity and cumulative glucocorticoid dose, suggesting that RA-related inflammation and treatment contribute to impaired nutritional status rather than inadequate diet (Gómez-Vaquero et al., 2001).

12.2.5 Cardiovascular disease

CVD is the leading global cause of death, with about 17 million deaths in 2008, and more women are affected than men. Risk score models, using multiple variables, offer a cost-effective way to identify high-risk individuals for prevention, especially in Asia, where CVD incidence is rising. Modifiable risk factors are increasingly common, and whereas they raise CVD risk across all groups, variations in their distribution among ethnicities may explain differences in overall risk (Dhaliwal et al., 2014).

12.2.5.1 Predictive models in women's cardiovascular disease and their nutritional impact

In a cohort of 4354 women aged 20–69 years from the Australian risk factor prevalence study, 10-year CVD risk was estimated using the Framingham model, systematic coronary risk evaluation (SCORE), and general CVD models. Compared with Caucasian women, Asian women generally showed lower predicted CVD risk, although some models produced similar estimates between Asian and Australian-born women. Findings align with national CVD prevalence data, supporting the use of SCORE low-risk charts and Framingham incidence models, while recommending inclusion of factors such as obesity, diet, and physical activity to refine risk prediction (Dhaliwal et al., 2014).

Several CVD risk models had been developed across Chinese and international cohorts with varying predictors and performance (Zhiting et al., 2022). Wang et al. used Chinese multiprovincial cohort study (CMCS) data (1992–2002) from 31,728 adults (35–64 years) to create a 10-year CVD model with predictors such as age, gender, cholesterol, BP, HDL-C, smoking, and fasting glucose. The Cox regression model achieved *C*-statistics of 0.78 (men) and 0.76 (women), with no calibration report or external validation (Wang & Zhao, 2003). Using similar CMCS data, Liu et al. developed a 10-year coronary heart disease (CHD) model ($n = 30{,}121$), including diabetes as a predictor, with slightly lower discrimination (0.76 men; 0.74 women) and Hosmer–Lemeshow calibration but no external validation (Liu et al., 2004). Wu et al. built a 10-year ICVD model from the USA–PRC cohort ($n = 9903$; follow-up 15.1 years), producing optimal and simplified Cox regression models with *C*-statistics up to 0.80; both were externally validated (Wu et al., 2006). Yang et al. introduced the China-PAR model ($n = 21{,}320$; 35–74 years) using expanded predictors, including WC, geography, family history, and urbanization; discrimination was 0.79–0.81 with internal cross-validation and external validation (Yang et al., 2016). Hu et al. modeled cardiovascular death in a Taiwanese cohort ($n = 381{,}963$; ≥ 20 years), achieving excellent discrimination (0.91) but no calibration report or external validation (Hu, Lee, Tsai, & Wen, 2017). Pylypchuk et al. created the New Zealand PREDICT equations ($n = 401{,}752$;

30–74 years), including deprivation index and TC/HDL ratio, with C-statistics of 0.73 and calibration slope assessment (Pylypchuk et al., 2018). Li et al. developed a Taiwanese 10-year risk prediction (COX-regression) model ($n = 2221$; ≥40 years, from Taichung Community Health study participants) incorporating marital status, physical activity, tobacco use, Estimated Glomerular filtration rate (eGFR, Albumin-to-Creatinine Ratio (ACR), and Ankle–Brachial Index (ABI), with C statistics of 0.88 and bootstrap validation (Li et al., 2020). Yang et al. developed a 3 year risk model targeting high-risk Zhejiang cohort ($n = 29930$ with high risk of CVD) and compared six modeling approaches, with RF performing best (0.82 men; 0.68 women) based on classification and regression tree (CART); no external validation (Yang et al., 2020). Huang et al. built the Guangzhou Biobank cohort study (GBCS) model ($n = 15,000$; ≥50 years) using age, SBP, smoking, diabetes, and antihypertensive use, yielding a better discrimination in both women (c-statistic 0.72, 95% CI 0.71-0.73) and men (c-statistic 0.68, 95% CI 0.67-0.70) as compared to the Framingham and China-PAR models, and no external validation (Huang et al., 2022). Wang et al. presented a Chinese multi-provincial cohort study (CMCS) lifetime risk model ($n = 21,953$; 35–84 years) using the modified Kaplan–Meier method. The lifetime CVD risk for men up to age 80 was 24.4%, and it was 20.2% for women at age 35. This risk reached 51.1% for men and 38.6% for women at the same age as before, with addition of two or more high-risk factors (Wang et al., 2015).

12.2.5.2 Dietary and biomarker predictors for cardiovascular disease risk

In the Golestan cohort study of 43,878 adults aged 37–80 years, an 8-year CVD mortality prediction model was developed and validated using nine predictors: age, physical activity level (MET minutes/week), waist-to-hip ratio, tea intake (cup/day), vegetable intake (g/1000 kcal/day), white meat intake (g/1000 kcal/day), salt intake (g/1000 kcal/day), dairy intake (cup/1000 kcal/day), and percentage of protein intake. The cohort was randomly split into derivation ($n = 28,930$) and validation ($n = 14,948$) sets. Using a Cox proportional hazards model the prediction tool achieved strong performance, with C-statistics of 0.76 in the derivation set and 0.77 in the validation set ($P < .001$), indicating good discrimination. Calibration was similarly robust in both datasets (0.81). To enhance clinical applicability a simple point-based dietary score was created from the model, enabling straightforward risk estimation in healthcare settings. This scoring system effectively translates complex dietary and lifestyle data into a practical tool for identifying high-risk individuals and guiding targeted lifestyle interventions to reduce future CVD mortality risk (Jabbari et al., 2025).

In a Canadian cohort of 12,130 adults followed from 2004 to 2018, conditional inference forest models using 61 nutrition and 14 nonnutritional variables identified supplement use, caffeine, and alcohol as key dietary predictors of CVD. Supplement use was linked to reduced risk, caffeine to increased risk, and alcohol showed a U-shaped association. The model achieved strong predictive performance (C-statistic = 0.821, 95% CI 0.801–0.842), supporting the potential of ML to enhance nutritional epidemiology in CVD risk prediction (Morgenstern et al., 2022). In the Women's Health Study of healthy women ≥45 years, adding hs-CRP to traditional risk factors improved

10-year cardiovascular risk classification—especially for those at intermediate risk, reclassifying up to 21% more accurately despite minimal change in *C*-statistic and outperforming individual lipid measures (Cook et al., 2006). In women from Fasa, Iran a theory of planned behavior–based educational intervention significantly improved attitudes, norms, control, intentions, and nutritional practices for CVD prevention, explaining 41.6% of behavior variance and highlighting mothers' key role in promoting healthy eating (Khani Jeihooni et al., 2021).

Lactate dehydrogenase (LDH) is a key enzyme in anaerobic metabolism, but its relationship with arterial stiffness (AS) and 10-year CVD (CVD10) risk remains unclear. A retrospective cross-sectional study analyzed 12,597 Chinese adults (6988 men, 5609 women; mean age 49.5 years) undergoing health examinations. AS was assessed using brachial–ankle pulse wave velocity (baPWV), and CVD10 risk was calculated with the Framingham model. Higher LDH levels were significantly associated with increased AS and CVD10 risk in both sexes (men: $\beta = 0.032$; women: $\beta = 0.025$; both $P < .001$). Individuals with high LDH ($\geq$172 U/L) had markedly elevated AS and CVD10 scores. Those with baPWV $\geq$1400 cm/s or higher CVD10 risk scores had significantly higher LDH compared to lower-risk groups (all $P < .001$). These findings suggest LDH may serve as a potential biomarker for AS and CVD10 risk in general health-check populations (Zhu et al., 2022). In the United Kingdom Biobank cohort of 468,885 adults free of CVD at baseline a higher fat-to-muscle mass ratio (FMR) was associated with greater CVD risk in women over 12.5 years of follow-up. Using bioelectrical impedance, total and regional (trunk, arm, leg) FMRs were calculated. In women, elevated total FMR predicted higher incidence of CVD (HR = 1.83), ischemic heart disease (HR = 1.81), myocardial infarction (HR = 1.49), and congestive heart failure (HR = 2.57). Cardiometabolites and inflammatory cells partially mediated these associations. FMR outperformed BMI in predicting CVD mortality, supporting its use for early risk stratification in women (Zhou et al., 2023). In postmenopausal women, adding five biomarkers (IL-6, d-dimer, factor VIII, von Willebrand factor, and homocysteine) to traditional risk factor models modestly improved 5-year CHD risk prediction (*C*-statistic 0.751 vs. 0.729) compared with traditional factors alone, whereas CRP added no benefit (Kim et al., 2010).

Overall, predictive models for women's CVDs are evolving with an emphasis on female-specific factors and the integration of nutritional data. Diet significantly impacts CVD risk and enhances model performance. The advent of AI and ML offers promising tools to refine these predictions and support personalized nutritional interventions to reduce cardiovascular risk in women. Further research is needed to incorporate female-specific and nutritional predictors more systematically into these models for better clinical outcomes.

12.2.6 Nutritional deficiency forecasting (anemia, vitamin D, iron, and folic acid deficiencies)

Underweight and overweight/obesity in pregnant women can be predicted with an accuracy of around 75% and an AUC near 0.85 using RF models with robust data transformation (Begum et al., 2024). Socioeconomic status, age, breastfeeding, and partner's education are consistently important predictors for nutritional outcomes in women of childbearing age (Khudri et al., 2023). Vitamin D deficiency prediction models achieve very high accuracy and AUC (near-perfect with XGBoost), with race, age, and BMI as top predictors (Bhimavarapu et al., 2025; Guo et al., 2024). Micronutrient deficiency risk is strongly associated with poverty, maternal education, media exposure, and geographic region, with an AUROC around 80% in RF models (Gebeye et al., 2024). Advanced feature selection (Boruta) and data balancing (SMOTE) techniques improve prediction performance for micronutrient supplementation status (Ngusie et al., 2024). The current state of ML applications in forecasting women's nutritional deficiencies, highlighting key predictive features and model performance metrics that can guide targeted nutritional interventions, is demonstrated in Table 12.3.

12.2.7 Cancers in women

12.2.7.1 Application of predictive models in breast cancer

Predictive models have emerged as transformative tools in breast cancer management, leveraging AI and ML to address various aspects of cancer care from early detection to treatment optimization. These models analyze diverse data sources, including medical imaging, genomic information, clinical variables, and pathological features, to provide actionable insights for clinicians and patients (Islam et al., 2024; Noman et al., 2025). Recent predictive modeling studies in breast cancer have demonstrated significant advances through diverse methodological approaches, from traditional ML to cutting-edge multimodal deep learning, as mentioned in Table 12.4.

12.2.7.1.1 Breast cancer and nutrition

Higher fruit and vegetable intake after breast cancer diagnosis was linked to lower overall mortality, but not breast cancer–specific mortality, in a study of 8927 women with stage I–III breast cancer identified during follow-up of the NHS (1980–2010) and NHS-II (1991–2011). Green leafy and cruciferous vegetables were particularly beneficial. Blueberry consumption was associated with reduced breast cancer–specific and all-cause mortality. In contrast, higher fruit juice intake, especially apple juice, was linked to increased mortality. Orange juice showed no such risk. These findings highlight the potential survival benefits of vegetable-rich diets and the risks of excessive fruit juice consumption among breast cancer survivors (Farvid et al., 2020).

12.2.7.2 Application of predictive models in cervical cancer and nutritional outcomes

Cervical cancer is a widespread disease among women worldwide. Like other major health conditions, medicine aims to develop tools for research and prevention. ML offers powerful support in this fight, particularly through clinical decision support systems (CDSS), which are increasingly used in healthcare. For example, Vidal et al. (2010) applied the analytic hierarchy process (AHP) in a CDSS to guide pharmacists in selecting cancer therapies, whereas Liberatore et al. (2003) used AHP to structure prostate cancer treatment protocols, showing the importance of expert-guided decision

Table 12.3 Key ML studies on forecasting women's nutritional deficiencies and associated risk values based on the latest research.

Source	Population and focus	Nutritional deficiency predicted	ML models used	Key predictors/features	Performance metrics	Risk values/important findings	Study
Begum et al. (2024)	Pregnant women in Bangladesh	Nutritional status: underweight, overweight/obese	RF, LR, SVM, ANN, etc.	Socio-demographic factors, pregnancy-related variables	RF accuracy: 74.75%, precision (underweight): 76.76%, *F*1-score (overweight): 83.78%, AUC up to ~0.85	Underweight and overweight were predicted with high precision; robust feature transformation improved results	ML prediction of nutritional status among pregnant women in Bangladesh
Khudri et al. (2023)	Women of childbearing age, Bangladesh	BMI classification and malnutrition risk (underweight, overweight, obesity)	SVM, KNN, combined predictors	Socioeconomic status, age, breastfeeding status, partner's education	High specificity, Cohen's kappa, *F*1-score, AUC (exact values not specified)	Socioeconomic and breastfeeding status are the top predictors; oversampling is used to address class imbalance	Predicting nutritional status for women of childbearing age from their economic, health, and demographic features: A supervised ML approach

(*continued on next page*)

Table 12.3 Key ML studies on forecasting women's nutritional deficiencies and associated risk values based on the latest research—cont'd

Source	Population and focus	Nutritional deficiency predicted	ML models used	Key predictors/features	Performance metrics	Risk values/important findings	Study
Guo et al. (2024)	General community population, United States	Vitamin D deficiency risk	XGBoost, RF, GB, LR	Race, age, BMI	XGBoost AUC: near-perfect (exact value not given), high accuracy	Race, age, and BMI are the strongest predictors; an online web calculator has been developed for rapid risk assessment	ML-based prediction of vitamin D deficiency: NHANES 2001–18
Gebeye et al. (2024)	Women and children in Ethiopia	Micronutrient deficiency risk	RF (RF), neural network, naïve Bayes	Region, wealth index, maternal education, media exposure, delivery location	RF AUROC: 80.01%, accuracy: 72.41%	Poorest wealth index and no maternal education increase risk; regional disparities are significant	Predictors of micronutrient deficiency among children aged 6–23 months in Ethiopia: An ML approach

(*continued on next page*)

Ngusie et al. (2024)	Pregnant women in East Africa	Micronutrient supplementation status	Boruta feature selection + various ML algorithms with SMOTE balancing	Number of children, residence, and other demographic variables	SMOTE balancing improved prediction performance (exact metrics not given)	Boruta algorithm identified key variables; data balancing is critical for model accuracy	Employing ML techniques for the prediction of micronutrient supplementation status during pregnancy in East African countries
Bhimavarapu et al. (2025)	Vitamin D status prediction	Vitamin D deficiency	Various ML models with explainability tools	Clinical and demographic features	High accuracy and clinical acceptability (exact metrics not specified)	Emphasis on explainability for clinical use	ML-driven prediction of vitamin D deficiency severity with hybrid optimization

ANN, artificial neural network; *AUC*, area under curve; *AUROC*, area under the receiver operating characteristic curve; *BMI*, body mass index; *GB*, gradient boosting; *KNN*, k-nearest neighbors; *LR*, logistic regression; *ML*, machine learning; *RF*, random forest; *SVM*, support vector machine

Table 12.4 Predictive modeling studies in breast cancer.

Source	Methodology	Dataset/cohorts	Algorithms/ architecture	Key features/variables	Evaluation metrics and results	Key findings	Study and model
Wang et al. (2024)	Multimodal integration of pathology images, molecular data (219 genes), and clinical data; WSIs preprocessed into 256 × 256 pixel patches with attention-based feature fusion	1020 patients: Training (741), Internal Validation (184), External Testing (95)	Multiinstance learning network with modified ResNet50 for feature extraction	Pathology images, molecular profiles, clinical data	Training AUC for DFS: 1-year 0.979, 3-year 0.957, 5-year 0.871; external AUC: 1-year 0.851, 2-year 0.878, 3-year 0.938; *C*-index: Training 0.925, validation 0.823, external 0.864; hazard ratios: Training 0.027, Validation 0.117, external 0.061 ($P <$ .0001)	Strong discriminative ability across cohorts; integration of multimodal data improved DFS prediction accuracy and robustness	DeepClinMed-PGM Model (2024)

(*continued on next page*)

Table 12.4 Predictive modeling studies in breast cancer—cont'd

Source	Methodology	Dataset/cohorts	Algorithms/ architecture	Key features/variables	Evaluation metrics and results	Key findings	Study and model
Mohammad and Ahmad (2025)	Retrospective analysis with demographics, laboratory values, clinical conditions; Bayesian network model using SPSS modeler 18.0; 70/30 train-test split	2995 breast cancer patients (2012–24)	Bayesian network	Demographics, hemoglobin, WBC, hypertension, diabetes	AUC 0.859; accuracy 96.7%; key predictors importance: WBC (0.19), diabetes and age (0.16), hemoglobin (0.13); outperformed other ML models	Bayesian networks showed high accuracy and interpretability; robust survival prediction using clinical and lab data	Bayesian Network Survival Prediction (2025)
Almarri et al. (2024)	LR, RF, DTs, SVM, neural networks; feature scaling, missing value imputation, K-fold cross-validation	Wisconsin Diagnostic Breast Cancer (569 samples, 30 features)	RF best performer	30 clinical and diagnostic features	RF: 92.55% accuracy; grid search CV improved accuracy to 92.6383%; 10-fold CV mean accuracy 95.5%	RF outperformed other algorithms, robust predictive performance on WDBC dataset	Breast Cancer Prediction Model (BCPM) (2024)

(continued on next page)

Islam et al. (2024)	Multiple ML algorithms with K-fold CV and SHAP interpretability; focus on morphological features such as perimeter, radius, texture	500 patients from Dhaka Medical College Hospital	XGBoost, RF, DT, LR, Naive Bayes	Morphological features: mean perimeter, radius, texture, smoothness, area	XGBoost: 97% accuracy, precision 0.94, recall 0.95, *F*1 0.96; RF: 96% accuracy; cross-validation: XGBoost 97.4%, RF 95.6%, LR 92.7%; SHAP: mean perimeter most important	XGBoost is the best performer; morphological features are highly predictive; interpretability via SHAP	XGBoost vs. Traditional ML Comparison (2024)
Tegaw and Asfaw (2025)	Ensemble models, including SVM, KNN, AdaBoost, GB, and RF; analyzing treatment impacts with SHAP	5000 samples from Kaggle	GB best performer	Clinical treatment variables: chemotherapy, hormone therapy, surgery, radiation	GB: Accuracy 97.2%, precision 97.3%, *F*1 97.3%, AUC-ROC 0.997; radiation therapy positive effect; hormone therapy negative effect	Ensemble methods with treatment data improve survival prediction; treatment impacts quantified; GB best	Ensemble Methods for Breast Cancer Survival (2022)

(*continued on next page*)

Table 12.4 Predictive modeling studies in breast cancer—cont'd

Source	Methodology	Dataset/cohorts	Algorithms/architecture	Key features/variables	Evaluation metrics and results	Key findings	Study and model
Al Tawil et al. (2024)	Comparison of CNN architectures on breast cancer medical images; preprocessing with normalization and augmentation	Medical breast cancer image datasets	VGG19, AlexNet, ResNet50	Image-based features	ResNet50 has the highest accuracy and *F*-score; AlexNet is the most computationally efficient; VGG19 has moderate performance	ResNet50 is recommended for accuracy and sensitivity; CNN choice impacts performance and efficiency	Convolutional Neural Networks Comparison (2024)
Noman et al. (2025)	Large multiconsortium data (METABRIC, MSKCC, Duke, SEER); models: LightGBM, XGBoost, RF; external validation with the Egyptian cohort	272,252 patients from multiple consortiums	LightGBM, XGBoost, RF	Clinical and genomic data; recurrence risk strategies	LightGBM: 92% AUC for recurrence prediction; *C*-index 0.837; XGBoost/RF 86% accuracy for recurrence type; external validation accuracy 74%–84%	Large-scale multimodal model shows high AUC and external validation accuracy; useful for recurrence prediction and stratification	Multi-Modal Survival Analysis (2025)

AdaBoost, adaptive boosting; *AUC*, area under curve; *CNN*, convolutional neural network; *DTs*, decision trees; *GB*, gradient boosting; *KNN*, *k*-nearest neighbors; *LR*, logistic regression; *ML*, machine learning; *RF*, random forest; *SVM*, support vector machine; *WSIs*, Whole Slide Images; *DFS*, Disease-Free Survival; *WBC*, White Blood Cell; *WDBC*, Wisconsin Diagnostic Breast Cancer.

counseling (Curia, 2021). In recent years, several studies have applied ML methods specifically to cervical cancer, producing valuable insights (Table 12.5).

12.2.7.2.1 Nutritional predictive models in cervical cancer

Recent studies have applied ML algorithms (e.g., deep learning and DTs) using large datasets of nutritional and nonnutritional factors (vitamins, minerals, fruit/vegetable intake, lifestyle, HPV status, etc.) to both predict risk and phase progression of cervical cancer. For instance, factors, such as zinc, iron, niacin, potassium, phosphorus, fiber, certain fruits, and vegetables, have shown beneficial links with reduced risk and progression, whereas high intake of salt, snacks, and milk correlated with higher risk. Models can achieve high accuracy and discrimination (e.g., AUC up to 0.993 for micronutrients) (Nazari et al., 2023). The PNI, calculated from serum albumin and lymphocyte count, is commonly used as a simple marker of nutritional status and immune competence. However, recent meta-analyses suggest PNI alone does not reliably predict overall or progression-free survival in cervical cancer patients, indicating a need for more comprehensive or alternative nutritional markers (Cao & Dong, 2024). Nutrients, such as folate, carotenoids, and vitamins C and E, have shown important roles for DNA repair and protection against oxidative stress, influencing both risk and treatment outcomes. Some studies recommend individualized nutritional interventions, especially for patients undergoing chemotherapy and radiation, to reduce toxicity and improve survival (Ifeanyi Obeagu, 2023).

12.2.7.3 Application of predictive models in ovarian cancer and nutritional outcomes

Ovarian tumor patients require appropriate management. Treatment in oncology centers improves prognosis, whereas benign cysts are common and may be managed conservatively or with surgery in general hospitals. Risk prediction models aid triage by estimating malignancy risk from key predictors (Ledger et al., 2023). Therefore assessing malignancy risk through various prediction models and cohort studies is essential for guiding ovarian tumor management. Table 12.6 summarizes the key methodological approaches, datasets, predictive features, model performances, calibration, and clinical utility, as well as main conclusions and limitations for the selected ovarian cancer prediction model studies.

12.2.7.3.1 Risk factors for ovarian cancer

A variety of lifestyle, surgical, and chemical factors have been tested and pooled via meta-analyses regarding their association with ovarian cancer risk.

Lifestyle factors—**Diet:** Seven studies (three case–control and two cohort) examined diet. A healthy diet showed an RR of 0.86 (95% CI: 0.73–1.00) in case–control studies and 1.33 (0.89–1.97) in cohort studies, indicating no statistically significant effect in either. An unhealthy diet yielded a RR of 1.27 (0.70–2.32) in case–control studies, also insignificant, but was associated with a modestly increased risk in cohort studies (RR: 1.46, 1.02–2.08). **Glycemic index (GI)/load**: Five case–control and three

Table 12.5 Recent cervical cancer predictive modeling studies.

Source	Year	Sample/data	Models used	Key metrics reported	Main results/performance
Devi et al. (2023)	2023	Pap smear, biopsies, multistage	DT, RF, LR, MLP, NB	Sensitivity, accuracy, AUC	LR: sensitivity 88%–94%, accuracy 84%–89%; DT similar accuracy, lower sensitivity; NB and LR highest AUC
Mohi Uddin et al. (2024)	2024	Patient demographics, clinical	SVM, NB, DT, KNN, RF, LR, GB, AdaBoost	Accuracy, *F*1-score	DT: accuracy 98.91%; *F*1 0.989; tuned SVM: accuracy 99.64%; *F*1 0.9963
Al Mudawi and Alazeb (2022)	2022	HPV and clinical data ($n = 132$)	DT, LR, SVM, KNN, AdaBoost, GB, RF, XGBoost	Accuracy	RF, DT, AdaBoost, GB: 100% accuracy; SVM: 99%
Aljrees (2024)	2024	Clinical data, KNN imputation	Ensemble (XGB, RF, ETC), RF, LR, SVC, GNB, etc.	Accuracy, precision, recall, *F*1	Ensemble showed improved metrics (accuracy, precision, recall, *F*1) vs. individuals
Pu et al. (2025)	2025	SEER registry	Survival Tree, RSF, GBSA, CoxPH, CoxTV	Concordance index, Brier score	GBSA: *C*-index 0.835, Brier 0.120; Tumor stage, surgery most important features

(*continued on next page*)

Table 12.5 Recent cervical cancer predictive modeling studies—cont'd

Source	Year	Sample/data	Models used	Key metrics reported	Main results/performance
Yuan et al. (2025)	2025	Chinese cohort ($n = 3900+$)	LASSO, Cox regression	*C*-index, ROC AUC, calibration, DCA	*C*-index 0.77–0.78; 1/3/5 years AUCs 0.76–0.82; outperformed FIGO staging
Li et al. (2024)	2024	SNPs + clinical ($n = 472$)	LR, SVM, RF, DT, XGBoost, DNN	Accuracy, sensitivity, specificity	The LR model with 6 SNPs + 2 variables is optimal; XGBoost/DNN has high accuracy but is less interpretable
Curia (2021)	2021	Small clinical datasets	SVM, C5.0 DT, extreme learning machine	Accuracy	C5.0 accuracy 67%–92% (varying context); social/behavioral features improved model

AdaBoost, adaptive boosting; *AUC*, area under curve; *DNN*, deep neural network; *DT*, decision tree; *ETC*, extra tree classifier; *GB*, gradient boosting; *KNN*, *k*-nearest neighbors; *LR*, logistic regression; *MLP*, multilayer perceptron; *NB*, naive Bayes; *RF*, random forest; *RSF*, random survival forest; *SVM*, support vector machine; *XGB*, extreme gradient boosting.

Table 12.6 The comprehensive study of ovarian cancer prediction models.

Source	Study/Model	Study design and dataset	Models compared	Predictors	Key metrics and results	Calibration and clinical utility	Conclusion and notes
Ledger et al. (2023)	Comprehensive Comparison of Multiclass Risk Models (2023)	Retrospective multicenter cohort; development $n = 5909$ (1999–2012), validation $n = 3199$ (2012–15)	Standard MLR, Ridge MLR, RF, XGBoost, NN, SVMs	Nine clinical and ultrasound features, with and without CA125 biomarker	Models with CA125: polytomous discrimination index ranged from 0.41 (SVM) to 0.55 (XGBoost); pairwise *C*-statistics >0.90 for some discrimination; AUROC ~0.92. Models without CA125 had similar AUROC	Best calibration observed for RF and XGBoost; worst for SVM. Clinical impact varied by model, affecting individual patient risk predictions	No single method consistently outperformed others. Individual risk estimates for same patient often varied by >20%. Model choice affects clinical decisions, highlighting the importance of interpretability and validation

(*continued on next page*)

Barreñada et al. (2024)	ADNEX Risk Model External Validation Meta-analysis (2024)	Systematic review and metaanalysis of 47 external validation studies (17,007 tumors)	ADNEX model	Clinical and ultrasound data, with and without CA125	Pooled summary AUC for benign vs. malignant discrimination was 0.93 with CA125 and 0.93 without. High consistency across populations	Well-calibrated across diverse populations. Estimated usefulness clinically: 95% (with CA125) and 91% (without CA125). High risk of bias present in many studies because of lack of calibration and data handling	ADNEX is robust for distinguishing benign vs. malignant adnexal masses worldwide, but calibration assessment needs improvement

(*continued on next page*)

Table 12.6 The comprehensive study of ovarian cancer prediction models—cont'd

Source	Study/Model	Study design and dataset	Models compared	Predictors	Key metrics and results	Calibration and clinical utility	Conclusion and notes
Breen et al. (2023)	AI and Deep Learning Models (up to 2023)	Systematic review of 45 studies covering 80 models; datasets 1–1375 histopathology slides (1–776 patients)	Mix of ML and deep learning: RF, SVM, DTs, neural networks, hybrids	Histopathology images and related data	Many models achieved >85% accuracy; RF often reported best; AUC up to 0.80. Performance is promising but variable quality	High risk of bias and generalizability issues noted; reproducibility is a critical challenge. No AI models currently in routine clinical use	Despite promise, AI models require validation, and clinical implementation hurdles remain
Asadi et al. (2025)	ML for Survival Outcome Prediction	Systematic review of ML models to predict ovarian cancer survival outcomes	RF, boosting, NN, traditional statistics	Clinical and molecular predictors	Improved accuracy over single predictors, but few were externally validated	Real-world utility and clinical adoption remain limited	ML models show potential but need larger validation and adoption
Wang et al. (2024)	Chemotherapy Response Prediction with ML	Systematic review of ML applications predicting platinum-based chemotherapy response	Various ML algorithms	Omics, imaging, clinical data	Some predictive power is seen but limited external validation	Not yet mainstream clinical use	Predictive ML models for chemotherapy response require further validation and acceptance

AI, artificial intelligence; *AUROC*, area under the receiver operating characteristic curve; *CA125*, cancer antigen 125 biomarker; *DTs*, decision trees; *LR*, logistic regression; *ML*, machine learning; *MLR*, multinomial LR; *NN*, neural networks; *RF*, random forest; *SVM*, support vector machine.

Table 12.7 Predictive models for women's postpartum depression, anxiety, stress-related disorders, and their nutritional status.

Source	Study, population, and focus	Predictive model type	Key predictors/features	Performance metrics	Nutritional status link	Notes
Qi et al. (2025)	PPD prediction (1138 perinatal women)	LR, ANN	History of mental illness, demographic, psychosocial, and physiological factors, postpartum care variables	AUC LR: 0.801–0.858; ANN: 0.787–0.844	Not directly focused on nutrition but includes physiological predictors	Early prediction tools for PPD with risk stratification and interpretability tools
Hosseinzadeh Kasani et al. (2023)	Depression and nutrition (4804 Korean adults)	ML (RF, XGBoost, etc.)	Nutritional markers: energy, protein, fat, carbohydrates, fiber; demographic and clinical data	Model-dependent; interpretability via SHAP and LIME	Strong negative correlation between dietary fiber, protein intake, and depression risk	Highlights nutrition as a modifiable risk factor for depression; interpretability varies by model
Khudri et al. (2023)	Nutritional Status Prediction in Women of Childbearing Age (Bangladeshi women)	Several supervised ML algorithms (RF, LR, etc.)	Socioeconomic status, breastfeeding practice, partner's education, residence, age	Variable importance rankings are used instead of direct metrics	Focus on predicting BMI and malnutrition risk	Breastfeeding practice and SES are important predictors of nutritional outcomes

(*continued on next page*)

Table 12.7 Predictive models for women's postpartum depression, anxiety, stress-related disorders, and their nutritional status—cont'd

Source	Study, population, and focus	Predictive model type	Key predictors/features	Performance metrics	Nutritional status link	Notes
Ndikumana et al. (2025)	Mental Health Predictive Modeling (Youth populations in multiple regions)	RF, SVM, GB, LR	Trauma experience, violence, family history, heavy drinking, BMI, physical activity	Accuracy up to 88.8%, AUC up to 83.59%	BMI and physical activity are included as predictors	Emphasizes environmental, behavioral, and nutritional factors in mental health
Saito et al. (2022)	Wearable Data for Mental Illness Prediction (General population with wearable data)	ML models using biometric and medical exam data	Sleep and activity data from wearables, medical examination records	AUC > 0.7	Indirect link via physiological health markers	Demonstrates feasibility of using physiological data for early mental illness prediction

ANN, artificial neural network; *AUC*, area under curve; *BMI*, body mass index; *GB*, gradient boosting; *LR*, logistic regression; *ML*, machine learning; *PPD*, postpartum depression; *RF*, random forest; *SVM*, support vector machine.

cohort studies analyzed these, finding no effect (GI RR: 1.08, 0.89–1.32; GL RR: 1.22, 0.95–1.56). **Cruciferous vegetable intake** was evaluated in six case–control and five cohort studies. Combined results indicated a small protective effect (RR: 0.90, 0.82–0.98); the effect was stronger in case–control studies (RR: 0.84, 0.75–0.94), but no effect in cohorts (RR: 1.00, 0.85–1.11). **Fish intake and green tea consumption** were also investigated. Green tea consistently showed a reduced risk (RR: 0.81, 0.73–0.89 across six studies), whereas fish intake showed no significant association. **Obesity (BMI > 30)**: Meta-analysis, including 30 case–control and 17 cohort studies, shows a modest increased risk (RR: 1.13, 1.06–1.20). **Physical activity**: Mixed results were observed. A meta-analysis of nine cohort studies found no significant association (RR: 1.01, 0.91–1.13). Pooled analysis from 10 case–control and 9 cohort studies found a possible reduction (RR: 0.92, 0.84–1.00), especially in case–control studies (RR: 0.86, 0.80–0.93), but no effect in cohort studies (RR: 1.03, 0.87–1.20). **Alcohol intake**: Multiple analyses (16 case–control, 4 cohort for light use; other subgroups) consistently reported no significant increase in ovarian cancer risk with light or moderate alcohol consumption (light intake RR: 0.98, 0.93–1.03; moderate RR: 1.03, 0.95–1.12). **Smoking**: Studies produced mixed results, with most analyses indicating no significant association in overall ovarian cancer risk but potentially increased risk for certain subtypes (21 case–control studies: RR: 0.89, 0.76–1.04; 32 case–control and 19 cohort: case–control RR: 1.08, 1.03–1.14; and cohort RR: 1.06, 1.01–1.11). **Breastfeeding**: Data from 35 case–control and five cohort studies show a substantial risk reduction (RR: 0.70, 0.64–0.76) (El-Sherif et al., 2021).

Surgical factors—Tubal ligation was associated with a significant decrease in ovarian cancer risk in a synthesis of 23 case–control and 7 cohort studies (RR: 0.70, 0.64–0.75), whereas hysterectomy also reduced risk (19 case–control, 5 cohort; RR: 0.74, 0.65–0.84) (El-Sherif et al., 2021).

Chemical factors—**Oral contraceptive** use was robustly associated with reduced ovarian cancer risk across 32 case–control and 13 cohort studies (RR: 0.73, 0.70–0.76). **Menopausal hormone** use showed an increased risk (52 cohort studies; RR: 1.14, 1.10–1.19). **Aspirin and NSAIDs**: The use of aspirin or NSAIDs across several studies did not show a significant effect on risk (Aspirin, 14 case–control and 6 cohort: RR: 0.93, 0.84–1.02; NSAIDs, 10 case–control and 6 cohort: RR: 0.94, 0.84–1.06) (El-Sherif et al., 2021).

12.2.8 Mental health predictions in women

Advanced ML approaches are revolutionizing the prediction and prevention of postpartum depression (PPD), anxiety, and stress-related disorders through sophisticated analysis of clinical, nutritional, and biological data. Current predictive models achieve remarkable accuracy rates of 73%–93% using ensemble methods, including RF, neural networks, and extreme GB (XGBoost) (Andersson et al., 2021; Lin & Zhou, 2025; Munk-Olsen et al., 2022; Qi et al., 2025). These models integrate multiple predictive factors ranging from prenatal mental health history and demographic variables to complex nutritional biomarkers and gut microbiome profiles. The application of predictive models for women's PPD, anxiety, stress-related disorders, and their nutritional predictive models is described in Table 12.7.

12.3 Conclusion

The application of AI and ML to healthcare data analysis represents a significant advancement. The area of predictive modeling in women's health is rapidly evolving, and its potential to revolutionize clinical practice is immense. ML and deep learning methods have shown promise in early disease diagnosis and prediction. ML techniques have been integrated to advance cervical cancer detection, where models analyze patient data to aid in early detection and prognosis. These models can uncover intricate relationships and predict individual risks, enabling healthcare providers to make informed decisions by analyzing complex datasets. Predictive models can also be used to identify women at high risk of pregnancy complications, allowing for timely interventions and improved maternal and infant outcomes. AI systems are increasingly used for disease detection, radiological imaging, genomics, and treatment planning, offering unprecedented diagnostic accuracy and efficiency. However, the successful implementation of predictive models requires careful consideration of ethical and practical challenges, including data privacy, model transparency, and potential biases. Recent developments in AI have enabled personalized treatment plans, which can significantly improve the standard of living for patients. Addressing these challenges will be crucial to realizing the full potential of predictive modeling in women's health and nutrition.

Ethical approval

Ethical approval was not required for this book chapter.

Declaration of competing interest

The authors declare that they have no known competing financial interests or personal relationships that could have appeared to influence the work reported in this chapter.

Acknowledgment

We are very much thankful to the Council of Scientific & Industrial Research (CSIR), Government of India, for providing a senior research fellowship (File no.—09/1035(18387)/2024-EMR-I) to S. Paul. The authors would like to acknowledge the Indian Council of Medical Research (ICMR) (File No.—5/13/59/2022/NCD-III), Government of India, for partly supporting the research to T. Parija.

References

Abualigah, L., Alomari, S. A., Almomani, M. H., Zitar, R. A., Saleem, K., Migdady, H., Snasel, V., Smerat, A., & Ezugwu, A. E. (2025). Artificial intelligence-driven translational medicine: A machine learning framework for predicting disease outcomes and optimizing patient-centric care. *Journal of Translational Medicine, 23*(1). https://doi.org/10.1186/s12967-025-06308-6.

Al Mudawi, N., & Alazeb, A. (2022). A model for predicting cervical cancer using machine learning algorithms. *Sensors, 22*(11), 4132. https://doi.org/10.3390/s22114132.

Al Tawil, A., Shaban, A., & Almazaydeh, L. (2024). A comparative analysis of convolutional neural networks for breast cancer prediction. *International Journal of Electrical and Computer Engineering (IJECE), 14*(3), 3406. https://doi.org/10.11591/ijece.v14i3.pp3406-3414.

Aljrees, T. (2024). Improving prediction of cervical cancer using KNN imputer and multi-model ensemble learning. *PLOS ONE, 19*(1), e0295632. https://doi.org/10.1371/journal.pone.0295632.

Almarri, B., Gupta, G., Kumar, R., Vandana, V., Asiri, F., & Khan, S. B. (2024). The BCPM method: Decoding breast cancer with machine learning. *BMC Medical Imaging, 24*(1), 248. https://doi.org/10.1186/s12880-024-01402-5.

Ameye, L. G., & Chee, W. S. (2006). Osteoarthritis and nutrition. From nutraceuticals to functional foods: A systematic review of the scientific evidence. *Arthritis Research & Therapy, 8*(4), R127. https://doi.org/10.1186/ar2016.

Andersson, S., Bathula, D. R., Iliadis, S. I., Walter, M., & Skalkidou, A. (2021). Predicting women with depressive symptoms postpartum with machine learning methods. *Scientific Reports, 11*(1), 7877. https://doi.org/10.1038/s41598-021-86368-y.

Asadi, F., Rahimi, M., Ramezanghorbani, N., & Almasi, S. (2025). Comparing the effectiveness of artificial intelligence models in predicting ovarian cancer survival: A systematic review. *Cancer Reports, 8*(3), e70138. https://doi.org/10.1002/cnr2.70138.

Asemi, Z., & Esmaillzadeh, A. (2015). DASH diet, insulin resistance, and serum hs-CRP in polycystic ovary syndrome: A randomized controlled clinical trial. *Hormone and Metabolic Research, 47*(03), 232–238. https://doi.org/10.1055/s-0034-1376990.

Ashinsky, B. G., Bouhrara, M., Coletta, C. E., Lehallier, B., Urish, K. L., Lin, P., Goldberg, I. G., & Spencer, R. G. (2017). Predicting early symptomatic osteoarthritis in the human knee using machine learning classification of magnetic resonance images from the osteoarthritis initiative. *Journal of Orthopaedic Research, 35*(10), 2243–2250. https://doi.org/10.1002/jor.23519.

Ba, D., Ba, S., & Md, M. (2023). What the world needs now: Lifestyle medicine for all women. *American Journal of Lifestyle Medicine, 17*(1), 97–107. https://doi.org/10.1177/15598276211028101.

Bachelot, G., Lévy, R., Bachelot, A., Faure, C., Czernichow, S., Dupont, C., & Lamazière, A.Alifert Collaborative Group. (2021). Proof of concept and development of a couple-based machine learning model to stratify infertile patients with idiopathic infertility. *Scientific Reports, 11*(1), 24003. https://doi.org/10.1038/s41598-021-03165-3.

Badawy, M., Ramadan, N., & Hefny, H. A. (2023). Healthcare predictive analytics using machine learning and deep learning techniques: A survey. *Journal of Electrical Systems and Information Technology, 10*(1). https://doi.org/10.1186/s43067-023-00108-y.

Barreñada, L., Ledger, A., Dhiman, P., Collins, G., Wynants, L., Verbakel, J. Y., Timmerman, D., Valentin, L., & Van Calster, B. (2024). ADNEX risk prediction model for diagnosis of ovarian cancer: Systematic review and meta-analysis of external validation studies. *BMJ Medicine, 3*(1), e000817. https://doi.org/10.1136/bmjmed-2023-000817.

Begum, N., Rahman, M. M., & Omar Faruk, M. (2024). Machine learning prediction of nutritional status among pregnant women in Bangladesh: Evidence from Bangladesh demographic and health survey 2017–18. *PLOS ONE, 19*(5), e0304389. https://doi.org/10.1371/journal.pone.0304389.

Bhimavarapu, U., Battineni, G., & Chintalapudi, N. (2025). Machine learning-driven prediction of vitamin D deficiency severity with hybrid optimization. *Bioengineering, 12*(2), 200. https://doi.org/10.3390/bioengineering12020200.

Breen, J., Allen, K., Zucker, K., Adusumilli, P., Scarsbrook, A., Hall, G., Orsi, N. M., & Ravikumar, N. (2023). Artificial intelligence in ovarian cancer histopathology: A systematic review. *npj Precision Oncology, 7*(1), 83. https://doi.org/10.1038/s41698-023-00432-6.

Brink, L. R., Bender, T. M., Davies, R., Luo, H., Miketinas, D., Shah, N., Loveridge, N., Gross, G., & Fawkes, N. (2022). Optimizing maternal nutrition: The importance of a tailored approach. *Current Developments in Nutrition, 6*(9), nzac118. https://doi.org/10.1093/cdn/nzac118.

Calcaterra, V., Magenes, V. C., Massini, G., De Sanctis, L., Fabiano, V., & Zuccotti, G. (2024). High fat diet and polycystic ovary syndrome (PCOS) in adolescence: An overview of nutritional strategies. *Nutrients, 16*(7), 938. https://doi.org/10.3390/nu16070938.

Cao, D., & Dong, Q. (2024). Predictive value of prognostic nutritional index for outcomes of cervical cancer: A systematic review and meta-analysis. *Experimental and Therapeutic Medicine, 28*(2), 316. https://doi.org/10.3892/etm.2024.12605.

Carvalho, F. R., & Gavaia, P. J. (2025). Enhancing osteoporosis risk prediction using machine learning: A holistic approach integrating biomarkers and clinical data. *Computers in Biology and Medicine, 192*, 110289. https://doi.org/10.1016/j.compbiomed.2025.110289.

Chavarro, J. E., Rich-Edwards, J. W., Rosner, B. A., & Willett, W. C. (2007). Diet and lifestyle in the prevention of ovulatory disorder infertility. *Obstetrics & Gynecology, 110*(5), 1050–1058. https://doi.org/10.1097/01.AOG.0000287293.25465.e1.

Clapp, M. A., Kim, E., James, K. E., Perlis, R. H., Kaimal, A. J., & McCoy, T. H. (2022). Natural language processing of admission notes to predict severe maternal morbidity during the delivery encounter. *American Journal of Obstetrics and Gynecology, 227*(3), 511.e1–511.e8. https://doi.org/10.1016/j.ajog.2022.04.008.

Cook, N. R., Buring, J. E., & Ridker, P. M. (2006). The effect of including C-reactive protein in cardiovascular risk prediction models for women. *Annals of Internal Medicine, 145*(1), 21–29. https://doi.org/10.7326/0003-4819-145-1-200607040-00128.

Curia, F. (2021). Cervical cancer risk prediction with robust ensemble and explainable black boxes method. *Health and Technology, 11*(4), 875–885. https://doi.org/10.1007/s12553-021-00554-6.

Deepak Kumar, K., Huntriss, R., Green, E., Bora, S., & Pettitt, C. (2023). Development of a nutrition screening tool to identify need for dietetic intervention in female infertility. *Journal of Human Nutrition and Dietetics, 36*(1), 154–168. https://doi.org/10.1111/jhn.13055.

Dejene, B. E., Abuhay, T. M., & Bogale, D. S. (2022). Predicting the level of anemia among Ethiopian pregnant women using homogeneous ensemble machine learning algorithm. *BMC Medical Informatics and Decision Making, 22*(1). https://doi.org/10.1186/s12911-022-01992-6.

Devi, S., Gaikwad, S. R., & Harikrishnan, R. (2023). Prediction and detection of cervical malignancy using machine learning models. *Asian Pacific Journal of Cancer Prevention, 24*(4), 1419–1433. https://doi.org/10.31557/APJCP.2023.24.4.1419.

Dhaliwal, S., Goh, L., Welborn, T., Thompson, P., Maycock, B., Kerr, D., Lee, A., Bertolatti, D., Clark, K., Naheed, R., Coorey, R., & Della, P. (2014). Cardiovascular disease risk score prediction models for women and its applicability to Asians. *International Journal of Women's Health, 259*. https://doi.org/10.2147/IJWH.S55225.

Du, Y., Almajalid, R., Shan, J., & Zhang, M. (2018). A novel method to predict knee osteoarthritis progression on MRI using machine learning methods. *IEEE Transactions on NanoBioscience, 17*(3), 228–236. https://doi.org/10.1109/TNB.2018.2840082.

El-Sherif, A., El-Sherif, S., Taylor, A. H., & Ayakannu, T. (2021). Ovarian cancer: Lifestyle, diet and nutrition. *Nutrition and Cancer, 73*(7), 1092–1107. https://doi.org/10.1080/01635581.2020.1792948.

Ende, H. B. (2022). Risk assessment tools to predict postpartum hemorrhage. *Best Practice & Research Clinical Anaesthesiology, 36*(3–4), 341–348. https://doi.org/10.1016/j.bpa.2022.08.003.

Erdélyi, A., Pálfi, E., Tűű, L., Nas, K., Szűcs, Z., Török, M., Jakab, A., & Várbíró, S. (2023). The importance of nutrition in menopause and perimenopause—A review. *Nutrients, 16*(1), 27. https://doi.org/10.3390/nu16010027.

Espinosa, C., Becker, M., Marić, I., Wong, R. J., Shaw, G. M., Gaudilliere, B., Aghaeepour, N., Stevenson, D. K., Stelzer, I. A., Peterson, L. S., Chang, A. L., Xenochristou, M., Phongpreecha, T., De Francesco, D., Katz, M., Blumenfeld, Y. J., & Angst, M. S. (2021). Data-driven modeling of pregnancy-related complications. *Trends in Molecular Medicine, 27*(8), 762–776. https://doi.org/10.1016/j.molmed.2021.01.007.

Farvid, M. S., Holmes, M. D., Chen, W. Y., Rosner, B. A., Tamimi, R. M., Willett, W. C., & Eliassen, A. H. (2020). Postdiagnostic fruit and vegetable consumption and breast cancer survival: Prospective analyses in the Nurses' Health Studies. *Cancer Research, 80*(22), 5134–5143. https://doi.org/10.1158/0008-5472.can-18-3515.

Fernandes, G. S., Bhattacharya, A., McWilliams, D. F., Ingham, S. L., Doherty, M., & Zhang, W. (2017). Risk prediction model for knee pain in the Nottingham community: A Bayesian modelling approach. *Arthritis Research & Therapy, 19*(1), 59. https://doi.org/10.1186/s13075-017-1272-6.

Garriga, C., Sánchez-Santos, M. T., Judge, A., Hart, D., Spector, T., Cooper, C., & Arden, N. K. (2020). Predicting incident radiographic knee osteoarthritis in middle-aged women within four years: The importance of knee-level prognostic factors. *Arthritis Care & Research, 72*(1), 88–97. https://doi.org/10.1002/acr.23932.

Gebeye, L. G., Dessie, E. Y., & Yimam, J. A. (2024). Predictors of micronutrient deficiency among children aged 6–23 months in Ethiopia: A machine learning approach. *Frontiers in Nutrition, 10*, 1277048. https://doi.org/10.3389/fnut.2023.1277048.

Gómez-Vaquero, C., Nolla, J. M., Fiter, J., Ramon, J. M., Concustell, R., Valverde, J., & Roig-Escofet, D. (2001). Nutritional status in patients with rheumatoid arthritis. *Joint Bone Spine, 68*(5), 403–409. https://doi.org/10.1016/S1297-319X(01)00296-2.

Gu, X., Li, Q., & Wang, X. (2025). Using life's essential 8 and heavy metal exposure to determine infertility risk in American women: A machine learning prediction model based on the SHAP method. *Frontiers in Endocrinology, 16*, 1586828. https://doi.org/10.3389/fendo.2025.1586828.

Guo, J., He, Q., & Li, Y. (2024). Machine learning-based prediction of vitamin D deficiency: NHANES 2001-2018. *Frontiers in Endocrinology, 15*, 1327058. https://doi.org/10.3389/fendo.2024.1327058.

Halilaj, E., Le, Y., Hicks, J. L., Hastie, T. J., & Delp, S. L. (2018). Modeling and predicting osteoarthritis progression: Data from the osteoarthritis initiative. *Osteoarthritis and Cartilage, 26*(12), 1643–1650. https://doi.org/10.1016/j.joca.2018.08.003.

Hejazi, J., Davoodi, A., Khosravi, M., Sedaghat, M., Abedi, V., Hosseinverdi, S., Ehrampoush, E., Homayounfar, R., & Shojaie, L. (2020). Nutrition and osteoporosis prevention and treatment. *Biomedical Research and Therapy, 7*(4), 3709–3720. https://doi.org/10.15419/bmrat.v7i4.598.

Hosseinzadeh Kasani, P., Lee, J. E., Park, C., Yun, C.-H., Jang, J.-W., & Lee, S.-A. (2023). Evaluation of nutritional status and clinical depression classification using an explainable machine learning method. *Frontiers in Nutrition, 10*, 1165854. https://doi.org/10.3389/fnut.2023.1165854.

Hu, W. S., Lee, J. H., Tsai, M. K., & Wen, C. P. (2017). A novel cardiovascular death prediction model for Chinese individuals: A prospective cohort study of 381,963 study participants. *Atherosclerosis, 264*, 19–28. https://doi.org/10.1016/j.atherosclerosis.2017.07.016.

Hu, Y., Sparks, J. A., Malspeis, S., Costenbader, K. H., Hu, F. B., Karlson, E. W., & Lu, B. (2017). Long-term dietary quality and risk of developing rheumatoid arthritis in women. *Annals of the Rheumatic Diseases, 76*(8), 1357–1364. https://doi.org/10.1136/annrheumdis-2016-210431.

Huang, Y. Y., Tian, W. B., Jiang, C. Q., Zhang, W. S., Zhu, F., Jin, Y. L., … Cheng, K. K. (2022). A Simple Model for Predicting 10-Year Cardiovascular Risk in Middle-Aged to Older Chinese: Guangzhou Biobank Cohort Study. *Journal of cardiovascular translational research, 15*(2), 416–426. https://doi.org/10.1007/s12265-021-10163-3.

Hussain, S., Ali, M., Naseem, U., Nezhadmoghadam, F., Jatoi, M. A., Gulliver, T. A., & Tamez-Peña, J. G. (2024). Breast cancer risk prediction using machine learning: A systematic review. *Frontiers in Oncology, 14*. https://doi.org/10.3389/fonc.2024.1343627.

Hyvärinen, M., Karvanen, J., Aukee, P., Tammelin, T. H., Sipilä, S., Kujala, U. M., Kovanen, V., Rantalainen, T., & Laakkonen, E. K. (2021). Predicting the age at natural menopause in middle-aged women. *Menopause, 28*(7), 792–799. https://doi.org/10.1097/GME.0000000000001774.

Ifeanyi Obeagu, E. (2023). Beyond conventional therapies: Exploring nutritional interventions for cervical cancer patients. *Cancer Research and Cellular Therapeutics, 8*(1), 1–6. https://doi.org/10.31579/2640-1053/180.

Islam, T., Sheakh, M. A., Tahosin, M. S., Hena, M. H., Akash, S., Bin Jardan, Y. A., FentahunWondmie, G., Nafidi, H.-A., & Bourhia, M. (2024). Predictive modeling for breast cancer classification in the context of Bangladeshi patients by use of machine learning approach with explainable AI. *Scientific Reports, 14*(1), 8487. https://doi.org/10.1038/s41598-024-57740-5.

Jabbari, M., Barati, M., Kalhori, A., Eini-Zinab, H., Zayeri, F., Poustchi, H., Pourshams, A., Hekmatdoost, A., & Malekzadeh, R. (2025). Development of a CVD mortality risk score using nutritional predictors: A risk prediction model in the Golestan cohort study. *Nutrition, Metabolism and Cardiovascular Diseases, 35*(1), 103770. https://doi.org/10.1016/j.numecd.2024.10.008.

Jamel, L., Umer, M., Saidani, O., Alabduallah, B., Alsubai, S., Ishmanov, F., Kim, T., & Ashraf, I. (2024). Improving prediction of maternal health risks using PCA features and TreeNet model. *PeerJ Computer Science, 10*, e1982. https://doi.org/10.7717/peerj-cs.1982.

Jeihooni, A. K., Hidarnia, A., Kaveh, M. H., & Hajizadeh, E. (2017). The predictors of osteoporosis preventive behaviors in women based on health belief model. *Journal of Research & Health, 7*(4), 971–978. https://doi.org/10.18869/acadpub.jrh.7.4.971.

Joseph, G. B., McCulloch, C. E., Nevitt, M. C., Neumann, J., Gersing, A. S., Kretzschmar, M., Schwaiger, B. J., Lynch, J. A., Heilmeier, U., Lane, N. E., & Link, T. M. (2018). Tool for osteoarthritis risk prediction (TOARP) over 8 years using baseline clinical data, X-ray, and MRI: Data from the osteoarthritis initiative. *Journal of Magnetic Resonance Imaging, 47*(6), 1517–1526. https://doi.org/10.1002/jmri.25892.

Kasartzian, D.-I., & Tsiampalis, T. (2025). Transforming cardiovascular risk prediction: A review of machine learning and artificial intelligence innovations. *Life, 15*(1), 94. https://doi.org/10.3390/life15010094.

Kaviani, E., & Passi, K. (2025). Forecasting cancer incidence in Canada by age, sex, and region until 2026 using machine learning techniques. *Algorithms, 18*(5), 265. https://doi.org/10.3390/a18050265.

Kerkhof, H. J. M., Bierma-Zeinstra, S. M. A., Arden, N. K., Metrustry, S., Castano-Betancourt, M., Hart, D. J., Hofman, A., Rivadeneira, F., Oei, E. H. G., Spector, T. D., Uitterlinden, A. G., Janssens, A. C. J. W., Valdes, A. M., & Van Meurs, J. B. J. (2014). Prediction model for knee osteoarthritis incidence, including clinical, genetic and biochemical risk factors. *Annals of the Rheumatic Diseases, 73*(12), 2116–2121. https://doi.org/10.1136/annrheumdis-2013-203620.

Khadidos, A. O., Saleem, F., Selvarajan, S., Ullah, Z., & Khadidos, A. O. (2024). Ensemble machine learning framework for predicting maternal health risk during pregnancy. *Scientific Reports, 14*(1). https://doi.org/10.1038/s41598-024-71934-x.

Khani Jeihooni, A., Jormand, H., Saadat, N., Hatami, M., Abdul Manaf, R., & Afzali Harsini, P. (2021). The application of the theory of planned behavior to nutritional behaviors related to cardiovascular disease among the women. *BMC Cardiovascular Disorders, 21*(1), 589. https://doi.org/10.1186/s12872-021-02399-3.

Khudri, M. M., Rhee, K. K., Hasan, M. S., & Ahsan, K. Z. (2023). Predicting nutritional status for women of childbearing age from their economic, health, and demographic features: A supervised machine learning approach. *PLOS ONE, 18*(5), e0277738. https://doi.org/10.1371/journal.pone.0277738.

Kim, H. C., Greenland, P., Rossouw, J. E., Manson, J. E., Cochrane, B. B., Lasser, N. L., Limacher, M. C., Lloyd-Jones, D. M., Margolis, K. L., & Robinson, J. G. (2010). Multimarker prediction of coronary heart disease risk. *Journal of the American College of Cardiology, 55*(19), 2080–2091. https://doi.org/10.1016/j.jacc.2009.12.047.

Kinds, M. B., Marijnissen, A. C. A., Vincken, K. L., Viergever, M. A., Drossaers-Bakker, K. W., Bijlsma, J. W. J., Bierma-Zeinstra, S. M. A., Welsing, P. M. J., & Lafeber, F. P. J. G. (2012). Evaluation of separate quantitative radiographic features adds to the prediction of incident radiographic osteoarthritis in individuals with recent onset of knee pain: 5-year follow-up in the CHECK cohort. *Osteoarthritis and Cartilage, 20*(6), 548–556. https://doi.org/10.1016/j.joca.2012.02.009.

Kraus, V. B., Collins, J. E., Hargrove, D., Losina, E., Nevitt, M., Katz, J. N., Wang, S. X., Sandell, L. J., Hoffmann, S. C., & Hunter, D. J. (2017). Predictive validity of biochemical biomarkers in knee osteoarthritis: Data from the FNIH OA biomarkers consortium. *Annals of the Rheumatic Diseases, 76*(1), 186–195. https://doi.org/10.1136/annrheumdis-2016-209252.

Landsmeer, M. L. A., Runhaar, J., Van Middelkoop, M., Oei, E. H. G., Schiphof, D., Bindels, P. J. E., & Bierma-Zeinstra, S. M. A. (2019). Predicting knee pain and knee osteoarthritis among overweight women. *The Journal of the American Board of Family Medicine, 32*(4), 575–584. https://doi.org/10.3122/jabfm.2019.04.180302.

LaValley, M. P., Lo, G. H., Price, L. L., Driban, J. B., Eaton, C. B., & McAlindon, T. E. (2017). Development of a clinical prediction algorithm for knee osteoarthritis structural progression in a cohort study: Value of adding measurement of subchondral bone density. *Arthritis Research & Therapy, 19*(1), 95. https://doi.org/10.1186/s13075-017-1291-3.

Lazzarini, N., Runhaar, J., Bay-Jensen, A. C., Thudium, C. S., Bierma-Zeinstra, S. M. A., Henrotin, Y., & Bacardit, J. (2017). A machine learning approach for the identification of new biomarkers for knee osteoarthritis development in overweight and obese women. *Osteoarthritis and Cartilage, 25*(12), 2014–2021. https://doi.org/10.1016/j.joca.2017.09.001.

Ledger, A., Ceusters, J., Valentin, L., Testa, A., Van Holsbeke, C., Franchi, D., Bourne, T., Froyman, W., Timmerman, D., & Van Calster, B. (2023). Multiclass risk models for ovarian malignancy: An illustration of prediction uncertainty due to the choice of algorithm. *BMC Medical Research Methodology, 23*(1), 276. https://doi.org/10.1186/s12874-023-02103-3.

Li, Q., Alfonso, Y. N., Wolfson, C., Aziz, K. B., & Creanga, A. A. (2025). Leveraging machine learning to predict and assess disparities in severe maternal morbidity in Maryland. *Healthcare, 13*(3), 284. https://doi.org/10.3390/healthcare13030284.

Li, T. C., Li, C. I., Liu, C. S., Lin, W. Y., Lin, C. H., Yang, S. Y., & Lin, C. C. (2020). Derivation and validation of 10-year all-cause and cardiovascular disease mortality prediction model for middle-aged and elderly community-dwelling adults in Taiwan. *PloS one, 15*(9), e0239063. https://doi.org/10.1371/journal.pone.0239063.

Li, X., Ning, R., Xiao, B., Meng, S., Sun, H., Fan, X., & Li, S. (2024). A multi-variable predictive warning model for cervical cancer using clinical and SNPs data. *Frontiers in Medicine, 11*, 1294230. https://doi.org/10.3389/fmed.2024.1294230.

Lim, J., Kim, J., & Cheon, S. (2019). A deep neural network-based method for early detection of osteoarthritis using statistical data. *International Journal of Environmental Research and Public Health, 16*(7), 1281. https://doi.org/10.3390/ijerph16071281.

Lin, Y., & Zhou, D. (2025). A method for predicting postpartum depression via an ensemble neural network model. *Frontiers in Public Health, 13*, 1571522. https://doi.org/10.3389/fpubh.2025.1571522.

Liu, B., Xia, H., Zhang, J., Hu, Y., & Wang, Q. (2024). Building personalized risk prediction models for polycystic ovary syndrome using machine learning techniques: A retrospective study. *SSRN*. https://doi.org/10.2139/ssrn.4865261.

Liu, J., Hong, Y., D'Agostino, R. B., Sr, Wu, Z., Wang, W., Sun, J., Wilson, P. W., Kannel, W. B., & Zhao, D. (2004). Predictive value for the Chinese population of the Framingham CHD risk assessment tool compared with the Chinese Multi-Provincial Cohort Study. JAMA, 291(21), 2591–2599. https://doi.org/10.1001/jama.291.21.2591.

Long, M. J., Papi, E., Duffell, L. D., & McGregor, A. H. (2017). Predicting knee osteoarthritis risk in injured populations. *Clinical Biomechanics, 47*, 87–95. https://doi.org/10.1016/j.clinbiomech.2017.06.001.

Mohammad, I. B., & Ahmad, M. M. (2025). Bayesian model prediction for breast cancer survival: A retrospective analysis. *European Journal of Breast Health*. https://doi.org/10.4274/ejbh.galenos.2025.2025-2-14.

Mohi Uddin, K. M., Sikder, I. A., & Hasan, M. N. (2024). A comparative study on machine learning classifiers for cervical cancer prediction: A predictive analytic approach. *EAI Endorsed Transactions on Internet of Things, 11*. https://doi.org/10.4108/eetiot.6223.

Morgenstern, J. D., Rosella, L. C., Costa, A. P., & Anderson, L. N. (2022). Development of machine learning prediction models to explore nutrients predictive of cardiovascular disease using Canadian linked population-based data. *Applied Physiology, Nutrition, and Metabolism, 47*(5), 529–546. https://doi.org/10.1139/apnm-2021-0502.

Munk-Olsen, T., Liu, X., Madsen, K. B., Kjeldsen, M.-M. Z., Petersen, L. V., Bergink, V., Skalkidou, A., Vigod, S. N., Frokjaer, V. G., Pedersen, C. B., & Maegbaek, M. L. (2022). Postpartum depression: A developed and validated model predicting individual risk in new mothers. *Translational Psychiatry, 12*(1), 419. https://doi.org/10.1038/s41398-022-02190-8.

Nazari, E., Hasanzadeh, M., Rezvani, R., Rejali, M., Badpeyma, M., Delaram, Z., Mousavi-Seresht, L., Akbari, M., Khazaei, M., Ferns, G. A., & Avan, A. (2023). Association of dietary intake and cervical cancer: A prevention strategy. *Infectious Agents and Cancer, 18*(1), 42. https://doi.org/10.1186/s13027-023-00517-8.

Ndikumana, F., Izabayo, J., Kalisa, J., Nemerimana, M., Nyabyenda, E. C., Muzungu, S. H., Komezusenge, I., Uwase, M., Ndagijimana, S., Twizere, C., & Sezibera, V. (2025). Machine learning-based predictive modelling of mental health in Rwandan Youth. *Scientific Reports, 15*(1), 16032. https://doi.org/10.1038/s41598-025-00519-z.

Ngusie, H. S., Enyew, E. B., Walle, A. D., Tilahun Assaye, B., Kasaye, M. D., Tesfa, G. A., & Zemariam, A. B. (2024). Employing machine learning techniques for prediction of micronutrient supplementation status during pregnancy in East African Countries. *Scientific Reports, 14*(1), 23827. https://doi.org/10.1038/s41598-024-75455-5.

Noman, S. M., Fadel, Y. M., Henedak, M. T., Attia, N. A., Essam, M., Elmaasarawii, S., Fouad, F. A., Eltasawi, E. G., & Al-Atabany, W. (2025). Leveraging survival analysis and machine learning for accurate prediction of breast cancer recurrence and metastasis. *Scientific Reports, 15*(1), 3728. https://doi.org/10.1038/s41598-025-87622-3.

Noormohammadi, M., Eslamian, G., Malek, S., Shoaibinobarian, N., & Mirmohammadali, S. N. (2022). The association between fertility diet score and polycystic ovary syndrome: A case-control study. *Health Care for Women International, 43*(1–3), 70–84. https://doi.org/10.1080/07399332.2021.1886298.

Ou Yang, W.-Y., Lai, C.-C., Tsou, M.-T., & Hwang, L.-C. (2021). Development of machine learning models for prediction of osteoporosis from clinical health examination data. *International Journal of Environmental Research and Public Health, 18*(14), 7635. https://doi.org/10.3390/ijerph18147635.

Pu, Y., Liu, J., & Chan, K. H. K. (2025). Comparative study of five-year cervical cancer cause-specific survival prediction models based on SEER data. *Scientific Reports, 15*(1), 22465. https://doi.org/10.1038/s41598-025-04540-0.

Pylypchuk, R., Wells, S., Kerr, A., Poppe, K., Riddell, T., Harwood, M., ... Jackson, R. (2018). Cardiovascular disease risk prediction equations in 400 000 primary care patients in New Zealand: a derivation and validation study. *Lancet (London, England), 391*(10133), 1897–1907. https://doi.org/10.1016/S0140-6736(18)30664-0.

Qi, W., Wang, Y., Wang, Y., Huang, S., Li, C., Jin, H., Zuo, J., Cui, X., Wei, Z., Guo, Q., & Hu, J. (2025). Prediction of postpartum depression in women: Development and validation of multiple machine learning models. *Journal of Translational Medicine, 23*(1), 291. https://doi.org/10.1186/s12967-025-06289-6.

Raeisi-Dehkordi, H., Kummer, S., Francis Raguindin, P., Dejanovic, G., Eylul Taneri, P., Cardona, I., Kastrati, L., Minder, B., Voortman, T., Marques-Vidal, P., Dhana, K., Glisic, M., & Muka, T. (2022). Risk prediction models of natural menopause onset: A systematic review. *The Journal of Clinical Endocrinology & Metabolism, 107*(10), 2934–2944. https://doi.org/10.1210/clinem/dgac461.

Ross, P. D., Wasnich, R. D., & Davis, J. W. (1990). Fracture prediction models for osteoporosis prevention. *Bone, 11*(5), 327–331. https://doi.org/10.1016/8756-3282(90)90088-G.

Saito, T., Suzuki, H., & Kishi, A. (2022). Predictive modeling of mental illness onset using wearable devices and medical examination data: Machine learning approach. *Frontiers in Digital Health, 4*, 861808. https://doi.org/10.3389/fdgth.2022.861808.

Shadick, N. A. (2006). C-reactive protein in the prediction of rheumatoid arthritis in women. *Archives of Internal Medicine, 166*(22), 2490. https://doi.org/10.1001/archinte.166.22.2490.

Shahid, R., Iahtisham-Ul-Haq, Mahnoor, Awan, K. A., Iqbal, M. J., Munir, H., & Saeed, I. (2022). Diet and lifestyle modifications for effective management of polycystic ovarian syndrome (PCOS). *Journal of Food Biochemistry, 46*(7). https://doi.org/10.1111/jfbc.14117.

Sheng, B., Huang, L., Wang, X., Zhuang, J., Tang, L., Deng, C., & Zhang, Y. (2019). Identification of knee osteoarthritis based on Bayesian network: Pilot study. *JMIR Medical Informatics, 7*(3), e13562. https://doi.org/10.2196/13562.

Simegn, G. L., & Degu, M. Z. (2025). Maternal health risk analysis, automated pregnancy risk level identification and status monitoring system based on multivariable clinical data. *Health Technology, 9*, 1. https://doi.org/10.21037/ht-23-10.

Sunyecz, J. (2008). The use of calcium and vitamin D in the management of osteoporosis. *Therapeutics and Clinical Risk Management, 4*, 827–836. https://doi.org/10.2147/TCRM.S3552.

Takahashi, H., Nakajima, M., Ozaki, K., Tanaka, T., Kamatani, N., & Ikegawa, S. (2010). Prediction model for knee osteoarthritis based on genetic and clinical information. *Arthritis Research & Therapy, 12*(5), R187. https://doi.org/10.1186/ar3157.

Tegaw, E. M., & Asfaw, B. B. (2025). Machine learning analysis of survival outcomes in breast cancer patients treated with chemotherapy, hormone therapy, surgery, and radiotherapy. *Scientific Reports, 15*(1), 24981. https://doi.org/10.1038/s41598-025-97763-0.

Teng, X., Liu, M., Wang, Z., & Dong, X. (2025). Machine learning prediction of preterm birth in women under 35 using routine biomarkers in a retrospective cohort study. *Scientific Reports, 15*(1). https://doi.org/10.1038/s41598-025-92814-y.

Tiulpin, A., Klein, S., Bierma-Zeinstra, S. M. A., Thevenot, J., Rahtu, E., Meurs, J. V., Oei, E. H. G., & Saarakkala, S. (2019). Multimodal machine learning-based knee osteoarthritis progression prediction from plain radiographs and clinical data. *Scientific Reports, 9*(1), 20038. https://doi.org/10.1038/s41598-019-56527-3.

Togunwa, T. O., Babatunde, A. O., & Abdullah, K.-R. (2023). Deep hybrid model for maternal health risk classification in pregnancy: Synergy of ANN and random forest. *Frontiers in Artificial Intelligence, 6*. https://doi.org/10.3389/frai.2023.1213436.

Toma, M., & Wei, O. C. (2023). Predictive modeling in medicine. *Encyclopedia, 3*(2), 590–601. https://doi.org/10.3390/encyclopedia3020042.

Tzimourta, K. D., Tsipouras, M. G., Angelidis, P., Tsalikakis, D. G., & Orovou, E. (2025). Maternal health risk detection: Advancing midwifery with artificial intelligence. *Healthcare, 13*(7), 833. https://doi.org/10.3390/healthcare13070833.

Van Oudenaarde, K., Jobke, B., Oostveen, A. C. M., Marijnissen, A. C. A., Wolterbeek, R., Wesseling, J., Bierma-Zeinstra, S. M. A., Bloem, H. L., Reijnierse, M., & Kloppenburg, M. (2017). Predictive value of MRI features for development of radiographic osteoarthritis in a cohort of participants with pre-radiographic knee osteoarthritis—The CHECK study. *Rheumatology, 56*(1), 113–120. https://doi.org/10.1093/rheumatology/kew368.

Wang, J., Shan, L., Hang, J., Li, H., Meng, Y., Cao, W., Gu, C., Dai, J., & Tao, L. (2025). Development and validation of a novel prediction model for osteoporosis: From serotonin to fat-soluble vitamins. *Bone & Joint Research, 14*(2), 111–123. https://doi.org/10.1302/2046-3758.142.BJR-2023-0409.R2.

Wang, Q., Chang, Z., Liu, X., Wang, Y., Feng, C., Ping, Y., & Feng, X. (2024). Predictive value of machine learning for platinum chemotherapy responses in ovarian cancer: Systematic review and meta-analysis. *Journal of Medical Internet Research, 26*, e48527. https://doi.org/10.2196/48527.

Wang, Wei, & Zhao, Dong (2003). Prospective study on the predictive model of cardiovascular disease risk in a Chinese population aged 35-64 Zhonghua xin xue Guan. *Bing za zhi, 31*(12), 902–908.

Wang, Y., Liu, J., Wang, W., Wang, M., Qi, Y., Xie, W., ... Zhao, D. (2015). Lifetime risk for cardiovascular disease in a Chinese population: the Chinese Multi-Provincial Cohort Study. *European journal of preventive cardiology, 22*(3), 380–388. https://doi.org/10.1177/2047487313516563.

Wang, Z., Lin, R., Li, Y., Zeng, J., Chen, Y., Ouyang, W., Li, H., Jia, X., Lai, Z., Yu, Y., Yao, H., & Su, W. (2024). Deep learning-based multi-modal data integration enhancing breast cancer disease-free survival prediction. *Precision Clinical Medicine, 7*(2), pbae012. https://doi.org/10.1093/pcmedi/pbae012.

Wu, Y., Liu, X., Li, X., Li, Y., Zhao, L., Chen, Z., ... Liu, K. (2006). Estimation of 10-year risk of fatal and nonfatal ischemic cardiovascular diseases in Chinese adults. *Circulation, 114*(21), 2217–2225. https://doi.org/10.1161/CIRCULATIONAHA.105.607499.

Yang, L., Wu, H., Jin, X., Zheng, P., Hu, S., Xu, X., ... Yan, J. (2020). Study of cardiovascular disease prediction model based on random forest in eastern China. *Scientific reports, 10*(1), 5245. https://doi.org/10.1038/s41598-020-62133-5.

Yang, X., Li, J., Hu, D., Chen, J., Li, Y., Huang, J., ... Gu, D. (2016). Predicting the 10-Year Risks of Atherosclerotic Cardiovascular Disease in Chinese Population: The China-PAR Project (Prediction for ASCVD Risk in China). *Circulation, 134*(19), 1430–1440. https://doi.org/10.1161/CIRCULATIONAHA.116.022367.

Yoshii, I. (2024). AB0583 prognostic nutritional index correlates with disease activity score after methotrexate initiation in patients with rheumatoid arthritis. *Annals of the Rheumatic Diseases, 83*, 1574. https://doi.org/10.1136/annrheumdis-2024-eular.1702.

Yu, K.-Q., Zhao, W.-Q., & Zhang, T. (2025). Comparative analysis of five obesity-related indicators for predicting infertility in U.S. adults. *Frontiers in Nutrition, 12*, 1593706. https://doi.org/10.3389/fnut.2025.1593706.

Yuan, L., Wen, B., Li, X., Lei, H., Zou, D., & Zhou, Q. (2025). A Chinese prospective cohort research developed and validated a risk prediction model for patients with cervical cancer. *Cancer Cell International, 25*(1), 142. https://doi.org/10.1186/s12935-025-03744-8.

Zad, Z., Jiang, V. S., Wolf, A. T., Wang, T., Cheng, J. J., Paschalidis, I. C., & Mahalingaiah, S. (2024). Predicting polycystic ovary syndrome with machine learning algorithms from electronic health records. *Frontiers in Endocrinology, 15*, 1298628. https://doi.org/10.3389/fendo.2024.1298628.

Zhang, P., Wu, J., & Xun, N. (2019). Role of maternal nutrition in the health outcomes of mothers and their children: A retrospective analysis. *Medical Science Monitor, 25*, 4430–4437. https://doi.org/10.12659/MSM.914679.

Zhang, R., Harun, Z., & Liu, L. (2025). Predicting maternal health risks using nutritional data and machine learning. *Journal of Neonatal Surgery, 14*(32S), 4097–4107.

Zhiting, G., Jiaying, T., Haiying, H., Yuping, Z., Qunfei, Y., & Jingfen, J. (2022). Cardiovascular disease risk prediction models in the Chinese population—A systematic review and meta-analysis. *BMC Public Health, 22*(1), 1608. https://doi.org/10.1186/s12889-022-13995-z.

Zhong, H., Miller, D. J., & Urish, K. L. (2016). T2 map signal variation predicts symptomatic osteoarthritis progression: Data from the osteoarthritis initiative. *Skeletal Radiology, 45*(7), 909–913. https://doi.org/10.1007/s00256-016-2360-4.

Zhou, R., Chen, H., Lin, Y., Li, F., Zhong, Q., Huang, Y., & Wu, X. (2023). Total and regional fat/muscle mass ratio and Risks of Incident cardiovascular disease and Mortality. *Journal of the American Heart Association, 12*(17), e030101. https://doi.org/10.1161/JAHA.123.030101.

Zhu, W., Ma, Y., Guo, W., Lu, J., Li, X., Wu, J., Qin, P., Zhu, C., & Zhang, Q. (2022). Serum level of lactate dehydrogenase is associated with cardiovascular disease risk as determined by the Framingham risk score and arterial stiffness in a health-examined population in China. *International Journal of General Medicine, 15*, 11–17. https://doi.org/10.2147/IJGM.S337517.

Zhu, Z., Otahal, P., Wang, B., Jin, X., Laslett, L. L., Wluka, A. E., Antony, B., Han, W., Wang, X., Winzenberg, T., Cicuttini, F., Jones, G., & Ding, C. (2017). Cross-sectional and longitudinal associations between serum inflammatory cytokines and knee bone marrow lesions in patients with knee osteoarthritis. *Osteoarthritis and Cartilage, 25*(4), 499–505. https://doi.org/10.1016/j.joca.2016.10.024.

Nutritional policies in war-affected countries

13

Surekha Routray and Shruti Senapati
R&D Department, Aashdit Nutritech Pvt. Ltd., Bhubaneswar, Odisha, India

13.1 Introduction

Micronutrients are essential elements, or components necessary in minute quantities to support healthy growth and development of living organisms. In other words, these are substances found in food that are vital for human health and are needed in small quantities (measured in milligrams per 100 g of food item). They contain essential vitamins and trace minerals such as iron, calcium, and zinc. Unlike macronutrients such as carbohydrate, protein, and fat, which are consumed in larger amounts, micronutrients are vital for supporting physical and cognitive development despite being required in smaller quantities.

Micronutrient deficiency refers to a shortage of vital vitamins and minerals crucial for proper bodily growth and development. Such deficiencies significantly contribute to the global disease burden, leading to higher rates of illness and death. Common deficiencies, including iron, vitamin A, and zinc, can result in severe and potentially life-threatening conditions. Approximately one-third of the global population is estimated to suffer from at least one form of micronutrient deficiency, which is highlighted as dramatic inequities in the burden of micronutrient deficiencies in the 2020 Global Nutrition Report by the World Health Organization (WHO) (Han et al., 2022). These deficiencies disproportionately affect children and pregnant women, underscoring significant global disparities. Food insecurity and malnutrition pose substantial global challenges. Food security is defined as the sustained access of all individuals to adequate, safe, and nutritious food, of sufficient quality and diversity, to meet dietary needs and support an active and healthy life, without the risk of future deprivation (Pinstrup-Andersen, 2009). This condition occurs when individuals face physical limitations in accessing food or lack the social and economic resources necessary to acquire sufficient and nutritious food.

Armed conflicts are closely linked to heightened vulnerability to nutritional insecurity, especially in low- and middle-income nations, where they are the primary drivers of malnutrition. Young individuals under 5 years of age residing in war-torn areas bear a disproportionate burden of malnutrition and related health issues. Over 112 million malnourished children reside in conflict-exposed regions (Carroll et al., 2017). Conflicts and natural disasters have led to food aid, leaving over 40 million individuals experiencing insufficient access to food, relying on humanitarian support in response to these crises.

Armed conflicts result in significant morbidity and mortality among women, as well as the displacement of populations. However, the vulnerable groups that do not

Nutritional Strategies, Predictive Models, and Sustainable Policies. DOI: https://doi.org/10.1016/B978-0-443-23671-6.00003-7

flee across international borders often remain unnoticed by the United Nations (UN) High Commissioner for Refugees (UNHCR). According to figures from the Internal Displacement Monitoring Centre the number of people internally displaced because of conflict and violence surged from around 25 million in 2009–10 to 45.7 million in 2019. Nearly 21 million, or 46%, were women and girls (IDMC, 2019, 2020).

The increasing worldwide refugee crisis has given researchers and policymakers a reason to divulge more and more about forced displacement in recent years. There were 65 million individuals who had been forcibly displaced worldwide in 2015. As the majority do not have the financial resources to travel long distances, they are compelled to migrate to nearby countries or relocate within their nation. Sub-Saharan Africa has seen a steady rise in the number of refugees since 2001, whereas the number of internally displaced people (IDPs) has subsequently varied annually between 6 and 12 million, contingent upon the intensity of conflicts, notably in nations such as the DRC, South Sudan, and Nigeria (Iacoella & Tirivayi, 2020). Forced displacement often exposes families to substandard and unhygienic living conditions, along with dysfunctional healthcare systems. This disrupts social and agricultural structures, including supply chains, affecting food production. Consequently, food insecurity rises, resulting in insufficient dietary consumption and, subsequently, malnutrition, particularly among vulnerable demographics such as children, women, and older people.

Yemen is the most severely impacted country in absolute numbers, with a minimum of 6 million individuals experiencing severe food insecurity, and those residing in the most affected regions may be on the brink of famine (Loewenberg, 2015). Several nations, including Sudan, Ethiopia, Nigeria, and parts of Central America and the Caribbean, are facing censorious circumstances primarily because of flooding, inadequate harvests, and conflict. Ethiopia, notably, ranks among the countries with the highest prevalence of child malnourishment rates.

Over the past decade, armed conflicts have been active in 38 countries, constituting approximately 19% of all nations. These conflicts, which are both internal and cross-border and prevalent in sub-Saharan Africa and Middle East countries, have caused significant harm to healthcare systems and food security and led to mass displacement (Fig. 13.1).

Food insecurity has not only contributed to social unrest but has also been exacerbated by conflict itself. This chapter explores the vulnerability experienced during wartime, prevalent micronutrient deficiencies in select conflict zones, and the policies aimed at addressing these global challenges. Further the chapter delves into nutritional burden because of conflict and policies adopted to commence sustainable change in countries such as Vietnam, Sri Lanka, and Ethiopia.

13.2 Spotlight on key micronutrient deficiencies in conflicted zones

The impact of armed conflict on the health and welfare of populations in conflict zones is multifaceted. War and famine are two significant causes of hunger challenges in

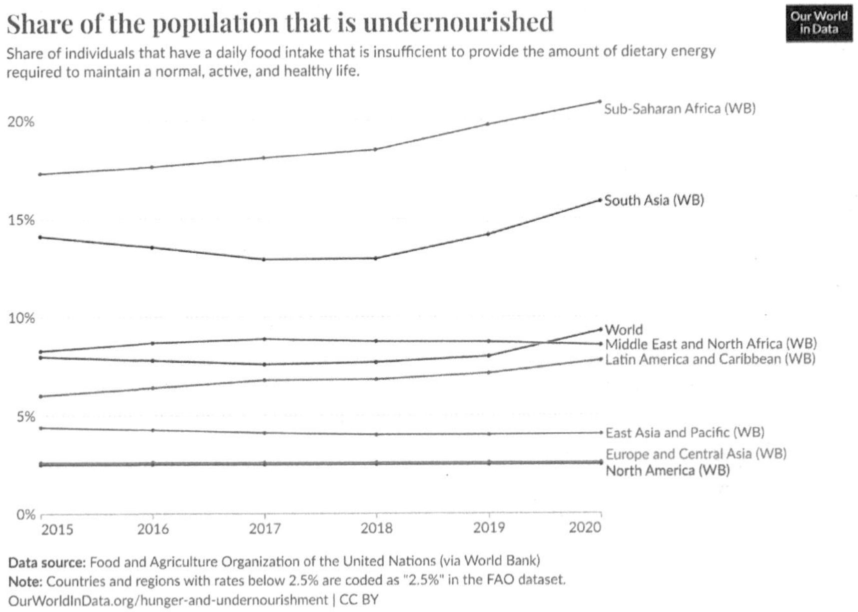

Figure 13.1 Region-wise prevalence of undernourishment (Han et al., 2022; Ritchie et al., 2023).

vulnerable areas. They disrupt food systems, destroy livelihoods, displace people, and leave those who do not flee terrified and uncertain about when to eat their next meal. Victims and survivors of war are vulnerable to food insecurity and malnutrition.

Governments and relief organizations have implemented various nutritional interventions in emergencies, which often arise from prolonged or abrupt environmental calamities, epidemics, civil unrest, financial instability, or the disintegration of social frameworks and institutions caused by conflict, governance breakdowns, and/or armed violence/warfare. The strategies adopted to address micronutrient deficiencies and malnutrition typically encompass comprehensive food distribution, broad supplementary feeding initiatives aimed at vulnerable populations, focused feeding programs, vital micronutrients, agricultural assistance, and tailored feeding programs for infants and young children. Evidence suggests that these nutritional strategies have shown efficacy in both steady and recovery phases of exigencies, particularly in refugee settlements, where their impact on malnutrition and deficiencies is evident through standard anthropometric measurements.

Research indicates that women in conflict zones are prone to stop breastfeeding, thereby depriving infants of the essential nutrients and protective benefits that breast milk provides. In addition, access to nutrition and safe drinking water continues to pose a significant challenge for forced migrants in warfare areas, leading to a heavy reliance on food imports. Refugees frequently resort to various coping mechanisms, such as reducing meal sizes and frequency, cutting back on food expenses, and borrowing food. The emphasis often shifts from food quality to the quantity of food available. In numerous conflict scenarios, hunger persists as food accessibility is often deliberately hindered as a strategy of warfare, stemming from the devastation of farming infrastructure and interference with the food production system. Children born in these circumstances are at heightened risk for serious long-term health issues, including acute undernutrition and mental health disorders such as post traumatic stress disorder (PTSD), anxiety, depression, and symptoms of dissociative conditions, all of which significantly impair their physical and cognitive development.

Malnutrition inhibits proper growth, deprives individuals of crucial vitamins and minerals, and increases their vulnerability to infections and chronic illnesses. Although the term "malnutrition" encompasses both undernutrition (e.g., moderate and severe acute malnutrition, stunting, underweight, and micronutrient deficiencies) and overnutrition, such as excessive weight gain and nutrition-related chronic illness, it signifies a disparity between the consumption of calories or nutrients and the body's physiological nutritional demands (Corley, 2021).

Globally the scope of micronutrient deficiency conditions is enormous. Besides the physiological effects of these deficiencies, food supply and consumption patterns also play a vital role. As internal and/or armed conflicts reduce food availability—i.e., the supply of food or the quality of food available to a given population—they significantly diminish accessibility to nutrition, meaning the availability of nutrients that can be taken up and utilized by a given population further diminishes beyond the availability of food. Some common micronutrient deficiencies are related to iron, zinc, iodine, vitamin A, vitamin D, and vitamin B6. Recent reviews have shown that the sub-Saharan Africa region has the highest rates of iron deficiency anemia (IDA), vitamin A deficiency (VAD), and zinc nutritional deficiency (Fig. 13.2) (Philipo et al., 2021).

The most common nutritional issue is iron deficiency. The majority of birth abnormalities are still caused by folic acid deficiency, and various micronutrient deficiencies continue to affect vulnerable populations already burdened by a sedentary lifestyle. The lack of vitamin D, which was once common among youngsters in developed nations, is now known to be incredibly common. It can cause osteoporosis/brittle bones and skeletal injuries, pose serious health risks, or result in permanent disability among older adults. Tables 13.1 and 13.2 showcase the micronutrient deficiency, i.e., mineral and vitamin deficiency conditions, and their worldwide prevalence.

Iron, a vital trace element, underpins numerous physiological functions, including DNA synthesis, cellular respiration, and immune competence. It plays a central role in hemoglobin and myoglobin, the oxygen-carrying proteins in blood and muscle tissue. IDA, the most common nutritional disorder globally, contributes to approximately 50%–60% of all anemia cases, with far-reaching implications for human development and survival.

IDA predominantly arises from chronic dietary iron insufficiency, heightened physiological demands, or impaired absorption. It is particularly prevalent during infancy, early childhood, and pregnancy, periods marked by accelerated growth and increased iron requirements. In conflict-stricken regions the convergence of food insecurity, health service disruption, and forced displacement exacerbates the prevalence of IDA. As per data from the WHO, around 40% of children aged 6–59 months, 37% of

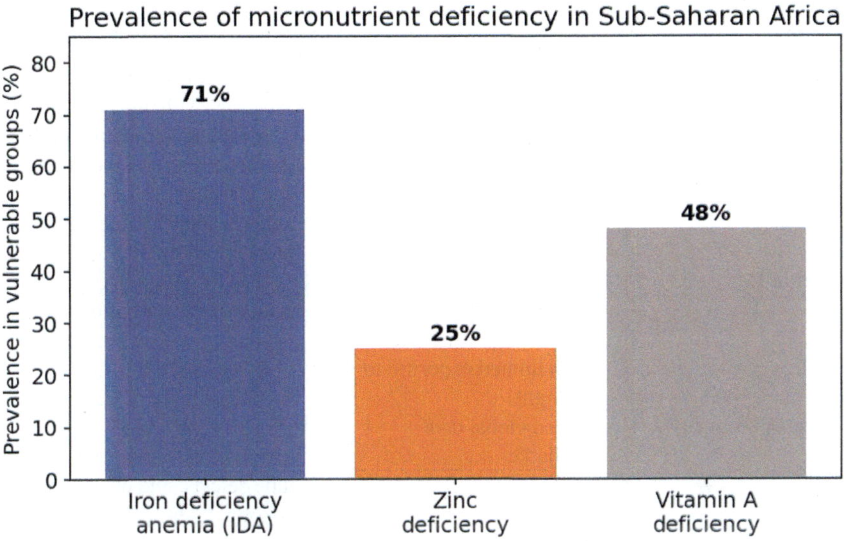

Figure 13.2 Prevalence of micronutrient deficiency in sub-Saharan Africa. The data shows IDA is most prevalent (71%) in vulnerable groups, whereas the prevalence of zinc (25%) and vitamin A (48%) deficiency was also high.

Table 13.1 Global prevalence of mineral deficiency disorder.

Mineral	Estimated prevalence of deficiency	Key health consequences
Iron	Affects over 2 billion people globally	Iron deficiency anemia, decreased cognitive and physical productivity, heightened maternal and neonatal mortality, and low birth weight in infants can result in iron deficiency anemia
Zinc	Prevalence is notably high in developing regions	Contributes to poor maternal outcomes, inhibited child growth (stunting), increased susceptibility to genetic disorders, and a weakened immune defense against infections
Iodine	Impacts around 2 billion individuals worldwide	Leads to thyroid-related conditions such as goiter and hypothyroidism, a rise in iodine deficiency disorders, increased risks of stillbirth and congenital disabilities, infant mortality, and reduced intellectual development

Table 13.2 Vitamin deficiency conditions and their prevalence worldwide.

Vitamin	Estimated deficiency prevalence	Primary health impacts
Vitamin A	Affects approximately 254 million children of preschool age	Associated with night vision impairment, xerophthalmia (severe dryness of the eyes), and elevated risk of mortality among young children and pregnant women
Vitamin D	Common across all demographics, particularly in individuals with limited exposure to sunlight	Can lead to rickets in children, osteomalacia and osteoporosis in adults, and has been linked to an increased risk of colorectal malignancies
Folate (Vitamin B9)	Limited global data available	Deficiency may result in megaloblastic anemia, neural tube defects, and other birth abnormalities, as well as cardiovascular conditions, cerebrovascular events (stroke), cognitive decline, and mood disorders such as depression

pregnant women, and 30% of women aged 15–49 globally are anemic, with iron deficiency as the leading cause. The African and Southeast Asian WHO regions report the highest burden, affecting an estimated 106 million adult females and 103 million minors in Africa, along with 244 million and 83 million women and children, respectively, across the Southeast Asia region (Harika et al., 2017; Walter et al., 1989).

The Syrian crisis, which has been going on since 2011, is a stark example. Prolonged conflict has decimated healthcare systems and food infrastructure, leading to a sharp decline in household access to iron-rich foods. Displacement, inflation, and market collapse have forced families to reduce consumption of iron-dense items such as meat, legumes, and fortified cereals, aggravating nutritional vulnerabilities among children and women of reproductive age (Albaroudi et al., 2018).

Heme iron—predominantly in animal-derived sources such as red meat, poultry, and seafood—offers high bioavailability (15%–35%). Nonheme iron, derived from plant sources such as lentils, beans, leafy greens, and fortified grains, is less bioavailable (2%–20%) and requires enhancers like vitamin C for effective absorption. Plant-based diets dominate many low-income conflict zones because of economic and cultural constraints, making vulnerable groups reliant on nonheme sources. Unfortunately, these are among the first food categories to become inaccessible during civil unrest and forced migration.

To combat IDA amid restricted availability of conventional sources, nutritional policy frameworks have explored several alternatives:

1. Iron-fortified staple foods: Fortifying flour, rice, and salt with iron compounds such as ferrous sulfate or NaFeEDTA is cost-effective. However, implementation is uneven. For example, whereas some East African nations have introduced mandatory fortification laws, others lack the institutional capacity to enforce standards, particularly during conflict.
2. Micronutrient powders (MNPs): These are single-serving sachets containing a blend of vitamins and minerals, including iron, intended for home fortification of children's meals. UNICEF has scaled MNP distribution in displaced populations, yet reach and compliance remain inconsistent because of logistical and behavioral barriers.
3. Biofortification: Breeding iron-rich crop varieties such as high-iron beans and pearl millet has shown promise in Rwanda and India. However, their availability remains limited in conflict zones because of restricted seed supply chains and a lack of awareness.
4. Iron supplementation programs: Oral iron tablets and syrups are often deployed via antenatal care programs. In war zones, however, healthcare access barriers significantly reduce program coverage and continuity.
5. Alternative protein sources: In areas where meat is unaffordable or unavailable, edible insects (e.g., mopane worms in Southern Africa) and seaweed have been explored as culturally acceptable and iron-rich alternatives. However, these have not yet been mainstreamed into national policy or emergency nutrition programs.

Zinc is a crucial trace mineral that plays a central role in human metabolism, catalyzing over 100 enzymatic reactions, facilitating protein folding, regulating gene expression, and supporting cellular immunity. It is indispensable for linear growth, immune competence, neurodevelopment, and wound healing. In populations exposed to chronic malnutrition and compromised gastrointestinal absorption—conditions prevalent in conflict zones—zinc deficiency becomes an acute public health concern. This deficiency has been acknowledged by the WHO as a key determinant in the burden of diarrheal diseases, skin disorders, growth retardation, and susceptibility to infectious diseases, particularly in low-resource and war-affected settings (Maxfield et al., 2023).

Zinc is primarily sourced from animal-derived foods such as beef, crab, and poultry. Dairy products, eggs, and fortified cereals also contribute moderately to zinc intake. Plant-based sources, including legumes, whole grains, and seeds, provide lower bioavailability because of high phytate content, which impairs absorption. In conflict-affected regions, livestock loss, seafood inaccessibility, and breakdown of cold chain logistics drastically reduce access to high-zinc foods. Simultaneously, phytate-rich staples such as maize and sorghum dominate diets, compounding bioavailability issues. Humanitarian food rations often lack targeted zinc-rich components, falling short of addressing the nutritional requirements of vulnerable populations, including young individuals, expectant mothers, and people living with chronic conditions like sickle cell disease (SCD). This nutritional gap persists because of weak policy mechanisms, inadequate dietary planning in aid packages, and minimal integration of culturally relevant zinc sources.

Zinc deficiency remains highly prevalent in sub-Saharan Africa and Central America, disproportionately affecting high-risk groups such as pregnant individuals, newborns, and those living with SCD. SCD, a genetic disorder requiring higher zinc turnover because of oxidative stress and chronic hemolysis, has an exceptionally high

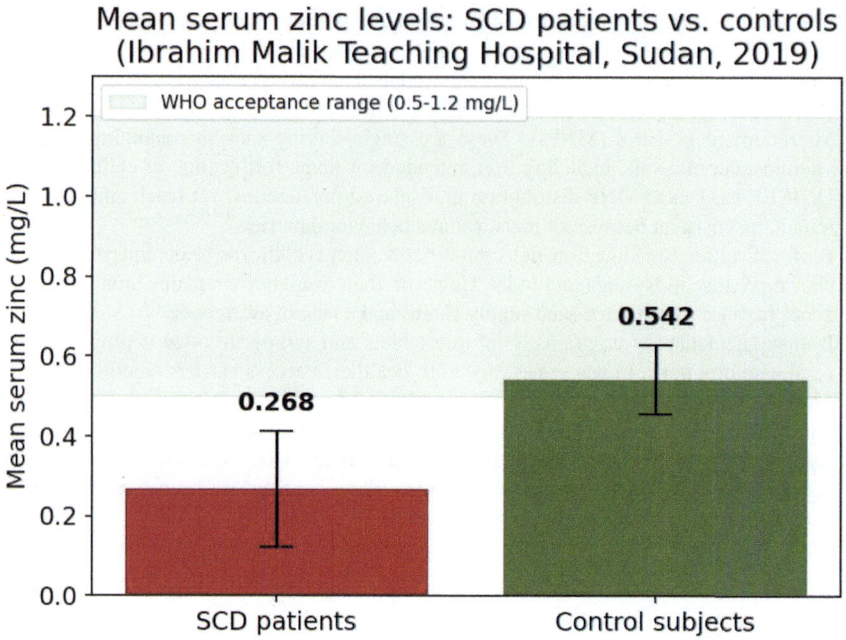

Figure 13.3 Mean serum zinc levels of the patients and the control as per the study conducted by the Paediatric Department of Ibrahim Malik Teaching Hospital, Sudan, in 2019.

mortality rate in sub-Saharan Africa—where 50%–90% of children born with the condition die before the age of 5 (Philipo et al., 2021).

A 2019 clinical study conducted at the Paediatric Department of Ibrahim Malik Teaching Hospital in Sudan reported critically low serum zinc levels among SCD patients, with a mean concentration of 0.268 ± 0.146 mg/L, in contrast to control subjects with 0.542 ± 0.087 mg/L—levels that hover close to the lower margin of the acceptance range (0.5–1.2 mg/L in children) (Fig. 13.3) (Abass et al., 2014; Suliman & Elamin, 2023). Such deficiencies exacerbate the disease burden, contributing to impaired immunity, poor appetite, and delayed wound healing.

Furthermore, zinc deficiency is strongly linked to low birth weight (LBW) in neonates, a pervasive issue in developing countries. In Sudan and similar regions, maternal anemia, compounded by zinc and iron deficiencies, significantly elevates the risk of obstetric complications. These include hypertensive disorders, prolonged labor, preterm birth, and increased maternal and neonatal mortality. The WHO estimates that zinc deficiency contributes to approximately 2.4% of all disease burden in sub-Saharan Africa, affecting 8.96 million individuals, many of whom reside in fragile, conflict-affected states.

Zinc deficiency interventions in conflict zones face structural and logistical hurdles. In Northern Nigeria, only 35% of children with diarrhea received WHO-recommended zinc treatment in 2022, hindered by broken cold chains and staff shortages

(Harika et al., 2017). In Chad and Central African Republic, flour fortification is non-operational because of inactive mills, whereas mobile units in Congo remain limited by insecurity. UNICEF clinics in Sudan reached 60,000 children with zinc-fortified ready-to-use therapeutic foods (RUTFs) in 2023, though distribution suffers from stockouts. Indigenous zinc-rich foods like mopane worms are nutritionally valuable but underutilized because of lack of policy support.

Vitamin A is a vital fat-soluble micronutrient crucial for preserving vision, supporting immune health, maintaining epithelial integrity, aiding reproduction, and facilitating cellular differentiation. Preformed vitamin A (retinol) is plentiful in animal-based foods such as liver (6582 μg RAE/100g), cod liver oil, eggs, and dairy, whereas provitamin A carotenoids (β-carotene) are found in dark leafy greens and fruits and vegetables such as carrots, mangoes, and sweet potatoes. However, the bioavailability of plant sources is significantly less and is affected by factors such as fat intake and gut health—both of which can suffer during food scarcity caused by conflict. VAD is a severe health issue for those in conflict zones, especially among preschool children and women of childbearing age, who are the most vulnerable. In war-torn areas, decreased agricultural output, livestock loss, limited market access, and low dietary diversity all contribute to nutritional deficiencies. These challenges, along with weakened healthcare systems and disrupted supplementation efforts, exacerbate rates of both clinical and subclinical deficiencies, leading to conditions such as xerophthalmia (which can cause childhood blindness), anemia, and compromised immune function, ultimately increasing vulnerability to infectious diseases and raising mortality risks.

There are specific barriers that cause the reduction in accessibility of vitamin A in Ethiopia. Low knowledge and awareness of VAD, low attention and motivation, and poor promotion of uptake of VAD programs and implementation schemes are the countable barriers. The two most prevalent demographic groups at risk of vitamin A insufficiency worldwide are women in their reproductive years and young children under 5. According to a 2009 assessment by the WHO, approximately one-third—about 190 million—of the world's children under 5 were at risk of developing xerophthalmia. Across the African continent, approximately 2% of children in the preschool age group suffer from night blindness, a rate that is quadruple that observed in Southeast Asia, with nearly half of affected children worldwide residing in Africa. It accounts for almost 6% of deaths among children under the age of 5 in Africa. Although the rate of subclinical VAD declined from 55.7% during 1990–2004 to 28.3% between 2005 and 2019, the reduction was not statistically meaningful. It is, hence, regarded as a significant public health issue within the community when it affects preschoolers with WHO-defined thresholds identifying the prevalence of Bitot's spots exceeding 0.5% and night blindness in children surpassing 1%. Preschoolers nationwide were the subjects of a clinical VAD survey in 2005, conducted by the Ethiopian Health and Nutrition Research Institute (EHNRI). The findings of the study showed that night blindness affected 0.7% of the population in the country. However, prevalence of Bitot's spots was reported at 1.7%, which is over threefold higher than the WHO-recommended threshold of 0.5%, indicating that although high-dose vitamin A supplementation (VAS) programs are occasionally offered in Ethiopia, vitamin A insufficiency remains a public health concern. Night blindness, typically the earliest clinical indicator of VAD, was projected to affect 1.2% of the population in 2020, whereas the occurrence of Bitot's spot, a clinical sign of VAD, was recorded at 0.8%. The total estimated rate of clinical insufficiency of vitamin A was 2.0% (Yisak et al., 2020).

To mitigate persistent VAD in conflict zones, WHO recommends biannual high-dose supplementation for children aged 6–59 months (100,000–200,000 IU) (Mulaw et al., 2023). Yet, in Ethiopia's Tigray region, coverage fell from 86% in 2011 to below 60% by 2021 because of conflict-related service interruptions. Food fortification initiatives, including vitamin A-enriched oil, sugar, and flour, remain limited—only 12% of cooking oil in IDP camps in Borno State, Nigeria, was fortified as of 2020. Though orange-fleshed sweet potatoes can meet a child's daily requirement in 100 g, adoption in conflict-affected Ethiopian regions remains below 10% because of weak supply chains and lack of program integration. Lipid-based nutrient supplements (LNS) have improved serum retinol levels in trials, such as in Burkina Faso, but scale-up is constrained by high costs and external sourcing. Culturally familiar, vitamin A-rich foods such as camel liver and dagaa (small dried fish) are nutrient-dense and shelf-stable yet remain excluded from most formal aid programs because of logistical barriers and policy oversight.

In Afghanistan, nutritional assessments have highlighted an alarming prevalence of VAD. According to the 2013 National Nutrition Survey, more than half of young children exhibited serum retinol levels below the threshold for adequacy (<0.70 μmol/L), suggesting widespread subclinical deficiency (Ministry of Public Health MoPH, 2013). Although large-scale data on visible signs such as night blindness or Bitot's spots remain sparse, localized studies in vulnerable provinces report these manifestations among severely malnourished children. VAS programs, supported by UNICEF, managed to reach over 9 million children in 2024, despite conflict-related disruptions (UNICEF, 2024a, 2024b). Nonetheless, Afghanistan lacks a robust fortification policy; whereas iodized salt is available, staple foods such as wheat flour and oil are not fortified with vitamin A (GAIN, 2023).

In Iraq, available evidence points to a moderate burden of clinical VAD, with WHO regional data indicating that around 4% of preschool-aged children may experience night blindness—a level of concern under international health guidelines (World Health Organization, 2009). Though vitamin A capsules are distributed via child health campaigns, consistent follow-up doses are often missed because of logistical barriers. Iraq began mandatory iron and folate enrichment of wheat flour in 2006 (FAO, 2006), but vitamin A fortification—especially in cooking oil—has not been legislated, despite earlier policy recommendations (FAO/WHO, 2000). This leaves key dietary gaps unaddressed, particularly in displaced populations.

13.3 The science and policy interface

An in-depth understanding of various branches of science, particularly those related to nutrition and food production, is crucial for formulating effective nutritional policies. It is essential to consider the nutritional abundance in locally available foods, as these can significantly influence dietary habits and overall health in communities. In addition, understanding food shelf life is vital; this knowledge helps minimize food waste and ensure that people can access nutritious options for extended periods. Moreover, the accessibility of these foods plays a key role, especially during political and administrative instability in the country, where reliable food sources may become scarce.

To alleviate the challenges of developing nutrition policies from scratch, international bodies such as the WHO have established comprehensive guidelines. These guidelines serve as a framework, enabling individual countries to tailor their nutritional policies according to local contexts and needs. By utilizing these guidelines, nations can adapt their strategies to improve food security and foster community resilience in times of crisis.

13.4 Why is nutrition important in emergencies?

- During emergencies, rates of malnutrition and death may increase substantially. Emergencies result in outcomes that can increase the risk of malnutrition, illness, and death, and it is critical to protect the nutritional status of those affected. People who suffer from acute malnutrition are far more likely to become sick and die. Malnutrition can negatively impact children's physical, cognitive, and social development. Moreover, people who become sick are more likely to be undernourished. This urgency should motivate us to act swiftly and effectively.

13.5 Food handling in emergencies

Disasters have an impact on food and nutrition conditions. Any crisis will cause disorganized social and economic routines, communications, and transportation networks. However, not every crisis results in food shortages that are severe enough to influence the impacted population's nutritional health significantly. The type of disaster, its duration, the size of the afflicted area, and the predisaster dietary state of the population all influence the sort of food and nutrition issues. Earthquakes typically do not significantly impact long-term food supplies. Hurricanes, floods, and tsunamis, on the other hand, directly impact food availability because they destroy stored food, ruin crops, and kill domestic animals and livestock. Food assistance is needed to prevent the disaster-affected population from going hungry. However, it is imperative to prepare for managing and treating malnutrition cases that were present before the crisis or have worsened and will be noticeable during relief efforts.

First the available food is computed to ensure a food assistance program works. Then the impacted population that needs to be fed is mapped. The food rations are calculated based on the population's characteristics and the anticipated length of the disaster's effects.

A food aid program's priority in times of crisis is in areas where there is or seems to be an immediate need, such as remote communities, institutions, hospitals, refugee camps, and among rescue teams and humanitarian workers, where food should be provided immediately. The impacted population's food requirements are calculated while considering its demographics. The distribution, storage, and transportation of food supplies (such as food aid groups and food stockpiles located throughout the nation) are determined and verified that the food and supplies received are appropriate and safe for the area. To guarantee safety and prevent the spread of disease through food, inspect the food that has been received, look for and dispose of any broken supplies, and ensure that the grain sacks or containers are in good condition. Reject items whose expiration date has passed and discard tins that are rusty, damaged, or bulging. Verify that no contaminated or dangerous goods have been transported in transportation units. Arrange food on stands that allow for proper air circulation and ensure that warehouses have adequate lighting and ventilation. To maintain a first-in/first-out distribution system, store food according to its entry date.

- As an immediate measure, any population group that is or appears to be at high nutritional risk is to be provided with 3 or 4 kg of food per person per week. The important thing at this stage is to provide sufficient energy, even if it is not a balanced diet. For a short period, 1700 kcal daily will prevent severe deterioration of nutritional status and famine. The quantity of food in a ration should depend on the stage of the crisis and available resources. For weeks or even months, and while the victims rely exclusively or almost exclusively on food aid, rations should aim to provide 1700–2000 kcal per person/day. A note must be made to ensure that the food provided is part of the population's food pattern. The food ration should be as simple as possible: a basic food (e.g., rice, corn, and wheat flour), a concentrated source of energy (oil or another fat), and a concentrated source of protein (e.g., dried or canned fish or canned meat). Along with the basic ration, vulnerable groups (children under 5, pregnant and breastfeeding women, and malnourished persons) need to receive a supplement.

Proposed composition of a food ration that provides approximately 1700 kcal is as follows:

Basic grain (e.g., rice): 400 g
A fat (e.g., oil): 15 g
Protein-rich food (e.g., dried fish): 45 g

13.6 WHO guidelines for nutrition in emergencies

The PAHO/WHO Institute of Nutrition of Central America and Panama (INCAP) prepared guidelines that are synchronized with those developed by UNHCR, UNICEF, World Food Programme (WFP), and WHO.

These jointly developed guidelines are a practical tool for assessing, estimating, and monitoring populations' food and nutrition needs in emergencies. Significant food shortages can be a primary feature of an emergency, such as droughts or floods that lead to famine, or they may be a consequence of war, economic disaster, or population displacement. The often severe protein-energy malnutrition and micronutrient deficiencies that inevitably follow such shortages significantly add to the burden of disease and mortality, slow—or even impede—socioeconomic recovery, and make intense additional demands on scarce resources. The guidelines are aimed at field staff involved in planning and delivering a basic general food ration for emergency-affected populations. They aim to promote timely, coordinated, and practical action through improved understanding of food and nutrition needs during emergencies.

The process of tailoring food requirements for a specific population requires several considerations. The initial planning figure for energy should be adjusted according to the environmental, demographic, and physiological criteria particular to the affected population. Food commodities are then selected to meet basic nutritional requirements. Finally, other factors are considered to ensure that the ration is appropriate to all population subgroups, such as infants and young children, pregnant and lactating women, and older persons. Food-management aspects and the underlying preconditions for ensuring adequate nutrition (such as the social and health situation or environmental issues) are also considered when estimating food and nutritional needs in emergencies.

The purpose of these guidelines is to provide practical tools for estimating the food and nutritional needs of populations in emergencies. In particular, these goals include the following:

- provide practical operational guidelines for UN and other agency staff involved in planning a basic general food ration for emergencies;
- estimate the food and nutritional needs for vulnerable groups;
- provide a clear outline of the main factors to take into consideration when planning an adequate ration; and
- provide a framework for training activities and/or supporting ongoing training activities related to planning food assistance.

13.6.1 Below is an overview of the process necessary to estimate emergency food and nutritional needs

Following the adoption of the initial planning figure of 2100 kcal/person/day, adjustments are made based on factors such as temperature, health, or nutritional status of the population, demographic distribution of the population, and activity levels.

Considering the initial planning figure (2100 kcal), food commodities that meet the affected population's basic energy, protein, fat, and micronutrient requirements must first be selected. An acceptable ratio also takes into consideration local dietary preferences.

Macronutrient (protein and fat) requirements: Energy needs are usually met through various commodities with ample protein content (cereal, blended food, and pulses). According to Food and Agriculture Organization (FAO)/WHO technical reports, protein should provide at least 10%–12% of total energy. At least 17% of energy in the ration should be provided as fat. However, with particular reference to the supplementary feeding program, the fat requirement for young children is between 30% and 40% of their energy requirements, and for pregnant and lactating women, at least 20%.

Once the per capita daily nutrient requirements have been established and basic food commodities are identified, the ration is refined to ensure that other specific requirements are covered.

In some emergencies, ready-to-eat meals may serve a useful temporary purpose, though their use should be carefully controlled. Examples of these types of food include high-energy/protein biscuits, humanitarian daily rations (HDRs), and meals ready to eat (MREs). These items should only be used as an immediate response at the outset of the emergency when no other foods/cooking facilities are available (e.g., when a population is in transit or fleeing).

13.7 Case studies: Bridging science and policy

Food policies are typically formulated at the national level, although they might also be established regionally depending on the level of alignment among countries within the region. These policies, set by local, state, and national governments, dictate agricultural practices and food consumption patterns. Ideally, they aim to ensure fair availability of healthy, cost-effective, and nourishing food for everyone while safeguarding natural reservoirs. Moreover, these policies strive to support farmers and workers in the food industry while maintaining stringent standards for the welfare of animals used in food production (Wilde, 2018).

Established in 1945 the FAO of the UN serves as the foremost global authority on food policy, tasked with the mission to improve dietary quality and quantity of life in member nations, boost the productivity and effectiveness of food and agricultural systems, enhance the welfare of rural communities, and promote global economic growth to eradicate hunger. Various international bodies also shape food policies by providing critical assessments of scientific research and evidence.

International organizations such as Codex Alimentarius (CODEX) have established numerous global standards and guidelines, primarily adopted by countries lacking their internal standards or those aiming to facilitate open trade with similar nations. The International Life Sciences Institute (ILSI) is a global nonprofit organization focused on advancing scientific research to improve human health and environmental protection. By fostering collaboration between industry and academia, ILSI develops critical scientific evidence to influence food policies, particularly in less developed regions. The WHO, under the UN, coordinates international health initiatives and supports member states in enhancing health outcomes. Similarly, organizations like Codex Alimentarius (CODEX) set global standards and guidelines, often adopted by nations without their own regulations or those seeking open trade. ILSI operates as a social enterprise/public benefit organization, driving collaboration to inform food policy based on scientific research.

Wars not only cause violent destruction through weaponry but also severely harm vital resources. Combatants often raid enemy food supplies and damage agricultural lands, livestock, and civilian infrastructure, leading to food shortages and economic disruption, threatening community survival. Conflict-induced displacement worsens conditions, disconnecting people from their livelihoods and increasing risks of malnutrition and disease. In addition, belligerents may besiege communities, trapping residents and depriving them of essential resources. Access to conflict zones for humanitarian aid is frequently obstructed, with relief efforts facing barriers and attacks from opposing parties.

During conflicts, nutritional policies adapt significantly to meet the challenges of war. Governments often implement rationing and provide food subsidies to ensure essential items are fairly distributed and affordable, responding to production and distribution disruptions. There is a heightened reliance on food aid, especially in conflict zones and among displaced populations. Nutrition programs focus on vulnerable groups such as children, pregnant women, and the elderly to combat malnutrition and its health risks. Strategies include food fortification, emergency feeding programs, and public health interventions to boost nutritional resilience. Effective monitoring and collaboration among government entities, humanitarian organizations, and international partners are vital to address changing dietary needs during wartime, striving to maintain food security and access to nutritious food for everyone.

13.7.1 Case study 1: Ukraine

The invasion of Ukraine by Russia has led to the most significant increase in global food insecurity resulting from military actions in over a century (Welsh, 2024). Despite fading from the headlines the repercussions persist. The conflict in Ukraine has brought about severe consequences for both its citizens and those worldwide reliant on its substantial grain exports. It has triggered one of the swiftest population displacements since World War II, with nearly 6 million Ukrainians currently living as refugees across Europe and another 4.9 million internally displaced. Many have faced the loss of their homes and sources of income. The agricultural sector has suffered an estimated $80 billion in damages and losses, profoundly impacting nearly a third of Ukraine's population employed in this crucial industry. As production and supply chains are disrupted, food prices continue to escalate, leaving numerous families in the eastern and southern regions without consistent access to nutritious food (Leal Filho et al., 2023; Welsh, 2024; World Food Programme, 2022).

Ukraine's economy has faced a sharp decline since the onset of the war, with Gross Domestic Product (GDP) dropping by an estimated 30%–35% in the first year, marking the deepest recession in its history. Although a minimal growth of 0.5% is projected for 2023, economic performance has been unstable over the past 6 years. The country saw moderate growth in 2017 (2.4%), 2018 (3.5%), and 2019 (3.2%), followed by a contraction of −3.8% in 2020 because of the COVID-19 pandemic and rising geopolitical tensions. A brief recovery occurred in 2021 with 3.4% growth, but GDP sharply fell again in 2022 by −29.1%, largely because of intensified conflict and instability (World Bank) (World Bank, 2022b) (Fig. 13.4).

The primary nutritional challenges affecting Ukrainian children include the following: (1) a possibly widespread incidence of iron deficiency, estimated to affect 40%–50% of the pediatric population. (2) A significant incidence of iodine deficiency, affecting approximately 35% of children. (3) A notable deficiency in vitamin C, affecting approximately 80%–90%, along with deficiencies in B-complex vitamins (B1, B2, B6, and folate) occurring at rates between 40% and 8%. Even before the onset of conflict, women faced greater vulnerability in accessing food and energy compared to men. The global gender disparity in food insecurity, which was at 1.7% in 2019, increased to over 4% by 2021. The prevalence of undernourishment in Ukraine

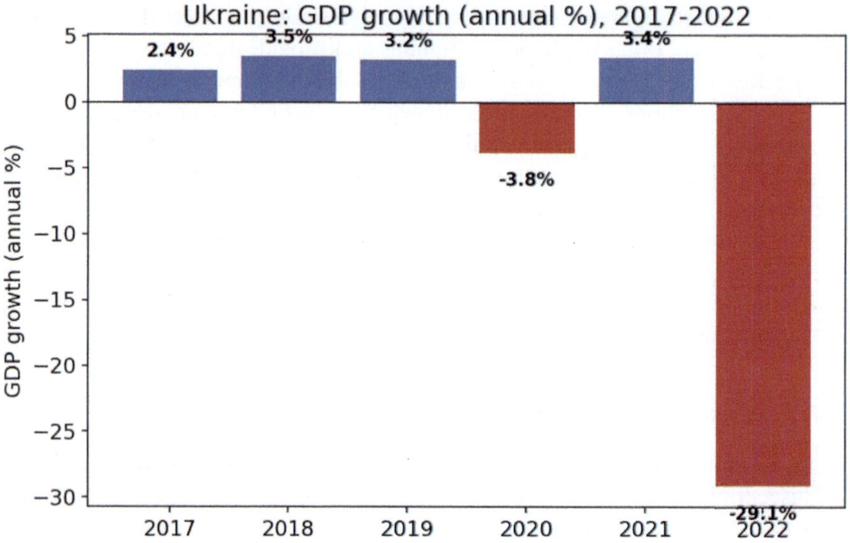

Figure 13.4 GDP growth of Ukraine from 2017 to 2022 (World Bank).

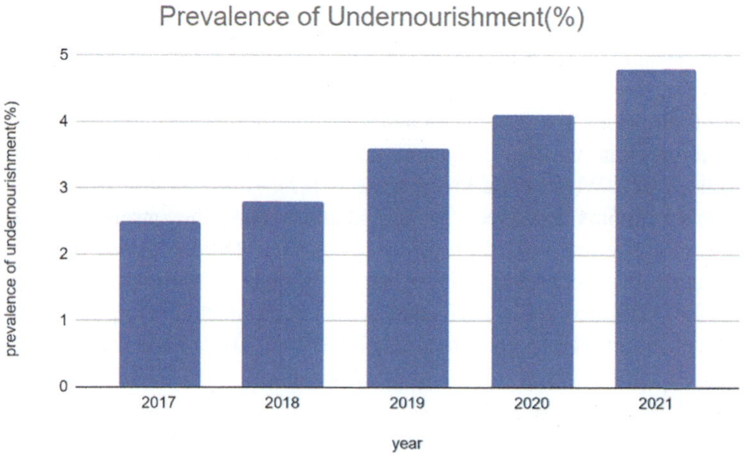

Figure 13.5 Prevalence of undernourishment in Ukraine from 2017 to 2021.

was reported at 4.8% in 2021, according to data from the World Bank (Fig. 13.5) (Trading Economics, 2026).

Out of Ukraine's total population, 1.5 million individuals experience prevalent undernourishment. According to FAO projections an estimated 11–19 million more people are expected to become undernourished in the coming year as a result of the ongoing conflict.

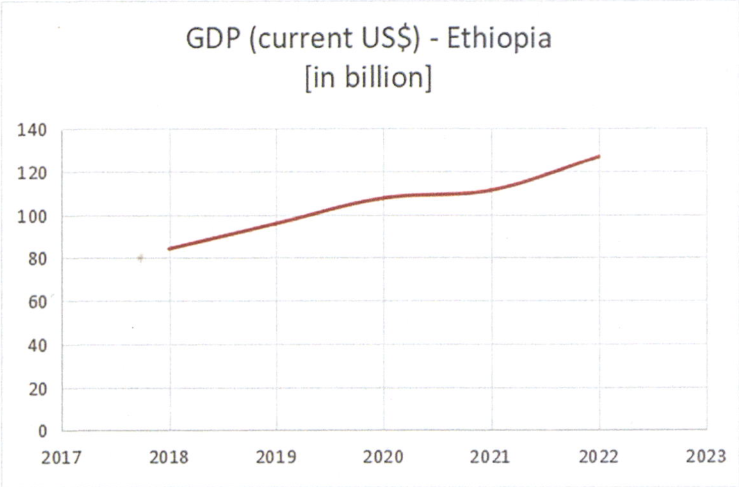

Figure 13.6 Ethiopia GDP in current US dollars.

13.7.2 Case study 2: Ethiopia

With a population of 123 million as of 2021, Ethiopia is the second largest nation in Africa according to the World Bank and is expected to experience significant population growth. With a 4.24 fertility rate, i.e., children per woman in 2020, it is estimated to be among the top eight nations with the highest population growth by 2050, reaching 205.4 million, as per the Population Reference Bureau. However, Ethiopia is currently facing challenges of sporadic violent conflicts and civil unrest across various regions, leading to instability and insecurity. Longstanding ethnic, political, and economic grievances have fueled tensions, resulting in outbreaks of violence, displacement of populations, and loss of life. The conflict in the Tigray region, ongoing since late 2020, has attracted international attention and exacerbated humanitarian crises, with significant numbers of IDPs and refugees fleeing to neighboring countries, as reported by the UN Refugee Agency (UNHCR) as of September 2023 (Gesesew et al., 2021).

Despite challenging circumstances, Ethiopia's GDP in current US dollars has consistently risen over the last 5 years. Beginning at $84.27 billion in 2018 the GDP surged to $95.91 billion in 2019 and further increased to $107.66 billion in 2020. Despite global adversities, such as the COVID-19 pandemic, Ethiopia's economic growth remained resilient, culminating in a GDP of $111.26 billion in 2021. This positive trajectory continued into 2022, with Ethiopia's GDP reaching $126.78 billion, according to the World Bank (Fig. 13.6) (World Bank, 2022a).

Ethiopia has made limited progress toward achieving targets related to diet-related noncommunicable diseases (NCDs). Among adults aged 18 and older, obesity affects 8.5% of women and 2.4% of men—figures that remain below the regional averages of 20.8% for women and 9.2% for men. Despite this, diabetes remains a notable concern, with 5.9% of women and 6.9% of men affected.

Malnutrition remains a significant public health issue in Ethiopia despite two decades of progress. Overall, 37% of children under 5 experience stunted growth, and 22% of reproductive-aged women are chronically undernourished (BMI < 18.5 kg/m^2). WHO classifies stunting as "very high" and wasting as "medium." Only 14% of children under 2 meet minimum dietary diversity standards. Micronutrient deficiencies often accompany chronic energy deficiency, compounding the complexities of the country's nutrition transition and changing dietary habits.

Undernutrition is more prevalent among children living in rural areas of Ethiopia compared to those in urban settings, with significant regional disparities in stunting and wasting rates. According to 2016 data from (Central Statistical Agency) CSA and ICF International the highest incidence of diarrhea occurs in children aged 6–35 months, ranging between 13% and 23%. This age range aligns with the period when complementary feeding is typically introduced, beginning at 6 months. However, in the absence of proper water, sanitation, and hygiene (WASH) practices, this critical stage of dietary transition can adversely affect children's nutritional health.

The etiology of spina bifida, a congenital defect characterized by incomplete closure of the neural tube during embryonic development, is intricately linked to multifactorial elements, encompassing both genetic predispositions and environmental influences, with a pronounced emphasis on maternal nutritional status, particularly folate intake (Mitchell et al., 2004). In Ethiopia the elevated incidence of spina bifida, approximately 40 cases per 10,000 births, starkly contrasts with global averages, underscoring the urgent need for comprehensive public health interventions (Zhang et al., 2019). This translates to a significant public health burden, with nearly 10,500 affected newborns annually, many of whom face delayed or inadequate surgical intervention, leading to increased rates of stillbirths and mortality in newborns and children under 5 (Gebrehiwot et al., 2018; Tesema et al., 2020)). The consequences of this birth defect extend beyond immediate mortality, often resulting in lifelong disabilities and imposing substantial burdens on families and healthcare systems. The imperative of ensuring adequate folic acid intake among women of reproductive age is further compounded by the fact that many pregnancies are unplanned, highlighting the limitations of relying solely on preconception supplementation strategies (Pal et al., 2023). This emphasizes the critical role of mandatory fortification programs (Molloy, 2002).

Research from institutions like the Center for Spina Bifida at Emory University underscores the potential of such fortification programs to avert thousands of stillbirths and under-5 deaths in Ethiopia annually. However, despite the proven effectiveness of this intervention, Ethiopia has not yet implemented mandatory food fortification for spina bifida prevention (Koning et al., 2023).

Ethiopia has shown a strong commitment to improving nutrition through a comprehensive framework of policies, strategies, and multisectoral initiatives. Key among these are the National Food and Nutrition Policy (NFNP) 2019–29, the Growth and Transformation Plan II (GTP II) for 2015/16–2019/20, and the Second National Nutrition Programme (NNP II) covering 2016–20. Foundational efforts are also guided by influential frameworks such as the 2015 Seqota Declaration, the Health Sector Transformation Plan (HSTP) 2016–20, and the Agriculture Sector Policy and Investment Framework 2010–20. The NFNP focuses on using evidence to guide decisions and encourages collaboration across different sectors to tackle child stunting and malnutrition. It presents seven key policy areas aimed at improving access to nutritious food, ensuring food safety, better managing food after harvest, and supporting nutrition at all stages of life. The Seqota Declaration aims to eliminate hunger and undernutrition by 2030. To implement these plans, Ethiopia has set up two main bodies: the National Nutrition Coordination Body (NNCB) and the National Nutrition Technical Committee (NNTC), along with similar structures in regional areas. The Ministry of Health leads the collaboration among sectors and works with development partners. As the Food and Nutrition Strategy is rolled out, the Food and Nutrition Council will play a crucial role in aligning and directing nutrition efforts across the nation.

13.7.3 Case study 3: Vietnam

Vietnam's experience with prolonged warfare—including the First Indochina War (1946–54), the Vietnam War (1955–75), and subsequent border conflicts—left deep scars on its socioeconomic fabric and food systems. The wars devastated agricultural infrastructure, led to massive population displacements, and introduced long-lasting ecological damage. The destruction of farmlands, exposure to chemical defoliants like Agent Orange, and loss of labor capacity all contributed to widespread food insecurity and malnutrition. Following reunification in 1975, Vietnam inherited a fractured food system characterized by inadequate caloric intake, poor diet diversity, and acute micronutrient deficiencies, especially among children and women.

The introduction of the Đổi Mới economic reforms in 1986 marked a turning point. These reforms liberalized agriculture, enabled private land use, and stimulated rural incomes. As a result of targeted investment in food security and social infrastructure, malnutrition rates steadily declined (World Bank, 2023).

From 2017 to 2019, Vietnam maintained robust annual GDP growth averaging over 7%. The COVID-19 pandemic led to a temporary slowdown, with growth dipping to 2.9% in 2020. However, the economy rebounded swiftly, reaching 8.0% growth in 2022—among the highest globally during the recovery period. The graph reflects this trend, highlighting Vietnam's economic resilience and the steady trajectory of its postconflict development (Fig. 13.7).

Despite these gains, undernutrition remains a significant concern, particularly among ethnic minorities in upland regions. National surveys indicate that stunting affected 23.4% of children under 5 in 2021, with wasting present in 6.5% of the same age group. Anemia affects approximately 30% of women of reproductive age, and VAD among children remains a persistent challenge (Mbuya et al., 2019).

The Government of Vietnam, in partnership with international agencies such as UNICEF, WHO, and the World Bank, launched multiple programs targeting maternal and child nutrition. These included food supplementation initiatives, vitamin A distribution campaigns, deworming, and growth monitoring. The National Plan of Action for Nutrition (NPAN), first introduced in 1995 and revised every 5 years, provided a strategic framework aligning with global nutrition targets. Fortification programs—particularly iodine in salt and iron in fish sauce—played a central role in addressing hidden hunger (Rocha et al., 2022).

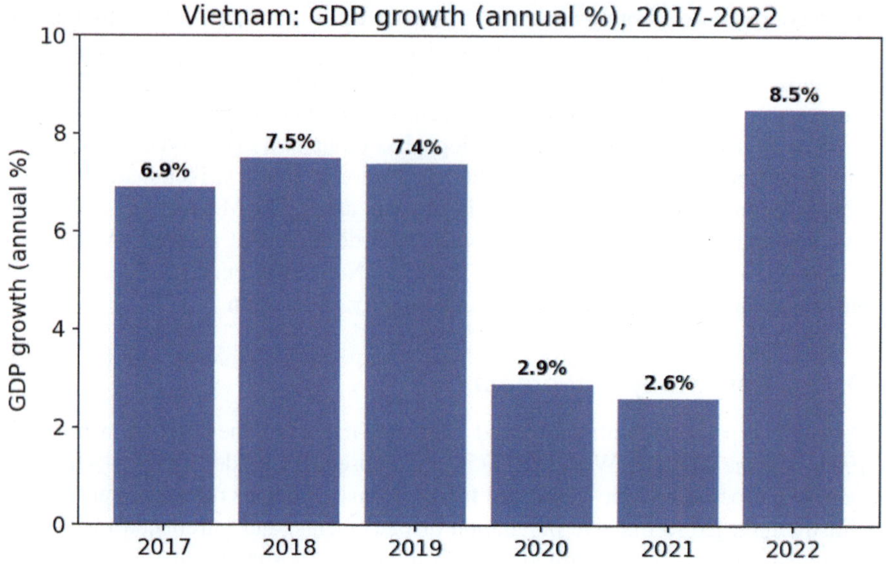

Figure 13.7 Vietnam's GDP growth rate from 2017 to 2022.

Vietnam's approach evolved into a food system model integrating agriculture, health, and social protection. The government prioritized local food production, clean water access, and sanitation—critical determinants of nutritional outcomes. The focus shifted from emergency relief to long-term sustainability through school meals, nutrition-sensitive agriculture, and community-based interventions (Harris et al., 2020).

According to the National Institute of Nutrition (NIN), annual national surveillance has guided evidence-based policy-making. A 2024 report emphasizes that food insecurity correlates with population mobility, economic transitions, and climatic events such as typhoons and droughts (Vaselli et al., 2024).

This chart shows a consistent decline in the proportion of undernourished individuals, from 9.3% in 2017 to 7.8% in 2022 (Fig. 13.8). These improvements are attributable to integrated nutrition programming, targeted social protection efforts, and large-scale food fortification policies spearheaded by the Ministry of Health in partnership with global agencies (FAO, 2021).

Efforts to address food insecurity were particularly crucial in remote provinces where infrastructure limitations and poverty restricted access to health and nutrition services. Here, community nutrition workers played pivotal roles in implementing household-level dietary changes and micronutrient supplementation strategies (Thi & Nhat, 2008). The above-shared graph is an indicator that the right strategic interventions at the policy level can have a large-scale, sustainable impact at the grassroots level, enabling the country to address the undernutrition challenges even in times of political and administrative instability (Fig. 13.9).

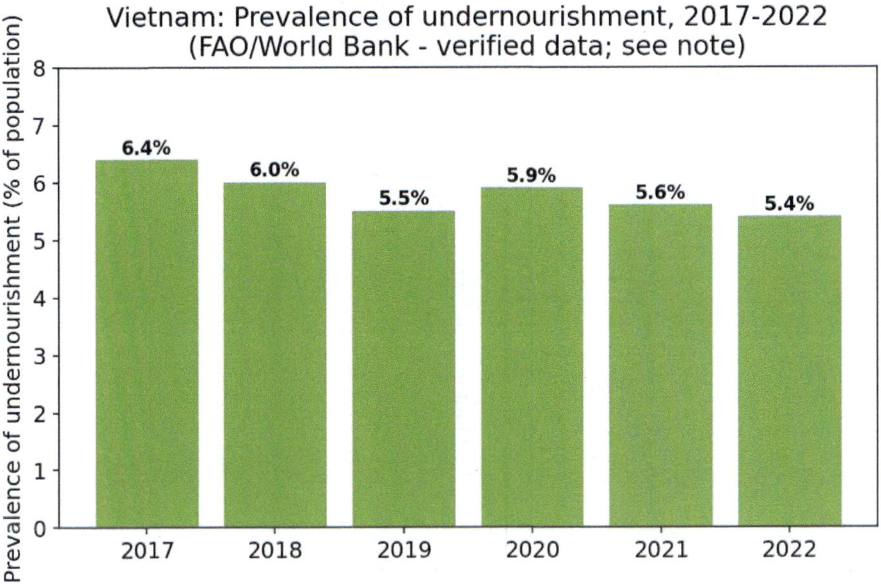

Figure 13.8 Prevalence of undernourishment in Vietnam (2017–22).

In comparing Ukraine, Ethiopia, and Vietnam, significant disparities emerge in various socioeconomic indicators. Although Ukraine boasts a smaller population of approximately 39.7 million compared to Ethiopia's sizable population of over 123 million, it exhibits a higher GDP of $161 billion. However, Ukraine experienced a negative GDP growth rate of −0.291% in 2022, contrasting with Ethiopia's positive growth rate of 0.0532%. Despite Ukraine's smaller population, it has a notably lower number of undernourished people at 1.5 million, constituting 4% of its population, whereas Ethiopia faces a substantial challenge with over 216 million undernourished individuals, accounting for 18% of its population. In addition, although both countries grapple with malnutrition, Ethiopia bears a higher burden with a malnutrition rate of 23%, compared to Ukraine's 25% (Table 13.3).

Vietnam occupies a unique middle ground. Although not currently facing active conflict, its postwar recovery over the past four decades offers a valuable lens into long-term policy-driven nutrition transformation. With a 2022 population of 98.2 million and a GDP of $409 billion, it achieved an impressive 8.0% growth—the highest among the three nations. Approximately 7.6 million people, or 7.8% of the population, remain undernourished. Although stunting persists in remote and ethnic minority regions, Vietnam has significantly reduced its overall malnutrition burden—estimated at 21%—through targeted policy reforms, widespread food fortification, and strong nutrition governance (Table 13.2).

Ukraine, Ethiopia, and Vietnam—despite their varied historical, economic, and political landscapes—have each contended with substantial nutrition and food security challenges. Yet, all three countries demonstrate a converging commitment to enhancing

Table 13.3 Comparative of Ukraine, Ethiopia, and Vietnam.

Country	Population (2022)	GDP (billion)	GDP growth	Undernourished people	Rate of malnutrition (%)	Burden of malnutrition (%)
Ukraine	39,701,739	$161	−0.291	1,500,000	4	25
Ethiopia	123,379,924	$127	0.0532	21,600,000	18	23
Vietnam	98,186,856	$409	8.0	7,600,000	7.8	21

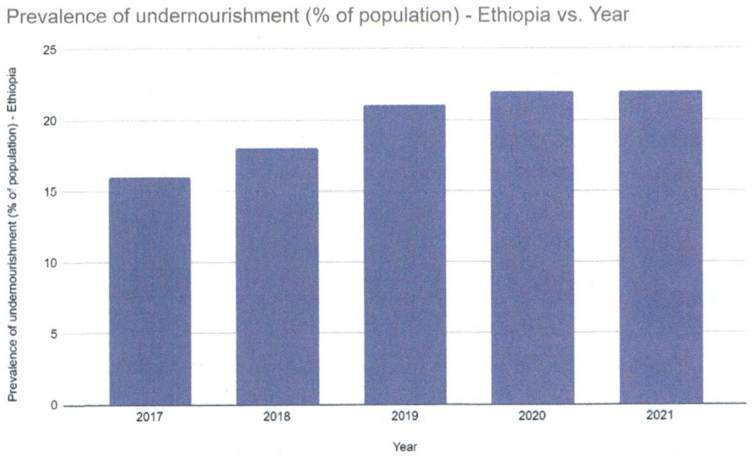

Figure 13.9 The prevalence of undernourishment in Ethiopia, as a percentage of the population, has seen a concerning upward trend in recent years. In 2017, it stood at 16%, followed by a slight increase to 18% in 2018. However, the situation worsened significantly in subsequent years, with the prevalence reaching 21% in 2019 and further escalating to 22% in both 2020 and 2021.

access to safe, nutritious, and affordable food through structured national responses. These efforts are anchored in data-driven policy development and strategic program implementation tailored to local contexts. Furthermore, each nation has prioritized robust institutional coordination and cross-sectoral governance, extending from national leadership to regional administrations, to effectively operationalize and sustain nutrition-focused initiatives.

13.8 Conclusion

Addressing malnutrition during emergencies requires more than rapid response—it calls for a strategic, data-driven approach. Key priorities include conducting comprehensive needs assessments that evaluate food access and the nutritional status of vulnerable groups such as children, pregnant and lactating women, older adults, and those with chronic illnesses. Food rations should meet both energy (2100 kcal/day) and micronutrient needs, with adjustments based on local conditions. Fortified foods and targeted supplementation are critical in low-diversity diets. Scaling up community-based management of acute malnutrition (CMAM) and supplementary feeding, particularly in displaced populations, enhances early treatment and supports optimal infant and young child feeding. Integrating health and WASH services is essential to tackle root causes and prevent recurrence. Strengthened monitoring systems, with regular data collection and evaluation, ensure responsiveness and accountability. Finally, preparedness through training, prepositioning supplies, and clear operational protocols is vital for timely and practical nutrition interventions.

In conclusion, safeguarding nutritional status during emergencies necessitates a comprehensive, adaptable, and rights-based approach. By adopting these recommendations, stakeholders can more effectively protect vulnerable populations, reduce the effects of crises, and establish a stronger foundation for recovery and resilience.

References

Abass, R. M., Hamdan, H. Z., Elhassan, E. M., Hamdan, S. Z., Ali, N. I., & Adam, I. (2014). Zinc and copper levels in low birth weight deliveries in Medani Hospital, Sudan. *BMC Research Notes, 7*(1), 1–5. https://doi.org/10.1186/1756-0500-7-386.

Albaroudi, I. N., Khodder, M., Saadi, T. A., Turk, T., & Youssef, L. A. (2018). Prevalence, diagnosis, and management of iron deficiency and iron deficiency anemia among Syrian children in a major outpatient center in Damascus, Syria. *Avicenna Journal of Medicine, 8*(03), 92–103. https://doi.org/10.4103/AJM.AJM_169_17.

Carroll, G. J., Lama, S. D., Martinez-Brockman, J. L., & Pérez-Escamilla, R. (2017). Evaluation of nutrition interventions in children in conflict zones: A narrative review. *Advances in Nutrition, 8*(5), 770–779. https://doi.org/10.3945/AN.117.016121.

Corley, A. G. (2021). Linking armed conflict to malnutrition during pregnancy, breastfeeding, and childhood. *Global Food Security, 29*, 100531. https://doi.org/10.1016/J.GFS.2021.100531.

Food and Agriculture Organization of the United Nation. (2021). *Food security and nutrition in the world the state of transforming food systems for food security, improved nutrition and affordable healthy diets for all.*https://doi.org/10.4060/cb4474en.

Food and Agriculture Organization of the United Nations. (2006). *The state of food and agriculture 2006*. FAO.

Food and Agriculture Organization of the United Nations, & World Health, Organization. (2000). *Human vitamin and mineral requirements*. Bangkok, Thailand: FAO.

Gebrehiwot, T., Fekadu, A., Abebe, S., et al. (2018). Malnutrition and associated factors among under-five children in Tigray, Northern Ethiopia: Evidence from the 2016 EDHS. *BMC Public Health, 18*, 1339. https://doi.org/10.1186/s12889-018-6265-2.

Gesesew, H., Berhane, K., Siraj, E. S., Siraj, D., Gebregziabher, M., Gebre, Y. G., Gebreslassie, S. A., Amdes, F., Tesema, A. G., Siraj, A., Aregawi, M., Gezahegn, S., & Tesfay, F. H. (2021). The impact of war on the health system of the Tigray region in Ethiopia: An assessment. *BMJ Global Health, 6*(11), 7328. https://doi.org/10.1136/BMJGH-2021-007328.

Global Alliance for Improved Nutrition (GAIN), Food Fortification Initiative (FFI), & Iodine Global Network, (IGN). *Global Fortification Data Exchange (GFDx): Afghanistan country profile*. https://www.fortificationdata.org.

Han, X., Ding, S., Lu, J., & Li, Y. (2022). Global, regional, and national burdens of common micronutrient deficiencies from 1990 to 2019: A secondary trend analysis based on the global burden of disease 2019 study. *EClinicalMedicine, 44*, 101299. https://doi.org/10.1016/j.eclinm.2022.101299.

Harika, R., Faber, M., Samuel, F., Mulugeta, A., Kimiywe, J., & Eilander, A. (2017). Are low intakes and deficiencies in iron, vitamin a, zinc, and iodine of public health concern in

Ethiopian, Kenyan, Nigerian, and South African Children and Adolescents? *Food and Nutrition Bulletin, 38*(3), 405–427. https://doi.org/10.1177/0379572117715818.

Harris, J., Nguyen, P. H., Tran, L. M., & Huynh, P. N. (2020). Nutrition transition in Vietnam: Changing food supply, food prices, household expenditure, diet and nutrition outcomes. *Food Security, 12*(5), 1141–1155. https://doi.org/10.1007/S12571-020-01096-x.

Iacoella, F., & Tirivayi, N. (2020). Child nutrition during conflict and displacement: Evidence from areas affected by the Boko Haram insurgency in Nigeria. *Public Health, 183*, 132–137. https://doi.org/10.1016/J.PUHE.2020.03.012.

IDMC. (2019). GRID 2019 | Global Report on Internal Displacement 2019. Retrieved May 19, 2025, from https://www.internal-displacement.org/global-report/grid2019/

IDMC (2020). Women and *girls in internal displacement*. https://doi.org/10.55363/IDMC.CYZB2861

Koning, M., Koning, J., Kancherla, V., O'Neill, P., Dorsey, A., Zewdie, K., Yesehak, B., Ashagre, Y., Woldermarium, M., & Biluts, H. (2023). A case study of ReachAnother Foundation as a change champion for developing spina bifida neurosurgical care and advocating for primary prevention in Ethiopia. *Child's Nervous System, 39*(7), 1783–1790. https://doi.org/10.1007/S00381-023-05932-1.

Leal Filho, W., Fedoruk, M., Paulino Pires Eustachio, J. H., Barbir, J., Lisovska, T., Lingos, A., & Baars, C. (2023). How the war in Ukraine affects food security. *Foods, 12*(21), 3996. https://doi.org/10.3390/FOODS12213996.

Loewenberg, S. (2015). Conflicts worsen global hunger crisis. *The Lancet, 386*(10005), 1719–1721. https://doi.org/10.1016/S0140-6736(15)00734-5.

Maxfield, L., Shukla, S., & Crane, J. S. (2023). Zinc deficiency. In *Causes and Management of nutritional deficiency disorders* (pp. 245–260). IGI Global. https://doi.org/10.4018/979-8-3693-2947-4.ch014.

Mbuya, N. V. N., Atwood, S. J., & Huynh, P. N. (2019). *Persistent malnutrition in ethnic minority communities of Vietnam: Issues and options for policy and interventions*. The World Bank https://doi.org/10.1596/978-1-4648-1432-7.

Ministry of Public Health (MoPH), Afghanistan. (2013). *National Nutrition Survey Afghanistan 2013*. Kabul: MoPH.

Mitchell, L. E., Adzick, N. S., Melchionne, J., Pasquariello, P. S., Sutton, L. N., & Whitehead, A. S. (2004). Spina bifida. *The Lancet, 364*(9448), 1885–1895. https://doi.org/10.1016/S0140-6736(04)17445-X.

Molloy, A. M. (2002). Folate and neural tube defects. Scandinavian Journal of Clinical and Laboratory Investigation, 62(Suppl. 234), 76–82. doi:https://doi.org/10.1080/003655102762377461

Mulaw, G. F., Masresha, S. A., & Feleke, F. W. (2023). Exploring barriers to Vitamin A supplementation uptake and program implementation among children aged 6–59 months in Ethiopia: A qualitative approach. *International Journal of Public Health, 68*, 1606167. https://doi.org/10.3389/IJPH.2023.1606167.

Pal, A., Seal, A., Kaur, P., et al. (2023). Micronutrient deficiencies in humanitarian settings: Evidence, gaps, and programmatic priorities. *The Lancet Global Health, 11*(5), e789–e801. https://doi.org/10.1016/S2214-109X(23)00001-0.

Philipo, M., Ndakidemi, P. A., & Mbega, E. R. (2021). Importance of common bean genetic zinc biofortification in alleviating human zinc deficiency in Sub-Saharan Africa. *Cogent Food & Agriculture, 7*(1). https://doi.org/10.1080/23311932.2021.1907954.

Pinstrup-Andersen, P. (2009). Food security: Definition and measurement. *Food Security, 1*(1), 5–7. https://doi.org/10.1007/S12571-008-0002-Y.

Ritchie, H., Rosado, P., & Roser, M. (2023). *Hunger and undernourishment*. Our World in Data https://ourworldindata.org/hunger-and-undernourishment.

Rocha, C., Mendonça, M., Huy, N. D, Phương, H. N., Hoa, D. T. B., Yeudall, F., Moraes, A., Brown, M. R., Yuan, Y. V., & Tenkate, T. (2022). A food-system approach to addressing food security and chronic child malnutrition in Northern Vietnam. *Journal of Agriculture, Food Systems, and Community Development, 11*(4), 273–292. https://doi.org/10.5304/jafscd.2022.114.019.

Suliman, O. S. M., & Elamin, H. A. M. (2023). Zinc level and effect of zinc supplementation on growth in a subset of Sudanese children with sickle cell disease. *Sudanese Journal of Paediatrics, 23*(2), 214–223. https://doi.org/10.24911/SJP.106-1638821311.

Tesema, G. A., Yeshaw, Y., Kebede, S. A., et al. (2020). Determinants of vitamin A supplementation among children aged 6–59 months in Ethiopia: A multilevel analysis of the 2016 EDHS. *BMJ Open, 10*(9), e037122. https://doi.org/10.1136/bmjopen-2020-037122.

Thi, T., & Nhat, H. (2008). Tackling household food insecurity: The experience of Vietnam. *Asian Journal of Agriculture and Development, 5*(2), 41–55. https://doi.org/10.22004/AG.ECON.198986.

Trading Economics. (2026). Ukraine—Prevalence *of u*ndernourishment (*%of p*opulation)—2025 data 2026 *f*orecast 1992-2022 *h*istorical. Retrieved May 19, 2025, from https://tradingeconomics.com/ukraine/prevalence-of-undernourishment-percent-of-population-wb-data.html.

UNICEF. (2024a). *Afghanistan* humanitarian situation report, *February 2024*. UNICEF Retrieved May 20, 2025, from https://www.unicef.org/documents/afghanistan-humanitarian-situation-report-february-2024 .

UNICEF. (2024b). *UNICEF IRAQ country programme document 2020-2024*. UNICEF. Retrieved May 20, 2025, from https://www.unicef.org/iraq/documents/unicef-iraq-country-programme-document-2020-2024

Vaselli, A., Nguyen, T. N., Savelli, A., Duong, T. T., Thi, P., Tuan, M., Truong, M. T., & Huynh, T. (2024). *Using Vietnam's National Nutrition Surveillance (NNS)* survey to explore the relationship between human mobility and food and nutrition security in *the Mekong Delta*. Bioversity International and International Center for Tropical Agriculture (CIAT) Retrieved May 20, 2025, from https://www.cgiar.org/funders/ .

Walter, T., De Andraca, I., Chadud, P., & Perales, C. G. (1989). Iron deficiency anemia: Adverse effects on infant psychomotor development. *Pediatrics, 84*(1), 7–17. https://doi.org/10.1542/PEDS.84.1.7.

Welsh, C. (2024, Februray 27). Russia, Ukraine, and global food security: A two-year assessment.Center for Strategic and International Studies(CSIS), https://www.csis.org/analysis/russia-ukraine-and-global-food-security-two-year-assessment.

Wilde, P. (2018). *Food policy in the United States: An introduction* (pp. 1–261). Routledge. https://doi.org/10.4324/9781315470337.

World Bank. (2022a). GDP (*c*urrent US$)—Ethiopia | data. Retrieved May 19, 2025, from https://data.worldbank.org/indicator/NY.GDP.MKTP.CD?end=2022&locations=ET&start=1981&view=chart

World Bank. (2022b). GDP *growth (annual %)*—Ukraine | data. Retrieved May 19, 2025, from https://data.worldbank.org/indicator/NY.GDP.MKTP.KD.ZG?end=2022&locations=UA&name_desc=false&start=2017

World Food Programme. (2022). Ukraine | World Food Programme. Retrieved May 19, 2025, from https://www.wfp.org/countries/ukraine

World Health Organization. (2009). *Global prevalence of vitamin A deficiency in populations at risk 1995-2005 : WHO global database on vitamin A deficiency*. World Health Organization Retrieved May 20, 2025, from https://iris.who.int/handle/10665/44110 .

Yisak, H., Elmneh, R., Taklual, W., Ewunetei, A., & Kefale, B. (2020). Prevalence and associated factors of clinical vitamin A deficiency among pre-school children 1–5 years of age in rural Kebeles in Farta district, South Gondar Zone, Ethiopia: A mixed methods study. *Journal of Multidisciplinary Healthcare, 13*, 1191–1201. https://doi.org/10.2147/JMDH.S279571.

Zhang, F., Chen, J., Pan, Z., & Chen, S. (2019). Large-scale food fortification operations: Implementation, monitoring, and quality control in low- and middle-income countries—A review. *Food Policy, 84*, 54–65. https://doi.org/10.1016/j.foodpol.2019.03.004.

Nutritional policies for Kenya: A critical examination of national and international interventions

14

Susan Atieno Onyango[a] *and Francis Aila Oketch*[b]
[a]Programmes, The Healthy Woman, Homa Bay, Nyanza, Kenya, [b]Department of Health, County Government of Homa Bay, Homa Bay, Nyanza, Kenya

14.1 Introduction

Kenya, like many developing countries, faces significant challenges in addressing malnutrition and food insecurity. The country suffers from the multifaceted crisis of malnutrition with high levels of undernutrition, a high prevalence of micronutrient deficiencies, and an ever-increasing rate of overnutrition (Demographic Health, 2022). The available nutrition interventions to tackle the heavy burden of malnutrition are greatly hampered by the siloed approach to handling the situation, instead of a more integrated approach to dealing with the multifaceted problem of malnutrition (Sibanda et al., 2023). The food systems in place lay much emphasis on food production with little regard for nutrition. The country is also faced with high burdens of various illnesses that exacerbate the malnutrition situation with a high prevalence of malaria, tuberculosis, and worm infestations, among other diseases of public health importance (Ministry of Health, 2024).

Climate change has also proved to be a complication in Kenya, with the disruption of the weather patterns and influence on food production, enhanced natural catastrophes such as floods and droughts, and changes in disease trends (Marigi, 2017). The Ministry of Health spearheads the delivery of nutrition services in the country, with much effort currently being laid on an all-inclusive approach to deliver nutrition to the population, though with several challenges given the weak multisectoral approach to tackling nutrition issues in the country (Ministry of Health, Republic of, 2018).

Despite progress made in the country in nutrition programming that has seen a reduction in malnutrition rates in recent years, the country continues to grapple with high rates of stunting, underweight, wasting (Demographic Health, 2022), and micronutrient deficiencies among children under 5 and women of reporductive age (KNBS, 2011). The incidence of overnutrition characterized by overweight and obesity has also been on the rise, with an upsurge in noncommunicable diseases (Wanjohi et al., 2021). Various policies and strategic plans are in place to address the poor health and nutrition situation with varied levels of success in their implementation (Sibanda et al., 2023). Key among the major challenges faced in the implementation of these policies and plans is the lack of an integrated monitoring and evaluation system that

Nutritional Strategies, Predictive Models, and Sustainable Policies. DOI: https://doi.org/10.1016/B978-0-443-23671-6.00001-3

encompasses all the players with a stake in nutrition in the country (Rifkin, 2023). This chapter provides an overview of Kenya's nutritional landscape and critically examines the existing national and international policies and strategies aimed at improving the country's nutritional status.

14.1.1 Current nutritional status in Kenya

The available food systems in Kenya lay more emphasis on food production with little regard to nutrition and nutrients. This has resulted in a focus on how much food the country can produce as opposed to what the food does in the human body, with increased land acreage for food being considered a great success regardless of the nutritional situation and outcomes in the country. Nutrition plays a critical role in human health, with adequate amounts of nutrients and quality of nutrients supporting the human body to regenerate and hence leading to a quality life (Keats et al., 2019). This is desirable if the country is to be productive, as a healthy population is beneficial to the economic growth of the country, with increased man-hours available to spur the economy and reduce expenditure on ill health. Access to nutritious foods and appropriate public health measures, therefore, determines the nutrition situation of the population.

Globally, close to 3 billion people suffer from various forms of malnutrition, with sub-Saharan Africa being the most affected region (UNICEF/WHO/World Bank Group, 2021). Global nutrition reports indicate that sub-Saharan Africa still faces a myriad of challenges in meeting the nutritional needs of its people, with large case loads of undernourished children being experienced in several countries in the region, women of reproductive age suffering from various forms of undernutrition, and an increasing population with overnutrition characterized by overweight and obesity and an upsurge of noncommunicable diseases (Development Initiatives, 2022). Various factors have occasioned this sorry state of affairs, key among them being climate change, instability because of wars, poor dietary choices, and poor food production systems, which result in minimal yield and the inability to exploit the region's full potential.

Kenya's nutritional situation remains a cause for concern, with persistent challenges across various health and nutrition indicators. Recent data from the demographic health survey show a marked improvement in malnutrition rates among the population, especially children under 5 years (Demographic Health, 2022). An analysis of the demographic health surveys for the past decade shows a steady decline in the country's undernutrition levels (Demographic Health, 2014). Despite this improvement, the rates of malnutrition are still high, representing a significant number of people at risk of ill health because of one or more nutritional deficiencies. Malnutrition in its various forms affects over 40 million Kenyans, posing a significant challenge to the country's growth and development. Other than undernutrition, overnutrition has also been on the rise in the country, posing additional challenges of noncommunicable diseases and putting a strain on the healthcare system that now seems overstretched following recent challenges with COVID-19, inadequate policy implementation, dwindling donor funding, and inadequate monitoring of the healthcare system (Government of Kenya, 2021).

14.1.1.1 *Stunting, underweight, and wasting*

Undernutrition, characterized by stunting, underweight, and wasting, is a leading contributor for morbidity and mortality among children under 5. Close to 50% of mortalities among children are associated with undernutrition; hence there is a need to identify the cause of undernutrition among children and the institutional measures to curb the situation (Black et al., 2008). Nationwide, 18% of children under 5 face developmental impairment, with this rate being a decline from the previous rate of 26% (Demographic Health, 2022). This represents approximately 10 million children at risk of not attaining their full potential because of developmental deficiencies associated with stunting. Despite this remarkable reduction in stunting rates, regional disparities within the country exist, with very high stunting rates in several counties, an indication that the great improvement in stunting rates was not in favor of the entire population. Kilifi, West Pokot, and Samburu counties have stunting rates of 37%, 34%, and 31%, respectively, with these counties being considered to have very high stunting rates. Another 11 counties have stunting rates of between 20% and 29%, an indication that the situation in Kenya is still not desirable for the optimal survival of children. From this demographic health survey, only two counties, Kisumu and Garissa, had low stunting rates at 9% each. In addition, undernutrition remains a concern in Kenya, impacting 10% of children, with 2% suffering from severe weight defficiencies, whereas 5% of children under the age of 5 years are classified as wasted. Despite the seemingly low wasting rates, regional variations show very high wasting rates in the northern parts of the country and major cities that are characterized by the presence of vast informal settlements.

This poor nutritional status among children has been attributed to diseases and poor diets among these age cohorts. This is mainly because of inadequate food and nutrition security among households, inadequate childcare practices, and various harmful social norms among community members. Infant feeding practices and access to health care contribute to the overall outcome of nutritional status among children. The country has experienced mixed results in maternal, infant, and young child nutrition (MIYCN) indicators, with the exclusive breastfeeding rates showing an upward trend before a slight dip. Close to 40% of children under the age of 6 months are not adequately breastfed, with their caregivers introducing complementary feeds earlier than expected. The minimum acceptable diet for children 6–23 months is generally low in the country, with many children missing out on essential nutrients during their crucial growth period. The insufficient introduction of complementary foods to children is attributed to insufficient knowledge among caregivers and a general lack of sufficient nutritious foods for most children.

The poor nutritional status of the country has major ramifications, with the country losing economically. The cost of hunger studies conducted in the country showed that malnutrition is a great threat to the economic growth of the country, with close to 7% of the gross development product being lost because of the current high levels of malnutrition. The amount of money projected as losses from this scenario is more than the budget allocated to the devolved units, which are mainly responsible for providing health care and agriculture services that are fundamental in ensuring that the population remains healthy and productive.

This dire situation has been occasioned by climate change that has resulted in droughts and floods in various parts of the country, causing disruptions in the normal food production and distribution systems and the poor living conditions in informal settlements that are characterized by overcrowding, poor dietary practices, and inadequate sanitation levels.

14.1.1.2 *Overnutrition*

In the recent past, Kenya has experienced an increasing trend in the cases of noncommunicable diseases (Masibo et al., 2020). Many predisposing factors, such as overweight and obesity, are on the rise, with about 4% of the overall population being overweight. The rates of overnutrition differ based on regional distribution and gender. The female gender was shown to be more prone to overweight and obesity compared to the male gender. Further, higher overweight levels were recorded within urban population as opposed to those in rural landscape. The higher overweight and obesity levels in the urban areas are attributed to changing lifestyles, with the population in urban setups generally leading a sedentary lifestyle with minimal or no physical activities and a shift in their dietary patterns to consuming more calories than their bodies can expend. Regionally, cases of noncommunicable diseases are more prevalent or elevated in central region of the country compared to other regions. Counties, such as Nyeri, Kirinyaga, and Muranga, have reported increased cases of noncommunicable diseases that are largely associated with overnutrition. In children under 5 years of age, the prevalence of overweight remained the same over time, with a sharp decline in the recent past.

14.1.1.3 *Micronutrient deficiencies*

Various micronutrients are considered of public health importance in Kenya, given their high levels of deficiencies and the health and economic impact that they pose to the population. Key among these micronutrient deficiencies of concern in the country are vitamin A, zinc, iron, and iodine. Hidden hunger or micronutrient deficiencies in Kenya have been reported across the country in different age cohorts. Table 14.1 highlights the micronutrient deficiencies in Kenya. Anemia (41.6%), iron deficiency (36.1%), and iron deficiency anemia (26%) are prevalent among pregnant women, negatively impacting maternal and fetal health. Despite the notable improvements in maternal health with reduced maternal deaths over the years, the average of 355 deaths per 100,000 live births remains significantly high compared to the global target of 70 per 100,000 live births. Some of the major causes of maternal deaths in the country are attributed to low hemoglobin levels among pregnant women. Other than poor maternal health, the lack of this essential nutrient also negatively impacts fetal outcomes, with mortalities recorded and low birth weights among women deficient in iron during pregnancy. The levels for these deficiencies in preschool children are 26.3%, 21.8%, and 13.3%, respectively. The high levels of iron deficiency among children negatively impact their growth and development and interfere with their cognitive ability, affecting their learning ability. Vitamin A deficiency affects children mainly under the age of

Table 14.1 Micronutrient deficiency levels in Kenya (KNBS, 2011).

Group/deficiency	Anemia	Iron deficiency	Iron deficiency anemia	Vitamin A deficiency (VAD)	Marginal VAD
Pregnant women	41.6	36.1	26	5.4	21.6
Men	9.3	3.6	2.9	0	0
Preschool children	26.3	21.3	13.3	9.2	52.6
School-aged children	16.5	9.4	4.9	3.6	33.9
Nonpregnant women	21.9	21.3	14	1.1	8.1

5, with 9.2% of preschool children being deficient in vitamin A, whereas 4.1% of the entire population was reported to be deficient in vitamin A. Marginal vitamin A deficiency was very high at 52.6% among preschool children.

Vitamin A plays a critical role in boosting immunity among children, along with other health benefits. Its deficiency, therefore, predisposes the children to morbidity and mortality that lead to the overall poor health indicators in the country. Iodine deficiency was reported at 22.1% in school-going children, while it was 25.6% among nonpregnant women. Iodine is critical for the development of children's intelligence quotient; hence its deficiency has an impact on the education sector. Zinc deficiency was the highest deficiency recorded during the last Kenya National Micronutrient Survey at 83.3% in preschool children and 82.3% in nonpregnant women. This high prevalence level of zinc deficiency predisposes a large population to a myriad of health problems, given that zinc plays a critical role in human health and nutrition of boosting immunity. A major gap still exists in the country in terms of accurate micronutrient deficiency data, as the available data that gives a national picture that was last collected over a decade ago. Despite this dearth of information, isolated studies have still revealed a high prevalence of micronutrient deficiencies among different population segments. Higher anemia prevalence was reported among Kenyan urban children (28%) compared to their rural counterparts (Evang et al., 2020). However, in the same population, the prevalence of iron deficiency was more significant among the rural inhabitants than their urban counterparts at 14% and 3%, respectively. This variation in micronutrient deficiencies across the country is a pointer to a possible high burden in different regions that require a multifaceted approach in addressing the gaps leading to this scenario.

14.1.1.4 Mortalities

Undernutrition contributes significantly to child mortality, with about 45% of all deaths among children under 5 attributed to one or more forms of undernutrition (Madewell et al., 2024). Kenya has, over the years, had a decline in child mortality rates, with the levels dipping from 96/1000 to 41/1000 for under 5 mortality over 20 years. The neonatal mortality declined from 26/1000 to 21/1000 live births during the same period (KNBS, 2019). Despite these great improvements, the mortality rates among children in the country are still way above the global targets. With these trends, it is highly unlikely that the country will meet the sustainable development goal (SDGs) targets, given that the country has less than 5 years to improve on these indicators. The drivers of child mortality in the country include malnutrition, poor sanitation, and high levels of diseases such as malaria and pneumonia.

14.1.2 National policies and strategies

Health and nutrition programming in Kenya is guided by various policies that take a stakeholder approach during their development. The country has about 20 policies and guidelines that are currently actively being used to guide the provision of nutrition services (Sibanda et al., 2023). These policies and guidelines address various aspects of nutrition that range from food production, food processing, food safety, and food utilization. The nutrition services geared toward supporting appropriate nutrition for the citizens of the country are coordinated under the Ministry of Health, which also has various divisions dealing with different health programs in the country. Despite being housed in the Ministry of Health, which majorly handles nutrition-specific issues, many other nutrition-sensitive programs are planned for and executed in sister sectors such as agriculture, water, social protection, education, trade, and industry.

The first document in Kenya that provides for the provision of health and nutrition services is the Kenyan Constitution 2010 (Constitution of Kenya, 2010). In schedule four of the constitution, provision of services between the central and county governments is stipulated, with health being a majorly devolved function, hence providing the onus to regional governments to discharge nutrition services to the citizens. The national government is primarily tasked with developing policies and building staff capacity. The Constitution of Kenya, 2010 provides for freedom from hunger for all and adequate nutrition for children. Specific sections of the constitution provide for this:

Article 43 (1c): Guarantees the right to be free from hunger and to have adequate food of acceptable quality.
Article 53 (1c): Guarantees the right of every child to basic nutrition (Constitution of Kenya, 2010). The Kenyan constitution, therefore, acts as the starting point for supporting nutrition for the citizens.

The Kenya Nutrition Action Plan (KNAP) 2023–27: This comprehensive plan aims to reduce the burden of malnutrition in its various manifestations across all age groups. It builds on the successes and lessons learned from the previous action plan (2018–22) and is the third action plan developed by the government (2018). This is the road map for the government in the delivery of nutrition services across the country and is domiciled in the Ministry of Health. Despite being anchored in the Ministry of Health the document takes a multisectoral approach in its implementation, given the multiplicity of nutrition needs in the country. This policy document is organized into key results areas, with the current KNAP having 14 key result areas. These result areas cover MIYCN; nutritional well-being of older children, adolescents, adults, and older people; mitigation and control of micronutrient deficiencies; administration of clinical nutrition and dietetic care at all tiers of healthcare system; sustained nutritional well-being of individuals and communities during emergencies and climate-related shocks; enhanced integration of nutrition into agriculture, livestock, and fisheries sectors; nutrition integration across all levels of the health sector; improved alignment of nutrition initiatives within the education sector; enhanced integration of nutrition within the water, sanitation, and hygiene (WASH) sector; nutrition integration across social protection programs; enhanced multisectoral nutrition governance, coordination, partnerships, advocacy, and community engagement; multisectoral systems for nutrition data, M&E systems, learning, research, and knowledge management; enhanced nutrition capacity for improved service provision; and strengthened supply chain management for nutrition-related supplies and tools/equipment. This national action plan is being implemented across the 47 counties, with the various regional governments focusing on nutrition-specific issues in their regions, which vary from region to region. A monitoring framework for this policy is available, and plans for mid- and end-term reviews are in place. A major gap in the implementation of the previous plans has been inadequate financing for the plans and insufficient monitoring of their implementation to better inform responses.

Food and Nutrition Security Policy (FNSP): This overarching framework encompasses diverse components of food security and nutrition advancement, recognizing the need for multisectoral involvement. The policy is based on the premise that food is a basic human right and there is shared responsibility in ensuring that the entire population is both food and nutrition secure. The FNSP focuses on the four prongs of food security: food availability, food access, food utilization, and food stability (2011). This policy document is anchored in the Ministry of Agriculture, with its implementation being shared across various government departments and agencies.

National MIYCN policy guidelines: These policy guidelines focus on the need to make the health facilities in the country baby friendly while promoting and protecting breastfeeding in the community. The policy guidelines have 19 policy steps that cover both the activities in the health facilities and the community level. The policy guidelines provide guidance on breastfeeding in the context of human immunodeficiency virus (HIV) and HIV testing services for pregnant women, lactating mothers, and their children.

Kenya Agri-Nutrition Strategy (2020–25): This strategy is anchored on the KNAP and addresses the production aspects of food in the country to address malnutrition from a production perspective. Its primary aim is to ensure access to safe, varied, and nutritious food platters by reinforcing both the national food chain and local food production systems and consumption of nutritious foods. In addition to supporting the rollout of the KNAP, this strategy provides a road map for the implementation of the agri-nutrition-related aspects of the FNSP. If well implemented, this strategy will promote dietary diversification in the various food chains available in the country.

Implementation framework for breastfeeding-friendly workplaces (2020–24): This roadmap coordinates interventions to support breastfeeding in both public and private sector workplaces. The goal of promoting and supporting breastfeeding is to ensure that all children receive the best form of nutrition as stipulated in the Kenyan Constitution, which advocates for basic nutrition for children. The framework was developed to secure safer breastfeeding practices at workplaces as a way of promoting infant and young child feeding and hence contributing to a reduction in morbidities and mortalities among children. This framework builds on several Acts of Parliament that seek to promote infant feeding, such as the Employment Act that provides for maternity and paternity leaves for parents to support breastfeeding and the Breastfeeding Substitutes Act that seeks to ensure the breastfeeding process is well protected by discouraging the promotion of the substitutes.

Scaling Up Nutrition (SUN) Business Network Kenya Strategy (2019–23): This initiative acknowledges the importance of the private sector ensuring the availability and affordability of safe, hygienic, wholesome, and nutritious food. The strategy was developed to provide an enabling environment for the private sector involved in food production, given their key role in working together with the government and other nongovernment actors to contribute to food and nutrition security in the country.

Kenya Universal Health Coverage Policy 2020–30: This health policy aims to ensure the population's access to essential quality healthcare services in the country without experiencing any financial hardships. Nutrition services in the country are largely coordinated by the Ministry of Health, under which the Kenya Health Policy is anchored. The policy addresses various critical issues that cut across various nutrition fronts. Key among issues being addressed by this policy are strengthening the human resources for health to ensure that the entire country has sufficient numbers and mix of the requisite healthcare providers, ensuring availability of the essential health products and technologies that include essential nutrition supplies, making use of the health information system to make critical decisions in the health sector, building and improving upon the existing health infrastructure to enhance quality healthcare services provision, and promoting uptake of research in the health sector to be able to link policy and implementation. This health policy has four objectives: ensuring access to health services by all citizens, provision of quality health services to the citizens of the country, protection of the community from financial risks, and a responsive healthcare system that adequately meets the health needs of the population.

School health policy: This policy was developed by the Ministries of Education and Health in Kenya to provide a platform for the delivery of comprehensive school health. The school health policy seeks to provide a platform for resource-efficient reduction of the consequences of both communicable and noncommunicable diseases; promote core values and life skills among beginners; improve WASH facilities with overall school infrastructure; meet the diverse nutrition and special needs of the learners; and mainstream gender issues in our education and health systems. Implementation of this policy takes a holistic approach from the two ministries, with various stakeholders involved. The policy takes care of a huge segment of the population, given the youthful nature of the Kenyan population. Its full implementation will, therefore, result in marked improvements in the nutritional status of the population.

Iron folic acid policy: Kenya has a policy guideline for the provision of combined iron and folic acid supplements during pregnancy. The goal of this policy is to promote healthy pregnancies and good pregnancy outcomes as a way of reducing maternal deaths and perinatal deaths and enhancing the overall quality of good health. The policy guideline provides for the content of the iron-folic acid supplements meant for use during pregnancy, provides for dosing, the target group, side effects, and how to manage them. The policy guideline assumes that these health products will be provided in all the health facilities, and hence, all the women seeking these services will benefit from them. The role played by iron and folic acid preconception and during pregnancy is critical. Hence the full implementation of this policy is necessary to support good health indicators in the country.

Vitamin A supplementation policy: This policy guideline provides for the dosage of vitamin A for children 6–59 months, the delivery platforms, and the handling of vitamin A capsules. The policy guideline is important in the health sector, given the public health importance of vitamin A in the Kenyan population. A key component of this policy is the delivery mechanisms for vitamin A supplements, with the country taking both facility and community approaches to reach all children.

Food fortification strategy: Kenya practices mandatory fortification of selected staple foods to prevent and control micronutrient malnutrition. The country has a food fortification strategy for 2023–27, whose aim is to provide overall guidance to the food industry on how to fortify staple foods adequately. The strategy provides for the food vehicles to be used, the dosaging rates, quality assurance measures to ensure adequate fortification, reporting on the fortification process, and monitoring of the entire process. This strategy provides the Ministry of Health with a strategic focus on preventing and controlling micronutrient deficiencies in partnership with agri, agritech, and food sectors whose actions impact health and nutrition.

Kenya's national strategy for the prevention and control of noncommunicable diseases: This strategy was developed by the Ministry of Health to aid in the response to the ever-increasing cases of noncommunicable diseases. The strategy focuses on strengthening the healthcare system to be able to respond to these conditions while promoting healthy lifestyles among community members. The strategy focuses on both preventive and curative aspects of noncommunicable diseases.

National School Meals and Nutrition Strategy: This strategic document was developed to guide the implementation of the school meals initiatives at both the preprimary and primary levels of schooling in line with the country's vision, which aims to transform the nation into a middle-income country while adhering to the tenets of the constitution that seeks to have all children attain basic nutrition. The strategy was developed by three sectors of education, health, and agriculture and livestock, building on relevant laws in these government ministries. The ultimate goal of this strategy is to have a government-owned and sustainable school feeding program that will promote the retention of children in schools and enhance learning among them.

National Guidelines for Healthy Diets and Physical Activity: Because of the increasing cases of morbidity among citizens as a result of sedentary lifestyles and poor dietary practices, the Ministry of Health, in collaboration with stakeholders, developed this dietary guideline to support in response to the increasing poor health of the populace. The guidelines cover nutrition assessment, food processing and preservation, and physical activities.

Kenya Nutrition Capacity Development Framework (KNCDF): The framework deals with the capacity of the nutrition workforce in the country to deliver quality nutrition services to its citizens. This framework looks at four aspects required to enable nutrition services delivery in the country. These are systemic, organizational, technical, and community. The framework guides the regional governments in assessing their ability to deliver nutrition services in the context of the four subthemes and provides room for improvement and upgrading of services based on the gaps identified during the assessment exercise. If well implemented, this framework can transform nutrition services provision, given its robustness and focus on all aspects required for quality nutrition services provision.

The Kenya Vision 2030: The country has a transformation blueprint that aims to improve its citizens' quality of life while raising the country's economic status to a middle-income level. This blueprint has three pillars: economic, political, and social, with each having particular targets to be attained by 2030. The implementation of

Vision 2030 is carried out through 5-year medium-term plans with an assessment every 5 years to assess the progress being made in the country. The social pillar harbors health, under which nutrition is anchored. The blueprint has seen the country grow from strength to strength, with health and nutrition indicators improving over the year, though the targets are yet to be met.

In addition, the country has the livestock strategic plan, National Agricultural Investment Plan livestock sector plan (LSP), and National FNSP-Implementation Framework domiciled at the Ministry of Agriculture. These strategies aim to increase food production in the country and ensure availability across the country to foster food and nutrition security.

With the ever-increasing cases of noncommunicable diseases in Kenya the Ministry of Health is in the process of developing front-of-pack labeling guidelines to curb the excess intake of ultra-processed foods that have been observed to result in these rising cases.

The Kenya Nutrition Monitoring and Evaluation Framework (KNMEF): Kenya has many health and nutrition policies that should be able to adequately address the current nutrition challenges experienced in the country. However, over the years, the gains made have not been commensurate with the number of available guidance documents because of many reasons. These include inadequate funding for the full rollout of these policies at scale to cover all the stipulated areas. In number the policy documents are partially implemented, and hence, the full anticipated benefits of the policies are never realized. A second reason for the ineffective implementation of the Kenyan policies is the siloed approach in their role, with policies being controlled by respective ministries, negating the need for a joint approach in their implementation. The lack of a robust monitoring and evaluation framework that encompasses all the government sectors makes it near impossible to wholly assess progress in the work being done and check on possible areas that need more focus for full-scale implementation. This is the greatest drawback in the implementation of the available policies.

14.1.3 International initiatives and their impact

Several international initiatives have played a crucial role in shaping Kenya's nutritional landscape. Kenya is a signatory to various international agreements that support human health and well-being.

SUN Movement: Kenya joined SUN in 2012, uniting national leaders, civil society, and international organizations in a collective effort to improve nutrition. The country has actively been involved in the SUN initiatives with the formation of various SUN chapters in the country, and great progress has been shown, with Kenya being among the 8 countries out of 194 worldwide on track to achieving four global nutrition targets of exclusive breastfeeding, stunting, overweight, and wasting.

Agenda 2063: Kenya is a member of the African Union and subscribes to the union's Agenda 2063. This agenda aims to transform the continent into a global powerhouse in the future. The Agenda 2063 has 20 goals, with 2 of them specifically touching on nutrition. Goal number 3 focuses on health and nutrition, with the ultimate goal being that the people of the continent will be healthy and well-nourished. Goal number 5 speaks to modern agriculture intending to have a productive continent able to meet the food needs of its citizens. Other than these two goals specific to food production and nutrition, some goals target economic empowerment of the population and resilience in the face of climate change. Kenya signed the Comprehensive Africa Agriculture Development Programme (CAADP), an Agenda 2063 initiative in 2010, demonstrating commitment to agricultural development and aligning with Africa-led efforts to reduce hunger and poverty.

Feed the Future: This US government initiative aims to facilitate extensive and inclusive growth in the agri and allied sector, combined with enhanced resilience, which would lead to the improvement of the nutritional status of the existing rural population with a primary focus on women and children (under 5 years).

14.1.4 Critical analysis of policy impact

Although Kenya has made progress in addressing malnutrition, the impact of these policies and initiatives has been mixed. Positive outcomes have been experienced in reducing undernutrition, with marked reductions in the levels of stunting among children under 5 years old. However, there have also been notable increases in overnutrition and noncommunicable diseases. These mixed results call for further scrutiny to better understand the roles played by the different policies and strategies in either combating malnutrition or exacerbating the situation.

14.1.4.1 Positive outcomes

- Reduction in child stunting from 35% in 2008 to 26% in 2014 and 18% in 2022. Over the years, Kenya has experienced an improved status of stunting among children under 5 years of age. This could be attributed to the many policies that have been developed and implemented, cutting across various sectors that have sought to work together in their efforts to reduce the stunting rates.
- Decline in child mortality rates since 2000, with a decline from 96/1000 to 41/1000 for under 5 infant mortality. The country has witnessed marked reductions in child mortality rates, and it is striving to achieve global mortality targets. However, the decline in the mortality rates indicates that the country may not meet the SDG targets by 2030.
- Improved coordination among different sectors and stakeholders in addressing nutrition issues. The country has witnessed great improvement in the coordination of nutrition work by bringing together different government sectors and stakeholders, especially during the development of the KNAP and its implementation. This coordinated approach has also been witnessed during the development of other policy documents, as witnessed by the multisector approach adopted by the country in the development of the policies.
- Anchoring of nutrition in key government policy documents. The inclusion of nutrition in the Kenyan Constitution and other policy documents has elevated nutrition in the country and contributed to its growth within the different government sectors. This recognition has played a critical part in mobilizing for resources to support the nutrition work and contributed to the gains observed in the sector.
- Increased food production: Over the years, Kenya has witnessed great government investments in food production to ensure food security. Subsidy programs have been introduced over the years for farmers to spur production and ensure an adequate supply in the country. Despite these efforts not fully yielding the desired effects the thought of subsidizing

production to cushion farmers shows that the country is going in the right direction to ensure that food and nutrition security is enhanced.

14.1.4.2 Persistent challenges

- Regional disparities in nutrition indicators persist, with some counties still experiencing severe levels of malnutrition. Despite the reported improvements in nutrition indicators in Kenya, some regions still have very high levels of malnutrition, with stunting levels up to twice the national average. These variations in malnutrition levels could be attributed to regional differences in the implementation of policies and strategies available in the country and the regional differences with regard to factors contributing to malnutrition.
- Recent increases in undernourishment rates are partly because of climate-related events like floods and droughts. The effects of climate change have been devastating in the country, with extremes in both floods and droughts. The country has witnessed recent cases of flooding, resulting in not only the displacement of families but also the destruction of food crops on the farms. These have aggravated the food and nutrition situation, leading to rescue efforts to support the affected families. On the other hand, other parts of the country have also been plagued by droughts, leading to crop failures and, hence, food insecurity.
- Urban food insecurity and undernutrition are emerging concerns requiring targeted interventions. Most urban areas are characterized by informal settlements, with the residents living on less than a dollar a day. These high poverty levels have witnessed poor household food security in these settlements, leading to high malnutrition levels. Despite the decline in malnutrition levels, overall in the country, these informal settlements are usually characterized by high levels of wasting because of inadequate food intake among children and poor sanitary conditions in these settlements.
- Increased cases of overweight and noncommunicable diseases. Kenya has, over the years, experienced an upsurge in nutrition, with females being more affected compared to males. The rates of overnutrition are also higher in urban areas compared to rural setups. This has been attributed to a change in dietary patterns in the urban setups with a focus on ultraprocessed foods as opposed to natural foods and a more sedentary lifestyle.
- The monitoring and evaluation of these policies have not been sufficient to ensure that all planned activities are undertaken to meet the set targets. Furthermore a fragmented monitoring system that exists with the different government sectors monitoring activities within their jurisdiction and the lack of an integrated monitoring system have led to slow implementation and attainment of the targets.
- Limited dietary diversity across different regions. The country has emphasized food production, with work yet to be done on food diversity. The government invests a lot in maize production, with the success of a good harvest being estimated from the tonnes of maize produced in a particular season. This reliance on maize as a staple has led the community to depend on its availability as a measure of food security, resulting in little diversification among the community members. Efforts are being made to educate the community on diversification, but more needs to be done to ensure that the community members consume the required food groups to promote adequate nutrition in the country.

14.1.4.3 Implementation gaps

- Despite comprehensive policies, implementation at the county level remains a challenge, with varying degrees of success across different regions. Differences in the operations of regional governments with little influence from the national government could derail the attainment of the set goals.

- Limited financial resources and capacity constraints hinder the full implementation of nutrition programs. Furthermore, there is an overreliance on development partners to fund nutrition initiatives such as capacity building and procurement of nutrition products, leading to a lack of sustainability in the initiatives initiated by the stakeholders. More often than not, when the support provided by the stakeholders runs out, the community is normally left vulnerable because of the inability of the government to continue with the initiatives uninterrupted.
- Inadequate community resilience to shocks in society, such as droughts, floods, and other disasters. The communities affected by shocks have often relied on donations, with little being done to make them resilient to the available shocks. This has resulted in a vicious cycle where resources have to be mobilized every time the shocks occur; this leads to slow response, leading to community suffering before help is finally provided.
- Delayed monitoring of progress is a result of the implementation of some key interventions, such as mitigation measures against micronutrient deficiencies. The monitoring and evaluation process for most of the policies and strategies relies on funding from the implementing partners and donors. With little or no investments in the monitoring process from the government, measurement of progress is usually delayed if funding from the other stakeholders is delayed. This leads to a delayed response if measures have to be put in place to turn around the situation.

14.1.4.4 Multisectoral approach

- Although policies recognize the need for multisectoral involvement, practical coordination between different ministries and sectors remains a challenge. Having a joint reporting framework with clear indicators being jointly tracked by the different sectors remains a pipe dream. This has been facilitated by the siloed approach to government operations, which has little or no integration of services.
- Establishing high-level coordination structures like the National Food Security and Nutrition Steering Committee (NFSNSC) is a step in the right direction, but their effectiveness needs further evaluation.
- Joint planning for nutrition interventions is still an existing gap, with the different government sectors conducting parallel planning and implementation initiatives for nutrition interventions. Despite attempts to develop some of the policy documents jointly, their implementation is largely skewed to the mother sector, with little or no collaboration after the initial document development.

14.1.5 Future directions and recommendations

To enhance the impact of nutritional policies in Kenya, several key areas require attention:

1. Strengthening implementation at the county level: Provide more support and resources to counties for implementing nutrition action plans, considering local contexts and challenges. In addition to availing the resources, an accountability framework needs to be put in place to ensure that the resources are well utilized and the targets are being met.

2. Addressing urban malnutrition: Develop targeted strategies to address the growing urban food insecurity and malnutrition issue. These should be accompanied by a resilient strategy to cushion the urban settlements from food insecurity shocks.
3. Climate resilience: Integrate climate-resilient approaches into nutrition and agriculture policies to mitigate the impact of climate-related events on food security.
4. Enhanced monitoring and evaluation: Implement robust monitoring and evaluation systems to track the progress and impact of nutrition interventions more effectively.
5. Private sector engagement: Strengthen partnerships with the private sector to improve the availability and affordability of nutritious foods and services.
6. Nutrition education: Scale up nutrition education programs, including those targeting fathers and grandmothers, to improve dietary practices at the household level.
7. Resource mobilization: Advocate for increased domestic and international funding for nutrition programs to ensure sustainable implementation of policies.
8. Joint planning across the different government sectors and stakeholders to enhance joint implementation and monitoring of nutrition initiatives in the country.
9. Regular monitoring of the implementation status of all the nutrition interventions in place.

14.2 Conclusion

Kenya has made significant strides in developing comprehensive policies and strategies to address malnutrition, with the policies and strategies spanning various sectors because of the multisectoral approach to tackling malnutrition in the country. However, the persistent nutritional challenges in implementing these policies and strategies highlight the need for continued efforts and innovative approaches to sustaining the gains made in improving the nutritional status. By addressing implementation gaps, strengthening multisectoral coordination, and adapting to emerging challenges such as urban malnutrition and climate change, Kenya can make substantial progress toward achieving its nutritional goals and contributing to the broader global agenda of zero hunger and improved nutrition for all.

References

Black, R. E., Allen, L. H., Bhutta, Z. A., Caulfield, L. E., de Onis, M., Ezzati, M., Mathers, C., & Rivera, J. (2008). Maternal and child undernutrition: global and regional exposures and health consequences. *The Lancet, 371*(9608), 243–260. http://www.journals.elsevier.com/the-lancet/. doi:10.1016/S0140-6736(07)61690-0.

Constitution of Kenya. (2010). Laws of Kenya. National Council for Law Reporting, February. https://www.parliament.go.ke/sites/default/files/2017-05/The_Constitution_of_Kenya_2010.pdf.

Development Initiatives. (2022). *Global Nutrition Report 2022: Stronger commitments for greater action*. Development Initiatives.

Evang, E. C., Habte, T. Y., Owino, W. O., & Krawinkel, M. B. (2020). The nutritional and micronutrient status of urban schoolchildren with moderate anemia is better than in a rural area in Kenya. *Nutrients, 12*(1). doi:10.3390/nu12010207.

Kenya Health. (2024). Information System. https://hiskenya.dha.go.ke/.

Kenya Demographic Health Survey. (2022). https://www.knbs.or.ke/kenya-demographic-health-surveys/.

Kenya Demographic Health Survey. (2014). https://www.knbs.or.ke/kenya-demographic-health-surveys/.

GOK. (2011). *National Food and Nutrition Security Policy 2011. II.* https://repository.kippra.or.ke/items/9fc6f96f-43de-4b56-8667-0f072d81253b.

Government of Kenya. (2021). *National strategic plan for the prevention and control of non-communicable diseases 2021/22–2025/26.*

Keats, E. C., Neufeld, L. M., Garrett, G. S., Mbuya, M. N. N., & Bhutta, Z. A. (2019). Improved micronutrient status and health outcomes in low-and middle-income countries following large-scale fortification: Evidence from a systematic review and meta-Analysis. *American Journal of Clinical Nutrition, 109*(6), 1696–1708. doi:10.1093/ajcn/nqz023.

KNBS. (2011). *The Kenya National Micronutrient Survey.* 1–150. http://www.nutritionhealth.or.ke/wp-content/uploads/Downloads/TheKenyaNationalMicronutrientSurvey2011.pdf.

KNBS. (2019). 2019 KPHC—Analytical report on mortality, Vol. VII. KNBS.

Madewell, Z. J., Keita, A. M., Das, P. M. G., Mehta, A., Akelo, V., Oluoch, O. B., Omore, R., Onyango, D., Sagam, C. K., Cain, C. J., Chukwuegbo, C., Kaluma, E., Luke, R., Ogbuanu, I. U., Bassat, Q., Kincardett, M., Mandomando, I., Rakislova, N., Varo, E., … Kotloff, K. L. (2024). Contribution of malnutrition to infant and child deaths in Sub-Saharan Africa and South Asia. *BMJ Global Health, 9*(12). gh.bmj.com/. doi:10.1136/bmjgh-2024-017262.

Marigi, S. N. (2017). Climate change vulnerability and impacts analysis in Kenya. *American Journal of Climate Change, 06*(01), 52–74. doi:10.4236/ajcc.2017.61004.

Masibo, P. K., Humwa, F., & MacHaria, T. N. (2020). The double burden of overnutrition and undernutrition in mother-child dyads in Kenya: Demographic and health survey data, 2014. *Journal of Nutritional Science, 9.* doi:10.1017/jns.2019.39.

Ministry of Health, Republic of Kenya. (2018). *Kenya Nutrition Action Plan 2018–2022.* https://familyhealth.go.ke/wp-content/uploads/2020/10/Kenya-Nutrition-Action-Plan-2018-2022.pdf.

Ministry of Health. (2024). Kenya Health. Information System. https://hiskenya.dha.go.ke/.

MOH. (2018). *Kenya National Nutrition Action Plan 2018–2022.* https://arua-ncd.org/wp-content/uploads/2022/10/Kenya-Nutrition-Action-Plan-2018-2022-POPULAR-VERSION.pdf.

Rifkin, M. E. (2023). Nutrition policy critical to optimize response to climate, public health crises. *Frontiers in Nutrition, 10.* doi:10.3389/fnut.2023.1118753.

Sibanda, S., Munjoma-Muchinguri, P., Ohene-Agyei, P., & Murage, A. W. (2023). Policies for optimal nutrition-sensitive options: A study of food and nutrition security policies, strategies and programs in Ghana, Kenya and South Africa. *Frontiers in Sustainable Food Systems, 7.* doi:10.3389/fsufs.2023.1088216.

Wanjohi, M. N., Thow, A. M., Abdool Karim, S., Asiki, G., Erzse, A., Mohamed, S. F., Pierre Donfouet, H. P., Juma, P. A., & Hofman, K. J. (2021). Nutrition-related non-communicable disease and sugar-sweetened beverage policies: a landscape analysis in Kenya. *Global Health Action, 14*(1). doi:10.1080/16549716.2021.1902659.

UNICEF/WHO/World Bank Group. (2021). *Levels and trends in child malnutrition.* https://www.who.int/publications/b/78252.

The paradox of progress: Examining the gap between policy and implementation in Ethiopia's nutritional reforms

15

Abebe Haile[a], *Shruti Senapati*[b] *and Surekha Routray*[b]
[a]Center for Food Security Studies, CDS, Addis Ababa University, Addis Ababa, Ethiopia, [b]Research and Development, Aashdit Nutritech Pvt. Ltd., Bhubaneswar, Odisha, India

15.1 Introduction

Ethiopia stands at the intersection of Africa's evolving nutritional policies, exemplifying the persistent challenges and emerging paradoxes that define the continent's public health landscape. This complexity becomes particularly visible when examining the country's nutritional profile, where gains in policy implementation are offset by structural and behavioral shifts. Ethiopia continues to confront a complex nutritional paradox. Despite decades of health and food policy interventions the country remains entangled in a dual burden of malnutrition, wherein undernutrition among children under 5 persists, even as overweight and obesity gradually emerge, especially in urbanized areas. This dichotomy reflects both long-standing structural deficits and recent shifts in dietary behavior, urban development, and socioeconomic inequality.

As of 2023 Ethiopia's population stood at an estimated 128.7 million, ranking it the 11th most populous country globally (Worldometer, 2023). Of this total, approximately 78.3% (~100.7 million) lived in rural areas, whereas 21.7% (~28 million) resided in urban centers, illustrating a predominantly agrarian demographic. The median age was 18.7 years, with a fertility rate of 3.99 births per woman, reflecting a youthful population structure. The gender split remained nearly even, with 50.2% female (~64.6 million) and 49.8% male (~64.1 million). Roughly 40% (~51.5 million) of the population was under the age of 15, and about 14.7% (~18.9 million) were children under 5.

15.2 Malnutrition burden

Nationally representative datasets from the Ethiopia Mini Demographic and Health Survey (EMDHS) and aligned international sources consistently report high rates of chronic child undernutrition. Stunting prevalence of 35.7% an estimated 6.75 million under-5 children were chronically undernourished: a condition indicative of long-term nutritional deprivation (FAO, 2024; UNICEF, 2023). Although this represents a modest

Nutritional Strategies, Predictive Models, and Sustainable Policies. DOI: https://doi.org/10.1016/B978-0-443-23671-6.00014-1

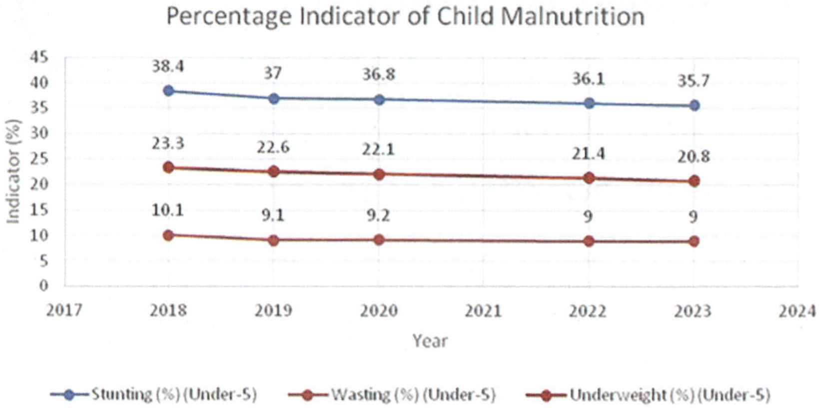

Figure 15.1 Trends in child malnutrition in Ethiopia (2018–2023) (FAO, 2024; UNICEF, 2023; WHO, 2023).

decline from 38.4% in 2018 (Fig. 15.1), the pace of reduction remains insufficient when compared to global targets under Sustainable Development Goal (SDG) 2.1. Regional disparities further exacerbate this burden; for instance the Afar region reports a wasting prevalence of 26%, whereas Addis Ababa reports only 4% (EPHI & ICF, 2019). Such variability reflects a broader spatial inequity in access to healthcare, dietary quality, and safe water. In addition, between 4.0 and 4.3 million women were estimated to be pregnant or breastfeeding—populations frequently underserved in nutrition planning and service delivery.

Acute undernutrition, measured by wasting, has shown minor fluctuations but remains persistent across drought-prone and food-insecure areas. The national wasting prevalence hovered around 9.0% between 2019 and 2023 (WHO, 2023; UNICEF, 2023). Underweight prevalence also saw a slight decline from 23.3% to 20.8%, underscoring incremental progress (Fig. 15.1).

Household-level data highlight strong correlations between food insecurity and child anthropometric failures. Studies from regions such as South Wollo and East Gojjam reveal that children from households with low dietary diversity or inconsistent meal patterns are significantly more likely to experience both stunting and wasting (Belayneh et al., 2021; Motbainor et al., 2015).

Furthermore, maternal nutritional status during pregnancy remains a strong predictor of child health outcomes. Poor maternal BMI, micronutrient deficiencies, and inadequate antenatal care are linked to low birth weight and impaired postnatal growth trajectories (Harper et al., 2023). The synergistic interaction between maternal undernutrition and child growth failure forms a vicious cycle that demands targeted, lifecycle-oriented interventions. Although child undernutrition remains the most visible face of Ethiopia's nutritional crisis, adult overnutrition is quietly on the rise. Increasing urbanization, income growth, and access to energy-dense foods have

Table 15.1 Comparative urban–rural adult obesity statistics (EDHS, 2016; WHO, 2023).

Location	Overweight (%)	Obese (%)
Addis Ababa	18.6	7.2
Other urban	13.2	4.9
Rural	5.8	1.1

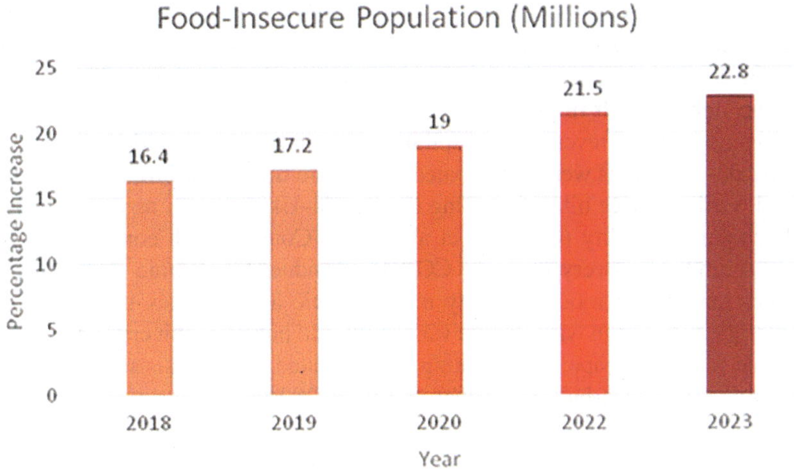

Figure 15.2 Food-insecure population in Ethiopia between 2018 and 2023.
Data from FAO (2024).

contributed to shifting dietary preferences, particularly among urban populations. In Addis Ababa, recent assessments estimate that 18.6% of adults are overweight, and 7.2% are obese, a contrast sharply with rural regions where overweight prevalence remains below 6% (Table 15.1) (Gezaw et al., 2023; WHO, 2023).

Food insecurity remains the critical underlying determinant that perpetuates malnutrition in both its forms. Between 2018 and 2023 the number of food-insecure individuals in Ethiopia escalated from 16.4 million to 22.8 million (Fig. 15.2) (FAO, 2024; World Bank, 2024). This sharp increase is attributable to a confluence of overlapping shocks, including the COVID-19 pandemic, the Tigray conflict, the Ukraine war, and recurrent droughts, which collectively destabilized livelihoods, markets, and national food systems. These events triggered inflation, disrupted agricultural value chains, and heightened fiscal imbalances.

The food security landscape further deteriorated in 2024. According to the USAID-supported Famine Early Warning Systems Network (FEWS NET), significant portions of northern and eastern Ethiopia were classified as IPC Phase 3 (Crisis) or Phase 4 (Emergency) between August and September 2024. The IPC framework categorizes food insecurity based on severity: households in Phase 3 face food consumption gaps or must deplete assets to meet minimum needs, whereas Phase 4 households experience large gaps, high acute malnutrition, or employ emergency survival strategies. Regions, such as Afar, Tigray, and Amhara, were among the hardest hit, with road blockades and administrative unrest compounding trade disruptions and market shortages. FEWS NET projected that these conditions would persist into early 2025, particularly in Afar. These developments underscore the geographic entrenchment of acute food insecurity, with profound implications for maternal and child nutrition (FEWS NET, 2024).

The **Tigray conflict alone displaced over 3 million people** and caused widespread infrastructure collapse across northern regions, leading to a reconstruction burden estimated at **$20 billion.** As humanitarian needs mounted, **15 million Ethiopians became reliant on food aid** by late 2023. The compounded crisis also contributed to Ethiopia's **sovereign debt default in late 2023**, a consequence of strained foreign reserves and declining government revenue amid spiraling humanitarian costs (Mathebula, 2025).

These developments were exacerbated by **double-digit inflation**, largely driven by fuel and fertilizer price hikes following the Russia–Ukraine war, as well as domestic macroeconomic fragility (Calderón et al., 2022). Coupled with continued displacement and limited recovery from the COVID-19-induced economic slowdown, these dynamics have made food insecurity more chronic and complex than ever before. The interaction between war, climate variability, and public health crises has reshaped Ethiopia's food landscape, necessitating an integrated, conflict-sensitive approach to recovery and resilience-building (Gejea & Tolesa, 2024).

Taken together the epidemiological profile of malnutrition in Ethiopia reveals a dynamic yet increasingly strained landscape. Although modest reductions in child stunting represent incremental gains, the persistence of acute undernutrition, the rise in adult overnutrition, and the deepening crisis of food insecurity exacerbated by conflict, economic instability, and climate shocks underscore the complexity of the current nutrition environment. Addressing this multifaceted burden demands more than targeted undernutrition strategies; it necessitates an integrated, equity-focused, and crisis-responsive policy approach. Future policy responses must be informed by disaggregated, real-time data and must address malnutrition in all its manifestations across age groups, geographies, and socioeconomic strata.

15.3 Drivers of the nutrition transition

In recent years, Ethiopia has witnessed a profound transformation in its food systems, lifestyles, and demographic structure, catalyzing what researchers and policy experts term the "nutrition transition." Although once predominantly characterized by food scarcity and undernutrition, the country is now grappling with a complex nutritional landscape that includes rising rates of overweight and obesity, particularly in urban settings.

Historically, rural diets in Ethiopia were dominated by *injera* (a fermented flatbread made from teff or sorghum), complemented by seasonal legumes (e.g., lentils and chickpeas), boiled greens, and occasional dairy. Urban diets, though modest, often included more diverse offerings such as spiced stews (*wot*), pasta, bread, eggs, and coffee-based beverages, reflecting urban trade exposure and cultural diversity (Mesfin et al., 2024). However, over the past decade, this traditional balance has been disrupted by overlapping crises, notably the Tigray war (2020–22), Oromia insurgencies (post-2018), and Amhara regional unrest (2022–23), alongside ongoing pastoralist conflicts in the Somali and Afar regions (Moyo & Blake, 2024; Muhyie et al., 2025).

As a consequence, food consumption patterns have shifted dramatically. In rural areas, instability has forced households to rely on emergency relief staples—mainly wheat flour, maize, and fortified blended flours—that offer limited micronutrient value. Meanwhile, urban populations have increasingly turned to low-cost, ultraprocessed foods, including packaged noodles, biscuits, fried snacks, and sugar-sweetened beverages (SSBs), driven by rising inflation and a shrinking middle class (Abay et al., 2022). Ethiopia's urban population exceeded 23 million in 2023 and continues to expand at an estimated annual rate of 4.3% (Desalegn et al., 2025). This demographic growth has fundamentally altered the urban food environment, shifting emphasis from quality to affordability and convenience. These developments have collectively reduced dietary diversity and protein intake while simultaneously increasing the prevalence of micronutrient deficiencies and obesity—particularly among women and adolescent girls.

The resulting decline in food quality and diversity has accelerated the nutrition transition across both rural and urban populations, deepening the national public health burden. Vulnerability to both under- and overnutrition now coexists within and across income groups, shaped by conflict exposure, fragmented markets, and growing dependence on food aid (Abay et al., 2023; Degfachew et al., 2025). This pattern is particularly evident in urban centers such as Addis Ababa, Bahir Dar, and Hawassa, where more than 30% of adults are now classified as overweight or obese (Glatzel et al., 2024).

The consequences of this dietary transformation became especially visible during the 2023 food crisis, one of the most severe in recent history. Over 22 million individuals faced acute food insecurity, including more than 4 million malnourished children and 1 million pregnant and breastfeeding women with acute malnutrition. This crisis was triggered by the worst drought in four decades, compounded by ongoing regional conflicts and escalating climate shocks that devastated agricultural output and strained already fragile food systems (Shekar & Okamura, 2024). The combined pressures widened nutritional inequities and hastened the nutrition transition, as both rural and urban households shifted further toward emergency-based, less diverse diets [urban and rural populations toward emergency-based and less diverse diets (Korir et al., 2024)].

Rural populations continue to bear the brunt of nutritional disadvantage. Stunting among children under 5 remains alarmingly high in regions such as Amhara, Afar, and Tigray—frequently exceeding 35%—compared to less than 15% in Addis Ababa and other urban zones (Haile & Legisso, 2024). A national analysis revealed that only 26.6% of rural children aged 6–23 months received a minimum acceptable diet (MAD), whereas that rate more than doubled to 52.7% among urban children (Mohammed et al., 2024). Although the government has made targeted commitments to reducing undernutrition through national policy frameworks and multisectoral coordination, it has struggled to adequately integrate strategies addressing rising urban obesity and noncommunicable diseases (NCDs). The 2024 National Food and Nutrition Strategy recognizes this evolving reality but underscores the importance of spatially differentiated policies that reflect Ethiopia's sociodemographic diversity (Desalegn et al., 2025). The nutrition transition in Ethiopia is neither linear nor homogeneous. It manifests across a stratified social landscape—urban centers contending with dietary excess and chronic disease risks, whereas rural areas remain locked in cycles of food insecurity and micronutrient deficiency. Effectively confronting this dual trajectory demands context-sensitive, data-driven policies that reimagine the national food system to foster health equity, nutritional resilience, and sustainability.

15.4 Evolution of Ethiopia's nutrition policy framework

15.4.1 From emergency relief to multisectoral strategies

Ethiopia's national approach to nutrition has evolved through a paradigm shift—from a reactive, emergency-oriented system to a proactive, multisectoral policy framework. This transition has been guided by changes in political will, donor alignment, and the increasing recognition of nutrition as a driver of human capital development.

In the 1980s and 1990s nutritional strategy was predominantly characterized by humanitarian interventions. Nutritional responses were driven by acute events such as droughts and displacement, with food aid serving as the primary mechanism of support. Institutions such as the Relief and Rehabilitation Commission (RRC) and the Emergency Nutrition Coordination Unit operated largely in isolation from the broader health and development infrastructure (FAO, 2005; UNICEF, 2019). During this era, nutrition was treated narrowly, primarily as a function of food availability rather than health, social protection, or structural poverty.

By the early 2000s this fragmented model came under increasing scrutiny as global research demonstrated the profound developmental consequences of early-life malnutrition. This intellectual shift catalyzed a transition in national thinking, from ad hoc nutritional responses to long-term, programmatic strategies. Nutrition began to be reframed within Ethiopia's Poverty Reduction Strategy Papers (PRSPs) and the Health Sector Development Program (HSDP), laying the groundwork for more integrated policy initiatives (World Bank, 2006).

Ethiopia's nutrition policy shifted from emergency relief to a coordinated, preventive, and lifecycle-based strategy. The National Nutrition Programme I (NNP I, 2008) introduced a multiagency framework for maternal, infant, and young child nutrition (MIYCN), emphasizing prevention and health system integration. NNP II (2016–20) expanded this with explicit performance targets for vulnerable groups (adolescents and pregnant women), formal governance structures such as the National Nutrition Coordination Body (NNCB), and cross-ministerial accountability beyond health to sectors such as education, agriculture, and water.

Aligned with global priorities, NNP II integrated guidelines from the Scaling Up Nutrition (SUN) Movement, the Global Nutrition Report, and SDG 2: Zero Hunger. Despite policy advances, challenges persisted: fragmented budgets, weak

Table 15.2 NNP II (2016–20) targets and performance indicators.

Indicator	Baseline (2016)	Target (2020)	Actual (2020)
Adolescent anemia prevalence (%)	30.0	15.0	~24.3
Pregnant women receiving ≥90 days of iron supplements (%)	7.0	50.0	11.0
Exclusive breastfeeding (0–6 months) (%)	58.0	70.0	60.3
Minimum dietary diversity (6–23 months) (%)	14.0	50.0	24.5

Ethiopia PSNP maternal health policy Korir et al. (2024); Ethiopia nutrition programming Ayele et al. (2022).
NNP, National Nutrition Programme.

monitoring, regional disparities, and uneven local ownership hindered implementation (Woldehanna et al., 2017; UNICEF, 2022).

Overall the evolution reflects Ethiopia's progression toward a resilience- and equity-focused system but highlights ongoing needs for stronger governance, localized accountability, and sustainable financing to translate strategic vision into effective ground-level results.

15.4.2 Key milestones: NNP II and NFNP 2018

The evolution of Ethiopia's nutrition governance can be traced through two landmark policy frameworks: the **NNP II (2016–20)** and the **National Food and Nutrition Policy (NFNP, 2018)**. These instruments not only introduced targeted interventions but also institutionalized cross-sectoral coordination and accountability mechanisms essential to addressing malnutrition in all its forms.

The launch of **NNP II** marked a transition from earlier fragmented efforts to a **cohesive, lifecycle-based model** that addressed nutritional needs from adolescence through adulthood. One of the most prominent objectives was the **reduction of adolescent anemia prevalence from 30% to 15%** by 2020, a target motivated by the high burden of micronutrient deficiency among adolescent girls (Federal Democratic Republic of Ethiopia FDRE, 2016).

The program also aimed to scale up coverage of maternal micronutrient interventions. However, **only 11% of pregnant women nationally received iron supplementation for the recommended 90 or more days** by the end of the program period (WHO, 2020), and breastfeeding improved modestly to 60.3%, still short of the 70% target. The dietary diversity among children aged 6–23 months improved to 24.5% (the target was 50%), reflecting ongoing challenges in access to diverse foods and caregiver education (WHO, 2020; UNICEF, 2022) (see Table 15.2).

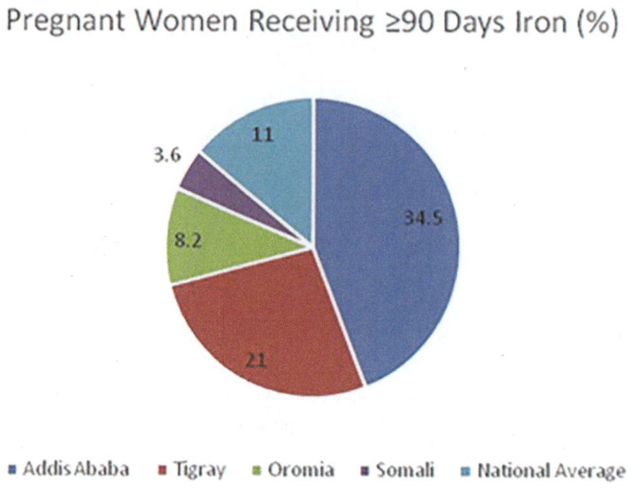

Figure 15.3 Regional disparities in maternal iron supplementation coverage in Ethiopia. Data from Federal Ministry of Health (2016), WHO (2020), UNICEF (2022).

Regional disparities were stark. For example, whereas **34.5%** of pregnant women in Addis Ababa received adequate supplementation, coverage was just **3.6%** in the Somali Region (see Fig. 15.3).

From an implementation standpoint, NNP II was operationalized through a multitiered coordination mechanism—anchored in the Ministry of Health, with delivery responsibilities delegated to regional health bureaus and woreda-level nutrition officers. The policy outlined service delivery platforms targeting underserved groups such as pregnant and breastfeeding women and children under 5, primarily through community health extension programs, maternal-child health (MCH) clinics, and school-based platforms for adolescent girls. Despite these structures, implementation varied significantly by region, and woreda-level bottlenecks—including weak logistics, low health workforce density, and limited outreach coverage—undermined impact. The recommended dietary interventions under NNP II were designed to combat widespread micronutrient deficiencies. These included the following:

- Iron-folic acid tablets to reduce anemia in adolescent girls and pregnant women.
- Lipid-based nutrient supplements (LNS) and fortified blended foods (like corn-soy blend) for children aged 6–23 months to address vitamin A, zinc, and protein-energy deficiencies.
- Promotion of nutrient-rich foods, such as eggs, dark green leafy vegetables, pulses (lentils and chickpeas), and orange-fleshed sweet potatoes, as part of household dietary diversification efforts.
- Therapeutic feeding (e.g., plumpy nut) for treatment of severe acute malnutrition (FA; UNIANDES, et al., 2021, WHO, 2020).

Table 15.3 NFNP 2018—Strategic policy directions.

Policy direction	Description
1. Diversified food consumption	Promote access to nutrient-dense, locally available foods
2. Food safety and quality	Implement standards, inspections, and labeling
3. Nutrition-sensitive social protection	Expand integrated food and cash support
4. Governance and coordination	Strengthen multisectoral nutrition bodies
5. Capacity building and institutional strengthening	Enhance training and management systems
6. Sustainable food systems	Promote climate-resilient, inclusive agriculture
7. Monitoring and evaluation systems	Institutionalize real-time data systems and reporting tools

Data from EPHI (2018); UNIANDES et al. (2021).
NFNP, National Food and Nutrition Policy.

Importantly, NNP II was introduced during a period of relative political fragility. Although Ethiopia was not in open war in 2016, the post-2015 political tensions and nationwide protests, particularly in Oromia and Amhara regions, created administrative and security challenges that hindered program rollouts in peripheral zones. These tensions culminated in the 2018 change of leadership, which created momentum for broader reforms—including the launch of the NFNP (Moyo & Blake, 2024).

The **NFNP** was launched in 2018 with the broader vision of achieving "**optimal nutritional status for all Ethiopians**" (FDRE, 2016). Unlike NNP II, which operated primarily through health system channels, the NFNP sought to transform the national food system by embedding nutrition within Ethiopia's economic development agenda.

NFNP is structured around **seven strategic policy directions** (see Table 15.3), with emphasis on building a resilient and inclusive food system. It broadened focus from acute undernutrition to include chronic hunger, micronutrient malnutrition, and emerging issues such as urban overweight and NCDs. A key implementation strategy involved expanding food-based approaches through agriculture, school feeding, and social protection schemes (EPHI, 2018; UNIANDES et al., 2021).

In terms of food-based deliverables, NFNP emphasized scaling up access to

- Biofortified staples (e.g., iron-rich teff and zinc-enriched maize) to address mineral deficiencies.
- School meals with legumes, oilseeds, fruits, and milk, aimed at improving child cognitive development and reducing hidden hunger.
- Homestead production of nutrient-dense foods (e.g., poultry, leafy greens, and orange fruits) through agri-nutrition programs.
- Food safety protocols, including market inspections and food labeling, to reduce consumption of unsafe street foods and adulterated products (Kennedy et al., 2023).

For implementation, NFNP established cross-sectral coordinating units, housed within the Ministry of Agriculture and the Prime Minister's Office, to integrate activities at federal and regional levels. It also included nutrition-sensitive budgeting frameworks, though resource limitations and security-related interruptions, particularly following the Tigray conflict in late 2020, have significantly slowed progress (Ayele et al., 2023).

Together, NNP II and NFNP 2018 illustrate Ethiopia's progression toward institutionalizing nutrition as a national development priority. Although NNP II created a vertical operational model through health platforms, NFNP redefined the paradigm to include food system transformation, social safety nets, and regulatory oversight.

15.5 Policy framing and sectoral integration

15.5.1 Framing of malnutrition in policy documents

Current nutrition policy frameworks heavily emphasize undernutrition, often at the expense of addressing the rising threat of **overnutrition and diet-related NCDs**. This disparity is evident in both programmatic content and the design of institutional response mechanisms.

The **NNP II (2016–20)** allocates more than **80% of its interventions to maternal and child undernutrition,** focusing on priorities such as stunting reduction, exclusive breastfeeding promotion, and micronutrient supplementation (FDRE, 2016). Meanwhile, overweight and obesity receive no quantified targets, cost estimates, or dedicated monitoring indicators. The NFNP (2018) outlined 56 objectives, but only two address diet-related chronic diseases, framed broadly under lifestyle goals (FDRE, 2016). National data show a growing NCD burden: urban female overweight reached 25.3% (2019) and hypertension 19.6% among adults aged 15–49 [EPHI & DHS Progra (UNIANDES et al., 2021)]. Longitudinal data confirm overweight among urban women nearly doubled from 11.2% (2000) to 24.8% (2016), whereas rural underweight stagnated, revealing a persistent dual burden of malnutrition (Tareke et al., 2024).

Surveillance systems remain child-focused. The HMIS monitors stunting, underweight, and vitamin A, but not adult BMI, waist measures, or NCD biomarkers. The last comprehensive chronic disease risk factor survey was the 2015 WHO STEPS report, with no updates since (WHO, 2016). Despite evidence of overnutrition, less than 3% of projected nutrition spending (2016–20) was allocated to related interventions, such as physical activity promotion or healthy food environments (UNICEF, 2022).

This framing gap is consistent with broader regional findings. A review across African nutrition plans identified a persistent trend: Although undernutrition is routinely articulated as a developmental emergency, NCDs are either absent or treated as secondary, future threats. In these contexts, donor influence, food aid history, and epidemiological inertia shape how malnutrition is defined and tackled (Weimann et al., 2021).

Policy scholars now call for a **"triple-duty" approach**—addressing undernutrition, micronutrient deficiencies, and overnutrition concurrently. For instance, interventions

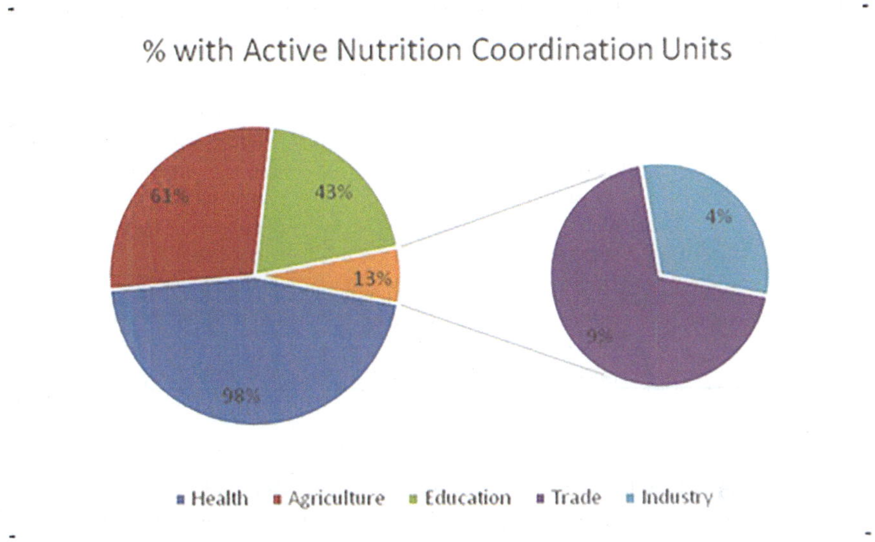

Figure 15.4 Data from Nutrition coordination metrics by sector (2022) (Haile & Singh, 2024). National Implementation Survey; Brhanu and Ayele (2023).

such as school feeding and maternal education could be reframed not only for child growth but also to **prevent adolescent obesity and intergenerational diet-related disease** (Jeyakumar et al., 2025).

15.5.2 Multisectoral coordination challenges

Despite clear commitments to collaborative governance in the national nutrition policy framework the actual integration of ministries into multisectoral nutrition programming is uneven and structurally imbalanced. These gaps are visible both in the design of institutional responsibilities and the functionality of coordination platforms.

The health sector remains the most institutionally embedded actor, managing nearly all nutrition-specific interventions and leading the majority of national coordination platforms. As of 2023, approximately **98% of regional and zonal health offices maintained active nutrition coordination units**, with health-based facilities collecting **monthly reports across 96% of woredas** (Brhanu & Ayele, 2023). The agriculture sector contributes mainly through food production and resilience programs, yet its engagement in coordinated planning is inconsistent. According to recent program reviews, **only 65% of agriculture offices implement nutrition-sensitive interventions,** and fewer than 40% include measurable nutrition indicators in their routine planning documents (Asirvatham et al., 2022). In practice, just **61% of regional agriculture bureaus operate active coordination mechanisms** with the health sector (see Fig. 15.4).

The education sector shows partial integration, with its largest contributions occurring through school feeding, water, sanitation, and hygiene (WASH) programs. Yet

Table 15.4 Sectoral integration of nutrition functions (2023) (Asirvatham et al., 2022; **Brhanu & Ayele, 2023;**Trübswasser et al., 2022).

Sector	Key contributions	Limiting factors
Health	Service delivery, budgeting, surveillance	Overconcentration, limited cross-sector synergy
Agriculture	Food systems, resilience programming	Lack of nutrition indicators in extension plans
Education	School meals, hygiene, limited curriculum	No standard nutrition curricula
Trade	Regulatory potential, import policy	Not included in coordination mandates
Industry	Food manufacturing and distribution	No reformulation policies or advertising rules

only **28% of schools deliver structured nutrition education** and locally adapted curriculum content. Only **43% of education bureaus participate in nutrition councils or interministerial platforms**, leaving gaps in adolescent-focused health promotion strategies (Trübswasser et al., 2022).

The national coordination survey found **less than 9% of trade offices and 4% of industry departments** participate in any form of nutrition-related planning (see Fig. 15.4). The absence of economic governance from nutrition policy has delayed meaningful progress in shaping consumer behavior and food system accountability (Desalegn et al., 2025).

These differences are summarized in Table 15.4, which captures both sectoral integration levels and key bottlenecks in the national implementation landscape.

The limited functionality of coordination bodies at subnational levels amplifies these sectoral disparities. A national implementation audit across 320 woredas revealed that **only 32% had active multisectoral nutrition task forces**, and **61% reported no joint planning activities within the last 12 months** (Haile & Singh, 2024). Fig. 15.4 illustrates these discrepancies in the prevalence of functional nutrition coordination across administrative levels.

Further hindering integration, data collection systems are highly fragmented. Only the health information system is robust, collecting monthly indicators on growth monitoring, anemia screening, and supplementation. The absence of cross-sector analytics precludes real-time evaluation and reinforces siloed policymaking (Tekle et al., 2023).

External donor programs contribute to coordination challenges. An estimated 46% of major nutrition initiatives in 2020–23 were implemented through vertical channels managed by nongovernmental partners. These often bypass government accountability systems and create parallel structures. For example, multiple overlapping feeding programs in northern districts failed to synchronize with regional health bureaus or agricultural platforms (Bach et al., 2020). Bridging these gaps requires structural and institutional reform. This includes establishing shared budgeting frameworks, integrating nutrition indicators into all sectoral plans, and developing interoperable monitoring systems.

Table 15.5 Target specificity—Undernutrition vs. overnutrition.

Metric	Policy target	2023 Value	Urban-specific action
Stunting (under 5)	37% → 26% by 2020	35.7%	Indirect
Adolescent anemia	30% → 15%	~22%–25%	Girls prioritized
Urban female overweight	Not defined	12.1% national; 25.3% in capital	None
Adolescent overweight (urban)	Not defined	~17%	Absent

Self complied.

15.6 Goal setting and equity considerations

15.6.1 Undernutrition vs. overnutrition targets

National nutrition strategies have historically prioritised the reduction of stunting as a core objective. A prominent benchmark aimed to lower the prevalence among children under 5 years from 37% to 26 %by 2020, supported by measurable indicators and structured tracking systems. As of 2023 the figure stands at 35.7%, reflecting limiting improvement despite substantial programming effors (Glatzel et al., 2024). Similarly the anemia reduction goal for adolescent girls from 30% to 15%has been supported through school based iron and folate supplementation and adolescent focused health services (Ali et al., 2024). These goals are embedded in policy frameworks and recieve regular performance assessments (see Table 15.5).

In contrast, strategies addressing overnutrition lack comparable precision. Although policy documents acknowledge the rise of diet-related NCDs, they do not specify targets, timelines, or geographic breakdowns to curb overweight and obesity. No structured objectives exist for BMI reduction, urban food regulation, or adolescent weight management—despite mounting evidence of their significance. For instance, 12.1% of urban women are overweight, with rates climbing to 25.3% in the capital, and adolescent overweight in urban schools nearing 17% (Abera et al., 2023; Haidar, 2024). Despite such data, existing policy instruments still portray overnutrition as a developing concern rather than an active policy priority (see Table 15.5).

Moreover, the food environments driving these trends—marked by increased access to calorie-dense, nutrient-poor foods—are insufficiently addressed. In urban areas, these environments remain unregulated, with little institutional oversight or cross-sector intervention despite their direct impact on dietary behaviors and health risks (Berhane et al., 2023).

This contrast in policy clarity reflects a broader strategic gap. Although efforts to combat undernutrition are guided by specific, time-bound benchmarks, the growing reality of overnutrition, especially in cities remains overlooked. The result is uneven resource allocation, limited surveillance, and weak institutional engagement across sectors.

A recent policy analysis underscores that urban dietary transitions and adolescent nutrition receive insufficient attention, leaving sectors such as education, trade, and municipal governance without mandates to engage in interventions such as restricting unhealthy food marketing or scaling up school-based activity programs (Desalegn et al., 2025).

To close this gap, future strategies must define SMART (specific, measurable, achievable, relevant, and time-bound) goals tailored to urban and adolescent overweight prevention. This includes BMI monitoring in school health systems, nutrition-sensitive urban planning, and cross-sectoral accountability mechanisms that reflect the full spectrum of malnutrition.

15.6.2 Gender and regional equity

Equity is a recurrent theme in national nutrition discourse, yet its translation into programming remains uneven—particularly along gender and geographic lines. Although adolescent girls have received targeted attention through school-based iron and folate supplementation and anemia prevention initiatives, deeper gendered determinants of nutritional vulnerability remain underexplored. The commitment to reducing anemia prevalence from 30% to 15% (see Table 15.5) among girls has led to some improvement, with recent estimates placing current levels at 22%–25% in intervention areas (Ali et al., 2024). However, this focus on adolescence is not matched by equivalent efforts addressing adult women's agency, economic access, or household influence.

Women's participation in household health and nutrition decisions is notably limited. According to Demographic and Health Survey (DHS) findings, only 35% of women independently determine their healthcare choices, and a mere 31% have input on food purchases or preparation. These deficits closely linked to maternal and child undernutrition are largely absent from national policy indicators or accountability frameworks (EDHS, 2019). Compounding these gender-based gaps are entrenched geographic disparities. In 2024 the Ministry of Health identified 219 "Priority 1" districts (woredas) marked by persistent malnutrition, limited infrastructure, and high food insecurity. These administrative units, predominantly located in Afar, Somali, Benishangul-Gumuz, and lowland parts of Oromia and Amhara, continue to face systemic exclusion from equitable service provision. In some of these zones, stunting exceeds 45%, whereas wasting levels remain above emergency thresholds. Expenditure data further reinforce these imbalances. A study found that per capita health financing in remote regions is up to 40% lower than in more centralized areas, impeding coverage of essential nutrition services. In addition, safety net schemes such as the Productive Safety Net Programme (PSNP) often fall short in addressing seasonal shocks or reaching nomadic populations in drought-prone zones (Yallew et al., 2022).

Despite a policy narrative that emphasizes inclusivity and cross-sectoral alignment, practical mechanisms for advancing equity remain limited. Monitoring systems typically report aggregate nutrition outcomes, masking disparities faced by specific subgroups. Gender-responsive nutrition programming must expand beyond adolescent health to encompass women's empowerment across the life course—including decision-making authority, income generation, and access to nutrition-sensitive agriculture. Likewise, regionally adaptive approaches must be prioritized through decentralized planning, local governance capacity-building, and performance-based equity metrics. Without such reforms, structural disparities in nutrition will persist—undermining the goal of inclusive, transformative development.

15.7 Policy instruments and implementation (this portion should be minimized)

15.7.1 *Dominance of educational tools*

Nutrition education has become the most widely applied instrument in Ethiopia's national nutrition policy portfolio. A policy content analysis reveals that nearly **71% of all strategic documents** rely primarily on behavior change and awareness tools to drive dietary improvements, with emphasis on breastfeeding promotion, infant and young child feeding (IYCF) counseling, and school-based learning platforms (Workicho et al., 2021). Community-level counseling remains a cornerstone of the approach. **Health extension workers (HEWs)** have been key agents of interpersonal communication across rural kebeles, delivering targeted messages on complementary feeding and exclusive breastfeeding. Despite broad outreach, the **coverage of IYCF counseling remains inconsistent**, with estimates ranging from **62% to 68% among mothers of children under 2**, often lower in more remote and underserved areas, i.e., 45% (Abiyu & Belachew 2020; Ahmed et al., 2021).

The reliance on education, whereas foundational, comes with critical shortcomings. Research shows that awareness does not always translate into behavior change. For example, although **breastfeeding initiation awareness is high**, exclusive breastfeeding rates remain suboptimal due in part to structural barriers such as maternal workload and weak postnatal support systems (Abdulahi et al. 2021; UNIANDES et al., 2021). Moreover, most messaging is targeted toward mothers, overlooking male caregivers and extended family members who often influence food-related decisions.

Urban–rural disparities further complicate reach. Many messages also lack cultural tailoring, reducing relevance among agro-pastoral or low-literacy populations. Although nutrition education remains a central pillar, its overemphasis can displace more systemic approaches—such as fiscal incentives, food labeling, or marketing restrictions—that address environmental drivers of malnutrition. Strengthening education must, therefore, occur alongside a more balanced toolkit of regulatory and structural measures.

15.7.2 *Regulatory and financial mechanisms*

Although Ethiopia's nutrition policy architecture includes some regulatory and economic instruments, their implementation remains uneven and often symbolic. However, critical policy levers—such as processed food regulation, mandatory labeling, and fiscal deterrents—remain underdeveloped.

Ethiopia has no enforceable regulation for **front-of-pack nutritional labeling**, and **no national restrictions exist on junk food advertising** targeting children and adolescents. This gap in regulatory action persists despite rising urban overnutrition and increasing consumption of processed foods. Without clear mandates on labeling

Table 15.6 Implementation status of nutrition-linked regulatory and economic tools (2024).

Instrument	Policy status	Implementation/compliance
Maternity protection for breastfeeding	Legal mandate (120 days paid leave)	~80% public sector, private unclear
Breast milk substitute marketing code	Adopted, weak oversight	Low enforcement
Food labeling (front-of-pack)	Not legislated	Absent
Junk food and SSB advertising controls	No national standards	Absent
Sugar-sweetened beverage tax	Discussed at MoF level	No implementation
PSNP IV (nutrition-integrated)	Active; ~8M recipients	~42% reach nutrition-specific add-ons
National nutrition budget share	<1% of health expenditure	Below global minimum

PSNP, Productive Safety Net Programme.

and marketing, consumer protection and dietary quality remain ungoverned in informal and commercial food environments (Ayele et al., 2022).

The **PSNP IV** is Ethiopia's flagship social protection intervention with nutrition-sensitive features. It currently covers approximately **8 million beneficiaries** through a combination of public works and direct support (see Table 15.6). Recent program design improvements included integration of maternal health checkups, nutrition behavior messaging, and local food procurement. However, inconsistencies in implementation across regions undermine its nutritional impact. Evaluations found that only **42% of PSNP recipients received any nutrition-linked service in 2023**, and most woreda offices lacked trained staff to deliver behavior change components (Korir et al., 2024).

Economic tools aimed at discouraging unhealthy food consumption—such as SSB taxation—have gained policy attention but remain theoretical. As of 2024 no legislation on sugar, salt, or *trans*-fat taxation has been enacted, nor has Ethiopia piloted a subnational version of these tools. This contrasts with peer countries in the region such as Kenya and Rwanda, where targeted fiscal reforms have already generated public health dividends.

Public investment in nutrition-specific programming remains minimal. **Less than 1% of the national health budget is allocated to nutrition**, significantly below the 3%–5% recommended by international benchmarks (see Table 15.2). This funding limitation constrains the expansion of legal enforcement structures and weakens the scale-up of preventive and community-based interventions (Ayele et al., 2022).

The policy landscape shows a heavy tilt toward voluntary and informational approaches, with modest uptake of regulatory or economic interventions that alter the food system's structure. Meaningful nutrition gains will require robust investment in policy enforcement, interagency coordination, and fiscal innovation to correct underlying consumption drivers and regional inequities.

Table 15.7 Status of organizational coordination mechanisms (2023–24).

Indicator	Value
Year of NFNGB establishment	2021
Ministries represented	9+ core ministries
Functional regional coordination bodies	4 out of 11
Dedicated NFNGB budget line	Absent
Percentage of planned activities funded (2022)	38%–40%
Frequency of multisectoral review meetings	Infrequent

NFNGB, National Food and Nutrition Governing Body. Data From UNIANDES et al. (2021)

15.7.3 Organizational reforms

Ethiopia established the **National Food and Nutrition Governing Body (NFNGB)** under the Prime Minister's Office to improve nutrition (UNIANDES et al., 2021). The NFNGB coordinates efforts across nine different ministries, including health, agriculture, and finance, to align them with the **NFNP**. Its main goals are to harmonize policies and manage national targets, specifically to reduce stunting and improve maternal nutrition. Regional bodies were also proposed to adapt these policies to local needs. The NFNGB faces significant challenges in its oversight role. As of 2023, only 4 of 11 regions had functioning nutrition coordinating committees (Table 15.7). The body suffers from inconsistent funding, with less than 40% of its activities fully funded in 2022. It also lacks a dedicated budget, relying instead on the Ministry of Health's funds or donor support. Other issues include overlapping responsibilities with older structures, limited enforcement power, and a lack of standardized metrics for joint reviews. These problems have been exacerbated by a high turnover in technical leadership and a lack of interagency agreements, hindering the integration of accountability frameworks. Although no public documentation discloses a specific budget for the NFNGB alone, Ethiopia's Food and Nutrition Strategy [FN (UNIANDES et al., 2021)] provides the clearest costing framework to date. A 2024 financial analysis estimates that full national implementation will require $2.55 billion over 10 years, or approximately $250 million per year. Of this total: $1.84 billion (72%) is earmarked for nutrition-sensitive interventions (e.g., water and sanitation, social protection, and school feeding); $704 million (28%) is planned for nutrition-specific interventions (e.g., micronutrient supplementation and treatment of severe acute malnutrition) (See Fig. 15.5) (Tadesse et al., 2024).

Source: Multisectoral Integration of Nutrition, Health, and Agriculture: Implementation Lessons From Ethiopia (Bach et al., 2020).

A major concern is the **disconnect between central coordination and local execution**. Regional health bureaus often operate independently of sectoral leads, and woreda-level nutrition task forces—despite being envisioned in NFNP—remain

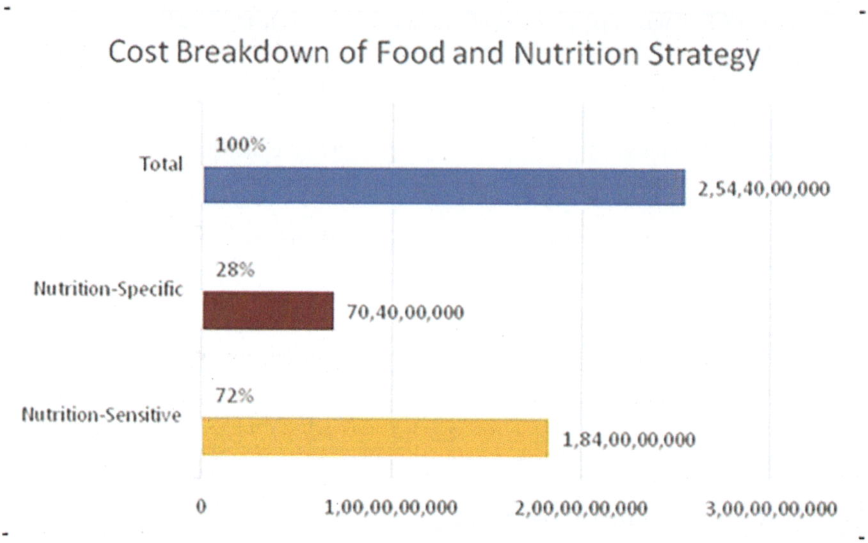

Figure 15.5 Estimated cost breakdown of Ethiopia's Food and Nutrition Strategy (2021–30). Data from Maru et al. (2024).

largely dormant. Decentralization lacks financial and technical scaffolding, leading to **variability in implementation quality between regions** (Kennedy et al., 2023).

To realize the ambitions of the NFNGB, several reforms are imperative. First, legal institutionalization through a standalone proclamation can formalize its authority across ministries. Second a dedicated and protected budget line must be embedded in the national planning framework to reduce dependency on donor cycles. Third, regional platforms need operational autonomy backed by trained focal persons, performance dashboards, and integration into regional development plans. Without these adjustments the NFNGB risks remaining nominal, unable to coordinate or enforce national nutrition priorities meaningfully.

15.8 Addressing the full spectrum of malnutrition

15.8.1 The rise of overnutrition and diet-related NCDs

Although undernutrition persists, Ethiopia is experiencing a nutrition transition, particularly in urban areas. The prevalence of overweight and obesity is rising, especially among women and school-aged children. In 2016 8% of women aged 15–49 were overweight or obese, up from 3% in 2000 (CSA & ICF, 2016). Urban areas show much higher rates: in Addis Ababa, 21% of women were overweight or obese (CSA and ICF, 2016).

Diet-related NCDs are also increasing (UNIANDES et al., 2021). A study found that the prevalence of hypertension among adults in Addis Ababa was 30%, with obesity as a key risk factor (Gebremariam et al. 2021; UNIANDES et al., 2021). The global burden of disease (IHME, 2022) study estimated that diet-related NCDs accounted for 22% of all deaths in Ethiopia.

The coexistence of under- and overnutrition, sometimes within the same household, constitutes the "double burden of malnutrition" (DBM). A 2023 cluster-randomized trial in Central Ethiopia found that 11% of households had at least one undernourished and one overweight member (Tadesse et al., 2023). This pattern is increasingly observed in urban and peri-urban settings, reflecting rapid changes in food systems and lifestyles. Recognition of the rising burden of overnutrition and NCDs is growing, but policy responses remain limited. The NFNP (2018) and the National Food and Nutrition Strategy [NFN (UNIANDES et al., 2021)] acknowledge the need to address overweight, obesity, and diet-related NCDs, but concrete targets, indicators, and interventions are still under development (MoH, 2018; UNIANDES et al., 2021).

15.8.2 Balancing under- and overnutrition: The need for integrated strategies

Current policies risk treating under- and overnutrition as separate issues, leading to fragmented interventions and missed opportunities for synergy. For example, school feeding programs may focus solely on caloric adequacy without addressing the quality of food or the risk of overweight. Similarly, agricultural policies may promote staple crop production for food security, inadvertently encouraging diets high in refined carbohydrates and low in diversity (UNIANDES et al., 2021).

Double-duty actions (DDAs) are interventions that address both under- and overnutrition simultaneously. Evidence from Ethiopia and other countries suggests that DDAs are cost-effective and efficient (WHO, 2017). Examples include the following:

- Improved complementary feeding: Promoting diverse, nutrient-rich foods for infants and young children can prevent both stunting and excessive weight gain (Dewey & Begum, 2011).
- Food system interventions: Policies that increase the availability and affordability of fruits, vegetables, and animal-source foods, whereas discouraging ultraprocessed foods can address multiple forms of malnutrition (Uccello et al., 2017; UNIANDES et al., 2021).

15.8.2.1 Evidence from Ethiopia

A 2023 cluster-randomized trial in Central Ethiopia implemented a package of DDAs, including nutrition education, physical activity promotion, and regulation of unhealthy foods in schools. The intervention reduced the prevalence of underweight by 6% and overweight/obesity by 4% over 12 months (Tadesse et al., 2023).

15.9 Policy coherence and multisectoral coordination

15.9.1 Institutional arrangements

Ethiopia has established multisectoral coordination mechanisms, including the NFNGB, the NNCB, and the National Nutrition Technical Committee (NNTC). These bodies bring together more than 14 ministries and agencies, including health, agriculture, education, water, and social protection (MoH, 2018).

15.9.2 Challenges to policy coherence

Despite these structures, policy coherence remains a challenge as ministries often pursue parallel strategies, with limited integration or shared accountability. They tend to operate in sectoral silos and sometimes may have conflicting objectives. For example, the agricultural policies may prioritize calorie production over dietary diversity, whereas trade policies may facilitate the import of ultraprocessed foods (UNIANDES et al., 2021).

The NFNP and NFNS advocate for a food systems approach, aligning agricultural, trade, and nutrition policies to promote healthy diets (MoH, 2018; UNIANDES et al., 2021). Developing common indicators for all forms of malnutrition and integrating them into national monitoring systems can facilitate alignment and accountability.

15.10 Implementation gaps and monitoring

15.10.1 Bridging the policy-implementation gap: Evidence-based challenges and solutions

Bridging the gap between Ethiopia's nutrition policy design and implementation remains a critical challenge, exacerbated by interconnected systemic barriers. Evidence highlights three primary constraints. Nutrition programs face severe funding deficits relative to needs, with recent crises intensifying gaps. The World Food Programme (WFP) suspended malnutrition treatment for 650,000 women and children in April 2025 because of funding shortages, jeopardizing life-saving interventions. Ethiopia faces a projected $70 million annual gap in nutrition-specific programming, hindering the implementation of the NNP II (Ministry of Health—Ethiopia, n.d.b). Only 50% of WFP's 2025 budget is funded compared to 2024, forcing ration cuts for 3.6 million vulnerable people.

Insufficiently trained professionals hinder service delivery. A national assessment found inadequate nutrition skills across health, agriculture, and WASH sectors, with most instructors lacking teaching skills. Education curricula lack nutrition-sensitive agriculture and WASH skills, limiting workforce readiness. Poor coordination among NGOs, government, and international agencies leads to fragmented community efforts and underutilized resources (Table 15.8).

Weak data infrastructure obstructs targeted action. Routine health data exhibit alarming inconsistencies: reporting completeness ranges from 50% to 100%, whereas timeliness scores fall below 80% in over half of the studies. Nutrition-specific data is particularly scarce, with national systems lacking disaggregated metrics for overweight/obesity and NCDs despite their urban prevalence rising from 11% (2000) to 21% (2016).

- DHIS2 platforms show internal consistency scores as low as 38.9%, undermining real-time decision-making.

Table 15.8 Evidence-based strategies and impact pathways.

Approach	Evidence-based strategy	Impact pathway
Funding coordination	Establish pooled funding mechanisms with multidonor commitments	Mitigate aid volatility
Workforce development	Revise preservice curricula to integrate nutrition/WASH competencies; scale skills labs	Address pedagogical gaps
Data systems	Deploy digital community-based monitoring with ICT infrastructure	Improve timeliness/completeness

Data From UNSDG (2016), UNIANDES et al. (2021).
ICT, information and communication technology; *WASH*, water, sanitation, and hygiene.

15.10.1.1 Integrated solutions for systemic improvement

Ethiopia's resource deficits, workforce gaps, and data limitations collectively undermine nutrition policy execution. Prioritizing integrated financing models, competency-based training, and digital surveillance could transform policy aspirations into measurable improvements in malnutrition outcomes.

15.10.2 Strengthening monitoring and evaluation

Robust monitoring and evaluation (M&E) systems are essential for tracking progress and identifying disparities. The National Food and Nutrition Survey (UNIANDES et al., 2021) provides a platform for collecting data on all forms of malnutrition, but further investments are needed to ensure regular, high-quality data collection and analysis [Mo (UNIANDES et al., 2021)].

15.10.2.1 Innovative approaches

- Digital health tools: The NFNP emphasizes the use of information and communication technology (ICT) for real-time monitoring and data-driven decision-making.
- Community-based monitoring: Engaging communities in tracking nutrition outcomes can enhance accountability and responsiveness.

15.11 Recommendations for comprehensive nutrition policy

A comprehensive nutritional policy must be inclusive, evidence-based, and adaptable to the diverse needs of Ethiopia's population. It should go beyond general dietary recommendations to address the specific requirements of different groups—normal, undernourished, and obese individuals—while also integrating the realities of a country's administrative, agricultural, and ecological landscape.

It should ensure the availability and accessibility of adequate, safe, and nutritious food for all Ethiopians at all times while striving to improve the quality and accessibility of nutrition and health services throughout the lifespan, with an emphasis on equity. The safety and quality of food along the entire value chain, from farm to table, should be enhanced while minimizing food and nutrient loss. Improvements in nutrition literacy and the promotion of healthy dietary practices will also strengthen the emergency risk management system and enhance resilience to nutritional crises. Some of the other key facets that should be considered are as follows:

15.11.1 Expand policy focus to all forms of malnutrition

- Set explicit targets: Develop clear, measurable targets for reducing overweight, obesity, and diet-related NCDs, alongside existing targets for undernutrition.
- Integrate DDAs: Systematically incorporate DDAs into all nutrition policies and programs.

15.11.2 Strengthen multisectoral coordination

- Clarify roles and responsibilities: Define clear mandates for each sector and establish shared accountability frameworks.
- Enhance authority and resources: Provide the NFNGB and NNCB with the authority, resources, and capacity needed to drive cross-sectoral action.

15.11.3 Improve implementation and monitoring

- Invest in workforce development: Expand training for nutrition professionals and community health workers.
- Strengthen M&E systems: Ensure regular, disaggregated data collection and use data to guide policy and program adjustments.
- Document and share best practices: Encourage learning across regions and sectors to accelerate progress.

15.11.4 Address food systems and the food environment

- Promote dietary diversity: Support the production and consumption of a variety of nutrient-rich foods through agricultural and market interventions.
- Regulate unhealthy foods: Implement policies to limit marketing of unhealthy foods to children, enhance nutrition labeling, and establish standards for food composition.
- Leverage social protection: Incorporate nutrition goals into social protection programs, such as the PSNP, to combat both under- and overnutrition among vulnerable populations (World Bank, 2020).

15.11.5 Challenges and future directions

Malnutrition in Ethiopia is largely a result of significant socioeconomic and regional inequalities. With the change in time and the consistent support from international bodies to address the issues of undernutrition, the urban centers are now seeing rising cases of overweight and NCD, whereas the rural areas still face the highest levels of undernutrition. Regions affected by conflict, such as Tigray and Amhara, experience severe food insecurity and high rates of wasting (FEWS, 2023). In the lowlands that experience extreme climate variability and repeated droughts, food security and nutrition are jeopardized and are always susceptible to the vagaries of nature. Incorporating climate resilience into nutrition strategies is vital for sustainable development (FAO, 2022). Rapid urban growth is altering food environments, increasing the availability of processed foods and promoting sedentary habits. Urban nutrition strategies need to respond to these shifts through regulation and behavioral change efforts (Popkin et al., 2020).

15.12 Conclusion

Ethiopia's nutrition policy landscape has undergone substantial evolution, transitioning from a narrow emphasis on undernutrition to a comprehensive, multisectoral framework. Nonetheless, the increasing prevalence of overnutrition and diet-related NCDs necessitates further modifications. Addressing the entire spectrum of malnutrition requires the following: (1) data-informed, dual-purpose interventions that concurrently address under- and overnutrition. (2) Cohesive policy formulation across the health, agriculture, education, and trade sectors. (3) Resilient systems for implementation and monitoring to ensure accountability and equity. By adopting these strategies, Ethiopia can accelerate its progress toward achieving SDG 2 (Zero Hunger) and improve the health and well-being of all its citizens.

References

Abay, K. A., Abay, M. H., Berhane, G., Chamberlin, J., Croke, K., & Tafere, K. (2022). Access to health services, food, and water during an active conflict: Evidence from Ethiopia. *PLOS Global Public Health, 2*(11), e0001015. doi:10.1371/JOURNAL.PGPH.0001015/OG_IMAGE.JPG.

Abay, K. A., Tafere, K., Berhane, G., Chamberlin, J., & Abay, M. H. (2023). Near-real-time welfare and livelihood impacts of an active war: Evidence from Ethiopia. *Food Policy, 119*. http://www.elsevier.com/inca/publications/store/3/0/4/1/9/index.htt. doi:10.1016/j.foodpol.2023.102526.

Abdulahi, A., Shibru, S., & Kassa, M. (2021). Dietary diversity and associated factors among children aged 6–23 months in Ethiopia: A systematic review and meta-analysis. *Italian Journal of Pediatrics, 47*(1), 126. Article https://doi.org/10.1186/s13052-021-01077-w .

Abera, M., Workicho, A., Berhane, M., Hiko, D., Ali, R., Zinab, B., Haileamlak, A., Fall, C., & Adhikari, C. (2023). A systematic review and meta-analysis of adolescent nutrition in Ethiopia: Transforming adolescent lives through nutrition (TALENT) initiative. *PLOS ONE, 18*(4), e0280784. doi:10.1371/journal.pone.0280784.

Abiyu, C., & Belachew, T. (2020). Effect of complementary feeding behavior change communication delivered through community-level actors on dietary adequacy of infants in rural communities of West Gojjam Zone, Northwest Ethiopia: A cluster-randomized controlled trial. *PLOS ONE, 15*(9), e0238355. doi:10.1371/JOURNAL.PONE.0238355.

Ahmed, K. Y., Agho, K. E., Page, A., Arora, A., & Ogbo, F. A. (2021). Interventions to improve infant and young child feeding practices in Ethiopia: A systematic review. *BMJ Open, 11*(8). http://bmjopen.bmj.com/content/early/by/section. doi:10.1136/bmjopen-2021-048700.

Ali, A. A., Adugna, D. T., Ayele, W. M., Tadesse, S. E., Mekonnen, T. C., & Wudu, M. A. (2024). Determinants of thinness among school adolescents in Legehida district, Amhara region, north east Ethiopia: An unmatched case-control study. *Frontiers in Adolescent Medicine, 2*, 1329731. doi:10.3389/fradm.2024.1329731.

Asirvatham, R., Demi, S. M., & Ezezika, O. (2022). Are sub-Saharan African national food and agriculture policies nutrition-sensitive? A case study of Ethiopia, Ghana, Malawi, Nigeria, and South Africa. *Agriculture and Food Security, 11*(1). https://agricultureandfoodsecurity.biomedcentral.com/. doi:10.1186/s40066-022-00398-x.

Ayele, B. Y., Megento, T. L., & Habetemariam, K. Y. (2022). The governance and management of green spaces in Addis Ababa, Ethiopia. *Heliyon, 8*(11), e09413.

Ayele, A., Belachew, T., & Tegegn, A. (2023). Dietary diversity, nutritional status and associated factors among Ethiopian population groups. *BMC Public Health, 23*(1), 1142. Article https://doi.org/10.1186/s12889-023-16051-x .

Bach, A., Gregor, E., Sridhar, S., Fekadu, H., & Fawzi, W. (2020). Multisectoral integration of nutrition, health, and agriculture: Implementation lessons from Ethiopia. *Food and Nutrition Bulletin, 41*(2), 275–292. doi:10.1177/0379572119895097.

Belayneh, M., Loha, E., & Lindtjørn, B. (2021). Seasonal variation of household food insecurity and household dietary diversity on wasting and stunting among Young children in a Drought Prone Area in South Ethiopia: A cohort study. *Ecology of Food and Nutrition, 60*(1), 44–69. doi:10.1080/03670244.2020.1789865.

Berhane, H. Y., Tadesse, A. W., Worku, A., Madzorera, I., Shinde, S., & Norris, S. A. (2023). Food environment around schools and adolescent consumption of unhealthy foods in Addis Ababa, Ethiopia. *Maternal & Child Nutrition, 21*(1), e13419.

Brhanu, G. A., & Ayele, Z. B. (2023). Policy and strategic responses to food and nutrition security in Ethiopia. *Indian Journal of Public Health Research & Development, 44*(4).

Calderón, C., Kambou, G., Zebaze, D., & Ianchovichina, E. (2022). The Ukraine war and rising commodity prices: Implications for developing countries. *Finance & Development, 59*(2), 16–19.

CSA and ICF. (2016). *Ethiopia Demographic and Health Survey 2016*. CSA and ICF https://dhsprogram.com/publications/publication-fr328-dhs-final-reports.cfm.

Degfachew, T. N., Dilnesaw, M. M., & Massa, M. M. (2025). Food security and dietary diversity status among rural households of Eastern Amhara, Ethiopia. *Discover Food, 5*(1). https://www.springer.com/journal/44187. doi:10.1007/s44187-025-00357-y.

Desalegn, P., Rezaei, M., & Alikhanova, S. (2025). *Understanding food systems policies for healthy diets in Ethiopia opportunities for urban inclusion*. ODI Global https://odi.org/en/publications/understanding-food.

Dewey, K. G., & Begum, K. (2011). Long-term consequences of stunting in early life. *Maternal & Child Nutrition, 7*(s3), 5–18. doi:10.1111/j.1740-8709.2011.00349.x.

EPHI & ICF. (2019). Ethiopia Mini Demographic and Health Survey. EPHI & ICF. https://dhsprogram.com/publications/publication-FR363-DHS-Final-Reports.cfm.

Ethiopia Demographic and Health Survey (EDHS) (2016). Addis Ababa, Ethiopia, and Rockville, Maryland, USA: Central Statistical Agency and ICF.

Ethiopia Mini Demographic and Health Survey (EDHS). (2019). *Final Report*. Rockville, Maryland, USA: EPHI and ICF.

Ethiopian Public Health Institute (EPHI). (2018). National food consumption survey (NFCS). *EPHI*.

FAO. (2024). *Food* Security and Nutrition in the W*orld*: Financing to end hunger, food insecurity and malnutrition in all its forms. FAO. doi:10.4060/cd1254en.

Federal Democratic Republic of Ethiopia (FDRE). (2016). *National Nutrition Programme II (NNP II), 2016–2020*. Addis Ababa: Federal Ministry of Health.

Federal Ministry of Health. (2016). *National Nutrition Programme II (NNP II): 2016–2020. Federal Democratic Republic of Ethiopia*. Federal Ministry of Health.

FEWS NET. (2023). Food access expected to improve for millions in October with Meher harvest: Key messages.

FEWS NET. (2024). Food access expected to improve for millions in October with Meher harvest: Key messages.

Food and Agriculture Organization of the United Nations (FAO). (2005). *The State of Food Insecurity in the World 2005: Eradicating world hunger — key to achieving the Millennium Development Goals*. Rome: FAO.

Food and Agriculture Organization of the United Nations (FAO). (2022). *The state of food security and nutrition in the world 2022: Repurposing food and agricultural policies to make healthy diets more affordable*. FAO, IFAD, UNICEF, WFP, & WHO.

Gebremariam, G., Mulugeta, A., & Tesfay, F. (2021). Maternal nutrition, dietary diversity and associated factors among women in Ethiopia. *PLOS ONE, 16*(4), e0250123. Article https://doi.org/10.1371/journal.pone.0250123 .

Gejea, Y. M., & Tolesa, S. F. (2024). The impact of national and international war on agriculture in Ethiopia: A review. *International Journal of Social Science, Management and Economics Research, 2*(3), 1–13.

Gezaw, A., Melese, W., Getachew, B., Belachew, T., & Cunningham, S. A. (2023). Double burden of malnutrition and associated factors among adolescent in Ethiopia: A systematic review and meta-analysis. *PLOS ONE, 18*(4), e0282240. doi:10.1371/journal.pone.0282240.

Glatzel, K., Ameye, H., Hülsen, V., & Qaim, M. (2024). *Changing food environments in Africa's urban and peri-urban areas: Implications for diets, nutrition, and policy*. https://www.econstor.eu/handle/10419/304435.

Haidar, J. (2024). Nutrition, food security and public health challenges in Ethiopia. *Ethiopian Journal of Health Development, 38*(1), 15–28. https://doi.org/10.4314/ejhd.v38i1.2.

Haile, T. G., & Singh, S. P. (2024). The whole-of-government approach to public policy integration from the Ethiopian experience: Policy analysis with a comparative focus on selected public policies. *International Journal of Public Sector Performance Management, 13*(4), 471–490. http://www.inderscience.com/ijpspm. doi:10.1504/IJPSPM.2024.138764.

Haile, Y. T., & Legisso, T. Z. (2024). Trends and determinants of child stunting in Ethiopia: A longitudinal analysis of sociodemographic factors and regional disparities. *BMC Public Health, 24*(1). https://bmcpublichealth.biomedcentral.com/. doi:10.1186/s12889-024-20962-3.

Harper, A., Rothberg, A., Chirwa, E., Sambu, W., & Mall, S. (2023). Household food insecurity and demographic factors, low birth weight and stunting in early childhood: Findings from a longitudinal study in South Africa. *Maternal and Child Health Journal, 27*(1), 59–69. doi:10.1007/s10995-022-03555-7.

Institute for Health Metrics and Evaluation (IHME). (2022). Global Burden of Disease Study 2019 (GBD 2019) results—country profile: Ethiopia. IHME.

Jeyakumar, A., Godbharle, S., Ravindran, S., & Zepeda, A. M. N. (2025). *The double burden of under and overnutrition: A Synopsis* (pp. 1–22). Springer Science and Business Media LLC. doi:10.1007/978-3-031-32047-7_39-1.

Kennedy, E., Alderman, H., & MaternalChild Nutrition Study Group. (2023). Evidence-based nutrition policy and programming: Progress, gaps, and priorities. *Food Policy, 118*, 102375.

Korir, J., Oldewage-Theron, W., Samuel, A., & Gichohi-Wainaina, W. N. (2024). Multisectoral approaches for sustainable food and nutrition security actions in Ethiopia. *African Journal of Food, Agriculture, Nutrition and Development, 24*(5), 26351–26376. doi:10.18697/ajfand.130.24180.

Maru, Y., Mesfin, F., Laillou, A., Noor, R., Adhikari, S. R., Zelalem, M., Darsene, H., Memire, S., Abie, A., & Chitekwe, S. (2024). Estimating the minimal cost of delivering nutrition-specific and nutrition-sensitive interventions in Ethiopia. *Maternal and Child Nutrition*. http://onlinelibrary.wiley.com/journal/10.1111/(ISSN)1740-8709. doi:10.1111/mcn.13758.

Mathebula, N. (2025). *Debt crises and sovereign risk in Africa* (pp. 1–106). Taylor and Francis. https://www.taylorfrancis.com/books/mono/10.4324/9781003569138. doi:10.4324/9781003569138.

Mesfin, A. H., Gebremedhin, K. G., Tefera, T., Chimsa, M. D., & Vonk, R. (2024). Pathways and policy options for food and nutrition gaps in arid agricultural farming systems in the Tigray Region, north Ethiopia. *Heliyon, 10*(7). https://www.sciencedirect.com/science/journal/24058440. doi:10.1016/j.heliyon.2024.e28213.

Ministry of Health (MoH) [Ethiopia]. (2018). *National Food and Nutrition Policy*. Addis Ababa, Ethiopia: Federal Democratic Republic of Ethiopia, Ministry of Health.

Mohammed, A., Tareke, A. A., Keleb, A., Kebede, N., Tsega, Y., Endawkie, A., Kebede, S. D., Mesfin Abera, K., Tilahun Abeje, E., Bekele Enyew, E., Daba, C., Asmare, L., Bayou, F. D., Endris, H., & Arefaynie, M. (2024). Urban–rural disparities in minimum acceptable diet intake among children aged 6–23 months in Ethiopia: A multivariable decomposition analysis of Ethiopian demographic and health survey 2019. *Frontiers in Public Health, 12*. http://journal.frontiersin.org/journal/public-health/section/public-health-education-and-promotion#archive. doi:10.3389/fpubh.2024.1361673.

Motbainor, A., Worku, A., Kumie, A., & van Wouwe, J. (2015). Stunting is associated with food diversity while wasting with food insecurity among Underfive children in East and West Gojjam Zones of Amhara Region, Ethiopia. *PLOS ONE, 10*(8), e0133542. doi:10.1371/journal.pone.0133542.

Moyo, M. M., & Blake, R. (2024). Pastoralist conflict in Ethiopia from 2015 to 2022: Climate change and food insecurity as exacerbating factors A mini-dissertation submitted in partial fulfilment of the requirement for the degree MASTER OF ARTS IN SECURITY STUDIES In the Department of Political Sciences, Faculty of Humanities at the UNIVERSITY OF PRETORIA.

Muhyie, J. H., Yayeh, D., Kidanie, S. A., Metekia, W. A., & Tilahun, T. (2025). Synthesizing the impact of armed conflicts on food security, livelihoods and social dynamics in Amhara region, Ethiopia. *BMC Nutrition., 11*(1). https://bmcnutr.biomedcentral.com/. doi:10.1186/s40795-025-01013-5.

Ministry of Health—Ethiopia. (n.d.b). *National Nutrition Program*. Retrieved June 28, 2025, from https://www.moh.gov.et/en/initiatives-4-col/Nutrition?language_content_entity=en.

National Food and Nutrition Policy (NFNP). (2018). *National Food and Nutrition Policy of Ethiopia*. Addis Ababa, Ethiopia: Federal Democratic Republic of Ethiopia.

Popkin, B. M., Corvalan, C., & Grummer-Strawn, L. M. (2020). Dynamics of the double burden of malnutrition and the changing nutrition reality. *The Lancet, 395*(10217), 65–74. http://www.journals.elsevier.com/the-lancet/. doi:10.1016/S0140-6736(19)32497-3.

Shekar, M., & Okamura, S. K. (2024). *Investment Framework for Nutrition 2024: An Update to the Investment Framework for Nutrition*. Washington, DC: World Bank.

Tadesse, M., Dawed, Y. A., Fentaw, Z., Endawike, A., & Adamu, K. (2023). Determinants of inappropriate complementary feeding among children 6–23 months of age in Dessie City, Northeast Ethiopia: A case-control study. *BMC Nutrition, 9*, 124. Article https://doi.org/10.1186/s40795-023-00779-w .

Tadesse, K., Seyoum, A., Baye, K., & Hirvonen, K. (2024). Estimating the minimal cost of delivering nutrition-specific and nutrition-sensitive interventions in Ethiopia. *International Journal of Health Planning and Management, 39*(6), 1531–1546.

Tareke, A. A., Alem, A., Debebe, W., & Zerfu, T. A. (2024). Sustained underweight in rural areas and emergence of overweight in urban Ethiopian women: A multivariate analysis of EDHS data 2000–2016. *Scientific Reports, 14*(1). https://www.nature.com/srep/. doi:10.1038/s41598-024-66409-y.

Tekle, D. Y., Rosewarne, E., Santos, J. A., Trieu, K., Buse, K., Palu, A., Thow, A. M., Jan, S., & Webster, J. (2023). Do food and nutrition policies in Ethiopia support the prevention of non-communicable diseases through population-level salt reduction measures? A policy content analysis. *Nutrients, 15*(7). http://www.mdpi.com/journal/nutrients/. doi:10.3390/nu15071745.

Trübswasser, U., Candel, J., Genye, T., Bossuyt, A., Holdsworth, M., Baye, K., & Talsma, E. (2022). Benchmarking policy goals and actions for healthy food environments in Ethiopia to prevent malnutrition in all its forms using document analysis. *BMJ Open, 12*(8), e058480. doi:10.1136/bmjopen-2021-058480.

Uccello, E., Kauffmann, D., Calo, M., & Streissel, M. (2017). *Nutrition-Sensitive Agriculture and Food Systems in Practice: Options for Intervention (revised edition)*. Rome: Food and Agriculture Organization of the United Nations (FAO).

UNIANDES, IFAD, & FAO. (2021). *Ethiopia: Building bridges between social and productive inclusion policies*. FAO https://openknowledge.fao.org/handle/20.500.14283/cb3278en.

United Nations. (2016). *The Sustainable Development Goals Report 2016*. United Nations, Department of Economic and Social Affairs, Statistics Division.

United Nations Children's Fund (UNICEF). (2019). *Improving child nutrition: The achievable imperative for global progress*. New York, NY: UNICEF.

United Nations Children's Fund (UNICEF). (2022). *Nutrition in Ethiopia: Situation analysis and programming priorities*. Addis Ababa, Ethiopia: UNICEF Ethiopia.

United Nations Children's Fund (UNICEF). (2023). *UNICEF Ethiopia Annual Report 2023*. Addis Ababa, Ethiopia: UNICEF Ethiopia.

Weimann, A., Shung-King, M., McCreedy, N., Tatah, L., Mapa-Tassou, C., Muzenda, T., ... Oni, T. (2021). Intersectoral action for addressing NCDs through the food environment: An analysis of NCD framing in global policies and its relevance for the African context. *International Journal of Environmental Research and Public Health, 18*(21), 11246. doi:10.3390/ijerph182111246.

WHO. (2016). 2015 STEPS Country Report Ethiopia. World Health Organization. https://www.who.int/publications/m/item/2015-steps-country-report-ethiopia.

WHO. (2017). *Double-duty actions for nutrition: Policy brief.* WHO Retrieved June 28, 2025, from https://www.who.int/publications/i/item/WHO-NMH-NHD-17.2.

WHO. (2020). *Global Nutrition Report 2020: Action on equity to end malnutrition*. Geneva: World Health Organization.

WHO. (2023). The state of food security and nutrition in the world 2023. Retrieved June 2, 2025, from https://www.who.int/publications/m/item/the-state-of-food-security-and-nutrition-in-the-world-2023.

World Bank. (2006). Repositioning nutrition as central to development : A strategy for large-scale action—overview. Retrieved June 3, 2025, from https://documents.worldbank.org/en/publication/documents-reports/documentdetail/185651468175733998/repositioning-nutrition-as-central-to-development-a-strategy-for-large-scale-action-overview.

World Bank. (2020). *In Ethiopia, the Second Agricultural Growth Project is improving nutrition outcomes*. Washington, DC: World Bank.

World Bank. (2024). *Investment framework for nutrition*. Retrieved June 2, 2025, from https://www.worldbank.org/en/topic/nutrition/publication/investment-framework-nutrition.

Woldehanna, T., Behrman, J. R., & Araya, M. W. (2017). The effect of early childhood stunting on children's cognitive achievements: Evidence from young lives Ethiopia. *Ethiopian Journal of Health Development, 31*(2), 75–84. http://www.ejhd.org/index.php/ejhd/article/download/1234/940.

Workicho, A., Biadgilign, S., Kershaw, M., Gizaw, R., Stickland, J., Assefa, W., Abuye, C., Woldegiorgis, B., Berhanu, L., & Kennedy, E. (2021). Social and behaviour change communication to improve child feeding practices in Ethiopia. *Maternal & Child Nutrition, 17*(4). doi:10.1111/mcn.13231.

Worldometer. (2023). *Ethiopia Population* https://www.worldometers.info/world-population/ethiopia-population/.

Yallew, W. W., Tadesse, A. W., Noor, A., Fawzi, W., & Berhane, Y. (2022). Stunting and thinness in school-attending adolescents in Addis Ababa. *BMC Nutrition, 8*(1). https://bmcnutr.biomedcentral.com/. doi:10.1186/s40795-022-00653-1.

Index

Page numbers followed by "*f*" and "*t*" indicate, figures and tables respectively.

9780443236716